Nuclear Cardiology and Correlative Imaging

Springer
New York
Berlin
Heidelberg
Hong Kong
London
Milan
Paris
Tokyo

Nuclear Cardiology and Correlative Imaging

A Teaching File

João V. Vitola, MD, PhD

Associate Professor, Department of Medicine, Federal University of Paraná Medical School; Director, Quanta Medicina Nuclear, Curitiba, Paraná, Brazil

Dominique Delbeke, MD, PhD

Professor and Director of Nuclear Medicine and PET, Department of Radiology and Radiological Sciences, Vanderbilt University Medical Center, Nashville, Tennessee

Editors

With Forewords by Joseph S. Alpert, MD, and E. Gordon DePuey III, MD

With 396 Illustrations, 117 in Full Color

With 143 Case Presentations

Springer

João V. Vitola, MD, PhD
Associate Professor
Department of Medicine
Federal University of Paraná
Medical School
and
Director
Quanta Medicina Nuclear
Curitiba, Paraná 80050-010
Brazil

Dominique Delbeke, MD, PhD
Professor and Director of Nuclear Medicine and PET
Department of Radiology and Radiological
Sciences
Vanderbilt University Medical Center
Nashville, TN 37232
USA

Library of Congress Cataloging-in-Publication Data
Vitola, João V.
Nuclear cardiology and correlative imaging: a teaching file / João V. Vitola, Dominique Delbeke.
p. cm.
Includes bibliographical references and index.
ISBN-13:978-1-4612-7392-9 e-ISBN-13:978-1-4612-2038-1
DOI: 10.1007/978-1-4612-2038-1

1. Heart—Radionuclide imaging. I. Vitola, João V. II. Title. 2003067334
RC683.5.R33D45 2004
16.1′207575—dc22

ISBN-13:978-1-4612-7392-9 Printed on acid-free paper

9 8 7 6 5 4 3 2 1 SPIN 10941805

Springer-Verlag is a part of *Springer Science+Business Media*

springeronline.com

Foreword I

The last 50 years have witnessed remarkable growth in our understanding of cardiovascular diseases. Furthermore, the ability of physicians to diagnose and treat patients with cardiovascular disorders has expanded in step with this enlarging knowledge concerning the pathophysiology of heart and vascular disease. Effective therapy for patients who have these disorders can occur only when an accurate diagnosis has been made. For example, starting in the early 1950s, invasive cardiac diagnostic ability and effective cardiac surgical intervention advanced together. Unfortunately, cardiac catheterization entails risk and morbidity that, although small, are nevertheless disconcerting to patients and physicians. The obvious solution to this conundrum was accurate, cost-effective, noninvasive diagnosis. The latter half of the twentieth century and the early years of the twenty-first century have seen explosive growth in our ability to perform such accurate and financially appropriate noninvasive diagnostic evaluations. Nuclear cardiology has emerged as a powerful diagnostic force in this arena, with a variety of modalities and protocols that define with exquisite accuracy the pathophysiologic features of many forms of cardiovascular disease.

In this regard, Drs. Vitola and Delbeke have assembled an impressive array of experts who have clearly and concisely reviewed the essential features of nuclear cardiologic diagnosis. Beginning with the principles of nuclear physics, the required instrumentation, and the most commonly employed radiopharmaceutical agents needed for nuclear cardiologic diagnosis, this book proceeds to cover the various techniques employed in nuclear cardiologic diagnosis. Didactic material is elegantly supplemented by beautifully illustrated case presentations. Stress and perfusion imaging techniques are described both in the nuclear cardiac laboratory and on the floors of the hospital. Evaluations of cardiac function and myocardial viability are explored, and correlations between nuclear techniques and MRI, CT, and echocardiography are examined. Pitfalls and artifacts in the various nuclear tests are clearly defined. Preoperative risk assessment by nuclear testing is also clearly demonstrated.

This book will be of great value to cardiology trainees and experienced cardiologists who desire a concise and well-illustrated source of information in the field of nuclear cardiac diagnosis. Drs. Vitola and Delbeke are to be congratulated on assembling an outstanding group of experts in the field and for bringing so much useful information together in such a visually and didactically outstanding fashion.

Joseph S. Alpert, MD
Robert S. and Irene P. Flinn Professor of Medicine
and
Head, Department of Medicine
University of Arizona Health Sciences Center
Tucson, Arizona

Foreword II

Over the past two decades, a wealth of information regarding the diagnostic accuracy and clinical applicability of nuclear cardiology procedures has emerged. Significant advancements in instrumentation and radiopharmaceuticals have greatly expanded our diagnostic and prognostic capabilities. At the same time, training programs in nuclear cardiology have increased, and there is a burgeoning number of physicians performing and interpreting nuclear cardiology studies. This book provides important insight into many vital facets of nuclear cardiology that directly impact on the clinical relevance of this rapidly growing field: the theory and scientific basis of a wide variety of applications of nuclear cardiology, the appropriate techniques by which these studies should be performed, a wealth of illustrative case examples, and detailed guidelines in evaluating and interpreting scans.

Nuclear cardiology now employs a pharmacopoeia of diagnostic agents. In this book, a wide variety of radiopharmaceuticals is highlighted, including ^{201}Tl, ^{99m}Tc sestamibi, ^{99m}Tc tetrofosmin, ^{18}F fluorodeoxyglucose, ^{13}N-ammonia, ^{82}Rb, and ^{99m}Tc-labeled red blood cells. Studies performed using a variety of stress modalities, including treadmill exercise, pharmacological chronotropic/inotropic stress, pharmacologic coronary vasodilatation, and a combination of these modalities, are described, and the potential pitfalls and limitations in their use are highlighted. Likewise, a variety of instrumentation developed to image these radiopharmaceuticals using SPECT and PET techniques is highlighted in case examples throughout the text. Moreover, analysis of left ventricular function by radionuclide ventriculography, gated perfusion SPECT, and gated PET are all described. Importantly, state-of-the-art technology, including combined PET/CT, is illustrated. Typical and atypical patterns of single-vessel and multivessel coronary artery disease are detailed in a manner by which they can be readily differentiated and by which readers can reinforce their diagnostic confidence. In addition, perfusion and functional abnormalities are characterized with regard to associated patient risk of subsequent cardiac events and the consequent impact of scan findings on patient management. Guidelines in both qualitative and quantitative analysis of both perfusion and function scans are offered. Importantly, scan artifacts that potentially decrease diagnostic specificity are emphasized, and the means to recognize and avoid such artifacts are illustrated in a variety of relevant case examples.

The use of nuclear cardiology studies in at-risk populations continues to expand and is now known to particularly benefit women, diabetics, and patients with congestive heart failure. These populations are described with regard to relevant image findings, as well as the cost-effectiveness of nuclear procedures. The evaluation of myocardial viability has been an intense area of interest and research in nuclear cardiology. In this textbook, a panoply of methods by which myocardial viability can be assessed, including ^{18}F FDG SPECT and PET, rest-redistribution ^{201}Tl SPECT, and ^{99m}Tc sestamibi imaging, are all described with regard to their significance as indicators of myocardial viability and implications with regard to patient management. The use of myocardial perfusion SPECT to evaluate patients presenting to the emergency department with acute chest pain is becoming an increasingly popular means to expedite patient diagnosis and care, as well as to decrease hospital length-of-stay and healthcare expenditure. The use of acute perfusion SPECT imaging with ^{99m}Tc sestamibi is illustrated in patients presenting with a variety of types of chest pain syndromes.

Just as nuclear cardiology has progressed, other noninvasive cardiac imaging modalities have advanced significantly in recent years. This book provides important insights into the complementary and possibly competitive applications of cardiac MRI, multislice CT, and stress echocardiography. Case examples are offered for review in which nuclear cardiology studies are directly correlated with those using other noninvasive techniques. Finally, a chapter is devoted to future directions in nuclear cardiology, highlighting potential new radiopharmaceuticals, instrumentation, and clinical applications.

In summary, this excellent book provides an exhaustive overview of the wide variety of radionuclide methods now available to evaluate cardiac perfusion and function and to diagnose, stratify risk, and follow patients with heart disease. Theoretical and practical explanations supplemented by numerous illustrative case examples derived from real clinical situations reinforce and update the knowledge and skills of physicians who have interpreted nuclear cardiology studies for many years, and also provide a thorough state-of-the art overview *from the ground up* for those just entering this exciting field.

E. Gordon DePuey III, MD
Professor, Department of Radiology
Columbia University College of Physicians and Surgeons
New York, New York

Contents

Contributors

Raed Al-Dallow, MD
Staff, Division of Cardiology, Rush Presbyterian-St Luke's Medical Center, Chicago, IL 60612, USA

Joseph S. Alpert, MD
Head, Department of Medicine, University of Arizona Medical Center, Tucson, AZ 85724, USA

Jeroen J. Bax, MD, PhD
Faculty, Department of Cardiology, Leiden University Medical Center, Leiden, 2333 ZA, The Netherlands

Daniel S. Berman, MD
Professor, Department of Medicine, University of California at Los Angeles School of Medicine, Los Angeles, CA 90095, USA; Director, Cardiac Imaging and Nuclear Cardiology, Cedars-Sinai Medical Center, Los Angeles, CA 90048-0750, USA

Sabahat Bokhari, MD
Assistant Clinical Professor, Department of Medicine, Nuclear Cardiology/Cardiology Stress Laboratory, Division of Cardiology, College of Physicians and Surgeons of Columbia University, New York, NY 10032, USA

Jean M. Cacciabaudo, MD, FACC
Associate Director, Nuclear Cardiology, Department of Medicine, North Shore University Hospital, Manhasset, NY 11030, USA

William Azem Chalela, MD, PhD
Chief, Cardiology Laboratory, Department of Nuclear Medicine and Molecular Imaging, Heart Institute (InCor), University of São Paulo Medical School, São Paulo, Brazil 05403-000

Carlos Cunha Pereira Neto, MD
Co-Director, Quanta Medicina Nuclear, Curitiba, Paraná, Brazil 80050-010

Seth Dahlberg, MD
Assistant Professor, Division of Nuclear Medicine, University of Massachusetts Memorial Medical Center, Worcester, MA 01655, USA

Jaydip Datta, MD
Radiologist, Division of Cardiac and Vascular Imaging, Quantum Radiology Northwest, Marietta, GA 30060, USA

Dominique Delbeke, MD, PhD
Professor and Director of Nuclear Medicine and PET, Department of Radiology and Radiological Sciences, Vanderbilt University Medical Center, Nashville, TN 37232, USA

E. Gordon DePuey III, MD
Professor, Department of Radiology, Columbia University College of Physicians and Surgeons, New York, NY 10025, USA

Tracy Faber, PhD
Associate Professor, Department of Radiology, Emory University School of Medicine, Atlanta, GA 30322, USA

Russell Folks, CNMT
Research Associate, Department of Radiology, Emory University School of Medicine, Atlanta, GA 30322, USA

Ernest V. Garcia, PhD
Professor and Vice Chairman, Department of Radiology, Emory University School of Medicine, Atlanta, GA 30322 USA

Guido Germano, PhD
Adjunct Professor, Artificial Intelligence in Medicine Program, Department of Medicine, Cedars-Sinai Medical Center, Los Angeles, CA 90048, USA

Gabriel Grossman, MD
Senior Research Associate, Department of Radiology, Emory University School of Medicine, Atlanta, GA 30322, USA

M. Reza Habibian, MD
Chief, Nuclear Medicine/Ultrasound Service, Veterans Administration Medical Center, Tennessee Valley Healthcare System, Nashville, TN 37212, USA

Rory Hachamovitch, MD, MSc
Faculty Attending, Division of Cardiovascular Medicine, Department of Medicine, Keck School of Medicine, University of Southern California, Los Angeles, CA 90089, USA

Sean W. Hayes, MD
Assistant Director, Department of Imaging and Medicine, Cedars-Sinai Medical Center, Los Angeles, CA 90048, USA

Gary V. Heller, MD, PhD
Director of Nuclear Cardiology, Hartford Hospital, Hartford, CT 06102, USA

Robert C. Hendel, MD
Associate Professor, Department of Medicine; Director, Nuclear Cardiology; Director, Cardiac Care Unit, Rush-Presbyterian-St Luke's Medical Center, Chicago, IL 60612, USA

Philipp A. Kaufmann, MD
Swiss National Science Foundation Professor of Nuclear Medicine and Cardiology, Department of Nuclear Cardiology, University Hospital Zurich, Zurich, CH-8091 Switzerland

Otávio J. Kormann, MD
Director, Stress Test Laboratory, Medicina Nuclear Alto da XV, Curitiba, Paraná, Brazil 80050-010

Marvin W. Kronenberg, MD
Professor, Division of Cardiovascular Medicine, Department of Medicine, Vanderbilt University Medical Center, Nashville, TN 37232, USA

Arnaldo Laffitte Stier, Jr., MD, MS
Head, Outpatient Cardiac Service, Departments of Internal Medicine and Cardiology, Federal University of Paraná Medical School, Curitiba, Paraná, Brazil 80050-010

Jeffrey A. Leppo, MD
Professor, Division of Nuclear Medicine, Departments of Radiology and Medicine, University of Massachusetts Memorial Medical Center, Worcester, MA 01655, USA

Mikhail Levin, CNMT
Technical Director, Nuclear Cardiology, Department of Cardiology, North Shore University Hospital, Manhasset, NY 11030; 279 Little Neck Rd., Centerport, NY 11721, USA

Vinícius Ludwig, MD
Faculty, Department of Nuclear Medicine, Centro de Medicina Nuclear do Paraná, Curitiba, Paraná, Brazil 80730-460

William H. Martin, MD
Associate Professor, Department of Radiology and Radiological Sciences, Vanderbilt University Medical Center, Nashville, TN 37232, USA

Luis E. Mastrocolla, MD, PhD
Director, Cardiology Group, Laboratório Fleury, São Paulo; Staff, Nuclear Medicine and Exercise Testing/Rehabilitation Section, Dante Pazzanese Institute of Cardiology, São Paulo, Brazil 04542-012

Wilson Mathias, Jr., MD
Staff, Department of Nuclear Medicine and Molecular Imaging, Heart Institute (InCor), University of São Paulo Medical School, São Paulo, Brazil 05403-000

José Claudio Meneghetti, MD, PhD
Director, Department of Nuclear Medicine and Molecular Imaging, Heart Institute (InCor), University of São Paulo Medical School, São Paulo, Brazil 05403-000

Jennifer H. Mieres, MD, FACP, FACC
Assistant Professor, Department of Medicine, New York University, Director of Nuclear Cardiology, North Shore University Hospital, Manhasset, NY 10030, USA

Kenneth J. Nichols, PhD
Medical Physicist, Department of Nuclear Medicine, Northwestern Memorial Hospital, Chicago, IL 60611, USA

James A. Patton, PhD
Professor of Radiology; Professor of Physics; Administrator, Radiology Academic Affairs; Program Director, Nuclear Medicine Technology, Department of Radiology and Radiological Sciences, Vanderbilt University Medical Center, Nashville, TN 37232, USA

Olímpio Ribeiro França Neto, MD
Staff Physician and Scientific Director, Chest Pain Unit, Emergency Department and Stress Testing Laboratory, Hospital Santa Cruz and Hospital do Coração, Curitiba, Paraná, Brazil 80050-010

Carlos Eduardo Rochitte, MD, PhD
Chief, Cardiovascular Magnetic Resonance and Computed Tomography Laboratory, Heart Institute (InCor), University of São Paulo Medical School, São Paulo, Brazil 05403-000

Martin P. Sandler, MD
Professor and Chairman, Department of Radiology and Radiological Sciences, Vanderbilt University Medical Center, Nashville, TN 37232, USA

Cesar Santana, MD, PhD
Assistant Professor, Department of Radiology, Emory University School of Medicine, Atlanta, GA 30033, USA

Heinrich R. Schelbert, MD, PhD
Professor, Department of Molecular and Medical Pharmacology, David Geffen School of Medicine, University of California, Los Angeles, Los Angeles, CA 90095, USA

Thomas H. Schindler, MD
George V. Tablin Professor, Department of Molecular and Medical Pharmacology, David Geffen School of Medicine, University of California, Los Angeles, Los Angeles, CA 90095, USA

Ronald G. Schwartz, MD
Associate Professor, Departments of Medicine and Radiology; Director, Nuclear Cardiology, University of Rochester Medical Center, Rochester, NY 14642, USA

Leslee J. Shaw, PhD
Director, Outcomes Research, Atlanta Cardiovascular Research Institute, Atlanta, GA 30342, USA

C. Andrew Smith, MD, BS
Fellow, Cardiovascular Medicine Division, Vanderbilt University Medical Center, Nashville, TN 37232, USA

David Townsend, PhD
Professor, Department of Medicine, University of Tennessee, Knoxville, TN 37920, USA

Gustav K. von Schulthess, MD, PhD
Director of Nuclear Medicine, Professor, Department of Radiology, Cardiovascular Center, University Hospital, 8006 Zurich, Switzerland

João V. Vitola, MD, PhD
Associate Professor, Department of Medicine, Federal University of Paraná Medical School; Director, Quanta Medicina Nuclear, Curitiba, Paraná, Brazil 80050-010

Jack A. Ziffer, MD, PhD
Director, Cardiac Imaging, Baptist Hospital, Miami Cardiac and Vascular Institute, Miami, FL 33176, USA

1
Diagnostic Tools to Approach the Cardiac Patient

João V. Vitola and Dominique Delbeke

It has been an exciting era for those working in the fields of cardiology and cardiac imaging. In the last few decades, numerous technological advances have provided innovative diagnostic tools for better identification and measurement of the extent of disease. A succession of new therapies for treating cardiac disease has impacted both cardiac morbidity and mortality. These new therapies include carvedilol, angiotensin-converting enzyme inhibitors, statins, and a new generation of stents, to mention just a few. In this text, the value of nuclear imaging is discussed in the context of other correlative imaging techniques to diagnose cardiac disease, to monitor the effects of therapy, and to better stratify patients into different risk categories for cardiac death or myocardial infarction. Ultimately, the optimal integration of nuclear imaging with the other diagnostic modalities will allow the most accurate identification of patients who may benefit from more aggressive treatments, such as myocardial revascularization or heart transplantation.

The impact of more accurate diagnosis and new therapeutic approaches has clearly benefited patients, but unfortunately the latest technological advances are often expensive and may not be universally available. While the delivery of optimal patient care is the ultimate goal, cost-efficient use of limited resources is a growing concern. The goal of avoiding the unnecessary use of expensive invasive procedures has focused more attention on the use of noninvasive or less invasive diagnostic and therapeutic modalities, including nuclear imaging. Ultimately, it is the treating physician's responsibility to rationalize the use of resources for optimal patient care at a reasonable cost.

In this chapter, an overview of the diagnostic modalities used for evaluation of the cardiac patient is presented, including resting electrocardiography (ECG), exercise testing or treadmill stress testing (TMT), echocardiography, computed tomography (CT), magnetic resonance imaging (MRI), and nuclear imaging using single photon emission tomography (SPECT) and positron emission tomography (PET). Before presenting this overview, it is imperative to review some concepts of the evolution of atherosclerotic plaque formation and its impact on coronary blood flow reserve.

The Atherosclerotic Process and Its Relationship to Coronary Blood Flow

Since the mid-19th century, there has been a near doubling life expectancy from 40 to more than 80 years.[1] This point is illustrated in Figure 1-1. Cardiovascular disease is the most important life-threatening illness affecting individuals, and—at least in the United States—5 out of 6 of the deaths attributed to cardiovascular disease occur in individuals older than age 65.[1] Human atherosclerosis is a dynamic process that begins even before birth and progresses throughout life. Early studies of young men who were victims of the Korean War (1950–1953) and the Vietnam War (1964–1973) demonstrated that atherosclerosis occurs quite frequently even at a young age. Stary[3] studied the coronary arteries of 691 American victims of violent death, including suicide and homicide. By age 39, approximately 90% of people had coronary artery lesions and 65% had lesions classified as intermediate to advanced by pathologic criteria. This point is illustrated in Figure 1-2. This fact does not take into account the presence of coronary risk factors, such as smoking, hypertension, hypercholesterolemia, diabetes, or a positive family history of coronary artery disease (CAD), but certainly their presence is known to accelerate the atherosclerotic process. Considering this high incidence of atherosclerotic plaques in the general population, independent of already having (documented or not) obstructive coronary lesions, all efforts should be directed at reducing risk factors, attempting to delay a process that already occurs early in members of Western societies. A comprehensive review of the process of atherosclerosis, plaque vulnerability, and coronary thrombi has been published by Burke et al.[4]

Considering this high incidence of atherosclerotic plaques, the active search for coronary lesions in the asymptomatic general population does not seem reasonable, as lesions will often be found, but will not necessarily be affecting myocardial blood flow (MBF). The fact that atherosclerotic lesions affect MBF is related to impairment of the dilatory capacity of the coronary arteries as well as to the number of collateral vessels at the microcirculatory level.

Atherosclerosis first causes narrowing of the coronary arteries, but without inducing ischemia. With progression, coronary stenosis first affects CBF that can be detected only with stress testing, before affecting MBF at rest. The relationship between the degree of narrowing of coronary arteries and MBF was first described by Gould et al.[5] Both myocardial metabolism and function change during severe myocardial ischemia at rest. During prolonged myocardial ischemia, irreversible cell damage and infarction occur first in the subendocardial tissue and then progress like a wave front toward the epicardium. Periods of ischemia

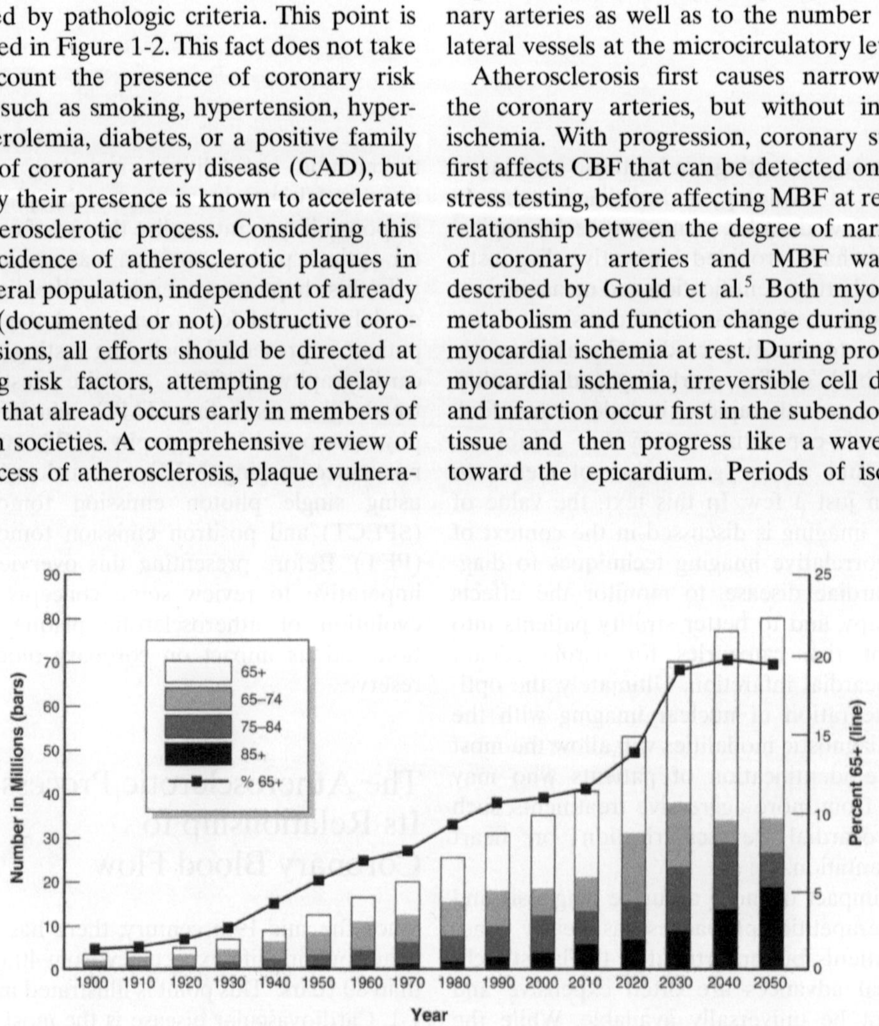

FIGURE 1-1. Growth of the elderly population (older than 65 years) between the years 1900 and 2050. A rapid expansion of the elderly in our population can be anticipated with the oldest (older than 85 years) of the elderly accounting for all the growth in the elderly population after the year 2030. (From US Bureau of the Census: Sixty-five Plus in America, pp 23–178 RV. Population projections of the United States are as of April 1, projections 2000–2050 are as of July 1.) (From Batchelor, Jollis, Friesinger [2], by permission of *Cardiol Clin.*)

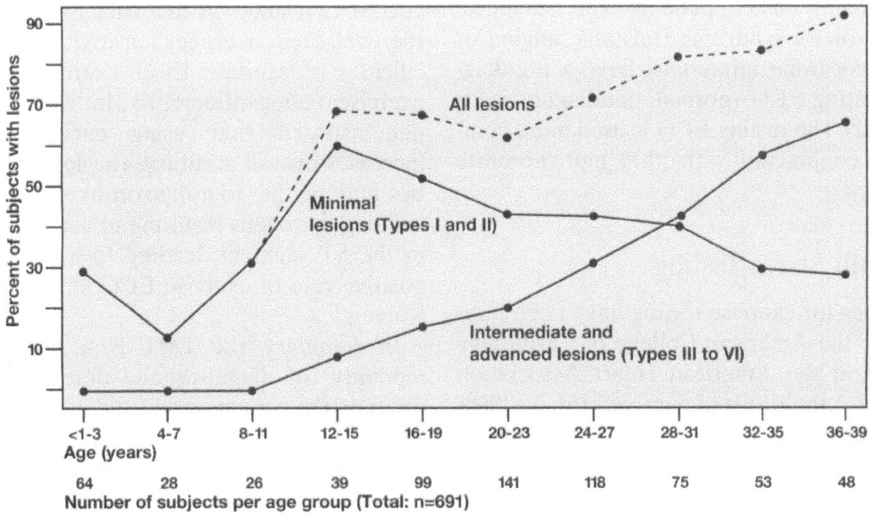

FIGURE 1-2. Atherosclerotic lesions have been classified histologically from type I to VIII. Type VI to VIII lesions have the strongest association with increasing symptoms and fatal outcome. This graph shows the percentages of all subjects with only minimal lesions (type I and II), or with pre-atheroma (type III) or advanced lesions (type IV–VI), plotted for successive 2-year or 4-year age groups. The data were obtained by autopsy microscopy of the LAD. At puberty, 69% and by the end of the fourth decade, 95% of the subjects have some type of coronary artery lesions. The years after puberty are marked by a rise in lesions of types III to VI, which develop from minimal lesions. Lesions type VII and VIII were not found in the coronary arteries of this relatively young population. (From Stary [3], by permission of Parthenon Publishing.)

lasting for more than 40 minutes cause irreversible injury. If the ischemic period is long enough to cause total necrosis (usually 6 to 12 hours), the infarct is transmural. Chronically ischemic myocardium, in which the blood supply is adequate to preserve viability but not to maintain normal cell function, can result in regional dyssynergy (hibernating myocardium). Revascularization procedures with restoration of normal blood flow to this tissue often lead to significant improvement in wall motion and ventricular function.[6]

An interesting observation is that the location of only 22% to 55% of future myocardial infarctions (MI) can be predicted on the basis of the most severe coronary stenosis by coronary angiography, and that most MIs do not occur at the sites of the most obstructing plaques.[7,8] Infarcts often occur due to the rupture of unstable or *soft* plaque with resultant occlusion of the coronary artery lumen.[9]

Modalities Available for the Evaluation of the Cardiac Patient

Electrocardiography

Since its early description by Einthoven[10] 100 years ago, the resting electrocardiogram (ECG) has been proven useful as a screening tool for heart disease. Despite the plethora of more sophisticated modalities available to evaluate the heart, none is so widely performed as a simple resting ECG. It is inexpensive; is universally available; can be performed in the physician's office; and provides information about heart rhythm, myocardial hypertrophy, conduction system abnormalities, myocardial injury and infarction, and in many cases acute or chronic ischemic changes. Of course, the resting ECG has its limitations. For example, approximately 50% of patients experiencing an acute coronary syndrome (unstable angina or acute myocardial infarction) have a nondiagnostic resting ECG (normal, nondiagnostic, or equivocal). The resting ECG is used more commonly in conjunction with other, more accurate modalities.

Treadmill Stress Testing

Guidelines for exercise testing have been published by the American College of Cardiology (ACC) and the American Heart Association (AHA).[11] A multitude of parameters have been studied and validated over the last 4 decades. Some useful parameters from the treadmill testing (TMT) include total exercise time, magnitude of increase in blood pressure and heart rate (indicative of good cardiac function), the magnitude of ST-segment shifts, the presence of chest pain on exertion, and the cardiac rhythm during exercise. In addition, the prognostic information obtained from a TMT is extremely important. Failure to achieve 85% of the age-predicted maximum heart rate and a low chronotropic index are predictive of adverse cardiovascular events.[12] The average sensitivity and specificity of TMT for the diagnosis of coronary artery disease (CAD) are 67% and 72%, respectively, according to two meta-analyses.[13,14] Unfortunately, the TMT also has additional limitations. The exercise ECG is noninterpretable in patients with left bundle branch block (LBBB) and pacemakers. In addition, some baseline ECG abnormalities make any additional changes during exercise poorly specific, such as those that may occur in left ventricular hypertrophy (LVH), with the use of some medications such as digitalis, and in the presence of Wolff-Parkinson-White syndrome or prior MI. Furthermore, the sensitivity of TMT is decreased, especially when related to a limited capacity to achieve an adequate increment of myocardial oxygen consumption, due either to limited exercise capacity or because of concurrent treatment with medications such as calcium channel blockers and beta-blockers.

TMT is less accurate in women than in men due to a higher number of false-positive exercise ECG results.[15] A metaanalysis determined the weighted average sensitivities and specificities of exercise ECG, exercise ^{201}Tl, and exercise echocardiography in women,[16] and demonstrated that using cardiac imaging increases overall accuracy. The lower specificities may be due to a digoxin-like effect of circulating estrogens resulting in varying changes in the ST segment, leading to a higher false-positive rate of exercise ECG stress testing in women.[17]

In summary, the TMT is a good proven modality for diagnosis and determination of prognosis in patients suspected of having CAD, but a wide variety of limitations restrict its utility, requiring the use of alternative or complementary modalities in many patients.

Echocardiography

Early in its development, echocardiography was mainly used at rest to evaluate cardiac structures and measure wall thickness, chamber volumes, heart valves, and global contractility. Technological improvements permitted the development of new applications. Regarding the detection of CAD, stress echocardiography using exercise or dobutamine stress has been widely used.[18] The occurrence of a transient contractile abnormality during dobutamine infusion is a very specific finding for the presence of CAD, and sensitivity is equally high. The limitations of the test include dobutamine intolerance in some patients, difficulties in acquiring high-quality images in some patients with a limited acoustic window, and difficulties in defining all the endocardial borders in some patients. Approximately 4% to 5% of patients have complex ventricular arrhythmias, such as ventricular tachycardia, during dobutamine infusion. Despite this, the overall safety profile of the test is considered good, as discussed in a review by Ehlendy et al.[19] Patients with previous MI and extensive scar tissue may already have significant wall motion abnormalities at rest, which impose a challenge for interpretation. Patients with preexistent ventricular dysrhythmia, poorly controlled atrial fibrillation, or concurrent beta-blockade are poor candidates for dobutamine stress.

Magnetic Resonance Imaging

Multiple applications for cardiac MRI have been developed during the last decade. Its major advantages over other technologies are its magnificent spatial resolution, good temporal resolution, high contrast between rapidly flowing blood and cardiac chambers, superior soft tissue contrast, and therefore excellent definition of cardiac structures. These advantageous aspects of MRI can be used to provide (1) superb three-dimensional definition of normal and pathologic anatomic details, allowing highly accurate measurement of wall thickness, volume, and mass; and (2) qualitative and quantitative assessment of the function of cardiac chambers and valves, with direct measurement of functional indices and wall-thickening dynamics. Phase contrast imaging can produce Doppler-like waveforms, allowing measurement of indices such as pressure gradients across stenosis or total blood flow through the aorta or pulmonary artery.

Technological developments have permitted progressive improvement in image quality and resolution. Recent MRI studies have demonstrated the possibility of defining thrombus age and monitoring the progression and regression of atherosclerotic lesions in experimental animal models.[20,21]

In addition to detailed evaluation of anatomy, dynamic contrast-enhanced MR angiography allows evaluation of myocardial perfusion in the resting state and during pharmacological stress[22] and allows for the accurate detection of stenosis of the proximal and middle segments of the coronary arteries.[23] Delayed contrast enhancement identifies areas of scarring and helps to differentiate scar from viable myocardium. A thorough discussion of the present and future applications of cardiac MRI is presented in Chapter 14.

Computed Tomography, Electron Beam Computed Tomography, and Computed Tomographic Angiography

A recent development in CT is the helical acquisition of multiple tomographic slices simultaneously, known as multiple-slice computed tomography (MSCT). Compared with single-slice CT, MSCT permits a large area to be scanned in a shorter time and in greater detail. With improved spatial resolution and ECG-gated acquisition, MSCT can assess cardiac function and congenital structural anomalies and perform high-resolution CT coronary angiography. In Chapter 15, the cardiac applications of MSCT are discussed in more detail.

Both helical CT and electron beam computed tomography (EBCT) allow quantification of coronary artery calcification using coronary calcium scoring. The calcium score correlates with the extent of coronary atherosclerosis, although only approximately 20% of atherosclerotic plaques are calcified.[24,25] Therefore, coronary calcium scoring has applications for early detection of coronary atherosclerosis, risk stratification, and monitoring the progression or regression of atherosclerosis with therapy, as outlined in the Expert Consensus Document on EBCT for the diagnosis and prognosis of CAD published by the ACC/AHA.[25] Coronary calcium scoring is discussed in more depth in Cases 9.9 and 18.11.

Contrasted Coronary Angiography and Intravascular Ultrasound

Both coronary angiography and intravascular ultrasound (IVUS) are invasive and costly techniques for evaluation of CAD. The technical advances of noninvasive imaging modalities allow early diagnosis of CAD, and coronary angiography can be reserved to evaluate the anatomical aspect of lesions and to plan therapy. Unfortunately, coronary angiography cannot predict the site of a subsequent MI in a patient with mild to moderate CAD,[7] illustrating that those lesions that are detected are not necessarily the lesions that put the patient at risk of adverse cardiac events. The development of IVUS has permitted exquisite assessment of coronary plaque morphology, helping to differentiate *hard* stable plaques from *soft* vulnerable plaques, as well as more accurate measurement of the stenotic area compared with contrast angiography alone. A rational integration of noninvasive techniques used to detect CAD and determine prognosis in CAD, with the invasive ones (coronary angiography and IVUS), to evaluate the detailed anatomical and morphological aspects of lesions, constitutes state-of-the-art practice of cardiology today.

Nuclear Cardiology

Nuclear medicine procedures allow evaluation of myocardial perfusion, viability, and function using SPECT, gated SPECT, PET, and radionuclide ventriculography (RVG). These techniques continue to evolve. Nuclear imaging of the heart is a valuable, widely used, noninvasive procedure that reveals important information about cardiac structure and physiology,[26,27] and is the major focus of this text. The indications for cardiac radionuclide imaging have been extensively reviewed and discussed in the guidelines published by a task force of the ACC/AHA.[28]

Myocardial perfusion imaging (MPI) is a nuclear medicine technique widely used to evaluate MBF. It provides the possibility of evaluating the coronary blood flow reserve, detecting ischemia, and providing risk stratification, including the degree, location, and extent to which CAD is affecting MBF. The prognostic and diagnostic value of MPI has been well established in the literature over the last three decades. MPI continues to grow, with 3.1 million patients in the United States undergoing MPI in 1996, 3.7 million in 1997, 4.1 million in 1998, 4.5 million in 1999, and 6 million in 2001 (according to industry sources of information). The number of ^{201}Tl administrations remained similar between 1998 and 2001, whereas the number of ^{99m}Tc-labeled radiopharmaceutical administrations doubled. At the time of this writing, approximately 30% of MPIs are performed using ^{201}Tl alone, 30% using ^{99m}Tc-MIBI alone, 20% using rest ^{201}Tl/stress ^{99m}Tc-MIBI, and 20% using ^{99m}Tc tetrofosmin, either alone or in combination with ^{201}Tl.[28]

The stress tests most commonly used for evaluation of coronary blood flow reserve include exercise, dipyridamole, adenosine, physical exercise combined with dipyridamole or adenosine, and dobutamine. These different stress protocols are discussed in Chapter 4. The most common indication for MPI, detection of CAD,[30] is addressed in Chapter 5, and more recently developed applications such as evaluation of acute coronary syndromes, evaluation of viability in myocardium at risk, evaluation of prognosis and risk stratification of patients with CAD,[31] and imaging the effects of therapy[32] are addressed in Chapters 6, 8, 9, and 10, respectively. Recent technological developments in nuclear imaging include improved software and hardware for better performance and interpretation of gated SPECT studies. These have been reviewed in a statement by the American Society of Nuclear Cardiology (ASNC).[33]

Evaluation of ventricular function is critical in many clinical situations, including patients with CAD and valvular diseases.[34] Both global and regional wall motion can be accurately evaluated with gated blood pool studies (RVG). In addition, ventricular size, right and left ventricular ejection fractions (RVEF and LVEF), and regurgitation indices can be calculated. The RVG technology and other nonperfusion applications in nuclear cardiology have been reviewed and summarized in a report by the task force of the ASNC.[35] Recent technical developments of SPECT technology applied to gated blood pool studies allow more accurate evaluation of ventricular function, especially right ventricular function and diastolic dysfunction. This is further discussed in Chapter 7. Alternative methods for these measurements include echocardiography, MRI, and contrast ventriculography.

Multimodality integrated imaging with integrated PET-CT and SPECT-CT systems offers the possibility for simultaneous evaluation of anatomy and function and is one of the most exciting new developments in imaging technology. Currently, most PET-CT imaging systems are equipped with a 2- or 4-slice CT scanner, but integrated PET-CT systems with a 16-slice CT scanner are becoming increasingly available for advanced cardiac applications. Case 1.1 illustrates an example of imaging atherosclerosis with ^{18}F fluorodeoxyglucose (FDG) and precise localization using an integrated PET-CT imaging system.

The choice of one of the tests discussed previously, to evaluate a specific patient, depends on several factors, including availability of technology, local experience with a given modality, and the pretest probability of disease, as well as patient-specific factors such as body habitus and resting ECG abnormalities.

Updated imaging guidelines for nuclear cardiology procedures have been published,[36] as well as guidelines for physician[37] and technologist[38] training in nuclear cardiology.

Choice of Tests Based on Prevalence of Disease

The appropriateness of noninvasive testing has to be considered in light of the Bayes theorem, which expresses the posttest likelihood of disease as a function of sensitivity and specificity of the test and the prevalence (or pretest probability) of disease in the population that is being tested. Algorithms used to evaluate patients for myocardial ischemia depend on the pretest probability for the presence of CAD. Patients can be classified into low, intermediate, or high pretest probability. Placing a patient into one or another category depends greatly on the physician's judgment, taking into consideration the patient's age, gender, coronary risk factors, and symptoms.

Diamond and Forrester[39] have reported the prevalence of CAD based on the patient's age, gender, and symptoms, after a review of the literature including 28,948 patients. With respect to symptoms, the patients were classified as having asymptomatic, nonanginal, atypical, and typical chest pain according to 3 characteristics of chest pain (substernal location, induction by exercise, relieved by nitroglycerin). When the 3 characteristics were present, the patients were classified as having typical chest pain. Their results demonstrated that the prevalence of CAD in the asymptomatic population ranges from 0% to 20%. As another example, the pretest likelihood of disease for men 30 to 60 years of age is much higher than that for women of the same age, of course, secondary to the influence of gender on CAD development. If symptoms of typical chest pain are present, as opposed to those of atypical chest pain, the pretest probability of CAD is markedly increased. Factors such as smoking; family history of CAD; sedentary life-style; or the presence of hypercholesterolemia, hypertension, or diabetes mellitus are known to contribute to the risk of CAD and to increase even further the pretest probability. The aggressiveness of further evaluation depends on the pretest probability.

Once the pretest probability of disease is estimated, an algorithm can be created to evaluate patients with chest pain. The posttest probability for CAD depends on the sensitivity and specificity of the test being performed. Figure 1-3 demonstrates the posttest likelihood of

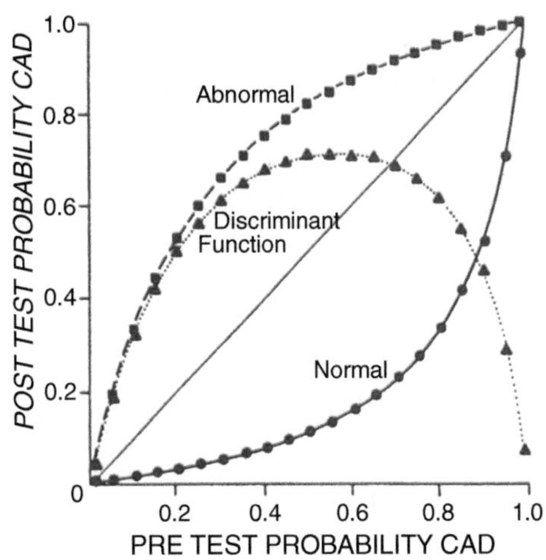

FIGURE 1-3. Probability of CAD and posttest probability of CAD for abnormal and normal results of quantitative ^{201}Tl stress imaging (sensitivity 90%, specificity 95%). The curve describes the difference between posttest probability of a normal and an abnormal test result, indicating the range of disease prevalence for which ^{201}Tl stress imaging discriminates most effectively between the presence or absence of disease. ^{201}Tl stress imaging is most useful when the pretest prevalence of CAD is 40% to 70%. For example, in a patient with a pretest probability of disease of 60%, a positive ^{201}Tl stress test increases the probability of CAD to 90%, while a negative test result decreases it to approximately 15%. Symbols: ■ = abnormal; ▲ = posttest probability difference; ● = normal. (From Hamilton, Trobaugh, Richie [40], by permission of *Semin Nucl Med.*)

CAD according to negative and positive ^{201}Tl studies in patients with different pretest likelihood of CAD.[40]

Patients with Low Pretest Probability of Coronary Artery Disease

According to Diamond and Forrester[39], a positive result obtained with MPI study or another method of evaluating myocardial ischemia (e.g., TMT and stress echocardiography) is more likely to be a false-positive result if the patient has a low pretest probability for CAD. This suggests that a positive MPI study result in asymptomatic patients with low risk factors (low pretest probability) does not necessarily establish the presence of CAD, while a negative test result effectively excludes the presence of CAD. Several studies do support that theoretical conclusion.[41,42] Therefore, the approach to the evaluation of patients with a low pretest probability is to begin with a resting ECG and a TMT. If there are abnormalities on the resting ECG, making it noninterpretable during a TMT, other options including imaging should be considered. MPI is one of the most sensitive and specific methods for the noninvasive evaluation of myocardial ischemia. Pooled data from 19 studies[43] have shown a sensitivity of 83% to 98% (with a mean of 92%) and a specificity of 53% to 100% (with a mean of 77%) for detecting ischemia.

Patients with Intermediate Pretest Probability of Coronary Artery Disease

MPI has optimal discriminative value in the patient population with an intermediate pretest probability of CAD in the range of 40% to 70%. This population includes: patients with nonanginal chest pain and a positive or nondiagnostic exercise ECG; asymptomatic patients with significant risk factors, abnormal resting ECG, or positive exercise ECG; patients with atypical chest pain; and patients with typical chest pain and a negative exercise ECG. For patients in this category, MPI may be more helpful as an initial evaluation than it would be in those with a low or high pretest probability. A positive result is more likely to be a true-positive finding in a patient with intermediate probability than in a patient with low probability. A negative result in a patient with intermediate probability is more likely to be a true-negative finding than in a patient with high pretest probability. This hypothesis was also supported by several studies.[44,45]

Patients with High Pretest Probability of Coronary Artery Disease

Patients with a high pretest probability should almost always be investigated more aggressively. According to the Bayes theorem, a negative MPI study in a patient with a high pretest probability for CAD—for example, symptomatic patients—is more likely to have a false-negative than a true-negative result. Coronary angiography is often used for the initial evaluation in these patients.

In some cases, the angiographic findings are already known, and the question is whether or not the lesions found compromise MBF, and to what extent. Information obtained with MPI allows accurate estimation of the prognosis. It is essential to remember that CAD is not synonymous with myocardial ischemia and that anatomic findings do not always provide information about the physiological significance of coronary lesions.

Conclusions

The evaluation of CAD involves a great deal of individual judgment by the physician. Before ordering any diagnostic test, it is essential to obtain a thorough medical history and perform a complete physical examination, formulating a diagnostic hypothesis and determining the pretest probability of disease. Nuclear cardiac studies and other complementary modalities are extremely helpful when well indicated and are invaluable diagnostic tools to evaluate the cardiac patient in today's practice of medicine.

Although MPI is more expensive than the TMT, its higher sensitivity and specificity for detection of myocardial ischemia can result in a more cost-effective evaluation, depending on the population being studied. MPI is also useful in patients who cannot perform exercise due to peripheral vascular disease or neurologic, orthopedic, or pulmonary problems. In these patients, MPI with pharmacological stress is an excellent alternative to exercise.

Case Presentation

Case 1.1

History

A 62-year-old man with no coronary risk factors, and no history of CAD or other known vascular disease was diagnosed with B-cell lymphoma. He had no cardiac symptoms, and his resting ECG was normal. He underwent bone marrow stem cell transplantation and was referred to PET-CT for restaging. An RVG, performed before therapy, demonstrated normal wall motion and an LVEF of 61%. Coronal and transaxial FDG PET, CT, and fusion images through the thoracic aorta obtained with an integrated PET-CT system are shown in Figure C1-1 A and B.

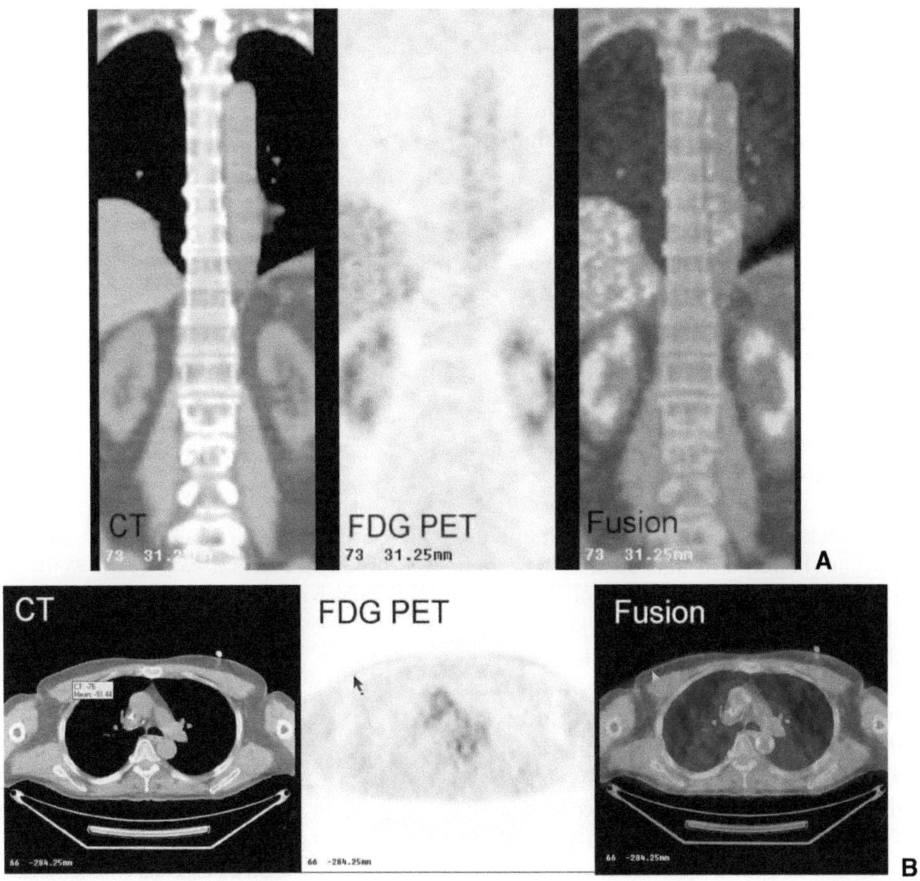

FIGURE C1-1. (A and B)

Findings

The images demonstrate FDG uptake in the walls of the ascending and descending thoracic aorta consistent with atherosclerosis, probably due to significant inflammatory activity in these atherosclerotic plaques.

Discussion

Inflammation contributes to atherosclerotic plaque remodeling, enlargement, and rupture. It has been reported that there is a high correlation between FDG uptake in the aorta and macrophage content of atherosclerotic lesions in an experimental rabbit model.[46] Histopathology confirmed that injured iliac artery had significantly higher intimal and medial cross-sectional area compared with uninjured artery. Injured artery also had significantly higher macrophage and smooth muscle cell density. Vascular uptake might be explained by smooth muscle metabolism in the media, subendothelial smooth muscle proliferation, and the presence of macrophages within the atherosclerotic plaque.

The frequency of FDG uptake in the large arteries has been correlated with age, atherogenic risk factors, and the presence of clinically known CAD. Among all risk factors, age was the most significant and consistent factor correlating with FDG uptake in large arteries. Vascular FDG uptake was present in 50% of the patients examined in a study of 133 patients referred for whole body FDG PET imaging, with an increased prevalence in older patients. When divided according to age, uptake of FDG in large arteries was present in 34% of patients younger than 40 years of age, 50% of patients between age 40 and 60 years, and 61% of patients over age 60.[47] The correlation with hypercholesterolemia seems consistent as well in a study of 156 patients.[48] A higher frequency of FDG uptake in the femoral arteries is present in patients with CAD compared with those without CAD. The positive correlation of arterial FDG uptake with the atherogenic risk factors suggests a promising role for FDG PET imaging in the diagnosis of atherosclerosis and follow-up after treatment intervention. Vascular uptake may also be seen in vasculitis, such as Takayasu's arteritis.[49,50]

A relatively recent study reports the ability of FDG PET to image carotid artery atherosclerotic plaque rupture and inflammation in eight patients.[51] Symptomatic plaques were visualized on FDG PET and the estimated net accumulation rate (plaque/integral plasma) was 27% higher in symptomatic than in contralateral asymptomatic lesions. Autoradiography of excised plaques confirmed accumulation in macrophage-rich areas of the plaque. Because FDG uptake is associated with the presence of macrophages, and the presence of macrophages contributes to plaque remodeling and eventual rupture, it has been postulated that FDG is a promising radiopharmaceutical for imaging soft plaques at risk of rupture.

Interpretation

Diffuse atherosclerotic disease demonstrated by FDG uptake in the aorta of an asymptomatic, 62-year-old man.

References

1. Dublin LI, Lorka LI, Spiegelman M. *Length of Life: A Study of the Life of the Life Table.* New York: Ronald Press; 1949.
2. Batchelor WB, Jollis JG, Friesinger GC. The challenge of health care delivery to the elderly patient with cardiovascular disease. *Cardiology Clinics.* 1999;17(1):1–17.
3. Stary HC (ed). *Atlas of Atherosclerosis: Progression and Regression.* New York: Parthenon Publishing; 1999.
4. Burke AP, Farb A, Kolodgie FD, et al. Atherosclerotic plaque morphology and coronary thrombi. *J Nucl Cardiol.* 2002;9:95–103.
5. Gould KL, Lipscomb K, Hamilton GW. Physiologic basis for assessing critical coronary stenosis. Instantaneous flow response and regional distribution during coronary hyperemia as measures of coronary flow reserve. *Am J Cardiol.* 1974;33:87–94.
6. Dilsizian V, Bonow RO. Current diagnostic techniques of assessing myocardial viability in patients with hibernating and stunned myocardium. *Circulation.* 1993;87:1–20.
7. Little WC, Constantinescu M, Applegate RJ, et al. Can coronary angiography predict the site of

a subsequent myocardial infarction in patients with mild to moderate coronary artery disease? *Circulation.* 1988;78:1157–1166.
8. Ambrose JA, Fuster V. The risk of coronary occlusion is not proportional to the prior severity of coronary stenoses. *Heart.* 1998;79:3–4.
9. Fuster V, Stein B, Ambrose JA, et al. Atherosclerotic plaque rupture and thrombosis. Evolving concept. *Circulation.* 1990;82(3 Suppl):1147–1159.
10. Einthoven W. Weiteres uber das electrokardiogramm. *Arch Ges Physiol.* 1908;172:517.
11. Gibbons RJ, Antman EM, et al. ACC/AHA 2002 guidelines update for exercise testing.
12. Lauer MS, Mehta R, Pashkow FJ, et al. Association of chronotropic incompetence with echocardiographic ischemia and prognosis. *J Am Coll Cardiol.* 1998;32:1280–1286.
13. Gianrossi R, Detrano R, Mulvihill D, et al. Exercise-induced ST depression in the diagnosis of coronary artery disease: a meta-analysis. *Circulation.* 1989;80:87–89.
14. Detrano R, Gianrossi R, Froelicker V. The diagnostic accuracy of the exercise electrocardiogram: a meta-analysis of 22 years of research. *Prog Cardiovasc.* 1989;32:173–206.
15. Miller TD, Roger VL, Milavetz JJ, et al. Assessment of the exercise electrocardiogram in women versus men using tomographic myocardial perfusion imaging as the reference standard. *Am J Cardiol.* 2001;87:868–873.
16. Kwok Y, Kim C, Grady D, et al. Analysis of exercise testing to detect coronary artery disease in women. *Am J Cardiol.* 1999;83:660–666.
17. Morise AP, Dalal JN, Duval RD. Value of a simple measure of estrogen status for improving the diagnosis of coronary artery disease in women. *Am J Med.* 1993;94:491–496.
18. Verani MS. Myocardial perfusion imaging versus two-dimensional echocardiography: comparative value in the diagnosis of coronary artery disease. *J Nucl Cardiol.* 1994;1:399–414.
19. Ehlendy A, Bax JJ, Poldermans D. Dobutamine stress myocardial perfusion imaging in coronary artery disease. *J Nucl Med.* 2002;43:1634–1646.
20. Corti R, Osende JI, Fayad ZA, et al. In vivo noninvasive detection and age definition of arterial thrombus by MRI. *J Am Coll Cardiol.* 2002;39:1366–1376.
21. Helft G, Worthley SG, Fuster V, et al. Progression and regression of atherosclerotic lesions: monitoring with serial noninvasive magnetic resonance imaging. *Circulation.* 2002;105:993–998.
22. Hartiala J, Sakuma H, Higgins CB. Magnetic resonance imaging and spectroscopy of the human heart. *Scand J Clin Lab Invest.* 1993;53:425–437.
23. Kim WY, Danias PG, Stuber M, et al. Coronary magnetic resonance angiography for the detection of coronary stenosis. *N Engl J Med.* 2001;345:1863–1869.
24. O'Rourke RA, Brundage BH, Froelicke VF, et al. American College of Cardiology/American Heart Association Expert consensus document on electron beam computed tomography for the diagnosis and prognosis of coronary artery disease. *J Am Coll Cardiol.* 2000;36:326–340.
25. O'Rourke RA, Brundage BH, Froelicke VF, et al. American College of Cardiology/American Heart Association Expert consensus document on electron beam computed tomography for the diagnosis and prognosis of coronary artery disease. *Circulation.* 2000;102:126–159.
26. Zaret BL, Wackers FJ. Nuclear cardiology, part 1. *N Engl J Med.* 1993;329:775–783.
27. Zaret BL, Wackers FJ. Nuclear cardiology, part 2. *N Engl J Med.* 1993;329:855–863.
28. Ritchie JL, Cheitlin MD, Garson A, et al. Guidelines for clinical use of cardiac radionuclide imaging: Report of the American College of Cardiology/American Heart Association Task Force on assessment of diagnostic and therapeutic cardiovascular procedures (Committee on Radionuclide Imaging), developed in collaboration with the American Society of Nuclear Cardiology. *J Am Coll Cardiol.* 1995;25(2):521–547.
29. Berman DS, Hayes SW, Germano G. Assessment of myocardial perfusion and viability with technetium-99m perfusion agents. In DePuey EG, Garcia EV, Berman DS (eds). *Cardiac SPECT Imaging.* Philadelphia: Lippincott Williams & Wilkins; 2001:179–210.
30. Iskandrian AS, Heo J, Kong B, Lyons E, Marsch S. Use of technetium-99m isonitrile (RP-30A) in assessing left ventricular perfusion and function at rest and during exercise in coronary artery disease, and comparison with coronary arteriography and exercise ^{201}Tl SPECT imaging. *Am J Cardiol.* 1989;64:270–275.
31. Brown KA. Prognostic value of ^{201}Tl myocardial perfusion imaging. *Circulation.* 1991;83:363–381.
32. Christian TF, Schwartz RS, Gibbons RJ. Determinants of infarct size in reperfusion therapy for acute myocardial infarction. *Circulation.* 1992;89:81–90.
33. Bateman TM, Berman DS, Heller GV, et al. American Society of Nuclear Cardiology posi-

tion statement on electrocardiographic gating of myocardial perfusion SPECT scintigrams. *J Nucl Cardiol.* 1999;6:470–471.

34. Johnson LL, Tauxe EL. Radionuclide assessment of ventricular function. *Curr Probl Cardiol.* 1994;19:590–635.
35. DePuey EG, Port S, Wackers FJ, et al. Nonperfusion applications in nuclear cardiology: Report of a task force of the American Society of Nuclear Cardiology. *J Nucl Cardiol.* 1998;5: 218–231.
36. DePuey EG, Garcia EV. Updated imaging guidelines for nuclear cardiology procedures. *J Nucl Cardiol.* 2001;8:G1–58.
37. Ritchie JL, Gibbons RJ, Johnson LL, et al. Task force 5: Training in nuclear cardiology. *J Am Coll Cardiol.* 1995;25:1–34.
38. Deman P, Eckdahl J, Folks R, et al. Guidelines for technologist training in nuclear cardiology. *J Nucl Cardiol.* 1997;4:422–425.
39. Diamond GA, Forrester JS. Analysis of probability as an aid in the clinical diagnosis of coronary artery disease. *N Engl J Med.* 1979;300: 1350–1358.
40. Hamilton GW, Trobaugh G, Richie JC, et al. Myocardial imaging with 201Tl: an analysis of clinical usefulness based on Bayes' theorem. *Semin Nucl Med.* 1978;8:358.
41. Uhl GS, Kay TN, Hickman JR Jr. Computer-enhanced thallium scintigram in asymptomatic men with abnormal exercise tests. *Am J Cardiol.* 1981;101:657–666.
42. Uhl GS, Kay TN, Hickman JR Jr, et al. Detection of coronary artery disease in asymptomatic aircrew members with thallium-201 scintigraphy. *Aviat Space Environ Med.* 1980;51:1250–1255.
43. Verani MS. Myocardial perfusion imaging versus two-dimensional echocardiography: Comparative value in the diagnosis of coronary artery disease. *J Nucl Cardiol.* 1994;1:399–414.
44. Melin JA, Piret LJ, Vanbutsele RJ, et al. Diagnostic value of exercise electrocardiography and thallium myocardial scintigraphy in patients without previous myocardial infarction: A Bayesian approach. *Circulation.* 1981;63:1019–1024.
45. Melin JA, Wijns W, Vanbutsele RJ, et al. Alternative diagnostic strategies for coronary artery disease in women: demonstration of the usefulness and efficiency of probability analysis. *Circulation.* 1985;71:535–542.
46. Lederman RJ, Raylman RR, Fisher SJ, et al. Detection of atherosclerosis using a novel positron-sensitive probe and 18-fluorodeoxyglucose (FDG). *Nucl Med Commun.* 2001;22:747–753.
47. Yun M, Yeh D, Araujo LI, et al. F-18 FDG uptake in the large arteries: A new observation. *Clin Nucl Med.* 2001;26:314–319.
48. Yun M, Jang S, Cucchiara A, et al. 18F FDG uptake in the large arteries: A correlation study with the atherogenic risk factors. *Semin Nucl Med.* 2002;32:70–76.
49. Meller J, Grabbe E, Becker W, Vosshenrich R. Value of F-18 FDG hybrid camera PET and MRI in early Takayasu aortitis. *Eur Radiol.* 2003; 13:400–405.
50. Hara M, Goodman PC, Leder RA. FDG PET finding in early-phase Takayasu arteritis. *J Comput Assist Tomogr.* 1999;23:16–18.
51. Rudd JH, Warburton EA, Fryer TD, et al. Imaging atherosclerotic plaque inflammation with [18F]-fluorodeoxyglucose positron emission tomography. *Circulation.* 2002;105:2708–2711.

2 Physics Principles and Instrumentation in Nuclear Cardiology

James A. Patton

For many years cardiac nuclear medicine procedures have been performed using a scintillation camera. Originally, multiple planar projections were acquired to provide diagnostic information, but more recently the techniques of single photon emission computed tomography (SPECT) have been used. During this time, the scintillation camera has evolved into a high-quality imaging device, and much of this evolution is due to the integration of digital technology into every aspect of the data acquisition, processing, and display processes.

Scintillation Camera

A block diagram of the modern-day scintillation camera is shown in Figure 2-1. This diagram has retained some of the nomenclature of early cameras to facilitate discussions of the methods by which the camera acquires an image. Today, as has been the case since the scintillation camera was first introduced, the detector of choice is a NaI(Tl) crystal. Since cardiac applications make use of low-energy radioisotopes (70 and 140 keV), the standard, rectangular, 3/8-inch-thick crystal is ideally suited due to its photopeak detection efficiencies of 100% and 90%, respectively, at these energies. When a photon interacts in the crystal, a flash of light (scintillation) is produced that is proportional to the energy the photon deposits in the crystal. The goal of the camera electronics is to measure accurately the location of the interaction in the crystal, determine if the photon is an unscattered photon (i.e., no interaction in the patient) that has been totally absorbed in the crystal, and display it in the image at a point corresponding precisely to the location of the interaction.

The location of the interaction in the crystal is determined in the following manner. An array of small photomultiplier tubes (PMTs) (55, 61, 75, and so forth, depending on the manufacturer) are either positioned in contact with the crystal or separated a small distance from it using a transparent Lucite light pipe. When scintillations are produced in the crystal as a result of photon interactions, the light is dispersed in all directions. The PMT closest to the point of interaction receives the most light, but many PMTs receive some light, the amount determined by their distance from the point of interaction. In the PMT, the visible light photons are directed to a light-sensitive material where electrons are liberated, the number determined by the number of light photons (intensity). The PMT amplifies the electron flow and integrates the charge to produce an analog voltage pulse whose height is a measure of the intensity of light detected and therefore a measure of the energy that the original photon deposited in the crystal. This pulse is shaped and amplified by a preamplifier and then transferred to an analog-to-digital converter (ADC) that converts the pulse to a number whose magnitude is proportional to the height of the analog voltage pulse. Thus, each PMT/preamplifier/ADC combination produces a number that is a measure of the light collected

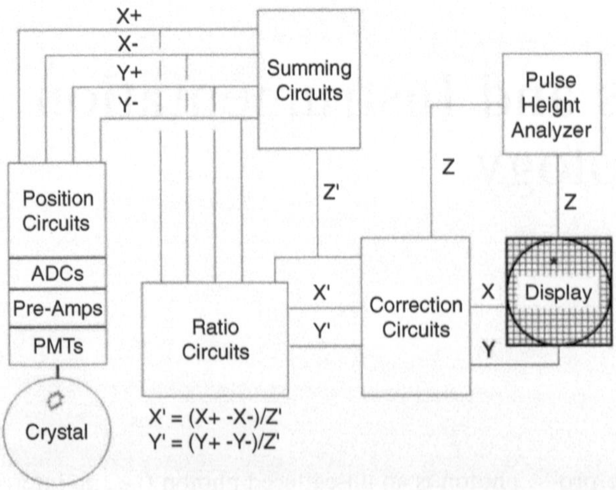

FIGURE 2-1. Block diagram of a state-of-the-art scintillation camera.

by each PMT in the camera head for each interaction in the crystal. A rectangular coordinate system can be established, with the origin at the center of the detector. The outputs of the ADCs can then be grouped depending on the quadrants in which the PMTs are positioned in relation to this coordinate system. For example, the outputs of all PMTs to the right of the Y-axis can be summed together using weighting factors determined by their distance from the Y-axis to produce a net positive X signal (X+). Similarly, X−, Y+, and Y− signals can be determined. The sum of these four signals yields a number that is proportional to the light produced in the crystal as a result of the scintillation process and is therefore a measure of the energy deposited in the crystal by the photon interaction. This signal is designated as Z′.

The four signals from the position circuit are also directed to a component designated as the ratio circuit. Here the X′ and Y′ coordinates of the location of the interaction are calculated:

$$[X' = (X+ - X-)/Z' \text{ and } Y' = (Y+ - Y-)/Z']$$

The division by Z′, the measure of total energy, is necessary to normalize the position measurements by eliminating the effects of different absorption energies on the magnitude of the signals. With this normalization, the absorption of photons of different energies at the same location in the crystal results in identical position calculations. Several years ago, manufacturers learned that improved spatial resolution at low energies could be obtained by reducing the thickness of the crystal and light pipe between the crystal and PMTs (or even eliminating the light pipe) and increasing the number of PMTs. Implementation of these improvements has resulted in scintillation cameras with bar pattern resolutions of approximately 2 mm at 140 keV. However, these changes increase the magnitude of the *nonuniformities* that are inherent in the imaging process. Specifically, there are errors in the measurement of energy and position that vary with the location of interactions in the crystal due to slight differences in absorption, scintillation production, and transmission to PMTs, and with the differences in gains of PMTs. These errors are corrected by digital circuitry to produce accurate measurements of energy and position.

An integral part of the scintillation camera system is the collimator that forms the image on the crystal before the detection process is performed. Parallel-hole collimators are almost universally used for nuclear cardiology applications. Each hole of the collimator permits a small region of the distribution being imaged to be measured by the portion of the crystal that is illuminated by that hole. Thus, this collimator forms a 2-dimensional image on the crystal with a one-to-one representation between object and image. Multiple low-energy collimators,

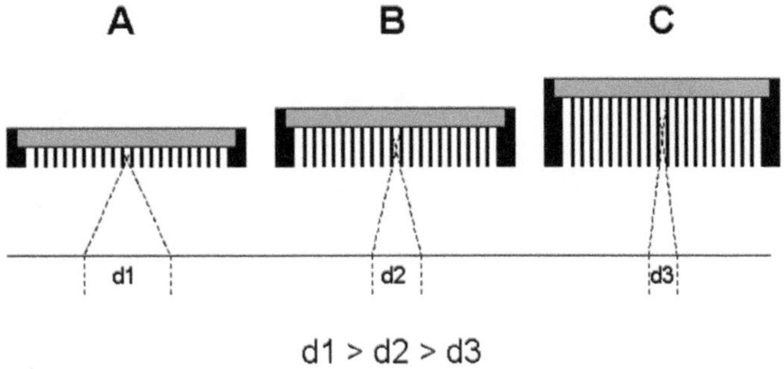

FIGURE 2-2. Low-energy, parallel hole collimators are generally classified as (A) high sensitivity, (B) general purpose, and (C) high resolution based on the relative length of the holes. Hole diameter can also be varied to produce the same results.

typically classified as high sensitivity, general purpose, and high resolution, are available from all manufacturers, as shown in Figure 2-2. High-sensitivity collimators are used only for first-pass studies in which resolution can be sacrificed for sensitivity. General-purpose and high-resolution collimators are used for routine static imaging and gated acquisition studies, with high-resolution collimators being the choice for multihead cameras in which collimator sensitivity can be sacrificed to improve spatial resolution.

Scintillation Camera Quality Assurance

To be certain that the scintillation camera is providing images that are of optimal quality, it is necessary to perform routine tests to evaluate the performance of the camera. Because most modern-day cameras are digitally based, it is generally assumed that measurements can be made at a single energy to verify the performance at all energies used for routine imaging procedures. Typically, a source of ^{57}Co is used because its energy (122 keV) is close to that of ^{99m}Tc (140 keV) and it has a relatively long half-life (240 days). Calibration sources of ^{57}Co in planar source configurations with uniform distributions that are accurate to 1% are commercially available and can be used for extrinsic (with the collimator on) measurements. At the beginning of each day, the peaking and uniformity of the camera should be verified. This is accomplished by placing the planar source in contact with the collimated camera, selecting the ^{57}Co window and peak settings, and evaluating the position of the pulse height analyzer window on the photopeak of the energy spectrum, as shown in Figure 2-3. The center of the window should be at the peak of the ^{57}Co spectrum. An image of the planar source is then acquired with sufficient counts to minimize statistical effects (typically 2 to 4 million counts, depending on the size of the camera detector). This flood image is then evaluated visually for nonuniformities and can be compared with a reference image made when the last tune-up was obtained and the camera was performing optimally. A calculation of integral uniformity can also be performed to

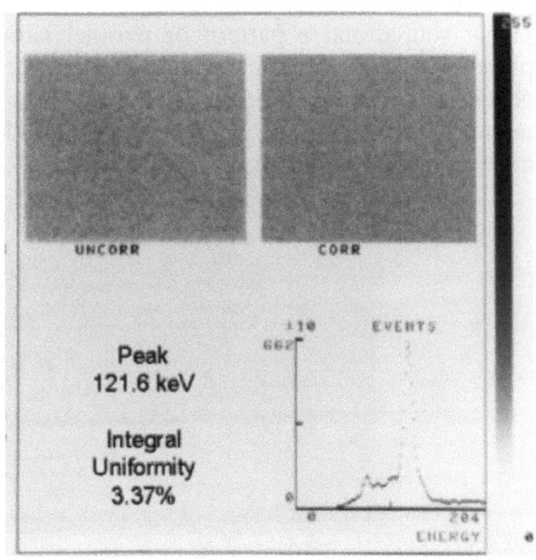

FIGURE 2-3. Example of a daily energy peak and uniformity check performed on a digital scintillation camera.

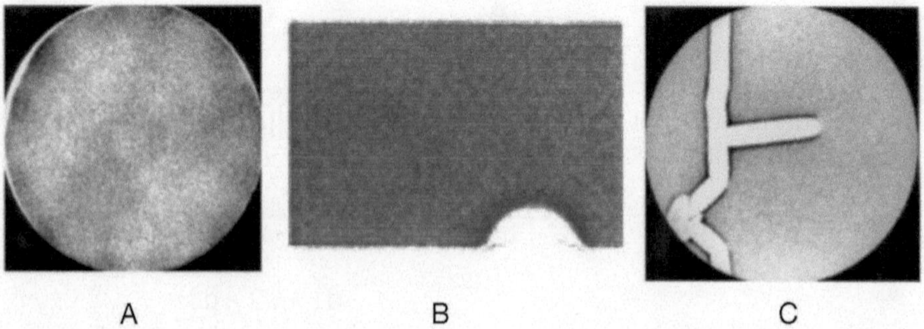

FIGURE 2-4. Examples of problems easily identified with a uniformity measurement. (A) Window off peak, (B) faulty photomultiplier tube, and (C) broken crystal.

numerically assess the uniformity of the image. Integral uniformity is defined as:

$$[(\max - \min)/(\max + \min)] \times 100$$

where max and min are the maximum- and minimum-intensity pixels in the image. This calculation actually provides a measure of the nonuniformity of the image, and modern-day cameras should have values of 2% to 4% when performing optimally. Figure 2-4 illustrates three problems that can be readily identified by performing a uniformity evaluation.

A weekly evaluation of spatial resolution and linearity should be performed using the ^{57}Co planar source and a pattern or parallel bars placed between the camera and the source acquiring an image with sufficient counts to minimize the effects of statistics as in the flood measurement, as illustrated in Figure 2-5. Ideally, this measurement should be performed intrinsically (with the collimator off) as shown in Figure 2-5A, but some laboratories choose to make this measurement extrinsically as shown in Figure 2-5B. If the latter method is chosen, it should be realized that spatial resolutions will be poorer than the intrinsic measurements due to the presence of the collimator. The bar pattern image should be visually evaluated for slight degradations in resolution and variations in linearity.

Single Photon Emission Computed Tomography

Cardiac nuclear medicine images of distributions of ^{201}Tl and ^{99m}Tc were originally obtained

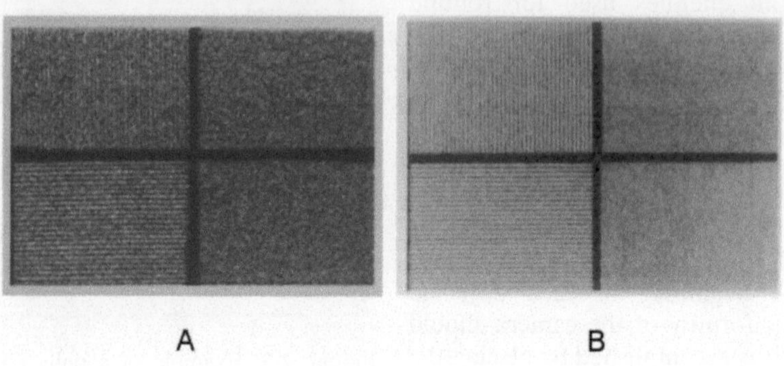

FIGURE 2-5. Examples of (A) extrinsic and (B) spatial resolution measurements performed on a scintillation camera.

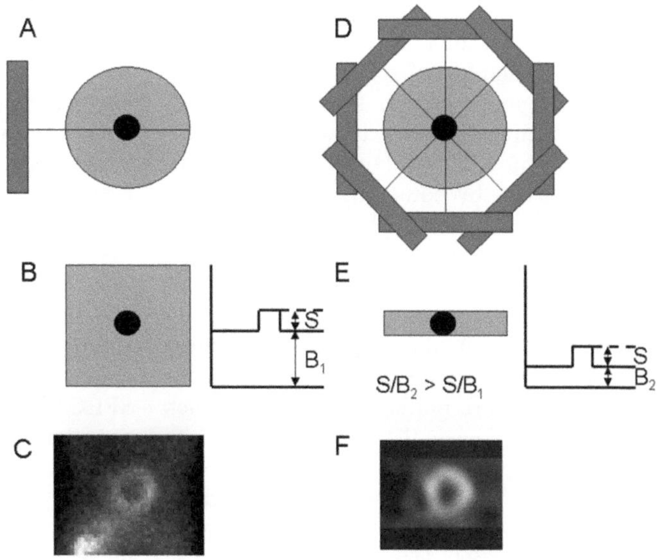

FIGURE 2-6. Planar images (A) are inherently low in contrast (B) due to contributions from activity above and below the region of interest. SPECT images reconstructed from multiple planar views (D) provide contrast (E) by eliminating contributions from activity outside the region of interest. Comparisons of planar and SPECT images of the myocardium are shown in C and F, respectively.

by conventional planar imaging techniques. But these images generally suffered from poor contrast due to the presence of overlying and underlying activity that interferes with imaging the region of interest. This is caused by the superposition of depth information into single data points collected from perpendicular or angled lines of travel of photons from the distribution being studied into the holes of the parallel-hole collimator fitted to the scintillation camera, as shown in Figure 2-6A. The resulting planar image, shown in Figures 2-6B and 2-6C, is low in contrast (S/B_1) due to the effect of the superposition of depth information. This effect can be reduced by collecting images from multiple positions around the distribution (Figure 2-6D) and producing an image of a transverse slice through the distribution, as shown in Figures 2-6E and 2-6F. The resulting tomographic image is of higher contrast (S/B_2) than the planar image due to the elimination of contributions of activity above and below the region of interest. This is the goal of single photon emission computed tomography (SPECT), i.e., to provide images of slices of radionuclide distributions with image contrast that is higher than that provided by conventional techniques.

SPECT Data Acquisition

Instrumentation

The development of the scintillation camera in the 1960s and its ultimate evolution into the imaging system of choice for routine nuclear medicine imaging applications resulted in a great deal of effort being expended toward the extension of the scintillation camera as a tomographic imaging device. The result of these efforts, along with the integration of computer systems, was the development of the modern-day SPECT system as a scintillation camera/computer system with 1, 2, or 3 heads and tomographic capability. The scintillation camera collects tomographic data by rotating around the region of interest and acquiring multiple planar projection images during its rotation. It is imperative that the region of interest be included in every projection image. If this is not the case, the resulting truncation of the images will produce artifacts in the final reconstructed images. The camera may move in a continuous motion during acquisition, but typically remains stationary during the acquisition of each projection image before advancing to the next position in a 'step-and-shoot' mode of operation. A complete 360-degree rotation of a scintillation camera with a rectangular field of view completely samples a cylindrical region of interest. Originally, camera systems were only capable of circular orbits. However, modern-day systems have elliptical orbit capability. This is accomplished by equipping the collimators with sensors that detect the presence of the patient and maintain the camera head(s) in close proximity to the patient as the orbit is completed. Since the spatial resolution of collimators used with the scintillation camera degrades with distance from the collimator face, the optimal resolution is obtained in each projection image when the camera is as close to the patient as possible.

Initial SPECT applications were performed with a single-head scintillation camera acquiring data from a 360-degree orbit as shown in Figure 2-7A. When interest in imaging the myocardium became prominent, experimental work demonstrated that acceptable images could be obtained using a 180-degree orbit (right anterior oblique to left posterior oblique).[1,2] Although this results in an incomplete sampling of the region of interest, the region of interest lies in the near field of view of the camera throughout the partial orbit where the spatial resolution is optimal, and images of acceptable quality are obtained. Early in the evolution of SPECT imaging it became evident that optimal counting statistics for many applications could not be obtained in a reasonable time frame that patients could tolerate. This situation was remedied by the development of multihead scintillation cameras. The first system to evolve was a dual-head camera in a fixed 180-degree geometry, permitting a 360-degree acquisition with only a 180-degree rotation of the gantry. This development provided a twofold increase in sensitivity for SPECT applications. However, this increase in sensitivity was not available for cardiac applications using 180-degree acquisitions. To address this problem, special-purpose, dual-head cameras were developed, with the camera heads fixed in a 90-degree geometry as shown in Figure 2-7B. This made a twofold increase in sensitivity available for cardiac imaging, and projections through 180 degrees could be acquired with a 90-degree rotation of the dual-head gantry. Since many scintillation cameras must serve multiple purposes in nuclear medicine departments, the next step was the development of dual-head, variable-angle scintillation cameras, as shown in Figure 2-7C.

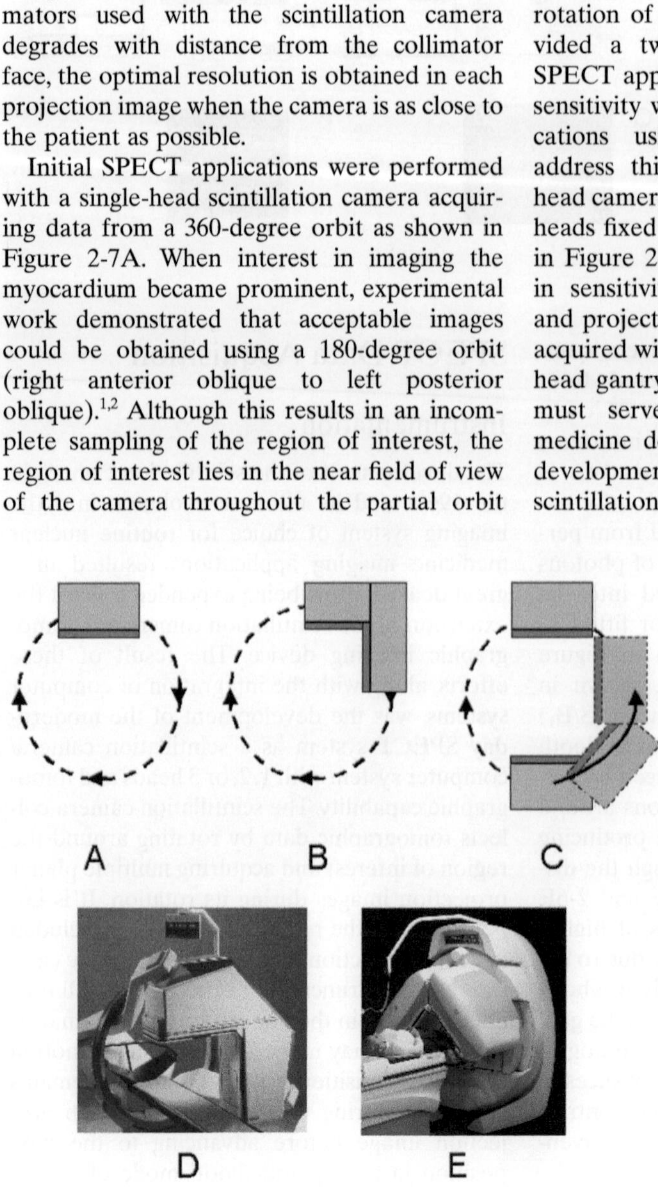

FIGURE 2-7. Scintillation cameras for cardiac nuclear medicine applications have evolved from single-head (A) to dual-head, fixed 90-degree geometry (B) and finally to dual-head, variable-angle multipurpose cameras (C). Examples of commercially available systems include dual-head, fixed 90-degree geometry (D) and dual-head, variable-angle (E) scintillation cameras. (General Electric Medical Systems, Waukesha, WI.)

These cameras can acquire images with the heads in a 180-degree geometry for routine 360-degree applications, and one head can be moved into a 90-degree geometry with the other head for 180-degree cardiac applications. Examples of commercially available systems are shown in Figures 2-7D and 2-7E.

Acquisition Parameters

Collimation

Early SPECT applications with a single-head camera were generally limited to the use of general-purpose, parallel-hole collimators when imaging low-energy radionuclides, due to the sensitivity limitations previously described. Thus, the resulting images typically exhibited poor spatial resolution. The emergence of multihead cameras and the resulting increase in sensitivity made it possible to improve spatial resolution by the use of high-resolution collimators, and these collimators are now the choice for most imaging applications.

Matrix Size

For cardiac SPECT, the acquisition matrix size for acquiring planar projection images is typically a 64 × 64 data point array. The decision is based on the size of the smallest object to be imaged in the distribution being studied. Sampling theory states that in order to resolve frequencies (objects) up to a maximum frequency (smallest object) at least two measurements must be made across one cycle. This maximum frequency is referred to as the *Nyquist frequency*. For example, using a camera with a 540-mm field of view and a zoom factor of 1.4 and a 64 × 64 acquisition matrix size would result in a pixel size of 6 mm, making it possible to image structures of 1.2 cm or larger. This is generally considered sufficient for cardiac SPECT.

Arc of Rotation

As previously stated, a 180-degree acquisition (right anterior oblique position to left posterior oblique position) is acceptable for cardiac imaging since the myocardium is always in the near field of the detector(s). Photons traveling in a posterior direction from the myocardium must travel significant distances through tissue, and therefore spatial resolution and sensitivity (due to attenuation) are degraded in posterior and right posterior oblique views. Thus, the data from the omitted projections are considered to be of poor quality and is generally not acquired.

Projections Per Arc of Rotation

The same sampling theory previously described also applies to the determination of the number of projection views that should be acquired throughout an arc of rotation. With current instrumentation, 120 views are typically obtained with a 360-degree acquisition, and therefore 60 views are generally acquired with a 180-degree acquisition when a dual-head system is used.

Time Per Projection

In general, SPECT techniques require the acquisition of as many photon events as possible to produce high-quality images. However, the limiting factor is typically the time that a patient can remain motionless during the acquisition. This time is typically 10 to 15 minutes and results in imaging times of 30 to 45 seconds for each projection when 60 projections are acquired in a 180-degree rotation with a dual-head camera in a 90-degree orientation.

SPECT Image Formation

Data Acquisition

SPECT data are acquired in the form of multiple projection images as the scintillation camera heads rotate about the region of interest, as illustrated by the 60 images shown in Figure 2-8. Each acquired image is actually a set of count profiles measured from different views with the number of count profiles determined by the number of rows of pixels in the acquisition matrix (e.g., 64 for a 64 × 64 matrix size). Using parallel-hole collimators, each pixel is the sum of measured photon events traveling along a perpendicular ray and interacting at a point

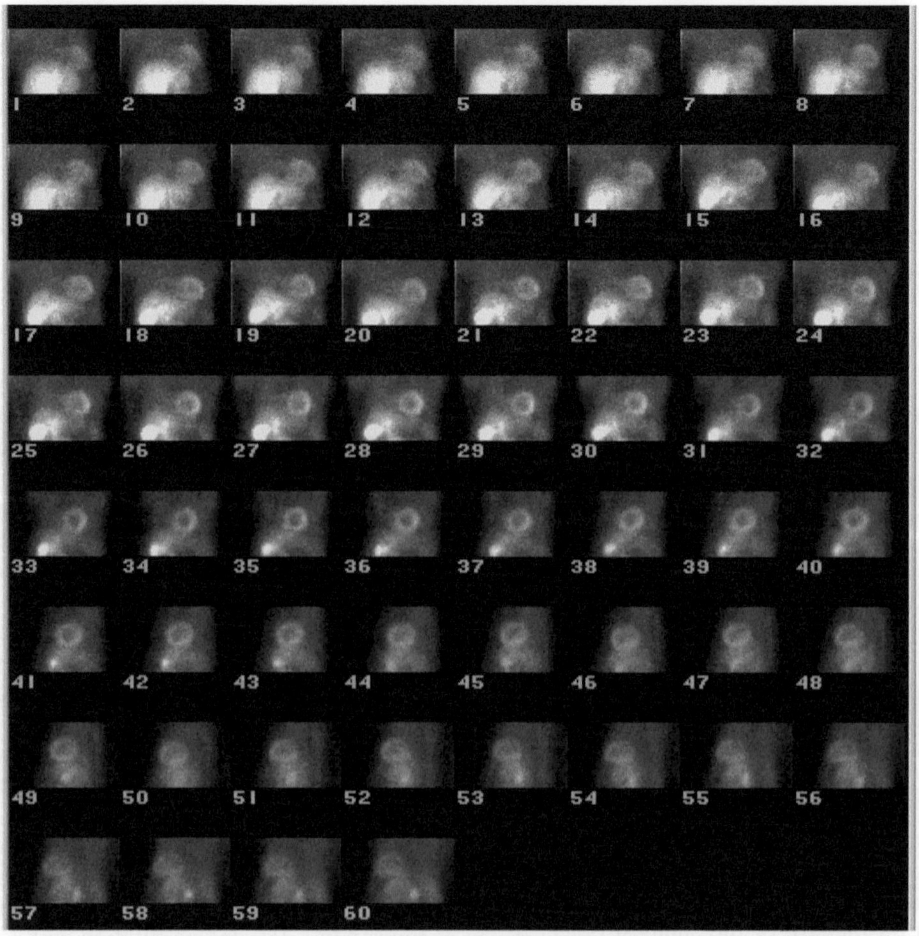

FIGURE 2-8. Sixty planar images acquired at 3-degree increments over 180 degrees.

in the detector crystal represented by the pixel location. For a 180-degree acquisition with 60 acquired projection arrays, 60 count profiles are acquired at 3-degree increments around the region of interest for each transaxial slice through the radionuclide distribution.

Image Reconstruction

An image of the transaxial slice through the distribution can be generated by sequentially projecting the data in each count profile back along the rays from which the data were collected and adding the data to previously backprojected rays. The mathematical term for this process is *linear superposition of backprojections*. Since there is no a priori knowledge of the origin of photons along each ray, the value of each pixel in the count profile is placed in each data cell of the reconstructed image along the ray. Representations of the images resulting from this process are shown in Figure 2-9. It should be noted that uniform projections are used in Figure 2-9 to illustrate the backprojection principle. In fact, the rays at the periphery of the sphere are of less intensity than at the middle. The classic *star effect* blur pattern inherent in backprojection images is evident in these images, with each ray of the star corresponding to one projection view. The importance of collecting the appropriate projections is evident from this diagram, since increasing the number

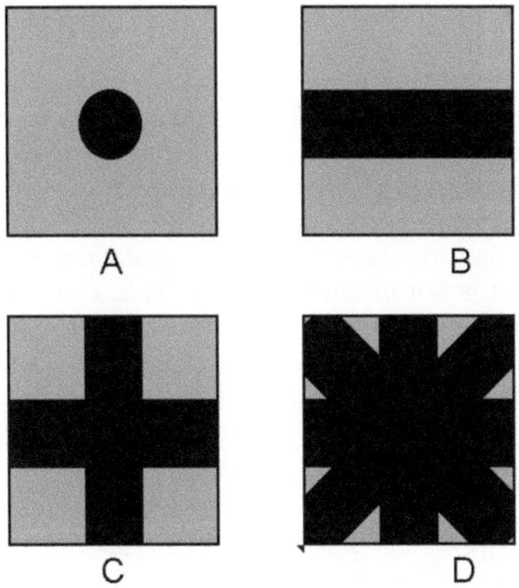

FIGURE 2-9. (A–D) Representations of the images resulting from linear superposition of backprojections are shown.

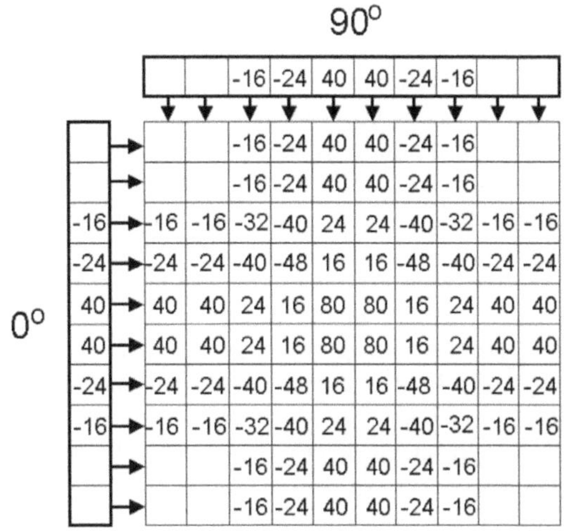

FIGURE 2-10. Two examples of filtered count profiles of data acquired at 90 degrees from a spherical source and the resulting image distribution after backprojection of the filtered profiles.

of projections enhances the image contrast and reduces the potential for artifacts from the star effect. This can be seen in Figure 2-9D, in which two additional sets of projection data at 45 degrees and 135 degrees are projected back into the image.

It is apparent from the data in Figure 2-9 that the blur pattern inherent in backprojection results in a significant background that reduces image contrast. To reduce these effects, and also to reduce the statistical effects of noise in the images, the mathematical technique of filtering is applied to the count profiles in the projection data before backprojection is performed. A filter is a mathematical function that is defined to perform specific enhancements to the profile data. In general, filters enhance edges (sharpen images) and reduce background. The effects of a simple edge enhancement filter (−1, 2, −1) are shown in Figure 2-10. In the application of this filter, each data point in the profile is replaced by 2 times its value and added to the negative of each adjacent data point. This process results in negative numbers being added to the count profiles. Figure 2-10 shows the backprojection of the filtered count profile at 0 degrees added to the filtered, backprojected count profile at 90 degrees. It can be observed that the negative data at the edges of one profile cancel unwanted data from other profiles. This effect is shown diagrammatically in Figures 2-11B

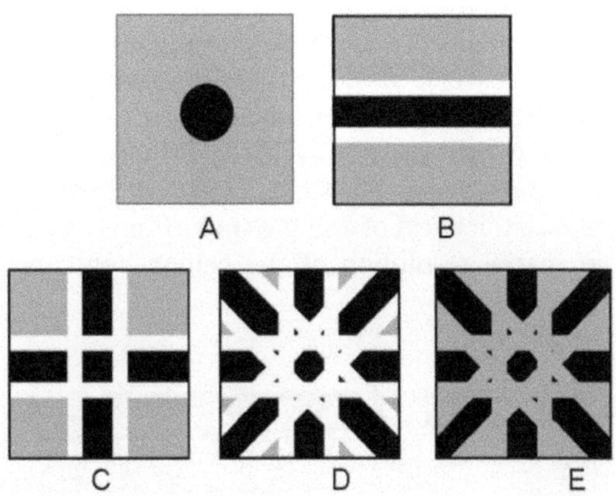

FIGURE 2-11. Demonstration of the blur pattern from a spherical source (A) resulting from filtered backprojection of a single view (B), two views at 0 and 90 degrees (C), and 0, 45, 90, and 135 degrees (D). In the final image (E), the negative values have been set to zero.

and 2-11C. As the number of projections is increased, this effect becomes more pronounced, as shown in Figure 2-11D, in which the filtered backprojections at 45 degrees and 135 degrees are added to the image. The final step is to set to zero each pixel in the reconstructed image that has a negative value, as shown in Figure 2-11E. The figure shows that the scanned object is now visible in the image, but many nonzero pixels remain. The addition of multiple projections removes these artifacts and further enhances the image of the actual measured distribution. This technique of linear superposition of filtered backprojections has been the image reconstruction algorithm of choice throughout most of the history of SPECT. Figure 2-11 also demonstrates the need to select an appropriate filter for each imaging application. If too many negative numbers are added to the image (overfiltering), valuable image data are removed. If not enough negative numbers are added to the image (underfiltering), unwanted data remain in the image, resulting in artifacts. The selection of the appropriate filter is probably the most significant factor in producing a high-quality image reconstruction. The effects of overfiltering and underfiltering are shown in the single reconstructed slice of the myocardium of a patient in Figure 2-12.

The techniques previously discussed were illustrated using data for a single transverse slice. In practice, it is possible to reconstruct as many transverse slices as there are rows in the acquisition matrix. For example, a 64×64 matrix provides 64 rows of data that can be used to reconstruct 64 slices. However, because the slice thickness of a single slice often exceeds the spatial resolution of the camera, and the data in a single slice are often statistically limited, it is common practice to add 2 or more adjacent slices to reconstruct thicker slices with improved statistics. The final result of the reconstruction process is a set of transverse slices. Images of sagittal and coronal slices can easily be generated from this data set by simply reformatting the data. Since the orientation of the heart is not in the traditional X, Y, Z orientation of the human body, it is necessary to reorient the axes to correspond to the long and short axes of the left ventricle. This is a straightforward procedure that can be accomplished automatically or manually under software control.

Filters

Routine methods for characterizing nuclear medicine images and data sets relate to the number of counts in a pixel. When data are referred to using this terminology, the data are defined as being in the *spatial domain*, and the simple filter previously used to illustrate the effects of filtering on image reconstruction was a *spatial filter*. In practice, filtering of projection data in the spatial domain is often cumbersome and time consuming. This problem can be overcome by working in the *frequency domain*. Here, the projection data may be expressed as a series of sine waves, and a frequency filter may be used to modify the data. The conversion of the projection data into the frequency domain is accomplished by the application of a mathematical function, the Fourier transform, and the result is that the projection data are represented as a frequency spectrum plotting the amplitude of each frequency in the data as shown in Figure 2-13A. In SPECT this fre-

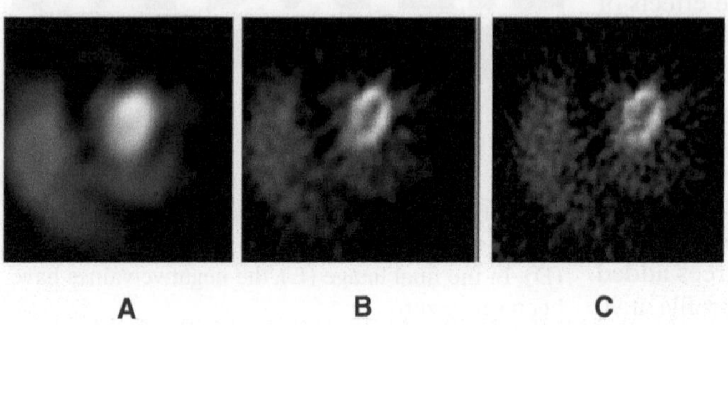

FIGURE 2-12. Single short-axis view of the myocardium with ^{99m}Tc-sestamibi demonstrating overfiltering (A), underfiltering (C), and optimal filtering (B).

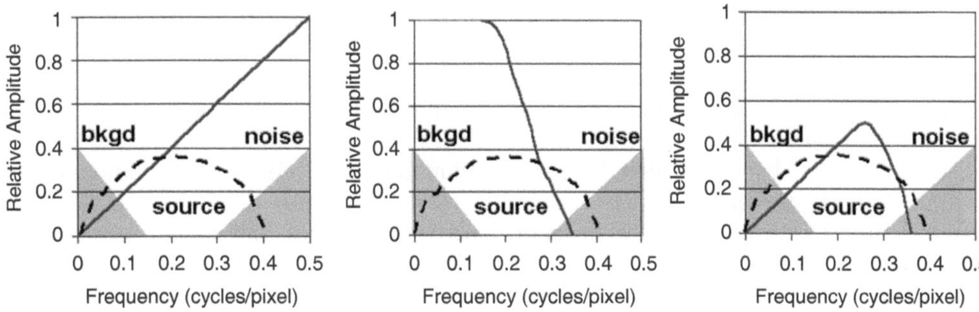

A B C

FIGURE 2-13. In the frequency domain, image data can be represented as a series of sine waves, and the data can be plotted as a frequency spectrum showing the amplitude of each frequency. Image data have three major components: background, source information, and noise (A). A ramp filter is used to eliminate or reduce the contribution of background to the reconstructed image (A). A low-pass filter reduces the contribution of noise to the image (B). Combining the 2 filters (C) creates a window or band-pass filter that accepts frequencies primarily from the source distribution.

quency spectrum has 3 distinct components. Background data (including the data from the star effect previously described) typically have very low frequencies and therefore are the main components of the low-frequency portion of the spectrum. Statistical fluctuations in the data (noise) generally have high frequencies and therefore dominate the high frequencies of the spectrum. True source data lie somewhere in the middle, while overlapping the background and noise components of the spectrum. Thus, the challenge in filtering SPECT data is clearly demonstrated in Figure 2-13A. The goal is to eliminate background and noise from the data while preserving as much of the source data as possible. It should also be noted that the frequency data in the figure are plotted as a function of cycles per pixel. In the discussion of matrix size previously presented, the concept of the Nyquist frequency was introduced. In the frequency domain, the highest frequency in a data set occurs when one complete cycle covers 2 pixels. Frequencies higher than this value cannot be imaged. This fact translates into a frequency of 0.5 cycle per pixel as the frequency limit and is defined as the Nyquist frequency. This is why the plot in Figure 2-13A terminates at 0.5 cycle per pixel. The pixel size used in a particular application can be introduced into this definition so that the Nyquist frequency for the application can be determined. For example, a pixel size of 0.5 cm would define a Nyquist frequency of 1.0 cycle/cm. And the smallest object size that could possibly be resolved in an image would be 1 cm.

The first step in filtering is to design a filter to remove or reduce the background. This typically is a ramp filter as shown in Figure 2-13A, a high-pass filter that reduces only the amplitudes of low-frequency data while having no effect on the midrange and high-frequency data, which contain the detail in the source (and also the noise). The second step is to define a filter to remove or reduce the noise while preserving the detail in the source data. This is accomplished using a low-pass filter as shown in Figure 2-13B, which accepts selected frequencies up to a certain value. There are a number of low-pass filters available for processing SPECT data. Some have fixed characteristics and others have flexibility in choosing the cutoff frequency and/or the slope of the filter. Some filters are optimized for image data with excellent counting statistics and others provide the capability for filtering data with poor statistics. Also, the amount of detail in an image and the object sizes to be resolved (spatial resolution) are important factors to be considered in the selection of a filter. In practice, the low-pass filter may be applied first to reduce the effects of noise, and then the ramp filter is applied to reduce background. The two filters may be combined as shown in Figure 2-13C to function as a band-pass filter. It can be seen in the latter figure that appropriate selection of the cutoff frequency eliminates much of the noise, and selecting an appropriate filter shape preserves most of the source data. The terms *underfiltering* and *overfiltering* were previously referenced, and examples were shown in Figure 2-12. From Figure 2-13C it can be observed that when a cutoff frequency is chosen that is too low, some of the source data are excluded from the final image, and this situation is referred to as *overfiltering*. Similarly, when too high a cutoff frequency is chosen, excessive noise is included in the final image and this is referred to as *underfiltering*. In clinical applications, most imaging systems provide the capability for trying different filters and filter parameters on a single slice of image data to select the appropriate processing algorithm for a specific patient study. Technologists and physicians in the clinical setting often prefer this method of trial and error.

Iterative Reconstruction

Filtered backprojection amplifies statistical noise, which adversely affects image quality. To address this problem, Shepp and Vardi introduced an iterative reconstruction technique in 1982[3] based on the theory of expectation maximization (EM), which has a proven theoretical convergence to an estimate of the actual image distribution that has a maximum likelihood of having projections most similar to the acquired projections. The initial implementation of these algorithms was very time consuming, with several iterations required to reach a solution, and extensive computer power was required. Since that time much effort has been expended in improving and testing algorithms based on this concept. Significant improvements in speed, signal-to-noise, and reconstruction accuracy have resulted from these efforts. In 1994 Hudson and Larkin[4] developed the technique of ordered sets expectation maximization (OSEM) for image reconstruction from 2-D projection data. This algorithm was based on the concept of dividing the projection data into small subsets (e.g., paired opposite projections in SPECT data) and performing the EM algorithm on each subset. The solution of each subset was used as the starting point for the next subset, with subsequent subsets being selected to provide the maximum information (e.g., choose the second subset of data to be orthogonal to the first subset). The advantage of this technique is that at the end of the first pass, the entire data set has been processed one time, but n successive approximations to the final solution have been made where n is the number of subsets. Thus, OSEM is n times faster than the original EM algorithm. Typically, only 2 to 3 passes through the data set (iterations) are required for the reconstructed image to converge to a final value that is essentially unchanged by further iterations. Correction for scatter and attenuation effects (topics that are discussed later) can be performed on the acquired projection data during the reconstruction process. The advantage of this technique is that the star effect inherent in filtered backprojection is virtually eliminated, since the acquired data is distributed within the body contour. Because of this result, signal-to-noise is generally improved. Filtering of the data can also be performed to further enhance the reconstructed images.

Factors Affecting Image Quality

The primary factors that affect image quality in SPECT are photon energy and attenuation. Earlier in this chapter it was stated that the position of the interaction of a photon in the NaI(Tl) crystal is measured by localizing the light (scintillations) produced in the crystal by the photon interaction. The intensity of the light produced is directly proportional to the energy absorbed in the crystal. Therefore, if a ^{201}Tl photon (70 keV) and a ^{99m}Tc photon (140 keV) are totally absorbed in the crystal, the light produced from the ^{99m}Tc photon absorption will be twice as intense as that for the ^{201}Tl photon. Thus, the measurement of the location

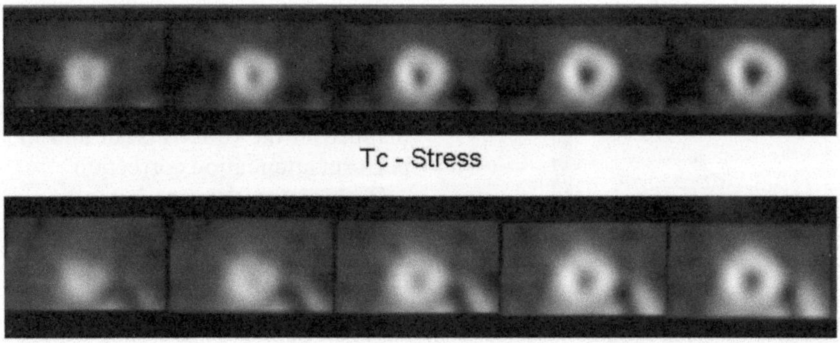

FIGURE 2-14. Short-axis views of a ^{99m}Tc-sestamibi distribution acquired after stress and a ^{201}Tl chloride distribution acquired at rest, demonstrating improved resolution and contrast in the ^{99m}Tc distribution due to higher photon flux and higher-energy photons.

of the ^{99m}Tc interaction will be more statistically accurate than that of the ^{201}Tl photon due to the increased light output. This translates into an improvement in intrinsic spatial resolution of approximately 0.5 mm for ^{99m}Tc for state-of-the-art scintillation cameras.

Photons are attenuated in the body due to photoelectric absorption and Compton scatter, with Compton scattering being the most predominant interaction in the diagnostic energy range. The probability of Compton scattering decreases with increasing energy. The effects of attenuation are significant, with approximately 62% of 70 keV photons and 54% of 140 keV photons being attenuated in 5 cm of tissue. Photoelectric absorption results in complete removal of the photon from the radiation field, while Compton scattering results in a change in direction with loss of photon energy, the magnitude of the loss being determined by the angle of scatter. Thus, Compton scattered photons enter the camera crystal with minimal or no information on their origins due to their change in direction within the patient. Pulse height analysis is used to prevent the counting of photons that have scattered through large angles (greater loss of energy), but small-angle scattered photons are counted. The use of a 20% window at 70 keV permits the acceptance of photons that have scattered through 0 to 79 degrees. At 140 keV, a 20% window permits the acceptance of photons that have scattered through 0 to 53 degrees, and a 15% window accepts photons scattered through 0 to 45 degrees.

Another factor to be considered is the flux of photons that are available for detection. Routine doses of ^{201}Tl used for diagnostic purposes are 2.5 to 4.0 mCi, whereas 20 mCi of ^{99m}Tc are routinely used. Thus, the photon flux from ^{99m}Tc is considerably higher than that for ^{201}Tl.

All of these factors result in SPECT images acquired from ^{99m}Tc distributions being superior in image quality to those obtained from ^{201}Tl distributions. This fact is evident in the SPECT images shown in Figure 2-14.

Attenuation Correction

Correction of cardiac images for attenuation effects is complicated by the broad range of tissue types (lung, soft tissue, muscle, and bone) in the vicinity of the myocardium, resulting in a nonuniform attenuation medium. Two commercial approaches to attenuation correction are currently available. The first makes use of line sources of ^{153}Gd as shown in Figure 2-15. These sources provide beams of 100 keV photons and are scanned in the longitudinal direction at each step of the SPECT acquisition to provide transmission maps of the region under study. Emission and transmission scans at each step can be acquired sequentially or simul-

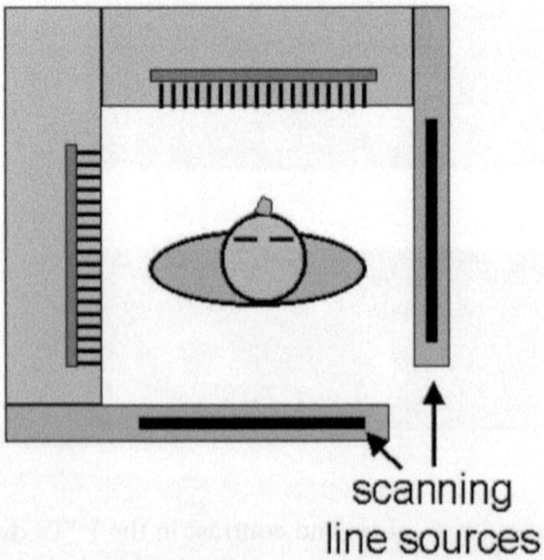

FIGURE 2-15. Scanning line sources mounted on a dual-head, 90-degree geometry scintillation camera for attenuation correction measurements.

taneously using synchronized energy windows, which move with the sources to acquire the transmission data. The transmission data are then used to correct the projection data prior to SPECT image reconstruction.

The second approach is the use of a low-output x-ray tube and linear array of detectors to acquire a nondiagnostic CT scan of the region of interest. A commercial version of this technology mounted on a dual-head scintillation camera is shown in Figure 2-16. The continuous rotation capability of the slip ring gantry on this camera makes it possible to acquire CT slices providing maps of attenuation coefficients that can be scaled to the photon energy being mapped in the SPECT scan and then used to perform attenuation correction.

Both of these methods tend to overcorrect for attenuation, and it is generally accepted that a scatter correction must also be performed. One solution to this problem is the simultaneous acquisition of a second set of planar projections using a scatter window positioned just below the photopeak energy being measured. This window is used to determine correction factors for the acquired planar projections prior to image reconstruction.

Gated Acquisition

Another problem that is inherent in cardiac SPECT and degrades image quality is the normal physiological motion of the heart during the acquisition. In routine planar imaging, physiological gating can be used to image segments of the cardiac cycle, as shown in Figure 2-17. In practice, an acquisition pulse (R-wave trigger) is generated from the R wave of the QRS complex measured by ECG. The time difference between R waves is measured and used to define the cardiac cycle. Typically, the first 85% to 90% of the cycle is used for acquisi-

Linear array of detectors

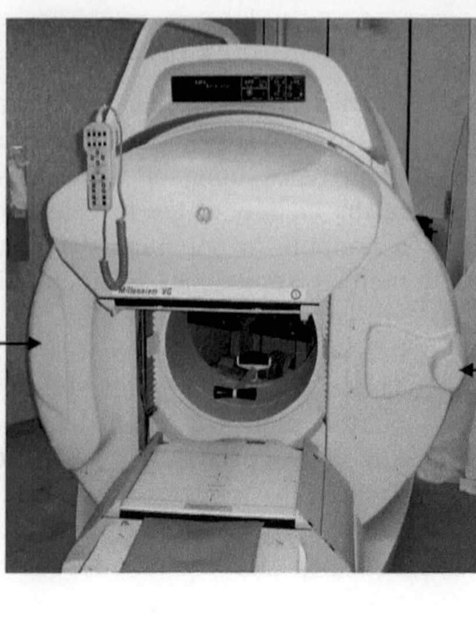

X-ray tube

FIGURE 2-16. X-ray tube and linear array of detectors (low-quality CT scanner) mounted on a dual-head scintillation camera for attenuation correction measurements. (General Electric Medical Systems, Waukesha, WI).

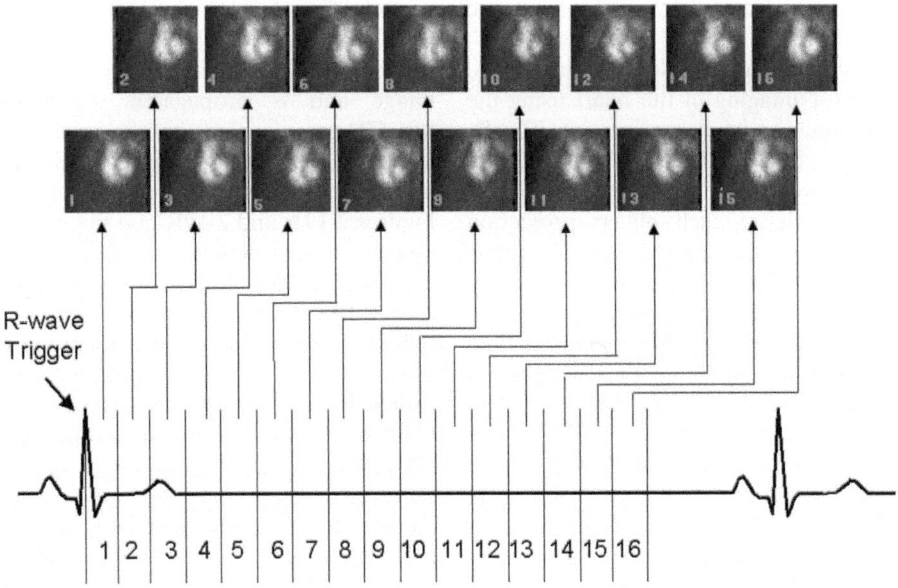

FIGURE 2-17. Diagram of the data collection process in a gated acquisition study using an R-wave trigger pulse from the ECG to control the acquisition process.

tion and divided into a number of equal time segments (e.g., 16). The R-wave trigger is then used to initiate acquisition into image frames, with the time duration determined by the length of each segment of the cycle. This process is repeated until sufficient data have been acquired to provide acceptable images of each segment of the cardiac cycle. These images can be displayed in cine mode to evaluate wall motion abnormalities. Digital data can be extracted from these images, as shown in Figure 2-18 to plot time activity curves measuring activity in the left ventricle as a function of time within the cycle. These data can then be used to

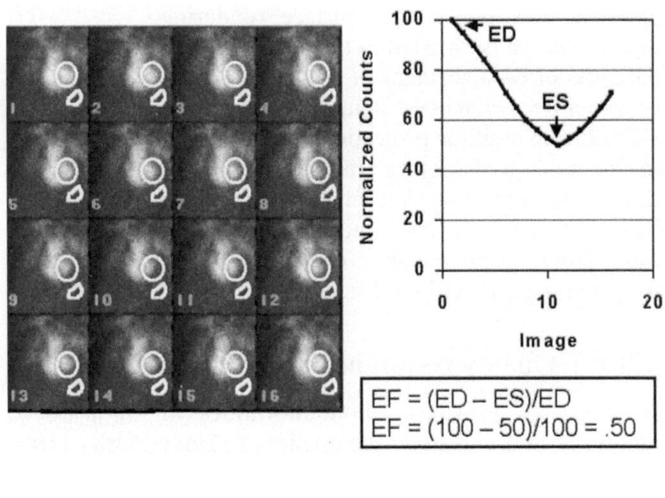

FIGURE 2-18. Regions of interest selected from images acquired in a gated acquisition study are used to create a time/activity curve from which the ejection fraction can be calculated.

calculate ejection fraction values, as illustrated in Figure 2-18.

Gated acquisition can also be performed during SPECT imaging of the heart using the same techniques as in planar imaging. The R-wave trigger pulse is used to initiate and control acquisition of a set of images representative of the cardiac cycle at each planar projection angle. Typically, a smaller number of cardiac segments (e.g., 8) are imaged than in routine planar imaging in order to obtain images of acceptable image quality in the limited time constraints imposed by the SPECT acquisition process. When the SPECT acquisition is complete, 60 data sets have been acquired, with each data set composed of a set of images (e.g., 8) that are representative of the cardiac cycle when viewed by the camera head at each angular projection position. Image reconstruction is accomplished as previously described for ungated SPECT. Attenuation and scatter correction can also be incorporated into the reconstruction algorithm. However, with this data set, it is possible to reconstruct a complete set of transverse slices for each segment of the cardiac cycle. Reformatting is accomplished as previously described to generate images of tomographic slices of short- and long-axis views of the left ventricle. The final set of images offers numerous possibilities for extracting diagnostic information. For example, it is possible to produce images of the standard long- and short-axis views that are the products of non-gated cardiac SPECT. It is also possible to view selected slices and orientations of the cardiac cycle in cine mode. Also, surface rendering algorithms can be applied to the 3-dimensional data sets of each segment of the cardiac cycle to generate volumetric images that can be viewed from multiple projections and reviewed in cine mode to access wall motion abnormalities. Ejection fraction determinations can also be performed from these data. Thus, a significant amount of information can be extracted from a single gated SPECT acquisition.

SPECT Quality Assurance

As discussed previously, nonuniformities in camera response degrade the quality of planar images. This fact is especially important in SPECT applications because a nonuniformity in response appears in each planar projection image and is propagated throughout the SPECT image reconstruction, resulting in ring artifacts in the final images. This potential problem is illustrated diagrammatically in Figures 2-19A and 2-19B, and the effect on the image reconstruction of slices through a uniform cylinder of activity is shown in Figure 2-19C. The proper implementation of a sensitivity correction eliminates artifacts of this type. This is accomplished by placing the planar source in contact with the collimated camera head and acquiring a high-count flood of 50 to 100 million counts. As shown in Figure 2-20, this acquired sensitivity map is used to calculate a correction factor for each pixel to force that pixel intensity to equal the average intensity of the flood. This flood correction is then used to perform a final uniformity correction on each acquired image before that image is used for SPECT reconstruction.

When acquiring SPECT data it is imperative that the center of the image matrix corresponds to the geometric center of rotation of the camera heads, as shown in Figure 2-21A. Errors in this correspondence result in degradations in reconstructed images because of misalignment of opposed views and can be detected as a cir-

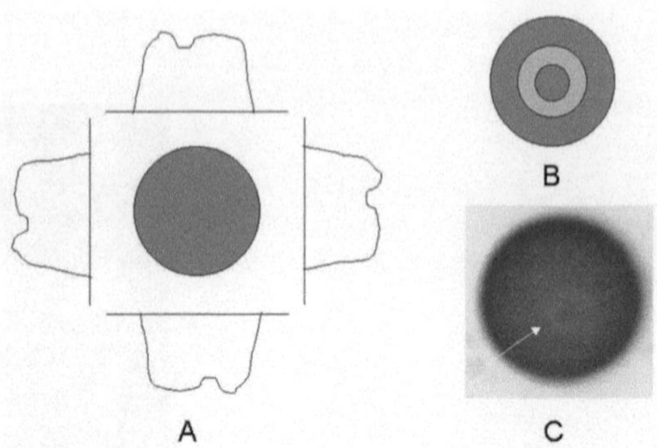

FIGURE 2-19. Four count profiles from a uniform distribution acquired with a scintillation camera exhibiting a uniformity defect (A). Reconstruction of images with this defect present results in a ring artifact (B and C).

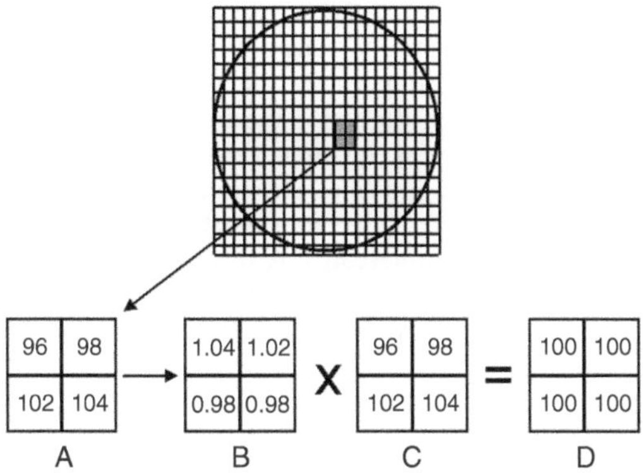

FIGURE 2-20. Data acquired from a high count flood (A) can be used to generate sensitivity correction factors (B) that can be applied to acquired SPECT planar projection images (C) to perform a uniformity correction (D) before the data are used for image reconstruction.

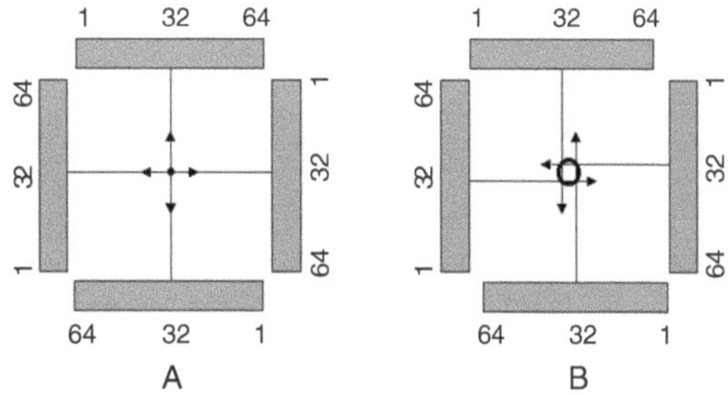

FIGURE 2-21. When the center of the acquired image corresponds to the center of rotation, all images are properly aligned for the image reconstruction process (A). If the center of the acquired image does not correspond to the center of rotation, images are misaligned, and the image reconstruction process results in a ring artifact about the center of rotation (B).

cular artifact about the center of rotation, as shown in Figure 2-21B. The accuracy of center of rotation alignment should be checked routinely (monthly) by placing a point source off center and acquiring a SPECT data set. The position of the centroid of the source is then plotted as a function of rotational angle and compared with a best-fit sine wave, as shown in Figure 2-22. Deviations from this fit should be less than half of a single pixel. These data can be used to correct for minor center of rotation errors, but major errors should be addressed because they are indications of mechanical or electronic problems. An example is shown in Figure 2-23. Image degradation suddenly appeared in routine dual-head SPECT images, and a center of rotation evaluation was performed. Figures 2-23A and 2-23B show plots of the X (transverse) and Y (longitudinal) differences between the measured positions of the point source and the best-fit sine wave. Serious errors in the X positions for head 1 are shown in Figure 2-23A. Examination of the camera head showed a mechanical failure resulting in a wobbling of the head during rotation. A center of rotation measurement performed after repair indicated acceptable deviations (Figures 2-23C and 2-23D).

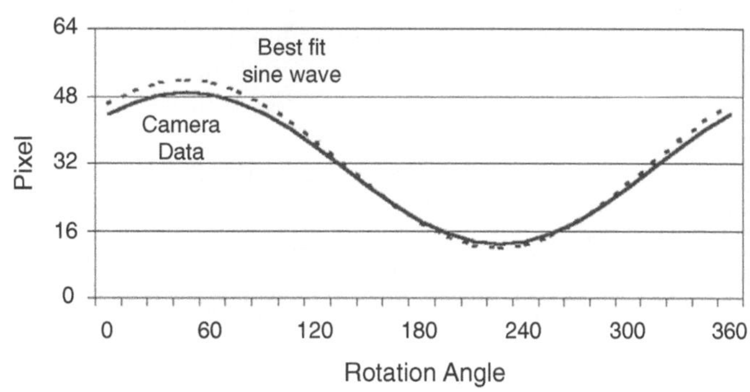

FIGURE 2-22. Plot of the centroid of a point source versus angle of rotation compared with a best-fit sine wave indicating a center of rotation error.

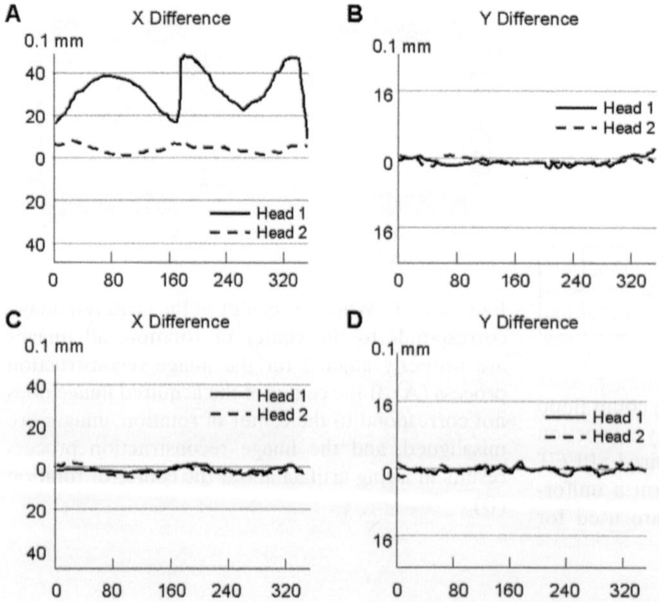

FIGURE 2-23. Plot of the difference between centroid of a point source and a best-fit sine wave versus angle of rotation in the transaxial (A) and axial (B) directions. The data in Part A indicates a large center of rotation error due to a mechanical problem with Head 1. A repeat of the center of rotation evaluation indicates that the problem has been corrected (C and D).

Positron Emission Tomography

Previous discussions have been related to the imaging of single photon emitting radionuclides using conventional scintillation camera systems. Another classification of radionuclides that has applications in nuclear cardiology is positron emitters that can be imaged using specially designed positron emission tomography (PET) systems. This technology has been previously described.[5,6] Positron-emitting radionuclides are distinguished by the unique method by which they are detected. The positron is a positively charged electron. When emitted from a radioactive nucleus, it travels only a short distance before losing all of its energy and coming to rest. At that instant, it combines with a negatively charged electron, and the masses of the two particles are completely converted into energy in the form of two 511-keV photons. This process is termed *annihilation*, and the 2 annihilation photons leave the site of their production at 180 degrees from each other. This process can be detected as shown in Figure 2-24 by using small, dual-opposed detectors connected by a timing circuit, termed a *coincidence* circuit, to simultaneously detect the presence of the two annihilation photons, a signature of the positron decay process. The timing window must be small, 7 to 15 nanoseconds, in order to reduce the possibility of detecting photons from two separate decay processes, i.e., random events. The spatial resolution of the imaging system is primarily determined by the size of the detectors, combined with the uncertainty due to the travel of the positron before

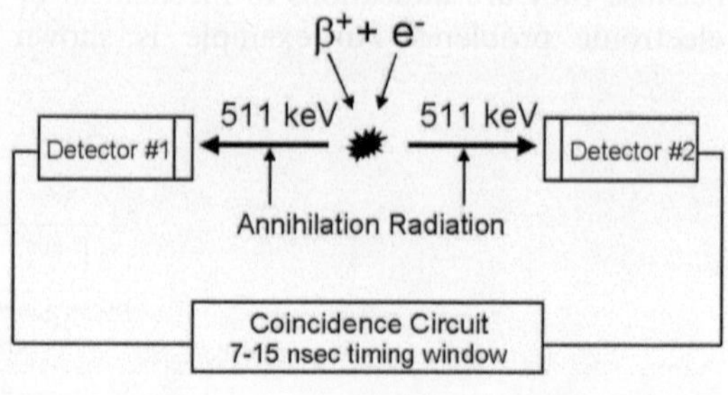

FIGURE 2-24. Block diagram of a 2-detector grouping with a coincidence timing window used to simultaneously detect the 2 photons resulting from the annihilation of a positron-electron pair using the technique of coincidence counting. (From Delbeke, Martin, Patton, et al. [6], by permission of Springer-Verlag.)

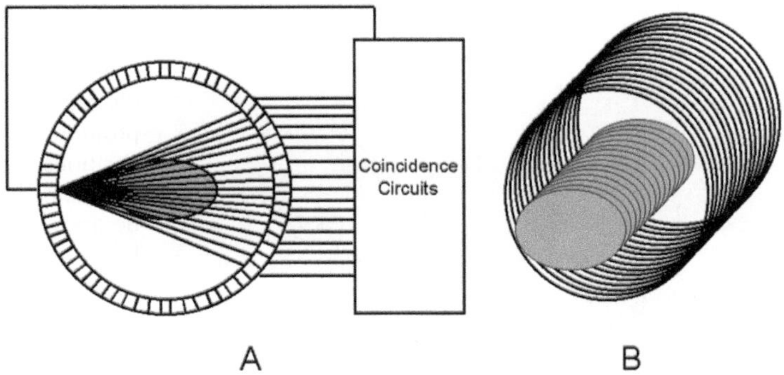

FIGURE 2-25. One ring of detectors from a multi-ring PET system. Many potential lines of coincidence are possible for each detector in the ring (A). Multiple rings of detectors are used to extend the axial field of view (B). (From Delbeke, Martin, Patton, et al. [6], by permission of Springer-Verlag.)

annihilation, typically less than 0.5 mm in tissue. In clinical imaging systems, many small detectors are used in multiple rings to provide high sensitivity for detection in the region being examined, as shown in Figure 2-25. A photograph of a dedicated PET scanner is shown in Figure 2-26.

Positron Emission Tomography Detectors

For many years the scintillation detector of choice for PET imaging has been bismuth germanate (BGO) instead of sodium iodide (NaI(Tl)), which is used in other nuclear medicine imaging devices. BGO is used because of its high density and high effective atomic number, which results in a high intrinsic detection efficiency for 511-keV photons. A 30-mm-thick crystal of BGO has an intrinsic detection efficiency of approximately 90% at 511 keV, and when two detectors are used in coincidence to simultaneously detect two 511-keV photons, the coincidence detection efficiency is the product of the efficiencies of the 2 detectors, or approximately 81%. Recently, a new scintillation material, lutetium oxiorthosilicate (LSO), has been introduced as a possible replacement for BGO. Although currently more expensive than BGO, LSO has the advantage of greater light output (factor of 6) and faster decay time (factor of 7.5), and these improvements can be used to advantage in increasing the count rate capabilities of modern-day systems. PET systems using LSO are now available from one manufacturer, (CTI, Knoxville, TN). More recently, another new scintillation detector material, gadolinium oxyorthosilicate (GSO) has been introduced with similar characteristics to those of LSO, but with improved energy resolution. PET systems using GSO detectors are now available from another manufacturer, (Philips Medical Systems, Andover, MA).

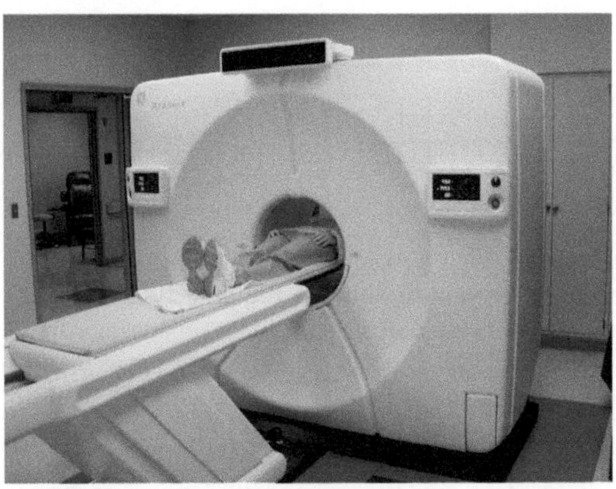

FIGURE 2-26. Photograph of a state-of-the-art, multi-ring PET scanner. (General Electric Advance.)

The high spatial resolution of these systems is accomplished by using a unique combination of small crystals and photomultiplier tubes. An example of this technology is shown in Figure 2-27. A rectangular solid crystal of detector material is modified by the addition of vertical and horizontal grooves partially through the volume to effectively create a block of many small discrete detectors (36 in the figure). Some manufacturers actually separate the discrete

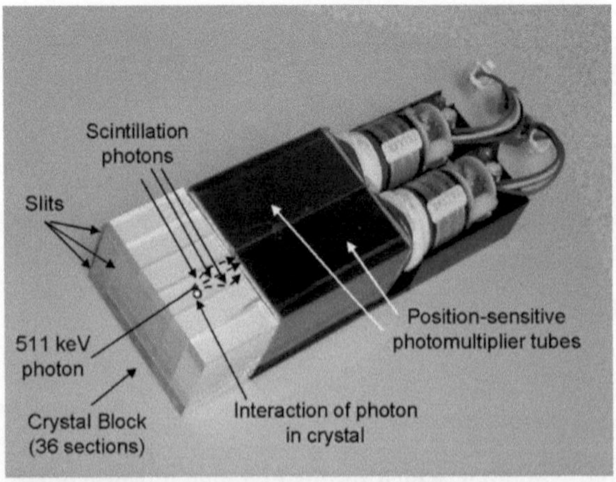

FIGURE 2-27. For high-resolution imaging, a block of crystal (bismuth germanate in this example) is segmented into many small, discrete detectors (36 in this example). Two position-sensitive photomultiplier tubes positioned at the back of the crystal block determine the detector in which an interaction occurs. (From Delbeke, Martin, Patton, et al. [6], by permission of Springer-Verlag.)

crystals entirely, creating pixilated detectors as in the figure. A photon interaction in one of the discrete crystals results in scintillations localized primarily in that crystal. The crystal in which the interaction occurred is then identified by photomultiplier tubes using conventional Anger logic and mounted on the base of the crystal block or by using position-sensitive photomultiplier tubes. In the detector block shown in Figure 2-27, the discrete crystals are 4 × 8 × 30mm deep, resulting in a transaxial spatial resolution of 4.6mm. Current systems have 18 to 32 rings of detectors providing axial fields-of-view of 15 to 18cm (Figure 2-25). Thus, the imaging of sections of the body greater than 15 to 18cm in the axial direction requires multiple acquisitions obtained by indexing the patient through the system using a movable imaging table under precise computer control.

Two-Dimensional versus 3-Dimensional Imaging

It is possible to reduce the effects of scatter and the possibility of random events by adding thin, one-dimensional collimators, termed *septa*, between adjacent rings of detectors to shield the detection of events in the axial direction, as shown in Figure 2-28A. These septa are typically constructed from tungsten with a thickness of 1mm and a spacing to match the axial width of each discrete crystal. They have the effect of creating 2-dimensional (2-D) slices from which events can be accepted in any transaxial direction. Thus, for a system with 18 rings of detectors, 18 direct imaging planes are established. To increase sensitivity, coincidence circuitry can also be used to record interactions occurring in 2 detectors in adjacent rings, resulting in the addition of a new acquisition plane positioned midway between the adjacent detector rings. Thus, in an 18-ring system, 17 new cross imaging planes can be added for a total of

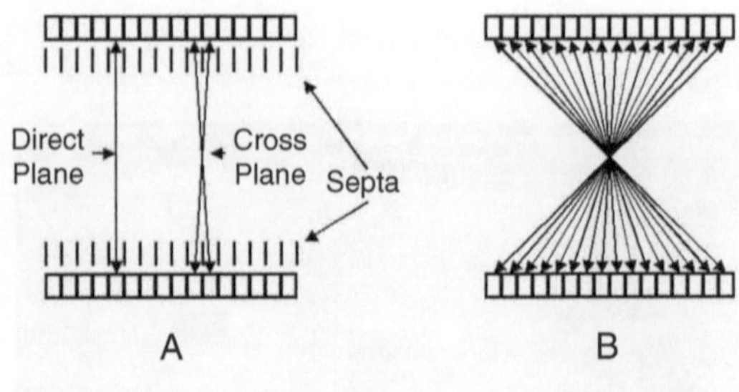

FIGURE 2-28. The use of septa collimators permits 2-D acquisition by limiting the detection of coincidence events to detectors within a single ring (direct planes) and detectors in adjacent rings (cross planes) (A). When the septa are withdrawn, 3-D acquisition is established by permitting the measurement of a coincidence event in 2 detectors in any 2 rings of the system (B). (From Delbeke, Martin, Patton, et al. [6], by permission of Springer-Verlag.)

35 imaging planes in this example. Additional sensitivity is obtainable by adding adjacent planes to this process. For example, 3 or 5 planes of detectors may be electronically grouped so that coincidence events may be measured in any 2 detectors within these groupings. The localization of the coincidence event in a transaxial imaging plane is typically determined by averaging the axial positions of the 2 detectors. The length of the septa limits the axial separation of any 2 rings that can actually be used in the measurement of the activity in a 2-D plane.

With the septa retracted, detector rings are opened to photons traveling in all directions, and a 3-dimensional (3-D) imaging geometry is established, as shown in Figure 2-28B. This increases the system sensitivity by a factor of 3 to 5 over that of 2-D imaging. However, the randoms rate and scatter fraction are increased with this geometry, resulting in images with reduced contrast. It is possible to limit the acceptance angle in the axial direction to reduce the effects of randoms and scatter, but this results in a reduction in sensitivity.

Data Acquisition and Image Reconstruction

As previously described, a coincidence event is recorded when 2 single events are simultaneously measured in 2 separate detectors. Thus, the coordinates of the 2 detectors determine the location of the coincidence event, as shown in Figure 2-29A. These coordinates are captured by calculating the perpendicular distance from the center of the scan field to a line connecting the 2 detectors (r), and measuring the angle between this line and the vertical axis (ϕ). These coordinates are then recorded as a data point in an (r, ϕ) plot or sinogram, as shown in Figure 2-29B. Each unit in the final sinogram consists of the total number of coincidence events recorded by a two-detector pair. The sinogram method of storage is used because it is more efficient than the storing of list mode data that record individual coordinates of detector pairs. In 2-D image acquisition there will be $(2n - 1)$ sinograms recorded, one for each direct plane and one for each cross plane, where n is the number of detector rings in the PET system. When the 2 detectors are in different detector rings, the event is recorded in the sinogram corresponding to the average

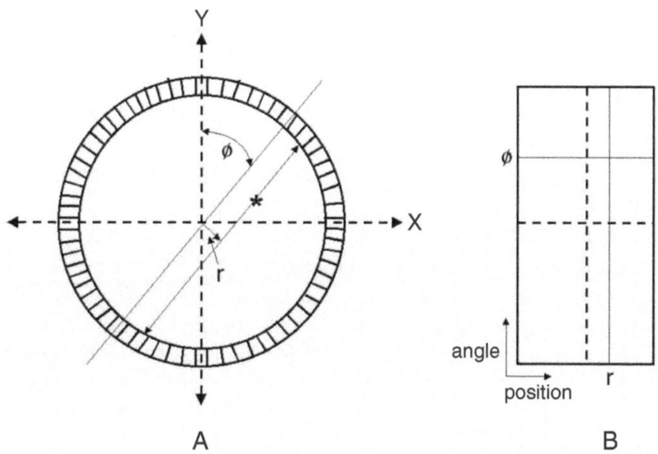

FIGURE 2-29. The coordinates of the 2 detectors involved in a coincidence measurement are captured by calculating the perpendicular distance from the center of the scan field to a line connecting the two detectors (r), and measuring the angle between this line and the vertical axis (ϕ) (A). These coordinates are then recorded as a data point in an (r, ϕ) plot or sinogram (B). Each unit in the final sinogram consists of the total number of coincidence events recorded by a 2-detector pair. (From Delbeke, Martin, Patton, et al. [6], by permission of Springer-Verlag.)

axial position of the two rings as previously stated.

Image reconstruction of the 2-D data is accomplished by first converting each sinogram of data into a set of planar projections. This can be accomplished in a straightforward manner from the sinograms, since each horizontal row of data in a sinogram represents events recorded at one angular position. It should also be noted that the events from each 2-detector pair are uniformly spread across the sinogram. A filtering algorithm is applied to each projection, after which the data are projected back along the lines from which they were acquired to generate the final image (i.e., filtered back-projection). Each sinogram of data is used in this fashion to generate an image corresponding to the activity distribution represented by the sinogram. Iterative algorithms that make use of ordered sets, or Ordered Sets Estimation Maximization (OSEM) can also be used in the 2-D reconstruction process to reduce noise and provide high-quality images.[4] The use of iterative algorithms also simplifies the process of adding corrections for effects such as attenuation and scatter.

The acquisition and reconstruction of 3-D data sets is more complicated than that for 2-D applications. First, it is not possible to perform the axial averaging of events recorded from 2 detectors in different detector rings. The origins of these data must be preserved in the acquisition process, and this results in a significant increase in the size of the acquired data set, since n^2 sinograms are now required to accurately acquire the data. In addition, the reconstruction process is complicated by the fact that it is necessary to use a true 3-dimensional volume algorithm to accurately locate detected events in axial as well as transverse directions. Iterative reconstruction algorithms, although time consuming and labor intensive, are well designed for this application. Currently available systems offer this technique as an option, and it has proven useful in brain imaging because the imaging volume is relatively small and count rates are relatively low. Because of the added sensitivity provided by 3-D imaging, a great deal of effort is currently being applied to develop accurate and efficient 3-D algorithms and techniques to correct for scatter to improve contrast. As improvements are made, it is anticipated that the use of 3-D techniques will become prevalent in the future.

Quantitative Techniques

Because of the block detector technology used with PET systems, there is a dead time associated with measurements of activity distributions, and corrections for this effect must be implemented so that the measurements are quantitatively accurate. When an interaction occurs in a crystal, a finite length of time is required to collect the light produced and process the resulting signal. If another event occurs in the same block while the first interaction is being processed, the light from the 2 events will be summed together by the photomultiplier tubes in that block, and the resulting signal will probably fall outside of the pulse height window. This effect will result in an erroneous measurement of count rate. Modern systems have dead time correction capability using correction factors determined for the system as a function of count rate. These correction factors adjust for errors in count rate but cannot add the lost events back into the acquired image.

A state-of-the-art PET scanner may have several thousand discrete crystals coupled to hundreds of photomultiplier tubes. Thus, there are inherent differences in sensitivity between detector pairs in the measurement process, and it is necessary to correct for these differences in order for measurements of coincidence events to correspond to the activity distribution being imaged. This correction is generally accomplished by exposing each detector pair to a uniform source distribution, typically created by a rotating rod source of ^{68}Ge, and measuring the response of each detector pair. This data set is called a *blank scan*. The blank scan can be used to create normalization factors that are stored away and used to correct data subsequently acquired in image acquisition. Blank scans must be acquired frequently (at least weekly) to monitor system parameters and adequately correct for small changes in detector responses.

A second factor to be considered is the exponential attenuation of photons within the body.

Photons are either absorbed or scattered by tissues based on the attenuation coefficients of these tissues and the distance of travel through the body. The attenuation effects are much more significant in coincidence imaging than in single photon imaging, since both photons from a single annihilation process must pass through the body without interaction in order to be detected and counted as a coincidence event. The probability of this occurrence is much less than that for a single photon emitted from the same location to escape the body without interaction. These effects result in nonuniformities, distortions of intense structures, and edge effects. Therefore, it is necessary to correct for attenuation to eliminate these effects, especially in the thorax and abdomen, where attenuation is nonuniform due to the presence of different tissue types. Since the brain is relatively uniform, it is possible to perform a calculated attenuation correction. This is accomplished by outlining the outer contour of the head, assuming uniform attenuation within this volume, and calculating correction factors to be applied to the raw projection data.

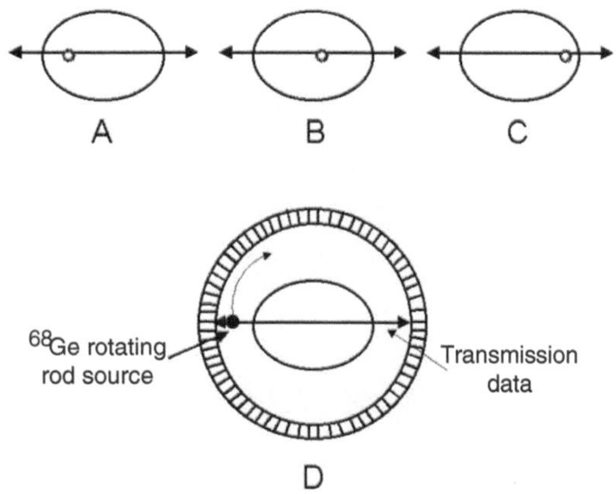

FIGURE 2-30. The attenuation of two annihilation photons is independent of the location at which the two photons were produced, since the photon pair must always travel the same distance within the patient and escape without interaction in order to be detected as a true event (A–C). Thus, attenuation can be measured using a rotating rod source of a positron emitter such as ^{68}Ge (D). (From Delbeke, Martin, Patton, et al. [6], by permission of Springer-Verlag.)

In the thorax and abdomen, because of the nonuniform attenuation, it is necessary to perform a measured attenuation correction. This approach is very accurate because attenuation of 2 annihilation photons from an annihilation event is independent of the location of the event, since the total distance traveled through the patient is constant, as shown in Figures 2-30A through 2-30C. It is therefore possible to measure the attenuation using an external source, as shown in Figure 2-30D. This is typically accomplished by transmission scanning using a rotating rod source of ^{68}Ge as in the acquisition of a blank scan for detector normalization, but with the patient present in the scan field. The transmission data can then be used to correct the raw projection data during the reconstruction process, and iterative reconstruction algorithms can be easily adapted to handle the attenuation correction process. Transmission scans with high counting statistics are required to prevent the addition of statistical noise in the corrected images. In the past, it was necessary to perform the transmission scan before administration of the radiopharmaceutical into the patient. This resulted in lengthened studies and the need for careful repositioning of the patient before acquiring the emission scan. Recent improvements in count rate capabilities have made it possible to acquire transmission scans after the patient has been injected with a radiopharmaceutical by increasing the activity in the transmission source. It has also been shown that it is possible to shorten the length of the transmission scan by using a process called *segmented attenuation correction*. In this process, attenuation coefficients are predetermined (based on certain tissue types) and limited in number. The measured attenuation coefficients from the transmission scan are then modified to match the closest allowed coefficients from the predetermined options. Figure 2-31 shows a single coronal view reconstructed from a set of transmission scans, the corresponding view reconstructed from emission data using filtered backprojection, and the same view reconstructed using an OSEM algorithm with attenuation correction.

The addition of transmission scanning permits accurate delineations of body contours. This fact limits image reconstruction to the

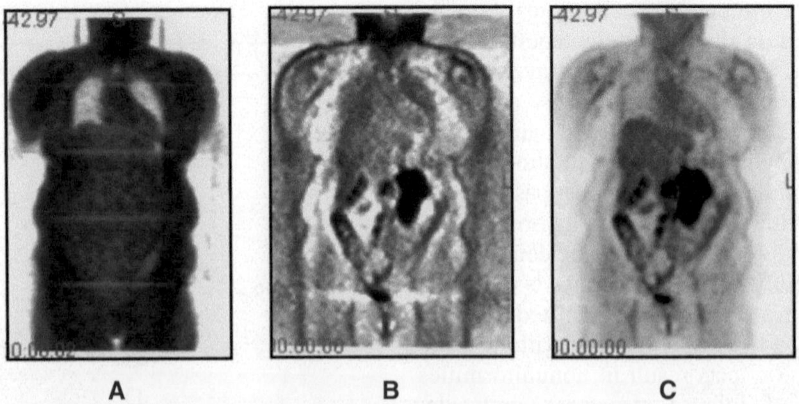

FIGURE 2-31 A coronal view of a transmission data set acquired from a multi-ring PET scanner (A). A coronal view of a patient with gastric cancer imaged with ^{18}FDG. (B) The image was reconstructed without attenuation correction using filtered back-projection. The same coronal view of the ^{18}FDG distribution reconstructed with attenuation correction from the transmission data set shown in (A) using an iterative reconstruction algorithm (OS-EM) (C). (From Delbeke, Martin, Patton, et al. [6], by permission of Springer-Verlag.)

areas defined by the contours. In addition, accurately knowing these contours permits the development of mathematical models for determining the contribution to the images of random and scatter events, and subsequently the implementation of correction methods to eliminate their effects. Work is currently ongoing in this area.

To make absolute measurements of activity in a region of the body, one additional calibration is necessary. A cylindrical phantom containing a very accurately known distribution of activity is scanned and total counts (after attenuation correction) are determined. A quantitative calibration factor is then determined by dividing the measured counts per unit time by the concentration of activity in the phantom. This results in a calibration factor of counts/sec/μCi/cc. To determine activity in a specific region, a region-of-interest is identified, the counts in the region are determined and converted to a count rate using the scan time, and the calibration factor is then used to calculate μCi/cc in the region. Current systems have the capability of measuring absolute activity to within 5%. In practice, it should be noted that the same acquisition and reconstruction algorithms (and filters) should be used in acquiring and processing the phantom data and the patient data in order to obtain accurate quantitative data. A quantitative measurement that has proven to be of use in clinical applications is the standard uptake value (SUV). This factor is determined by normalizing the measured activity in a region to the administered activity per unit of patient weight. Using the SUV, regions of abnormal uptake can be compared with those of normal regions, and lesion uptake in serial scans can be compared.

Categories of PET Systems

In this text, the high-end dedicated PET system has been used to describe the physical principles of coincidence detection. This system, as has been described, consists of multiple complete rings of small crystals with 2-D imaging with septa in place, and 3-D imaging with the septa retracted. Some systems use 3-D imaging only. However, other, less expensive midrange dedicated PET systems are commercially available, as shown in Figure 2-32. One approach to reducing cost is to reduce the number of detectors and detector rings and eliminate the septa, as shown in Figure 2-32B. This is the approach that has been taken with the Siemens-CTI ART system. This system consists of 24 rings of dual-opposed arcs (60 degrees) of detectors. Crystal thickness is reduced to 20mm, and complete sampling in transaxial planes is accomplished by rotating the detector rings at 30rpm. Since the septa have been eliminated, only 3-D acquisition and image reconstruction is used with this system.

Another approach is to replace the discrete crystals with large-area, camera-type NaI(Tl) detectors as shown in Figure 2-32C. To increase detection efficiency, the crystal thickness has been increased to 1 inch compared with 3/8 inch for conventional single photon camera systems. To improve system sensitivity, 6 detector heads are used in a hexagonal arrangement to completely surround the patient. Complete sampling in transaxial planes is accomplished by rotating the system during image acquisition. Septa are not used with these systems, and therefore these systems are limited to 3-D acquisitions. Since large-area, camera-type detectors are used, the axial field of view is increased over that of ring-type systems. The first of these systems to be commercially available is the C-PET system manufactured by ADAC/Philips. The C-PET uses a unique curved crystal design to improve the acquisition geometry. Count rate capability is enhanced by the use of a parallel processing technique provided by limiting the measurement of light produced by a photon interaction to the photomultiplier tubes closest to the interaction and clipping of the voltage pulses that result from this measurement. This process is made possible by the relatively large amount of light produced from a 511-keV photon interaction in the crystal and permits the simultaneous measurement of multiple photon interactions in different locations of the crystal. A review of currently available PET imaging systems was presented by Tarantola et al.[7]

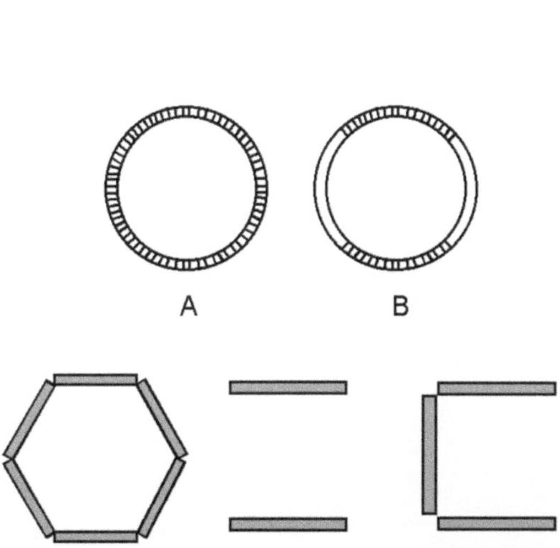

FIGURE 2-32. Positron emission tomography can be accomplished using (A) systems with complete rings of detectors, (B) systems with partial rings of detectors, (C) camera-type systems with multiple large-area detectors (D–E). In addition, multihead scintillation cameras used for routine single photon imaging to which coincidence detection circuitry has been added (hybrid cameras) can also be used for this purpose. (From Delbeke, Martin, Patton, et al. [6], by permission of Springer-Verlag.)

In recent years, the capability for coincidence imaging has been made available on multihead scintillation camera systems used for routine nuclear medicine imaging procedures (Figures 2-32D and 2-32E and Figure 2-16).[8] To make these hybrid systems possible, conventional camera systems have been modified by the addition of detector shielding, the extension of the pulse height energy range, the implementation of high-energy sensitivity and linearity corrections, and a significant improvement in count rate capability. Coincidence circuitry has been added to establish a possible line of coincidence between any 2 positions in opposing heads. To increase sensitivity, crystal thicknesses have been increased to $^{5}/_{8}$ or $^{3}/_{4}$ inch, the maximum crystal thickness that can be used while preserving spatial resolution in the conventional single photon energy range. Even with $^{5}/_{8}$-inch-thick crystals, the photopeak detection efficiency is only increased to approximately 17%, and the coincidence photopeak detection efficiency is 2.9%. This limitation in sensitivity has severely hampered the clinical utility of hybrid camera systems for positron imaging, and even with the recent introduction of 1-inch grooved crystal technology, dedicated PET systems are still the systems of choice for these applications.

Case Presentations

Case 2.1

History

An elderly gentleman with a history of chest pain was administered 20 mCi of ^{99m}Tc-sestamibi for a rest perfusion SPECT study. The patient was not able to place his arms above his head for the study as routinely required. The acquired planar images are shown in Figure C2-1. A very bright spot was noted in many of the planar images that made it impossible to reconstruct clinically acceptable images of the myocardium.

Findings

The patient had his arms crossed over his abdomen and the artifact (hot spot) in the planar images was determined to be due to residual activity in the injection site in the arm.

Discussion

This case illustrates the importance of having the arms out of the field of view during cardiac SPECT acquisition, not only to eliminate attenuation effects but also to prevent activity in the injection site from interfering with the study.

If the patient is not able to place his arms above the head, holding the arms along the side as posteriorly as possible does limit attenuation artifacts. A study of 41 patients concluded that arm positioning (assuming there is no dose infiltration) does not influence the interpretation of ^{99m}Tc-sestamibi SPECT myocardial perfusion imaging with regard to image quality or defect location and extent.[9]

Interpretation

Left arm in the field of view over the abdomen and dose infiltration prevented reconstruction of clinically acceptable images.

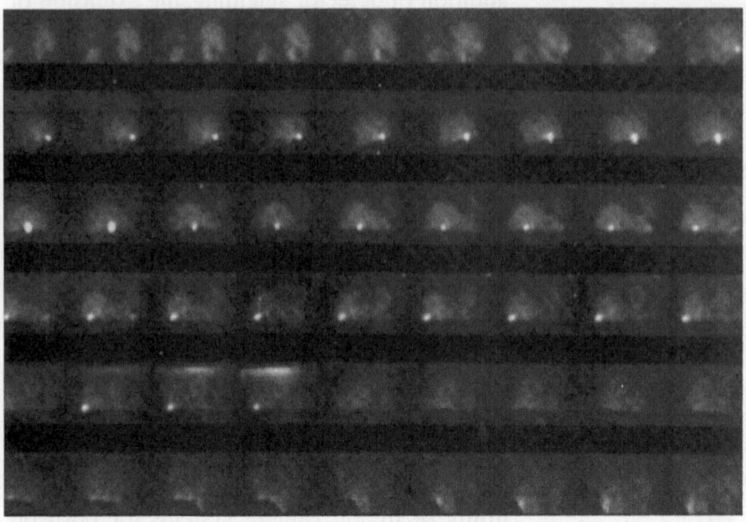

FIGURE C2-1.

Case 2.2

History

A middle-aged woman with a history of breast cancer presented for evaluation of cardiac function before chemotherapy. The patient was first administered a dose of *cold* pyrophosphate followed 30 minutes later with 20 mCi of ^{99m}Tc-pertechnetate to accomplish in vivo labeling of the patient's red blood cells. Acquisition of a gated blood pool data set was then accomplished. The acquired images are shown in Figure C2-2.

Findings

A large area of decreased activity was noted at the apex of the left ventricle. On examination of the patient, it was determined that the patient was wearing a prosthetic bra with metal beads in it. The bra was removed and the study was successfully completed.

Discussion

This case illustrates the importance of evaluating the clothing of the patient before performing a nuclear cardiology procedure and removing any articles that may attenuate the radiation from the patient and affect the quality of the diagnostic study.

Interpretation

Prosthetic bra with metal beads created an artifact at the apex of the heart on the radionuclide ventriculogram.

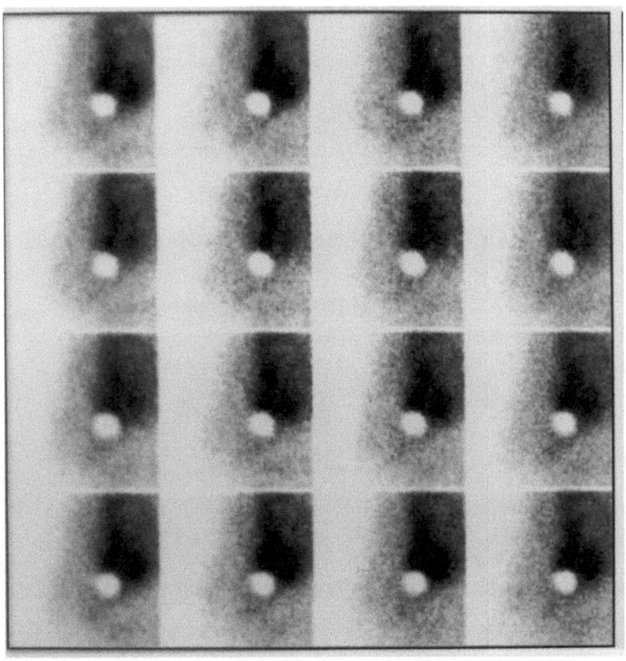

FIGURE C2-2.

Case 2.3

History

A middle-aged man with a history of coronary artery disease was studied in the supine position using the standard rest ^{201}Tl chloride, stress ^{99m}Tc-sestamibi SPECT protocol. Figure C2-3 shows a selected short-axis view of the stress and 24-hour redistribution images.

Findings

A large inferior wall defect is noted in the stress study that did not fill in on the redistribution images, consistent with a myocardial infarction. An area of activity is also noted at the periphery of the anterior wall in the redistribution images. Review of the planar images acquired for the redistribution study indicated that the patient was positioned such that the left ventricle was at the edge of the camera field of view in some of the images (Figure C2-2B). Thus, the activity distribution was truncated in some of the images, resulting in an inadequate data set for image reconstruction.

Discussion

It is imperative that the region of interest under study using SPECT techniques be centered in the field of view in all images so that a complete data set is acquired with no truncation.

Interpretation

Truncation artifact.

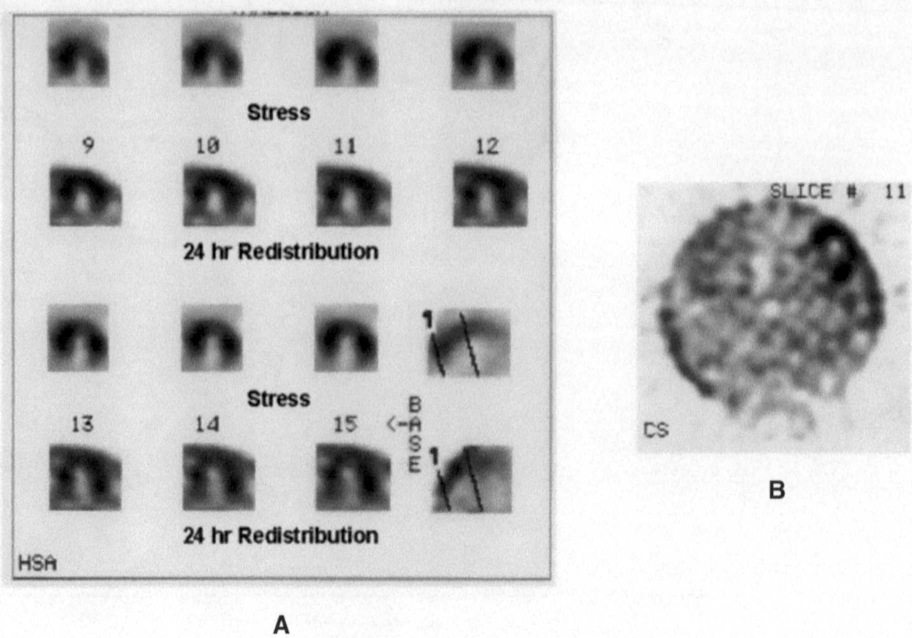

FIGURE C2-3. (A and B)

Case 2.4

History

An elderly man with a history of chest pain was studied in the supine position using the standard rest ^{201}Tl, stress ^{99m}Tc-sestamibi SPECT protocol. In each acquisition, 60 images were acquired over 180 degrees using a dual-head camera with a 90-degree orientation. Selected short axis views from this study are shown in Figure C2-4A.

Findings

The rest images showed decreased uptake in the inferior wall, but the stress sestamibi images were impossible to interpret because of significant distortions in the reconstructed images. Distortions of reconstructed data sets such as seen in the stress images are often indicative of patient movement during the acquisition process. A tool that is helpful in evaluating patient motion is a sinogram. This image is generated by displaying one line of data, typically from the center, from each acquired planar projection image. With no motion, this image should be a smooth sinusoid with no discontinuities. However, the sinogram shown in Figure C2-4B shows discontinuities at the midportion of the data set from each camera, indicating movement of the patient.

Discussion

It is virtually impossible to correct for horizontal movement, as was the case in this example, and it was necessary to repeat the acquisition. Vertical movement, *upward creep*, can be assessed by viewing a cineloop display of the acquired projection images with a cursor placed at the upper edge of the left ventricle. In some instances it is possible, using correction algorithms, to translate images and achieve an acceptable reconstruction.

Interpretation

Motion artifact was seen.

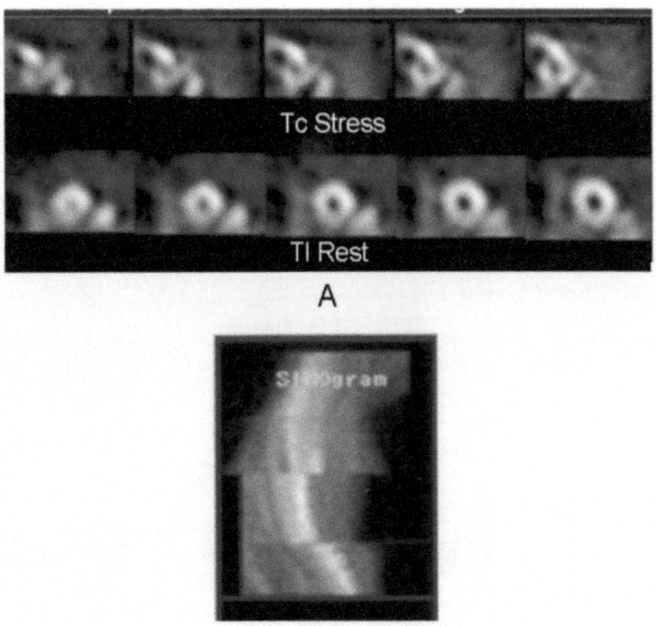

FIGURE C2-4. (A and B)

Case 2.5

History

A 61-year-old man with atypical chest pain was evaluated for ischemia with SPECT imaging at rest after administration of 8 mCi of ^{99m}Tc-tetrofosmin and after adenosine-induced stress after administration of 23 mCi of ^{99m}Tc-tetrofosmin. In each acquisition, 60 photopeak images and 60 scatter images (scatter window positioned below the photopeak) were acquired over 180 degrees using a dual-head camera with a 90-degree orientation with the patient in the supine position. CT-based transmission maps (GE Hawkeye) were also acquired sequentially in each study with no patient movement in order to perform attenuation corrections. Five short-axis views of the myocardium without corrections at rest and after stress are shown in Figures C2-5A and C2-5C, respectively, and the corresponding views after attenuation and scatter correction are shown in Figures C2-5B and C2-5D, respectively. The patient was also imaged in the prone position after stress using the same acquisition protocol, and the corresponding views from this acquisition are shown in Figure C2-5E without corrections and Figure C2-5F with attenuation and scatter correction.

Findings

The rest and stress images acquired in the supine position without attenuation correction showed a mild inferoseptal wall defect (Figures C2-5A and C2-5C). Since many inferior wall defects are due to diaphragmatic attenuation of photons emitted from this region, the patient was imaged in the prone position. In this position, the heart is often elevated away from the diaphragm so that attenuation effects are

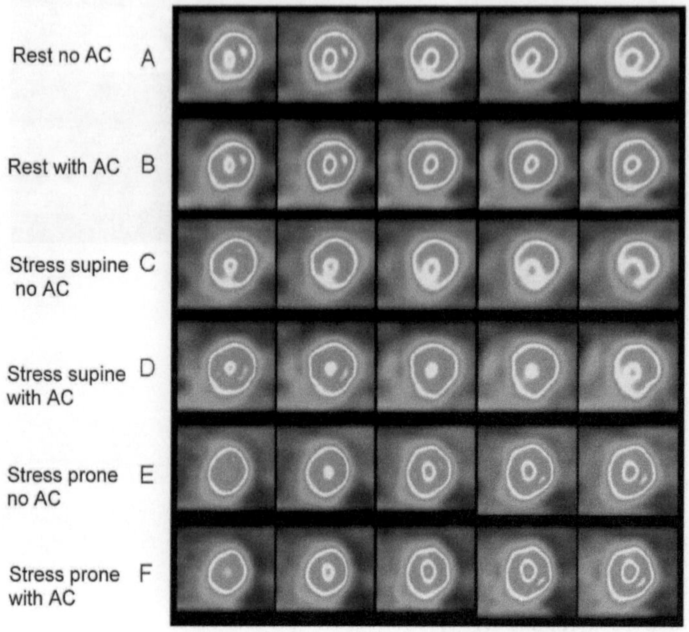

FIGURE C2-5. (A–F)

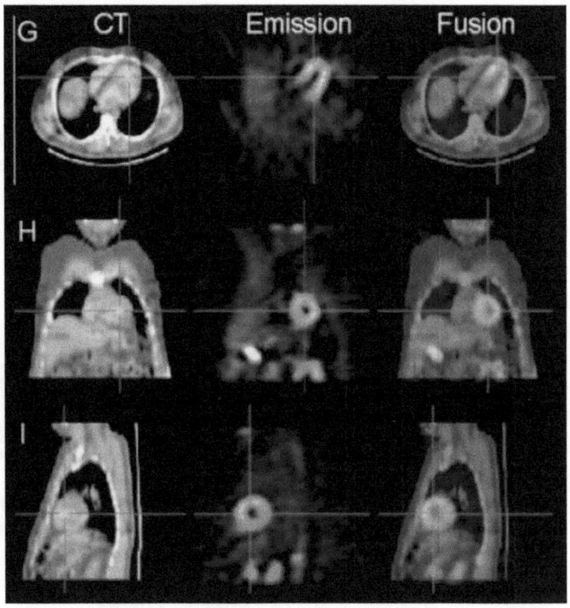

FIGURE C2-5. (G–I)

reduced. This was the case in this patient, since the prone views were normal (Figure C2-5E). The application of attenuation and scatter corrections to the supine views resulted in normal distributions (Figures C2-5B and C2-5D). Attenuation and scatter corrections applied to the prone images did not change the appearance of the radionuclide distribution (Figure C2-5F). Figures C2-5G through C2-5I show 3 transverse, sagittal, and coronal views from another patient with similar findings showing the emission scans (center) and the CT attenuation maps corresponding to these views (left). Fused images of these 2 data sets are shown on the right. The complex nonuniform tissue distribution in the vicinity of the myocardium, along with the location of the myocardium in relation to the diaphragm in this patient is shown in the fused images on the right. These images illustrate the importance of having a high-quality attenuation map to perform an accurate attenuation correction.

Interpretation

Inferoseptal wall defect resolved both with prone imaging and with attenuation correction resulted in a normal study. ECG, ejection fraction, and wall motion evaluations confirmed this normal finding.

Case 2.6

History

A middle-aged woman with a history of chest pain was studied in the supine position using the standard rest ^{201}Tl, stress ^{99m}Tc-sestamibi gated SPECT protocol. In each acquisition, 60-image data sets were acquired over 180 degrees using a dual-head camera with a 90-degree orientation. Attenuation correction was not available. Selected short-axis views of the stress and rest images acquired in the supine position are shown in Figures C2-6B and C2-6C. The patient had large breasts, and therefore stress images were also acquired with the patient in the prone position, and the short-axis views are shown in Figure C2-6A. From the gated SPECT data acquired in the supine position after stress, 4 views of 3-dimensional surface renderings of the left ventricle at end systole and end diastole were constructed and are shown in Figure C2-6D.

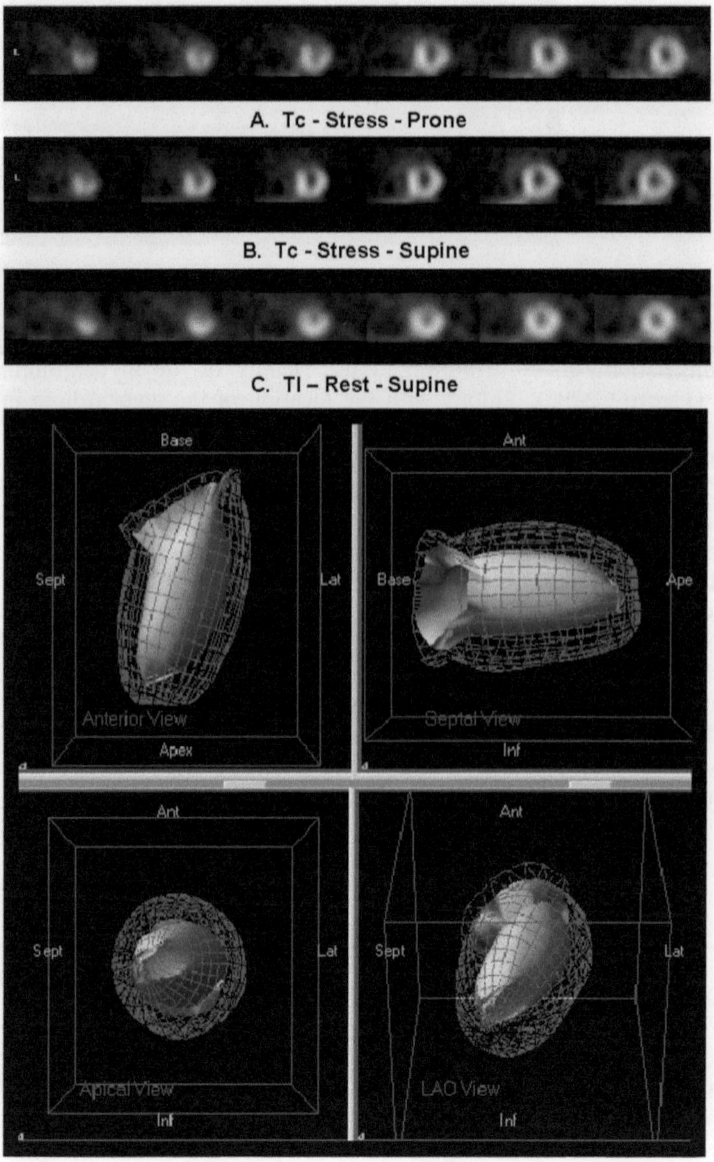

D

FIGURE C2-6. (A–D)

Findings

The rest and stress studies acquired in the supine position indicated an anterior wall defect. Since the patient had large breasts, there was concern that the defect was actually due to breast attenuation. Therefore, the patient was imaged in the prone position, and these images also demonstrated a defect in the same location as in the supine views. The 3-D surface renderings were viewed in cine mode to evaluate wall motion, and it was concluded that there were no wall motion abnormalities that could be identified. The patient's ejection fraction calculated from this data set was also normal. Thus, the study was read as normal with an anterior wall defect due to breast attenuation.

Interpretation

Anterior wall defect due to breast attenuation.

Case 2.7

History

A middle-aged man underwent an oncological evaluation with ^{18}FDG PET/CT for carcinoma of the lung. A single coronal slice of the diagnostic CT performed for attenuation and image registration is shown in Figure C2-7A. The corresponding coronal slice of the ^{18}FDG distribution is shown in Figure C2-7B, and fusion of the 2 images is shown in Figure 2-3C. A single transverse CT slice through the lungs and heart is shown in Figure C2-7D, and the corresponding ^{18}FDG distribution is shown in Figure C2-7E. Fusion of the CT and ^{18}FDG distribution is shown in Figure C2-7F.

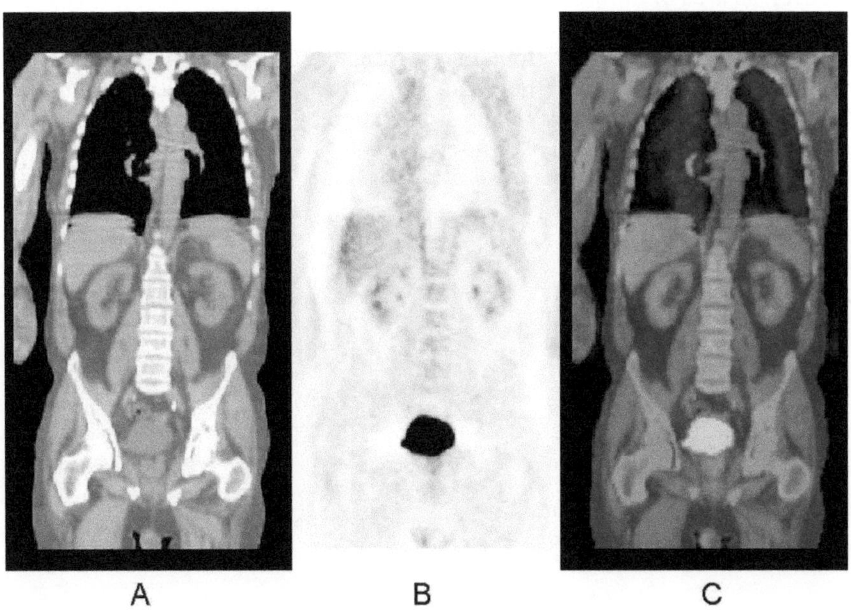

FIGURE C2-7. (A–C)

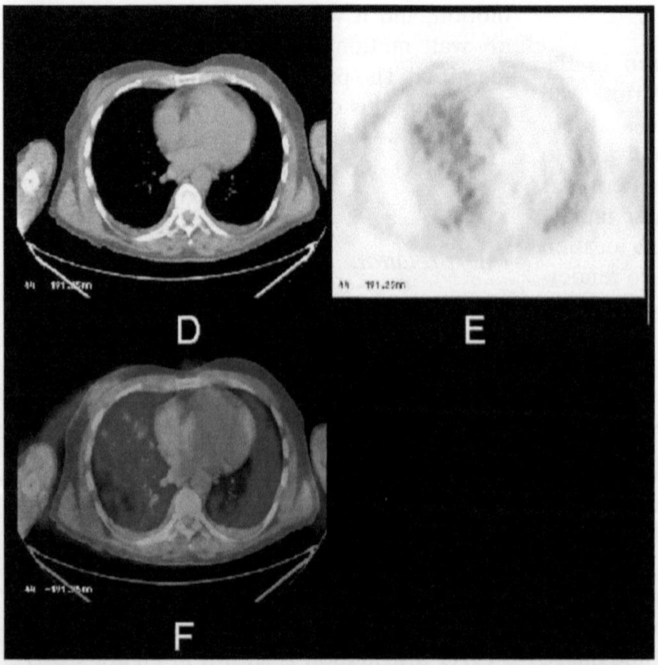

FIGURE C2-7. (D–F)

Findings

No focal areas of increased activity were noted in the ^{18}FDG images to indicate the presence of cancer. However, an area of diffuse uptake was noted medially from apex to base in the right lung (Figure C2-7B) that extended from the anterior to the posterior wall of the lung (Figure C2-7E). The fused images (Figures C2-7C and C2-7F) show that this area of diffuse activity is probably due to heart and mediastinal activity that is misregistered due to patient motion.

Interpretation

Normal PET study with patient movement after the CT scan resulting in a misregistration of anatomy and radionuclide distribution in the chest.

Case 2.8

History

A middle-aged man with a history of head and neck cancer underwent an oncological evaluation with ^{18}FDG PET for tumor reoccurrence. A single transverse slice of the attenuation-corrected ^{18}FDG distribution through the chest and heart is shown in Figure C2-8A, and a single medial sagittal slice through the body is shown in Figure C2-8B.

Findings

A band of decreased activity is noted through the chest from left to right in the transverse slice (Figure C2-8A), and a similar finding is noted vertically through the sagittal slice (Figure C2-8B). A failure of a detector block was suspected, and removing the patient and performing a blank scan to evaluate the detector normalization verified this problem.

Interpretation

Artifact due to detector block failure.

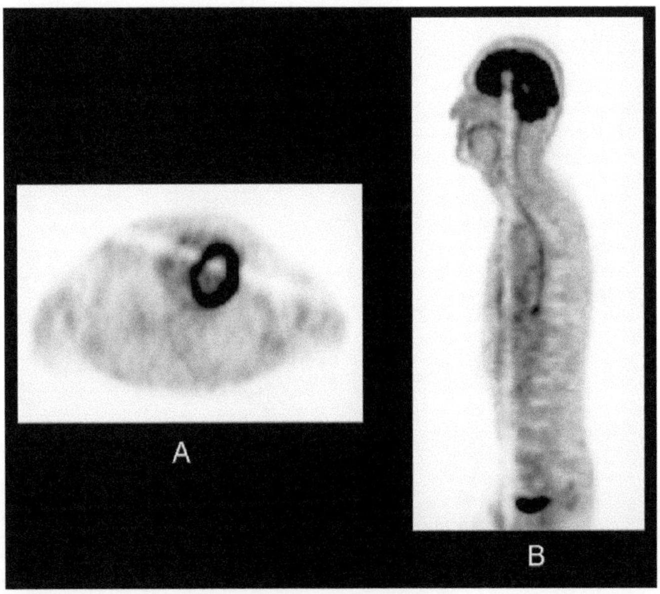

FIGURE C2-8. (A and B)

References

1. Galt JR, Germano G. Advances in instrumentation for cardiac SPECT. In DePuey EG, Berman DS, Garcia EV (ed). *Cardiac SPECT Imaging.* New York: Raven Press; 1995:91–102.
2. Garcia EV (ed). Imaging guidelines for nuclear cardiology procedures, part I. *J Nucl Cardiol.* 1996;3:G3–45.
3. Shepp LA, Vardi Y. Maximum likelihood reconstruction for emission tomography. *IEEE Trans Med Imag.* 1982;MI-1:113–122.
4. Hudson HM, Larkin RS. Accelerated image reconstruction using ordered subsets of projection data. *J Nucl Med.* 1994;13:601–609.
5. Phelps ME. History of PET. In Delbeke D, Martin WH, Patton JA, Sandler MP (eds). *Practical FDG Imaging: A Teaching File.* New York: Springer-Verlag; 2002:1–17.
6. Patton JA. Physics of PET. In Delbeke D, Martin WH, Patton JA, Sandler MP (eds). *Practical FDG Imaging: A Teaching File.* New York: Springer-Verlag; 2002:18–36.
7. Tarantola G, Zito F, Gerundini P. PET instrumentation and reconstruction algorithms in whole-body applications. *J Nucl Med.* 2003;44:756–769.
8. Patton JA. Instrumentation for coincidence imaging with multihead scintillation cameras. *J Nucl Med.* 2000;30:239–254.
9. Toma DM, White MP, Mann A, et al. Influence of arm positioning on rest/stress technetium-99 mm labeled sestamibi tomographic perfusion imaging. *J Nucl Cardiol.* 1999;6:163–168.

3 Radiopharmaceuticals and Protocols in Nuclear Cardiology

Dominique Delbeke, João V. Vitola, and William H. Martin

The basic procedure for cardiac imaging in nuclear medicine is the same for all studies. A radiopharmaceutical agent or radioisotope, in the case of thallium 201 chloride (^{201}Tl), is injected intravenously, and the emitted gamma rays are detected by a nuclear gamma camera as the radiolabeled agent enters the myocardium, circulates in the cardiac blood pool, or both. These signals are then collected and transformed by a computer into an image that depicts the regional distribution of the radiopharmaceutical in the body. Studies continue to become more sophisticated and accurate as new techniques and radiopharmaceuticals are developed. The principal advantages of nuclear imaging of the heart and central circulation are its noninvasiveness and its ability to assess quantitatively or semiquantitatively myocardial blood flow (MBF), metabolism, and ventricular function. Its main disadvantages are its relative cost and the special expertise required for accurate interpretation of the study.

Myocardial Perfusion Imaging

Under normal physiologic conditions, the coronary vessels receive 4% of the cardiac output. Stenotic lesions in these vessels may significantly reduce the blood flow, leading to ischemia and jeopardizing cellular survival. Such lesions cause diminished distribution of perfusion radiopharmaceuticals in the affected vascular territory, especially evident during periods of increased myocardial oxygen demand, induced by stress testing with exercise or pharmacological agents. Typically, imaging radioactive tracer distribution can demonstrate relative regional perfusion differences but does not directly measure absolute MBF. Quantitation of MBF requires attenuation correction (AC), scanner calibration, kinetic analysis, and compartmental modeling possible only by utilizing the technology of positron emission tomography (PET). The mass of myocardium and the degree of flow reduction required to detect a relative regional difference in perfusion are related to the sensitivity of the camera system used to perform the study and to the extraction efficiency of the radiopharmaceutical.

For detection of stress-induced ischemia, the optimal time for intravenous injection of a perfusion agent is during the peak level of exercise in exercise stress testing or at the point of maximum coronary hyperemia in pharmacological stress testing. Areas of diminished perfusion or ischemia have decreased or unchanged uptake of the radiopharmaceutical, whereas regions supplied by patent coronary arteries demonstrate increased relative perfusion. The stress-induced study is then compared with a study with the patient in the resting state. A fixed perfusion defect is characteristic of myocardial infarction (MI), whereas a reversible abnormality is typical of ischemia.

Ideal Perfusion Radiopharmaceutical and Linearity with Flow

The characteristics of a perfusion radiopharmaceutical depend on the physical characteristics of the radiotracer and the biological properties of the pharmaceutical. An ideal perfusion agent should have a high first-pass extraction (close to 100%) and should exhibit a linear relationship between the degree of myocardial uptake and MBF over a wide range of MBF, considering that MBF can rise up to fivefold above baseline flow with pharmacological stress using vasodilators such as adenosine. The relationship between myocardial uptake and MBF for perfusion radiopharmaceuticals is shown in Figure 3-1A. Cationic ^{99m}Tc-labeled perfusion agents such as ^{99m}Tc-methoxy-isobutyl-isonitrile, also known as ^{99m}Tc sestamibi (MIBI), and tetrofosmin have a relatively low first-pass extraction fraction (24% to 39%) compared with ^{201}Tl and lipophilic neutral agents (approximately 75%).[1] For most radiopharmaceuticals there is overestimation of blood flow at low flow rates and underestimation at high flow rates (roll-off). The threshold at which roll-off occurs varies among the different radiopharmaceuticals. The linearity of uptake with flow rates occurs over the widest range of flow rates for lipophilic neutral ^{99m}Tc radiopharmaceuticals (^{99m}Tc-NOET and ^{99m}Tc-teboroxime), followed by ^{201}Tl (linear range: 0.3 to 2.5 ml/min/g), followed by the lipophilic cationic ^{99m}Tc radiopharmaceuticals (MIBI and tetrofosmin: 0.3 to 2.0 ml/min/g).[2] Early roll-off in hyperemic segments of the myocardium can potentially result in underestimation of perfusion abnormalities with lower grades of coronary stenosis, especially with pharmacological stress,[3,4] resulting in false-negative studies for ischemia.

In addition, ideal perfusion radiopharmaceuticals should have stable myocardial retention, and the hepatic and gastrointestinal uptake should be minimal with exercise as well as with pharmacological stress and resting studies. Hepatic and gastrointestinal uptake (bowel loops with activity can be adjacent to or abut or overlap the inferior wall of the heart) can interfere with image interpretation as discussed in Case 3.10.

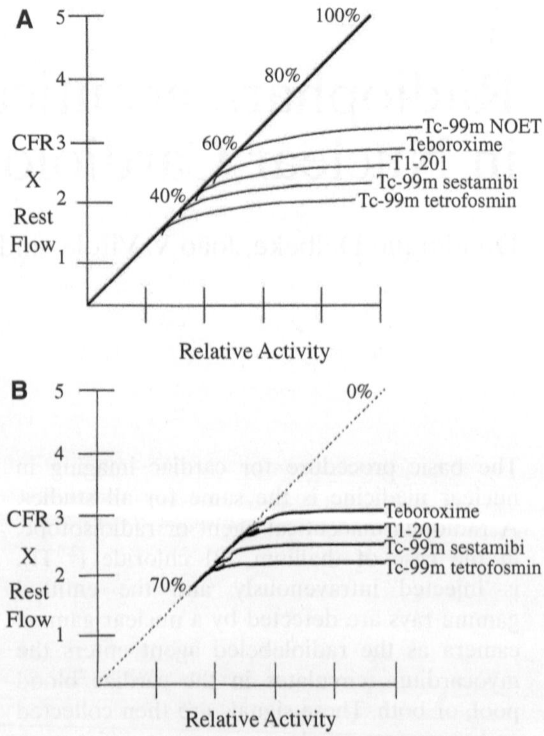

FIGURE 3-1. Linearity of uptake of different radiopharmaceuticals in relation to myocardial blood flow. (A) The line of linearity is labeled with the percentage of the CBF reflected by a linear flow relationship at any given level. (B) The approved perfusion agents are similarly plotted, but the range of percent stenosis related to CBFR is approximated. All agents have a high sensitivity for hemodynamically significant stenoses. (Self-Study Program III: Nuclear Medicine Cardiology Topic 5. In Botvinick E (ed). *Myocardial Perfusion Scintigraphy-Technical Aspects.* Reston, VA: Society of Nuclear Medicine, 2001. Used by permission.)

Radiopharmaceuticals and Imaging Protocols

The perfusion imaging agents most commonly used clinically are ^{201}Tl and ^{99m}Tc-MIBI and ^{99m}Tc-tetrofosmin. The properties and imaging protocols of these agents are discussed in the case presentations.

^{99m}Tc-Labeled Agents

Several groups of ^{99m}Tc-labeled agents have been developed including ^{99m}Tc-isonitriles (e.g., ^{99m}Tc-MIBI),[5,6] boronic acid adducts of technetium oximes (BATO compounds, e.g., ^{99m}Tc-teboroxime) and diphosphine compounds (e.g., ^{99m}Tc-tetrofosmin).[7] Isonitriles and diphosphines are lipophilic cationic agents, whereas teboroxime is a lipophilic neutral agent.

In 1990, ^{99m}Tc-MIBI and ^{99m}Tc-teboroxime became available for clinical use in the United States, and there is now widespread use of ^{99m}Tc-MIBI. A few years later, ^{99m}Tc-tetrofosmin became commercially available and is now used almost as commonly as ^{99m}Tc-MIBI.

The mechanism of uptake for ^{99m}Tc teboroxime is not well understood and may be due to nonspecific binding to cell membrane due to its lipophilicity. Its advantages are its high first-pass extraction and its linear relationship between myocardial uptake and MBF over a wide range of perfusion rates (0–4.5 ml/min). However, because of its rapid clearance from the heart, image acquisition must be completed within 5 to 6 minutes postinjection, which is technically challenging. For this reason, clinical use of ^{99m}Tc-teboroxime is limited, and ^{99m}Tc-teboroxime is no longer available commercially. This subject is further discussed in Case 18.1.

More recently, two more promising ^{99m}Tc-labeled agents have been evaluated, ^{99m}Tc-N-ethoxy, N-ethyl dithiocarbamato nitrido V (NOET)[8] and ^{99m}Tc-nitromidazole.[9] The agent ^{99m}Tc-NOET is a neutral lipophilic compound with high myocardial extraction fraction and the highest linear relationship with flow among all the agents evaluated to date. The extraction fraction is in a similar range as that of teboroxime. The lipophilic properties and consequently large permeability/surface area product explain the high extraction fraction. Structural membrane integrity is important in myocardial retention of ^{99m}Tc-NOET. ^{99m}Tc-NOET remains tightly bound to the hydrophobic components of the cell, and therefore the cell membranes are the most probable subcellular localization site of ^{99m}Tc-NOET. Its clearance from the blood pool is slower compared with the cationic agents. The lung uptake is initially high but decreases faster than cardiac uptake with a heart-to-lung ratio of 1.04 at 5 minutes and 1.84 at 1 hour postinjection. The liver uptake remains constant over time. ^{99m}Tc-NOET redistributes to the myocardium in a manner similar to that of ^{201}Tl. If flow is normalized after the initial uptake, redistribution is virtually complete within 90 minutes.[10,11] The agent ^{99m}Tc-NOET (Scherring Diagnostics, Berlin, Germany) is currently in phase II trials in the United States and phase III trials in Europe. This subject is further discussed in Case 18.2.

^{99m}Tc-nitromidazole shows promises for a *hot spot* imaging agent to identify ischemic and viable myocardium. Tissue hypoxia occurs in ischemia due to an imbalance between oxygen supply and demand. Tracers developed to image hypoxia have a low redox potential. They become reduced by receiving electrons from disturbed mitochondrial electron transport chains in hypoxic cells with abnormal electron flow. The reduced complexes are trapped intracellularly. Nitroimidazoles have been used in therapeutic doses as radiation sensitizers and as antibiotics.[12] The mechanism of retention in therapeutic doses probably involves covalent intracellular binding. When administered in tracer amounts for imaging, the retention mechanism of the labeled product is unknown. Various compounds have been investigated in animal models.

Current limitations of SPECT perfusion radiopharmaceuticals include (1) inefficient stress/rest protocols because of the relatively long half-lives of the SPECT emitters; (2) dosimetry concerns limiting the dose that can be administered and the count density; (3) attenuation artifacts leading to *false-positive images*; and (4) inability to quantitate absolute MBF. Some of these limitations can be overcome with PET perfusion radiopharmaceuticals: ^{82}Rubidium (^{82}Rb) and ^{13}N-ammonia. The PET perfusion agents are discussed in Case 3.8.

Image Acquisition and Processing

Presently, planar cardiac perfusion imaging is performed only rarely. Each image in the computer memory is divided into small squares and cubes of information called *pixels* and *voxels*, respectively. Each pixel records signals from one area of the organ being imaged. If there is a higher concentration of radiotracer in one wall of the heart than in the other walls, the number of signals originating from that wall will be high and the number of counts in the pixels corresponding to that wall will also be high. This area will have increased count density on the images created by the computer.

SPECT imaging provides three-dimensional images with better localization and visualization of small or mild perfusion defects in the heart than planar images. The left ventricle (LV) is viewed in tomographic sections in the transverse plane (short axis) or longitudinal plane (vertical and horizontal long axis) as shown in Figure 3-2. Myocardial segmentation and nomenclature for tomographic imaging of

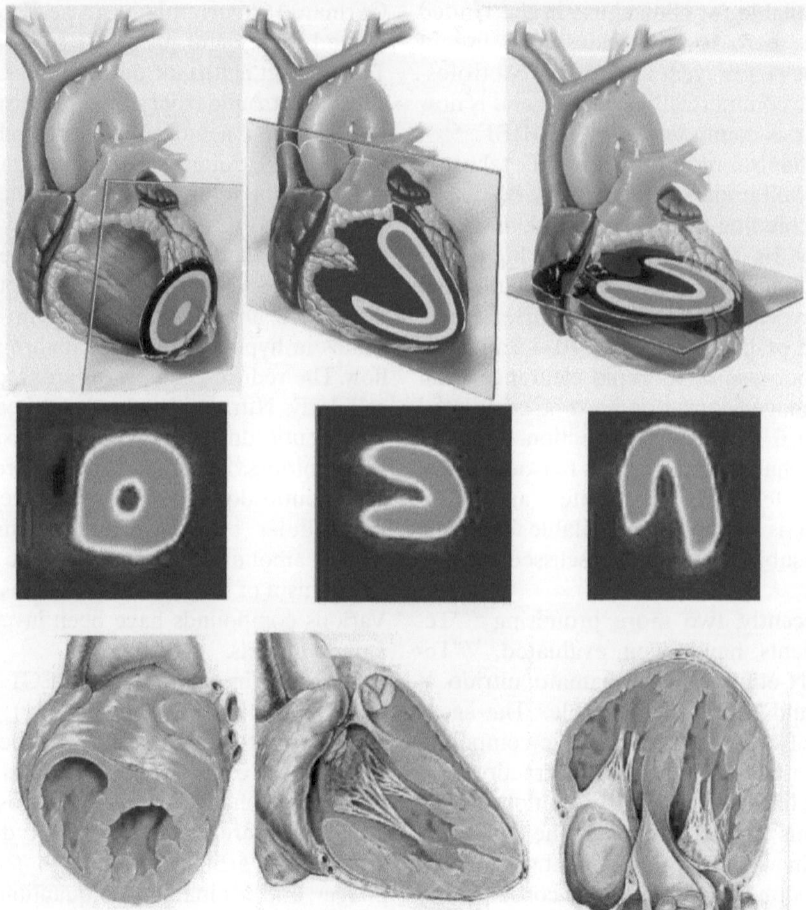

FIGURE 3-2. Schematic representation of tomographic sections through the heart along the short axis, vertical long axis, and horizontal long axis.

the heart is discussed in detail in a position statement of the ASNC.[13]

The protocols for image acquisition are discussed in detail in the Guidelines for MPI published by the ASNC.[14] A series of projection images is acquired for 20 to 30 seconds each over 360- or 180-degree arcs from the right anterior oblique (RAO) to the left posterior oblique (LPO) projection. Each projection image is first corrected for nonuniformity. The images are then filtered and reconstructed using the filtered back projection technique or an iterative algorithm. The images are normalized to the area of highest myocardial uptake and reoriented in three orthogonal projections related to the axis of the LV (Figure 3-2). Acquisition of transmission maps for attenuation correction is available on some SPECT gamma camera systems. Iterative reconstruction algorithms can be used instead of filtered back projection together with attenuation and scatter correction.

SPECT images display in the three orthogonal planes for review, and semiquantitative analysis of perfusion is available with most commercial software. The semiquantitative analysis is typically displayed in a polar map format with comparison with a normal database according to the patient's age and gender as well as the protocol used for MPI. This is further discussed in Case 3.7.

ECG-Gated Myocardial Perfusion Imaging

For clinical purposes, gated SPECT acquisition has replaced the first-pass technique for evaluation of LV function. It is much less demanding technically and can also provide evaluation of regional LV wall motion and thickening, as well as both regional and global LVEF both at rest and after stress. The principle of gated acquisition as well as the impact of the number of gates and count rate on measurements of the LVEF is described with the technique of gated blood pool radionuclide ventriculography (RVG) in Chapter 7.

Processing of a gated acquisition is similar to a nongated acquisition. All the temporal frames in each projection are collapsed (*de-gated*) into one static image. This new image set is equivalent to the image set that would have been acquired without gating and processed as an ungated image set.

The display of the gated SPECT study includes a 3-D rendering of the beating heart in various projections as well as a 2-D display of selected beating short-axis and long-axis slices. Quantitative polar plot displays of regional wall motion, thickening, and LVEF are provided as well as estimates of the end diastolic (EDV) and systolic volumes (ESV) and global LVEF. The LVEF quantitation by gated SPECT provided by several commercially available software programs has been validated using echocardiography, RVG, and MRI, with correlation coefficients of approximately 0.9. However, the gated measurements are algorithm-dependent; for example, for patients with a low likelihood of CAD, the average LVEF, LVEDV, and LVESV are smaller using QGS/QPS^R than the ECTtoolbox.[15]

The accuracy of the technique for LVEF measurement depends on the definition of the endocardial borders at end-systole and end-diastole. In patients with small ventricles, the LVEF can be overestimated because of underestimation of the ESV due to poor spatial resolution and scatter. The limited sampling rate can lead to underestimation of the LVEF in patients with slow heart rate (HR) due to the associated prolonged diastolic phase. Gating abnormalities (variable R-R interval, peaked T-waves, pacer spikes, and so forth) can also lead to inaccurate measurements of the LVEF. Ideally, the same number of cardiac cycles should be acquired for each projection, meaning that the actual acquisition time (number of cycles x cycle length) is the same for each projection. Technical factors may also impact the measurement of LVEF, for example, 8-frame gating results in LVEF 3 to 4 percentage points lower than 16-frame gating.

Image Interpretation

SPECT perfusion images are viewed on a computer monitor and interpreted visually and by using semiquantitative analysis. Regional abnormalities are determined to be *fixed*, i.e., unchanged at rest as compared with stress, or *reversible*, i.e., normal or significantly improved on the rest images as compared with the stress images. Reversible abnormalities are typically related to ischemia, whereas fixed defects are characteristic of myocardial scarring or attenuation artifacts.

Accurate interpretation requires integrating (1) clinical data from the patient's history, stress hemodynamics, and stress ECG; (2) inspection of raw projection data (patient's motion, soft tissue attenuation, extracardiac uptake, lung uptake, and hepatic/gastrointestinal uptake); and (3) assessment of perfusion and segmental analysis and assessment of function.

Evaluation of Myocardial Viability

Evaluation of myocardial viability using both SPECT (^{201}Tl and ^{99m}Tc-labeled agents) and PET (^{18}F-fluorodeoxyglucose [FDG] and labeled fatty acid analogs) radiopharmaceuticals is discussed in Chapter 8, specifically addressing myocardial viability.

Imaging Apoptosis and Necrotic Cell Death

Although necrosis and apoptosis are two distinct forms of cell death, their boundaries are not well defined, especially in myocardial cell death.[16,17] Necrosis occurs after exogenous insult such as ischemic or inflammatory injury leading to cell swelling and rupture, denaturation and coagulation of cytoplasmic proteins, disintegration of subcellular organelles, and release of intracellular contents. Necrosis is followed by an inflammatory reaction and later by fibrosis. Apoptosis is a programmed cell death in response to various stimuli leading to chromatin condensation and fragmentation, followed by cellular shrinkage and breakage into small apoptotic bodies. The apoptotic bodies are removed with minimal disruption of the normal tissue architecture. Apoptosis is part of a normal process to remove unwanted damaged cells but can also occur in pathologic conditions of the heart. Excessive apoptosis or lack of appropriate apoptosis can play a role in various disease processes; for example, impaired apoptosis can lead to oncogenesis.

During prolonged myocardial ischemia, irreversible cell damage and infarction occur. It is becoming increasingly clear that cell death may begin as apoptosis and not as necrosis, although necrosis occurs after a finite amount of time.[18] Because apoptosis is a programmed sequence of intracellular events, it can possibly be manipulated and reversed.[19] Therefore, noninvasive detection of apoptosis may be important in the identification of potentially salvageable myocardium. Now that thrombolytic agents and angioplasty are available, CBF can be reestablished relatively soon after the patient arrives at the hospital with an acute coronary syndrome, and the number of transmural infarctions has decreased. Determining the location of the infarct and estimating its extent has important prognostic and therapeutic implications.

Scintigraphic agents such as ^{201}Tl or FDG, and eventually ^{99m}Tc-agents, can be used to differentiate viable tissue from scarring related to infarction, as discussed previously. Infarct-avid agents are radiopharmaceuticals that bind to recently infarcted tissue, identifying tissue undergoing necrosis. These include ^{99m}Tc-pyrophosphate, ^{111}In-antimyosin, and ^{99m}Tc-glucarate. ^{99m}Tc-annexin is a marker of apoptosis. Noninvasive detection of cell death has been reviewed and discussed in a relatively recent editorial by Narula and Baret.[20]

^{99m}Tc-Pyrophosphate

During the process of irreversible injury that follows prolonged ischemia, there is a marked influx of calcium to the cytosol and mitochondria. This influx peaks 24 to 72 hours after an MI. ^{99m}Tc-pyrophosphate accumulation in infarcted areas gradually diminishes over 5 to 7 days but in large infarcts may persist for weeks. The 24- to 72-hour lag time between vessel occlusion and development of a positive scan obviates the use of pyrophosphate in the emergency department. In the past, ^{99m}Tc-pyrophosphate was frequently used for bone scanning, because it adheres to tissues undergoing significant calcium deposition. After irreversible myocardial injury, this agent can be used to evaluate the extent and location of infarction. There is somewhat diminished specificity because pyrophosphate will also interact with severely ischemic but viable myocardium in the patient with unstable angina. This subject is further discussed in Case 6.6.

^{111}In-Antimyosin

Recent infarction can also be evaluated with ^{111}In-antimyosin, which is the radiolabeled Fab fragment of a monoclonal antibody that binds to the exposed heavy chains of myosin following disruption of the myocyte membrane during infarction. Myosin is the major intracellular myocardial protein. Although uptake of the radiopharmaceutical into damaged myocardial cells occurs immediately after the onset of infarction, imaging must be delayed for 24 to 48 hours to allow blood pool clearance. In contrast to ^{99m}Tc-pyrophosphate scintigraphy, ^{111}In-antimyosin images may remain positive for as long as 12 months following the clinical event. Thus, the value of a negative scan result is more useful in excluding infarction over the prior 6 months than with ^{99m}Tc-pyrophosphate. Increased cardiac uptake of ^{111}In-antimyosin occurs not only in acute MI but also in acute myocarditis, doxorubicin-induced cardiotoxicity, and acute or chronic rejection of a transplanted heart. Clinical use of infarct-avid agents is uncommon today because other techniques have been developed to detect and localize MI, and because other radiopharmaceutical agents are superior in estimating myocardial viability and the extent of infarction. The occasional patient with a suspected intraoperative infarction or with delayed presentation may benefit from infarct-avid imaging. ^{111}In-antimyosin is no longer commercially available in the United States.

^{99m}Tc-Glucarate

^{99m}Tc-glucarate is a derivative of a sugar that is the physiologic end product of uridine diphosphoglucose metabolism. It localizes in areas of acute necrosis, and imaging its myocardial distribution appears to combine rapid evaluation with high diagnostic accuracy. In experimental acute MI, 75% of intracellular ^{99m}Tc-glucarate is localized to the nucleus and 83% of the nuclear fraction is associated with nucleoproteins (histones).[21,22] It has been hypothesized that intracellular accumulation of ^{99m}Tc-glucarate is associated with disruption of the cell and nuclear membranes, allowing free intracellular diffusion and electrochemical binding to histones. When full necrosis and cell death occur, nuclear histones are released and ^{99m}Tc-glucarate can no longer accumulate. Images are obtained 2 to 3 hours following the administration of 25 to 30 mCi of ^{99m}Tc-glucarate to allow for blood pool clearance. A study of 28 patients presenting to the emergency department with symptoms suspicious for MI suggests that ^{99m}Tc-glucarate localizes in acute myocardial necrosis when injected within 9 hours of onset of infarction.[23] ^{99m}Tc-glucarate (Amiscan, Draximages, Inc, Kirkland, Quebec, Canada; and Molecular Targeting, Inc, West Chester, PA) is in phase II trials in the United States. This subject is further discussed in Case 18.4.

^{99m}Tc-Annexin

Annexin V is a naturally occurring human protein with high affinity for membrane-associated phosphatidylserine (PS). PS is normally located on the inner layer of the cell membrane (not accessible for annexin V binding) but is transported to the outer layer early during apoptosis. Annexin V can also gain access to PS as the result of the membrane fragmentation associated with necrosis. Scintigraphic studies in humans using ^{99m}Tc-annexin V have demonstrated the feasibility of imaging cell death in acute MI and ischemia,[24] in acute allograft rejection after transplantation,[25,26] in tumors with a high apoptotic index, and in response to anti-tumor chemotherapy of various tumors.[27] Apoptosis can also be detected in heart failure but the exact mechanism is still unclear.[28,29] The agent ^{99m}Tc-annexin (Apomate, North American Scientific, Inc, Chatworth, CA) is in phase I/II trials for applications in oncology. This subject is further discussed in Case 18.3.

Imaging the Autonomous Nervous System

The sympathetic innervation of the heart plays a major role in the regulation of myocardial function, HR, and MBF. Sympathetically mediated vasoregulation plays a major role in the regulation of MBF at rest and during stress. Denervation may occur in various conditions such as myocardial ischemia, MI, diabetes, or heart transplantation. Myocardial sympathetic innervation can be assessed with ^{123}I-metaiodobenzylguanidine (^{123}I-MIBG), an analog of the false neurotransmitter guanethidine that is taken up by adrenergic neurons in a similar fashion to norepinephrine but does not undergo intracellular metabolism.

The poor count statistics seen with ^{131}I-MIBG prohibit its use in cardiac imaging. To perform MIBG imaging, planar images are acquired immediately after intravenous administration of 4 mCi of ^{123}I-MIBG and again 4 hours later. The early images reflect receptor density; washout over time is a reflection of adrenergic activity.

For semiquantitative interpretation, the heart-to-mediastinum ratio can be calculated on both sets of images. SPECT images can be acquired to give a better topographic regional distribution in the myocardium, and SPECT images can be analyzed the same way as perfusion images. Both sets of SPECT perfusion and MIBG images can be compared in terms of matched and mismatched pattern of perfusion and presence and extent of denervation.

A recent review summarizes data of multiple studies that have reported the potential role of ^{123}I-MIBG imaging in ischemic heart disease, diabetes mellitus, congestive heart failure (CHF) and cardiomyopathy, heart transplantation, and arrhythmia.[30] A variety of clinical conditions associated with increased sympathetic tone have demonstrated enhanced washout of MIBG, defined as more than 25% over a period of 15 minutes to 3 to 4 hours compared with <10% in control patients.[31,32] These conditions include dilated cardiomyopathy, hypertrophic cardiomyopathy, ischemic heart disease, essential hypertension, and hypothyroidism. The level of myocardial MIBG washout seems to be related to the severity of CHF as measured by the New York Heart Association classification.[33] Cardiac adrenergic innervation seems to be affected in asymptomatic subjects with very early stage CAD.[34] In addition, an abnormal heart-to-mediastinum ratio at 4 hours on planar images seems to be the best predictor of survival and was demonstrated to be an independent predictor of death.[35–37] MIBG imaging is promising for early detection of autonomic neuropathy in patients with diabetes mellitus and for investigation of the pathophysiology of certain types of arrhythmias. A major drawback to the more widespread use of MIBG imaging is the lack of a source of commercially available radiopharmaceutical. In addition, MIBG is not yet approved by the FDA for cardiac imaging in the United States. This subject is further discussed in Case 18.8.

Case Presentations

Case 3.1

History

A 48-year-old man with no previous cardiac history presented with 3 weeks of progressive weakness, nausea, and chest pain. His cardiac risk factors included hypertension, tobacco abuse, and a family history of CAD. The patient exercised on a treadmill with a standard Bruce protocol for 9 minutes, reached 85% of maximum predicted HR, and remained asymptomatic. His baseline ECG showed LV hypertrophy, and with exercise there were no changes consistent with ischemia. The exercise/reinjection ^{201}Tl SPECT images are shown in Figure C3-1A and a planar anterior image in Figure C3-1B.

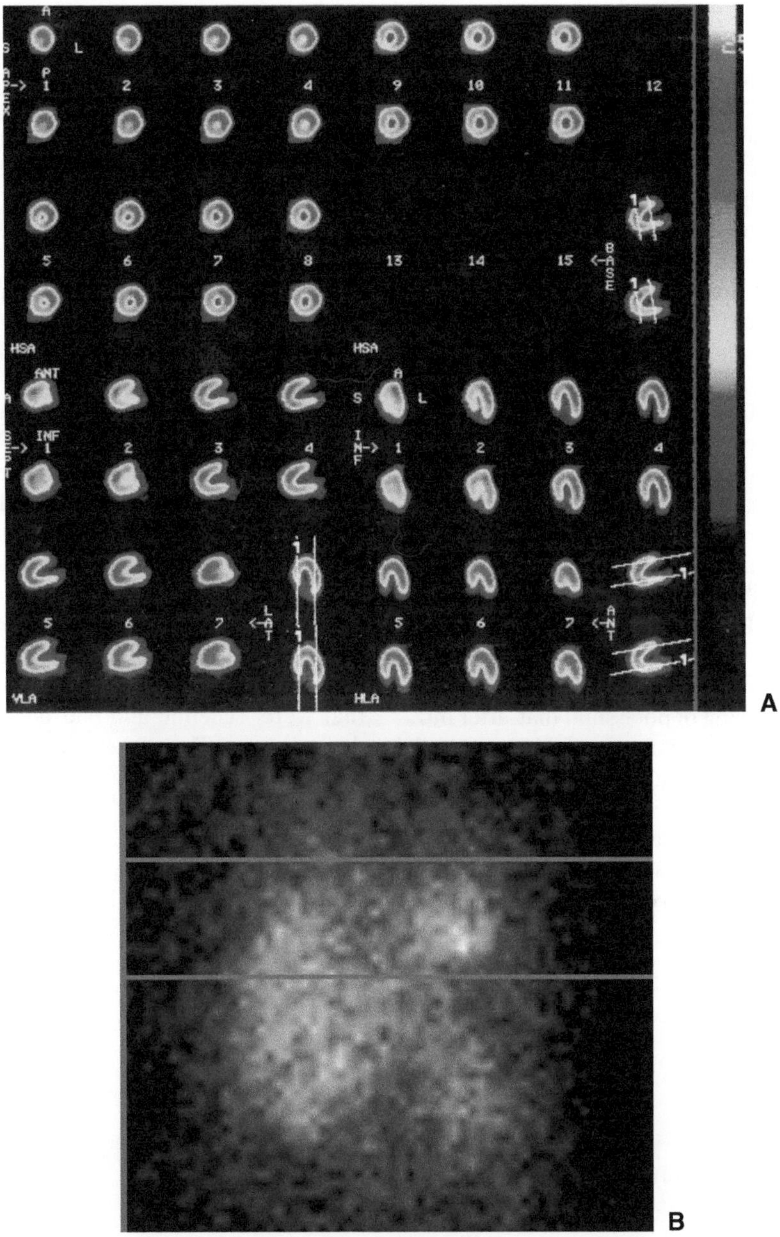

FIGURE C3-1. (A and B)

Findings

There is normal myocardial perfusion images during exercise and rest after reinjection of ^{201}Tl. On the anterior planar image (Figure C3-1B), the typical biodistribution of ^{201}Tl is seen with predominantly renal excretion, whereas ^{99m}Tc-MIBI and tetrofosmin are predominantly excreted by the hepatobiliary system (see Case 3.2).

Discussion

Normal perfusion refers to homogeneous uptake of ^{201}Tl throughout the myocardium at rest and with stress. This patient's pretest probability of myocardial ischemia is moderate because of his age, numerous cardiac risk factors, and symptoms. The scintigraphic images of an exercise myocardial perfusion study should be interpreted in conjunction with the exercise capacity of the patient and whether or not 85% maximum predicted HR response was achieved. Sensitivity for detection of ischemia by exercise MPI is diminished if the target HR is not achieved by the patient. There is more limited sensitivity of exercise MPI to detect CAD if the patient does not reach target HR. This is further discussed in Chapter 4.

A normal exercise/rest myocardial perfusion scan with ^{201}Tl scan predicts an excellent prognosis and a very low risk (<1%) of MI or cardiac death occurring over the next year.[38,39] This is further discussed in Chapter 9.

^{201}Tl is an analog of potassium that, after intravenous (IV) injection, enters viable myocardial cells by passive diffusion and also by an active mechanism involving the sodium-potassium adenosine triphosphatase pump.[40] Only 4% to 5% of the injected dose, usually 2.0 to 3.5 mCi, concentrates in the myocardium, the remainder being distributed to skeletal muscle and other tissues. The physical half-life of ^{201}Tl is approximately 72 hours, but the half-life in the myocardium is significantly less. During its decay, ^{201}Tl emits low-energy x-rays of approximately 70 keV. ^{201}Tl is usually administered at peak stress and then distributes in the myocardium proportionally to blood flow at stress.

One of the most clinically important characteristics of ^{201}Tl is its redistribution over time. Redistribution is a phenomenon by which an agent dynamically crosses the cell membrane, recirculates into the coronary vessels, and becomes concentrated in the myocardium proportionally to resting blood flow. This property forms the basis of stress-redistribution imaging protocols used to diagnose CAD with ^{201}Tl. With ^{201}Tl, redistribution is significant, and acquisition of stress images should begin soon after the isotope is injected, preferably within 10 to 20 minutes. The longer the redistribution time, the more likely ^{201}Tl will redistribute within viable cells with an intact cell membrane that were ischemic and had decreased uptake during stress. Therefore ^{201}Tl is often used to differentiate viable tissue from scar tissue. The pharmacokinetics of ^{201}Tl have been investigated and discussed by Krahwinkel et al.[41] Protocols for ^{201}Tl imaging are shown in Figures C3-1C, C3-1D, and C3-1E.

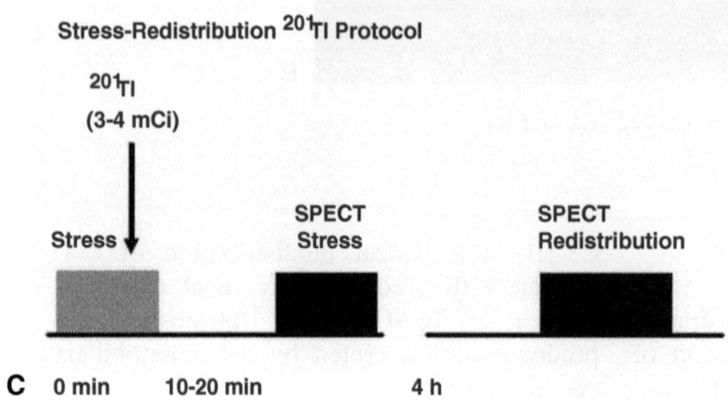

FIGURE C3-1. (C)

FIGURE C3-1. (D and E)

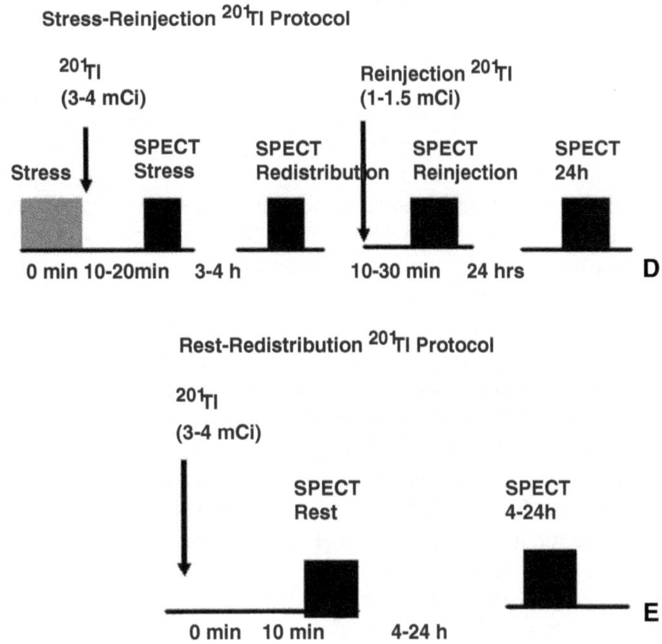

^{201}Tl migrates intracellularly and begins to be redistributed approximately 20 minutes after its injection. Regions of the myocardium that had decreased uptake of the radiotracer on the post-stress images, but that are viable, appear normal on resting redistribution images. Areas of nonviable cells resulting from previous MI have decreased uptake of ^{201}Tl on both the post-stress and resting images. These are matched, or fixed, defects. With the stress-redistribution protocol (Figure C3-1C), 3 to 4 mCi of ^{201}Tl is injected at peak stress and the images are acquired after 10 to 20 minutes. The redistribution images are then acquired after a 3- to 4-hour interval. Because this protocol overestimates the number of fixed defects by as much as 50%, the reinjection protocol has become the standard. With the reinjection protocol (Figure C3-1D), a second dosage of the tracer (1 to 1.5 mCi) is given 2 to 3 hours after the stress testing is completed. After 10 to 30 minutes, a second set of images, called *reinjection images*, is acquired. In extremely ischemic cells, significant uptake of ^{201}Tl into these segments may be seen only when a longer period (24 hours) of redistribution is allowed.[42] Often patients evaluated for viability cannot be stressed due to clinical constraints because of symptoms of CHF. For these patients, viability can be evaluated using the rest-redistribution ^{201}Tl protocol (Figure C3-1E). ^{201}Tl (3 to 4 mCi) is injected at rest and images are acquired 4 and sometimes 24 hours later. Protocols for evaluation of myocardial viability are discussed further in Chapter 8.

Interpretation

Normal ^{201}Tl myocardial perfusion study and noncardiac chest pain.

Case 3.2

History

A 55-year-old woman presented with episodes of left chest discomfort radiating to the shoulder blades occurring at rest and resolving spontaneously after 10 to 15 seconds. She had no history of CAD and no cardiac risk factors. The resting ECG was normal. A low-dose rest/high-dose exercise ^{99m}Tc-MIBI SPECT 1-day protocol was performed. She exercised 11 minutes using a standard Bruce protocol and reached 85% of her maximum predicted HR. No chest pain occurred during exercise, and the stress ECG was negative for myocardial ischemia. The rest/exercise SPECT images are displayed in Figure C3-2A, the functional stress images in Figure C3-2B, and a planar anterior image in Figure C3-2C.

Findings

Distribution of the radiopharmaceutical is homogeneous throughout the myocardium on both sets of images, compatible with normal perfusion at both stress and rest. The polar plots reveal similar normal perfusion. Gated images demonstrated normal wall motion and thickening of the myocardium. The global LVEF is 66% and the ESV and EDV are normal at 14 and 43 ml, respectively. The anterior planar image (Figure C3-2C) demonstrates the typical distribution of ^{99m}Tc-MIBI with prominent hepatobiliary excretion. The cineloop display of the planar projections should be inspected to assess motion artifact and possible soft tissue attenuation artifacts due to the body habitus of the patient.

A

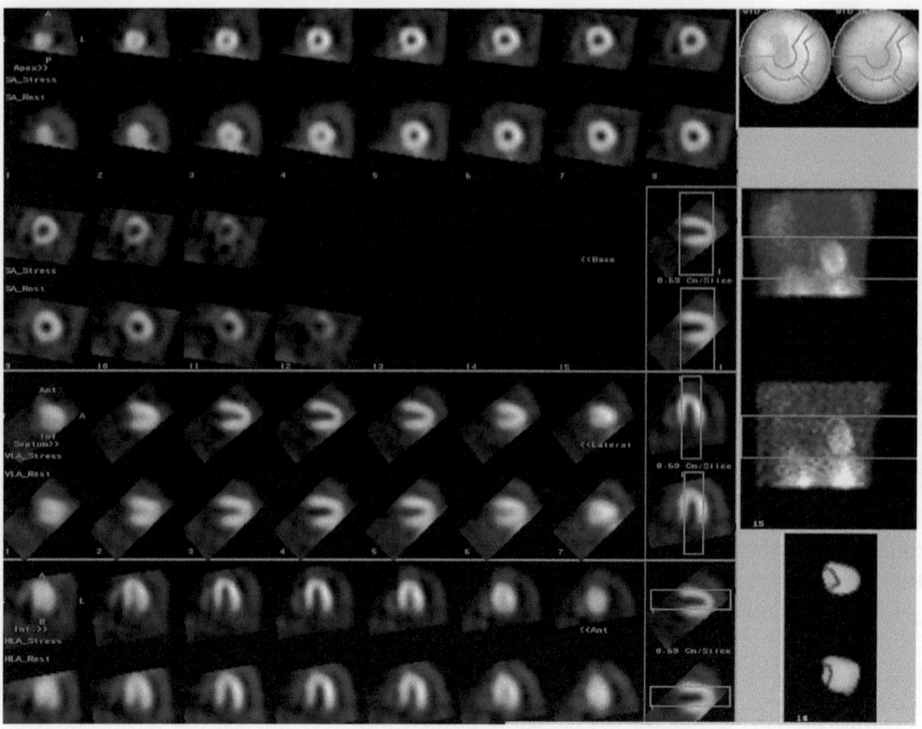

FIGURE C3-2. (A)

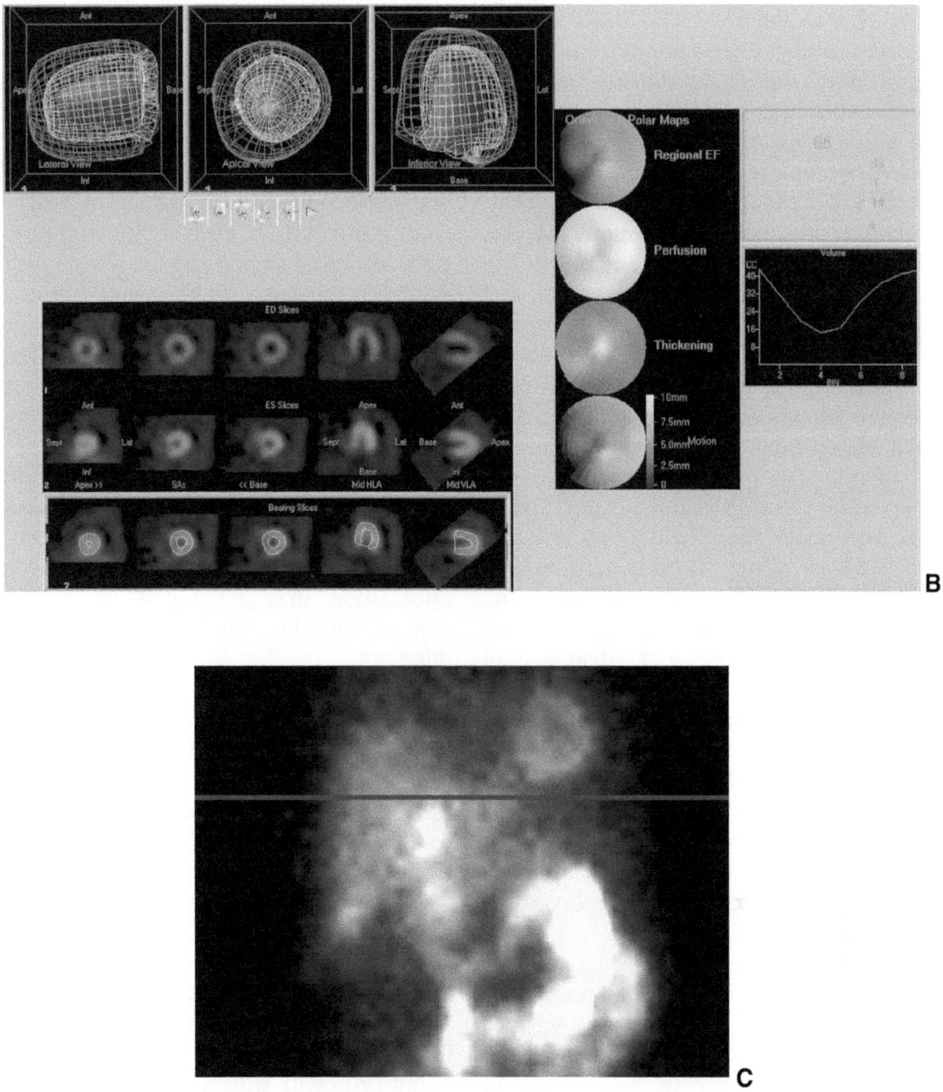

FIGURE C3-2. (B and C)

Discussion

The normal myocardial perfusion images are indicative of an excellent prognosis, even in the presence of an abnormal ECG or abnormal coronary arteriogram.[43] A study of 652 patients who had a normal stress SPECT study alone and were followed for 2 years demonstrated that the overall cardiac event rate in these patients was <1%.[44]

Cellular uptake of cationic perfusion agents, such as MIBI and tetrofosmin, is mediated by a nonspecific charge-dependent transfer of lipophilic cations across the sarcolemma but is independent of Na^+/K^+ channels. Therefore, cellular uptake is not affected by cation channel inhibitors. Intracellularly, ^{99m}Tc-MIBI appears to bind to the mitochondria in myocardial cells. Damaged nonviable cells do not maintain membrane potential, so MIBI does not accumulate within nonviable cells.

^{99m}Tc-MIBI rapidly clears from the blood pool with a peak activity at 1 minute postinjection and 95% clears the plasma 5 minutes postinjection. Myocardial uptake is 1% of the injected dose following a resting injection and 1.4% following an injection during exercise. ^{99m}Tc-MIBI has a slow clearance rate from the heart. Effective half-life is 3 hours. After it binds to the mitochondria, there is little redistribution, approximately 2% after 1 hour and 5% after 6 hours. Images can be acquired up to 6 hours postinjection. This allows evaluation of patients with acute chest pain syndrome and patients with evolving MI in whom thrombolytic therapy is planned. Although the kinetics of ^{99m}Tc-MIBI are affected by cell metabolism and viability,[45] a disadvantage of the labeled isonitriles is underestimation of the extent of viable myocardium in comparison with ^{201}Tl studies using a reinjection or 24-hour redistribution protocol. The gold standard for evaluating myocardial cellular viability is evaluation of glucose metabolism with FDG. A significant disadvantage of ^{99m}Tc-MIBI is prominent excretion into the bowel via the hepatobiliary system.

^{99m}Tc-tetrofosmin is used as commonly as ^{99m}Tc-MIBI. The myocardial uptake is approximately 1.2% of the injected dose both at rest and during exercise. Mitochondrial membrane potential plays a major role in myocardial uptake and retention of tetrofosmin, as it does for MIBI.[46] Blood clearance is rapid and hepatic excretion is rapid as well, an advantage over ^{99m}Tc-MIBI. Therefore, ^{99m}Tc-tetrofosmin causes less hepatic artifact but the myocardial uptake plateaus at a slightly lower flow rate than ^{99m}Tc-MIBI.

The isotope ^{99m}Tc is widely used in nuclear medicine because the detectors and electronics of conventional gamma cameras are optimized for the 140 KeV photons emitted by ^{99m}Tc. In addition ^{99m}Tc is inexpensive and readily available. The short 6-hour half-life of ^{99m}Tc permits it to be given in higher dosages than ^{201}Tl, resulting in higher count statistics with resultant better image resolution and quality and less attenuation by intervening soft tissues. The higher count rate also allows high-quality gated images to be acquired to assess wall motion and ventricular function simultaneously with perfusion. Due to the absence of significant redistribution, both supine and prone (or right lateral) imaging can be accomplished in instances in which diaphragmatic attenuation artifact may pose a problem.

The energy emitted by the various isotopes may affect the choice of agent. For example, in patients with a large body habitus, it may be wise to use a higher energy tracer such as ^{99m}Tc-MIBI because there is less soft tissue attenuation than with a lower energy-emitting tracer such as ^{201}Tl. Due to the lower dose used (usually) for the rest study, more soft tissue attenuation may be noted on the resting images; usually this presents no clinical dilemma.

The disadvantages of ^{99m}Tc-MIBI and tetrofosmin compared with ^{201}Tl are reduced linearity with flow, increased hepatic and splanchnic uptake, and diminished reliability of lung uptake as an indicator of LV dysfunction. Protocols for ^{99m}Tc-MIBI and tetrofosmin are shown in Figures C3-2D, C3-2E, and C3-2F.

Two separate administrations of radiopharmaceutical are necessary for the stress-induced and resting images because they are retained in the myocardium without redistribution over time. Ideally, rest and stress studies are performed on two different days (Figure C3-2D: 2-day protocol) with a 25-mCi dose for each study, but this is practical for neither patients nor referring clinicians. If a 1-day protocol (Figures C3-2E and C3-2F) is used, a lower dose is administered for the first study (typically 8 to 10 mCi), and the second study can be performed 1 hour later with a threefold higher dose (25 to 30 mCi). Images are typically acquired 30 to 60 minutes after administration of the radiopharmaceutical at rest and 15 to 30 minutes after physical exercise. After pharmacological stress using vasodilators, vasodilation of the splanchnic circulation increases liver uptake, so a longer waiting period of 45 to 90 minutes before acquisition of the images

FIGURE C3-2. (D–F)

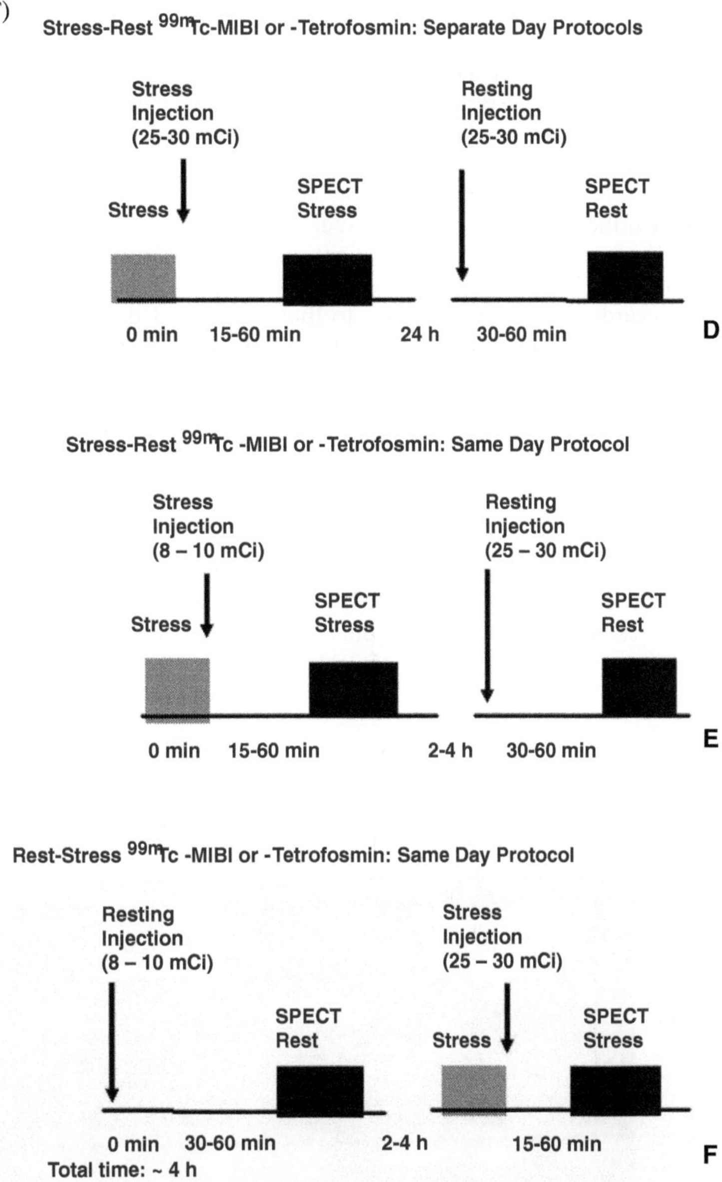

reduces interference of hepatic and bowel uptake with the inferior wall of the myocardium. Longer intervals may be necessary in individual cases.

In the rest/stress protocol, there is no contamination on the rest study from the previous ^{99m}Tc-MIBI injection. Despite some limitations of the same day compared with separate day protocols, the rest/stress same day ^{99m}Tc-MIBI protocol provides a high diagnostic accuracy for detection of CAD.[47] If the low-dose stress/high-dose rest sequence is used, there may be some contamination from the previous ^{99m}Tc-MIBI injection due to cross talk from the stress study present in the rest images. If stress imaging is performed first and is normal, rest imaging may not be necessary, an advantage of the stress/rest sequence. If a 2-day rest/stress protocol is used with the higher dose (25 to 30 mCi) of ^{99m}Tc-MIBI, performance of the resting study may be unnecessary if the stress images are normal.

The overall sensitivity, specificity, and accuracy of ^{99m}Tc-MIBI SPECT for the detection of myocardial ischemia is similar to that of ^{201}Tl imaging. No clinically significant difference between stress/rest and rest/stress ^{99m}Tc protocols has been reported.

Protocols using ^{99m}Tc-labeled radiopharmaceuticals for evaluation of myocardial viability are discussed in Chapter 8.

Interpretation

Normal myocardial perfusion scintigraphy using rest/exercise ^{99m}Tc-MIBI gated SPECT 1-day protocol, consistent with noncardiac chest pain.

Case 3.3

History

A 32-year-old man with chronic back pain and peptic disease presented with left-sided chest pain radiating to the arm. A dual isotope rest ^{201}Tl/exercise ^{99m}Tc-tetrofosmin gated myocardial perfusion study was performed (Figures C3-3A and C3-3B). He exercised for 9 minutes using a standard Bruce protocol and reached 85% of predicted maximum HR. He complained of chest pain with deep inspiration but had no ECG changes suggestive of ischemia.

A

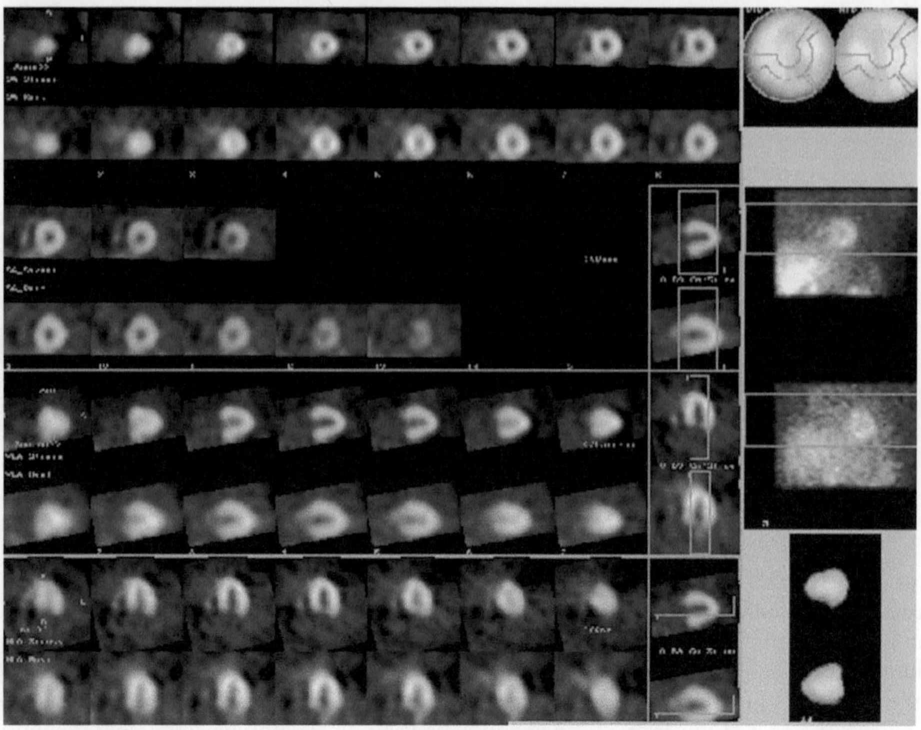

FIGURE C3-3. (A)

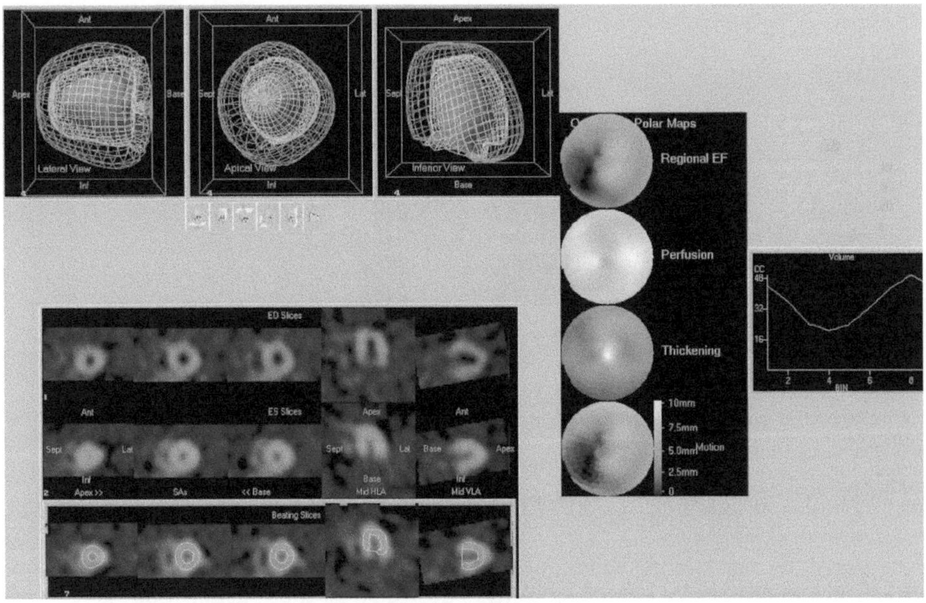

B

FIGURE C3-3. (B)

Findings

Homogenous myocardial perfusion is seen on both stress and rest images. The gated images revealed normal wall motion and wall thickening. The LVEF was 58% and the EDV and ESV were 49 and 20 units, respectively, both of which are within normal limits.

Discussion

When images obtained with radiopharmaceuticals labeled with isotopes of different energies are compared, such as ^{99m}Tc and ^{201}Tl, the interpreter must take into account the technical differences in the image quality. The ^{99m}Tc images have a better resolution than the ^{201}Tl images; therefore, the ^{201}Tl images appear fuzzier, the walls of the myocardium are not as well defined and appear thicker, and the LV cavity appears smaller than on the ^{99m}Tc images. For the same reason, a perfusion defect may appear smaller on ^{201}Tl compared with ^{99m}Tc images and partially reversible defects on dual isotope studies are sometimes a diagnostic challenge. When semiquantitative analysis of perfusion and motion are performed, normal reference data are different for different isotopes, and the appropriate ones must be selected for accurate interpretation. Different reference values for LVEF, ESV, EDV, and transient dilatation of the LV must also be taken into account.

Differential attenuation of isotopes of different energies by soft tissues such as diaphragm and breast can also be challenging and cause partially reversible defects that can be confused with ischemia. Imaging in both supine and prone positions is often helpful to assess the persistence or not of a defect when the source of attenuation projects differently over the myocardium.

The comparison of gated-SPECT data on rest and stress images acquired with radiotracers of different energies is more challenging as well. LVEF is usually accurate but wall motion analysis is less often interpretable with ^{201}Tl than with the ^{99m}Tc-agents. A common protocol for dual isotope perfusion scintigraphy is displayed in Figure C3-3C.

The resting study is acquired 10 to 20 minutes following administration of 3 mCi ^{201}Tl, after which the patient can be immediately stressed

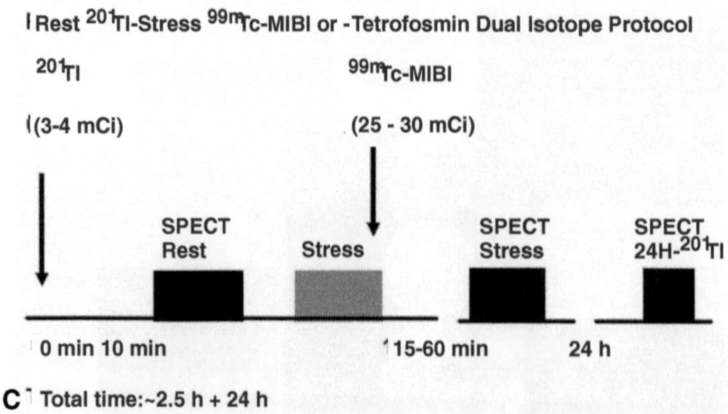

FIGURE C3-3. (C)

and the ^{99m}Tc-labeled agent (25 to 30 mCi) is administered at peak stress.

Advantages of the dual isotope technique for MPI include faster protocol for rest/stress study increasing throughout and the possibility of acquiring 24-hour delayed ^{201}Tl images for assessment of viability if fixed perfusion defects interpreted as MI are present.

The disadvantages include (1) the difference in resolution of the images; and (2) differential attenuation related to the lower peak energy of ^{201}Tl compared with ^{99m}Tc, making the interpretation of the images more difficult, especially in obese patients. In addition, the dual isotope protocol requires different filters and separate acquisition of the images. Simultaneous dual-isotope acquisition is complicated by cross-talk of ^{99m}Tc photons in the ^{201}Tl energy window.

Interpretation

Normal dual-isotope rest ^{201}Tl/exercise ^{99m}Tc tetrofosmin myocardial perfusion study results. The atypical chest pain was thought to be of gastrointestinal origin.

Case 3.4

History

A 59-year-old man with no risk factors for CAD and no chest pain was referred for a treadmill test as a precaution before initiating an aerobic exercise program. His exercise ECG was positive for ischemia. He was then referred to the nuclear laboratory for cardiac risk stratification. A 1 day rest/exercise stress ^{99m}Tc-MIBI protocol was performed. He exercised 9 minutes and 30 seconds on a standard Bruce protocol without chest pain. His hemodynamic response to exercise was normal and his target HR was exceeded. Although the patient was referred because of a positive TMT, the exercise ECG performed in the nuclear laboratory showed only borderline changes. The rest/stress MPI are displayed in Figure C3-4A and a right anterior oblique projection planar image in Figure C3-4B.

Findings

The rest/stress SPECT images demonstrated homogenous perfusion of the myocardium both at rest and during stress. On the planar image, a focus of uptake is noted in the right lung field adjacent to the heart, suggestive of a lung tumor.

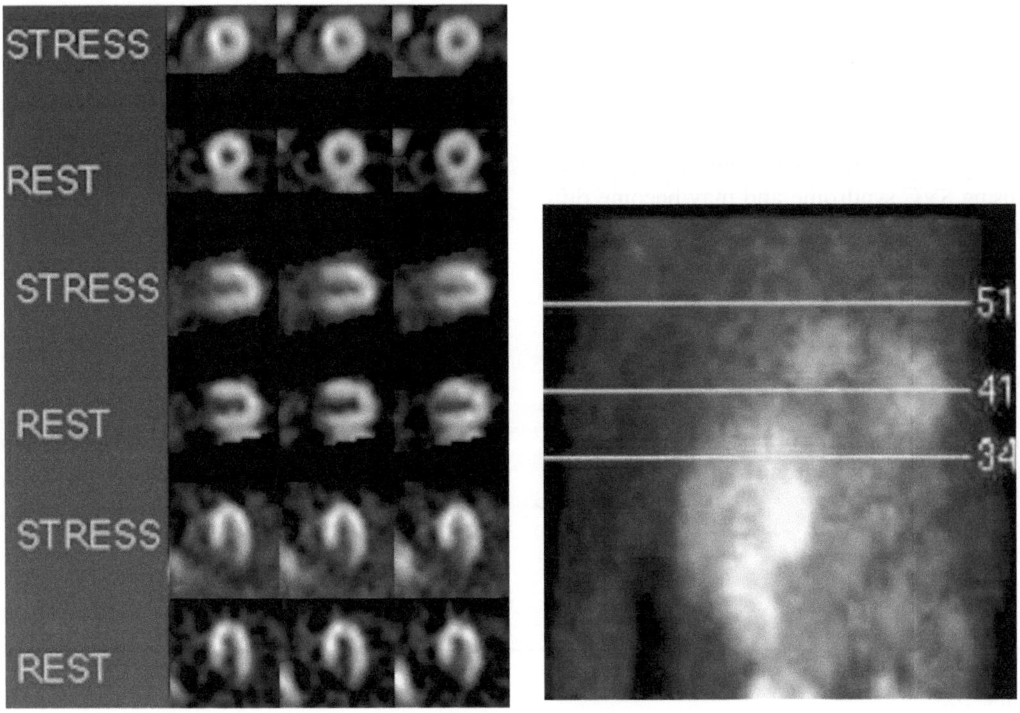

A B

FIGURE C3-4. (A and B)

The finding of abnormal uptake in the right lung triggered the referral for a chest CT scan shown in Figure C3-4C adjacent to the corresponding transaxial slice of the ^{99m}Tc-MIBI image (Figure C3-4D).

Discussion

The CT scan showed a right middle lobe lung mass adjacent to the superior vena cava (SVC). The patient was referred for lobectomy, and a

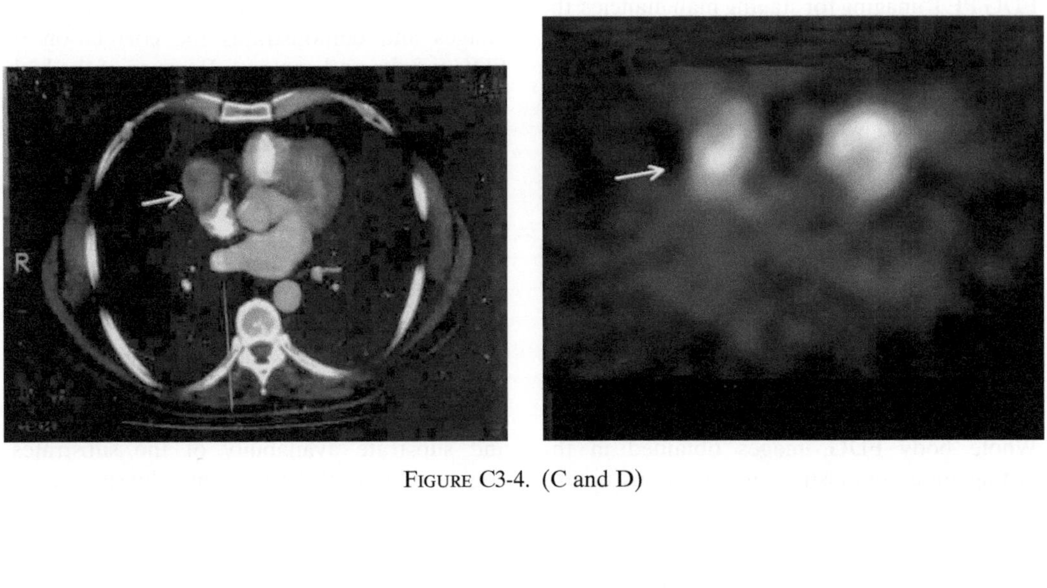

C D

FIGURE C3-4. (C and D)

thymoma was diagnosed at pathology. Approximately 30% of patients with thymomas have no symptoms. Surgery is indicated to avoid compression, erosion, or invasion of important vascular structures located in this region. Occasionally, thymomas may compress the SVC causing SVC syndrome and may become difficult to resect.

^{99m}Tc-MIBI does accumulate in some neoplastic processes and has been investigated as an agent for tumor imaging. As the chest is partially in the field of view of cardiac imaging studies, screening for abnormal foci of uptake in the mediastinum and lung fields should be part of the evaluation of myocardial perfusion studies. Incidental finding of chest or breast tumors is not uncommon. Bilateral uptake in the mammary glands is seen in breast-feeding women.

The sensitivity of the exercise ECG for detecting ischemia is approximately 60% to 70% with a similar specificity. In the absence of exercise-induced perfusion defect, the prognosis of these individuals is no different than those without ECG findings.

Interpretation

1. Incidental diagnosis of thymoma.
2. No evidence of exercise-induced myocardial ischemia; false-positive exercise ECG result.

Case 3.5

History

A 77-year-old man underwent an FDG PET study for initial staging of non-small cell lung carcinoma. His risk factors for CAD included diabetes mellitus, hypertension, and tobacco use. A stress dobutamine echocardiogram, performed for risk stratification of CAD before lobectomy, was normal with no evidence of ischemia. As per protocol for the whole body FDG PET imaging for staging malignancies, the patient had been instructed to fast for 12 hours. His blood glucose level was normal at the time of FDG administration. FDG images of his heart obtained with a dedicated PET tomograph with full rings of BGO detectors (Discovery LS, General Electric Medical Systems, Milwaukee, WI) and reconstructed with iterative reconstruction and segmented attenuation correction using CT attenuation maps are displayed in Figures C3-5A and C3-5B.

Findings

Whole body FDG images obtained in the fasting state demonstrate homogenous uptake throughout the myocardium, which is not uncommon. These images illustrate the exquisite resolution that can be obtained with state-of-the-art high-resolution PET systems. The papillary muscles and all chambers of the heart can be identified, right ventricle and atria as well as LV. No abnormalities are present. Figure C3-5B displays CT transmission (left), FDG emission (center), and fusion (right) transaxial images and demonstrates the correlation of FDG uptake and anatomy. Because of the high resolution of the PET images, uptake in the wall of the right ventricle and atria is commonly seen.

Discussion

FDG is an analog of glucose allowing noninvasive evaluation of glucose metabolism. The myocardium can use several other substrates for energy production, most notably fatty acids. How much of each substrate is used depends on a variety of factors including hormonal status and substrate availability of the substrates. High insulin levels accompanied by suppressed

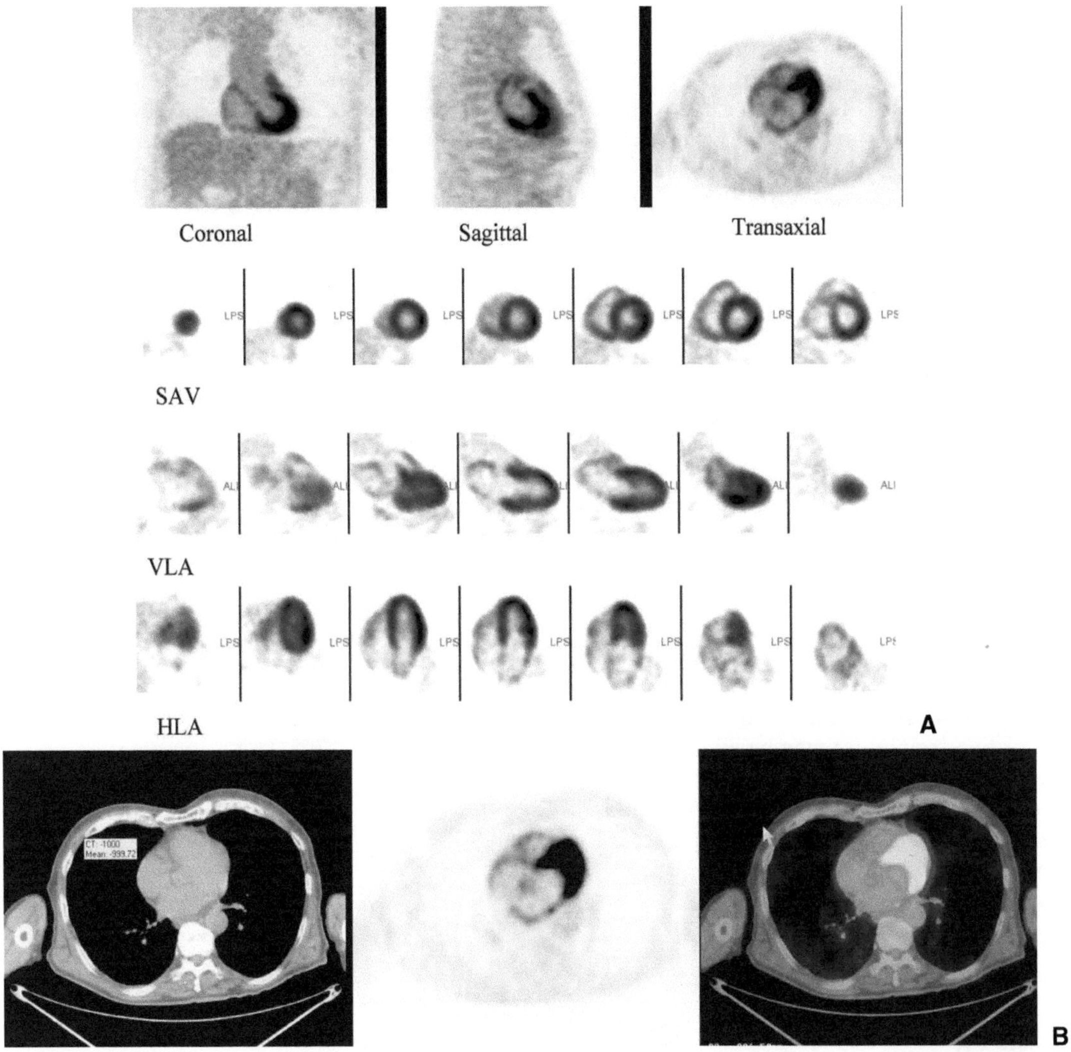

FIGURE C3-5. (A and B)

FFA levels promote FDG uptake, whereas high FFA levels inhibit FDG uptake. For these reasons, in the fasting state the distribution of FDG is often quite heterogenous, even in the normal myocardium. The low insulin levels and elevated FFA levels seen in fasting patients result in uninterpretable FDG images in approximately 50% of fasting patients. Therefore, interpretation of myocardial images should not be attempted on whole body FDG studies performed in the fasting state for oncological purposes. The presence of *defects* may just reflect heterogeneity of myocardial metabolism in the fasting patient.

For evaluation of myocardial viability using FDG, the circulating substrate and hormone levels need to be manipulated to favor utilization of glucose by the myocardium. The metabolic conditions during FDG imaging are extremely important; they determine myocardial FDG uptake and thus image quality.

Several protocols are available to promote cardiac FDG uptake. Oral glucose loading is the most commonly used approach, although it often results in uninterpretable images in patients with impaired glucose tolerance or diabetes mellitus (i.e., fasting serum glucose >115 mg/dl). This is usually accomplished by loading the patient with glucose following a fasting period of at least 6 hours to induce an endogenous insulin response. A shorter fasting time may depress this physiological response. Generally, an oral load of 25 to 100g or an intravenous load is adequate for nondiabetic patients. The IV route avoids potential problems due to variable gastrointestinal absorption times or inability to tolerate oral dosage. If the patient is on medications that may either antagonize or potentiate the effects of insulin, these should be taken into account by the physician.

The hyperinsulinemic euglycemic clamp allows near-perfect regulation of metabolic substrates and insulin levels, ensuring excellent image quality in all patients. However, the procedure is laborious and time-consuming.

Acipimox is not currently available in the United States, but has been used successfully in Europe. Oral administration of a nicotinic acid derivative (acipimox) may be an alternative to clamping; acipimox inhibits peripheral lipolysis, reducing plasma free fatty acid levels, and indirectly stimulating cardiac FDG uptake. Initial data suggest that good image quality can be obtained using this approach.

Diabetic patients pose a challenge as they have either limited ability to produce endogenous insulin or their cells are less responsive to insulin stimulation. For this reason, the simple fasting/oral glucose-loading paradigm is often not effective in diabetic patients. Unfortunately, CAD is a complication of diabetes and sometimes patients are evaluated for CAD before a diagnosis of diabetes has been established. The methods used for loading nondiabetic patients with glucose have been modified to optimize myocardial glucose utilization in diabetic patients with variable success. The reference method, euglycemic hyperinsulinic clamp, provides excellent image quality in most patients, especially in patients with non-insulin-dependent diabetes mellitus. This topic is further discussed in Chapter 8, which addresses myocardial viability with references to the literature.

Interpretation

Normal myocardial FDG uptake in a fasting patient.

Case 3.6

History

A 37-year-old G_1P_1 woman without known heart disease but with a past history of non-Hodgkin's lymphoma was referred for FDG PET imaging 6 weeks postpartum for a newly palpable inguinal lymph node. She did not wish to cease breast-feeding her infant. After a 12-hour fast, 10mCi of FDG was administered intravenously and whole-body PET images acquired. Attenuation correction was performed using the transmission maps obtained with rotating sources of ^{68}Ge. The maximum intensity projection image is displayed in Figure C3-6.

Findings

No FDG uptake is seen in the inguinal region, indicating a benign etiology. No FDG uptake is seen in the myocardium in this fasting patient. Bilateral and symmetric activity is noted in the breasts due to lactation.

Discussion

The bilateral activity in the anterior chest is related to physiologic uptake within the lactating breasts. Because of the short half-life of FDG (110 minutes), discontinuation of breast-feeding is recommended for 24 hours.

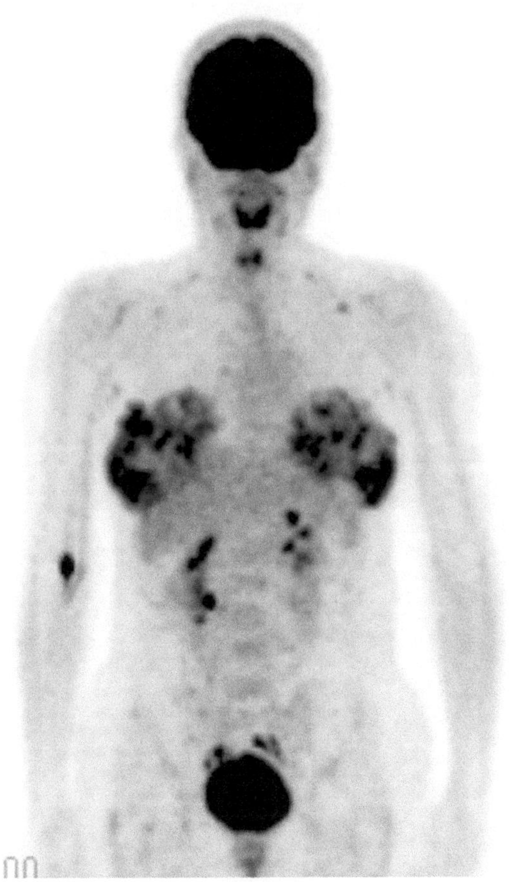

FIGURE C3-6.

Although, this patient was referred for evaluation of lymphoma with FDG PET imaging, myocardial perfusion studies are occasionally indicated in young women of childbearing age potentially breast-feeding. The choice of perfusion tracer is important if the patient wishes to continue breast-feeding.

With ^{201}Tl, the whole body equivalent effective dose is 10 to 15 times higher than with ^{99m}Tc-labeled agents, with the thyroid gland, kidneys, and gastrointestinal tract receiving the higher radiation dose. ^{201}Tl is excreted in the breast and because of the 72-hour half-life, cessation of breast-feeding is recommended for 3 weeks after a 3-mCi dose of ^{201}Tl.[48]

With ^{99m}Tc-MIBI, the intestinal tract receives the highest radiation exposure with both rest and stress dosing, but exposure will not exceed 5 rads even when 30 mCi is administered. There is accumulation of ^{99m}Tc-MIBI in the mammary glands but minimal transfer to milk.[49] If a nursing mother must undergo MPI imaging, the ^{99m}Tc-agents are much preferred over ^{201}Tl. With ^{201}Tl administration, women must discontinue nursing for 2 to 3 weeks, whereas with ^{99m}Tc-MIBI no interruption of breast-feeding is required but close contact should be restricted for 24 hours.

Other etiologies of extracardiac thoracic uptake of ^{201}Tl or ^{99m}Tc-MIBI include a variety of neoplasms, both benign and malignant, and including benign thyroid and parathyroid lesions, hiatal hernia, inflammatory processes, and recent radiation therapy.

Interpretation

Puerperal breast uptake of FDG.

Case 3.7

History

A 73-year-old woman with a family history of CAD presented with atypical chest pain. She underwent a low-dose rest/high-dose exercise ^{99m}Tc-tetrofosmin gated SPECT study. She exercised 9 minutes on a standard Bruce protocol achieving 85% of the predicted maximum HR. She denied chest pain and there were no ECG changes. The study was processed using the ECTtoolbox software and the summary page is displayed in Figure C3-7A.

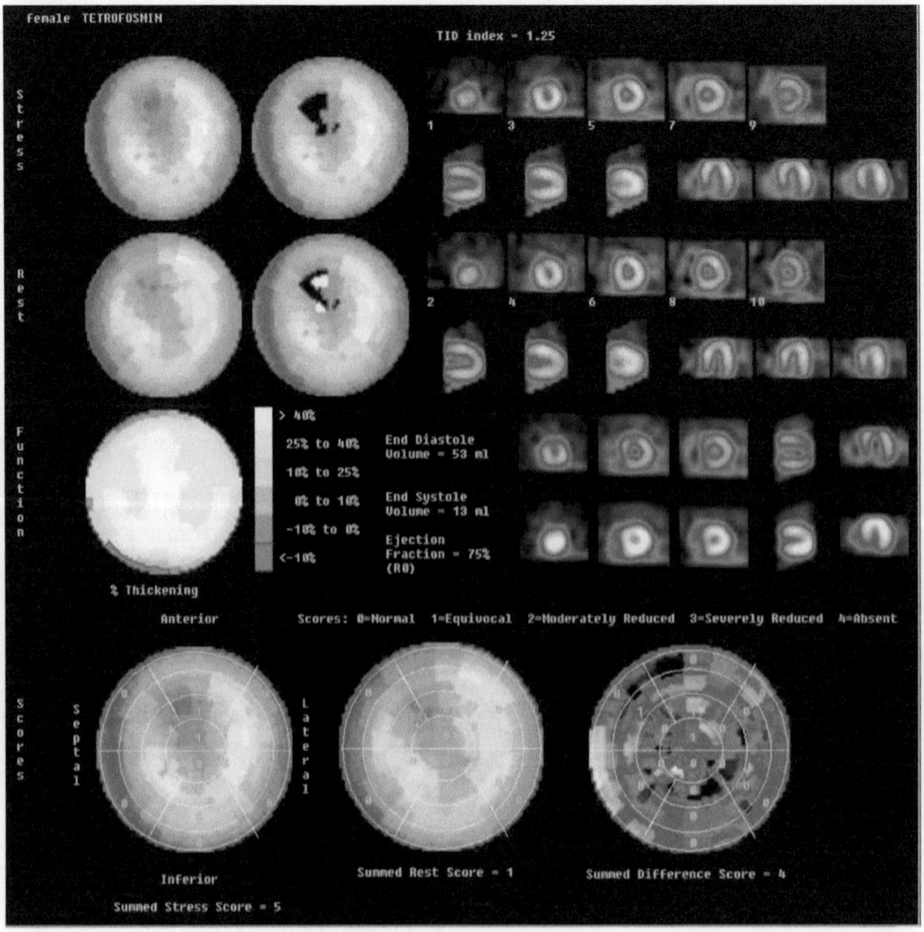

A

FIGURE C3-7. (A)

Findings

The SPECT slices displayed along the short axis and the vertical and horizontal long axis of the heart (right upper corner) and the polar maps (left upper corner) demonstrate homogenous uptake both on the post-stress and the resting images, except for a small defect in the anterior wall, slightly worse on the stress than the rest images, probably due to breast attenuation artifact.

The functional data of the gated study is summarized in the middle panel and demonstrated an EDV of 53 ml, ESV of 13 ml, and LVEF of 75%. The display of the end-diastolic and end-systolic frames (right middle panel) and the polar map display of function (left middle panel) demonstrate normal thickening throughout the myocardium, confirming a breast artifact as the cause for the small fixed anterior perfusion defects seen on the SPECT slices.

The bottom panel displays the polar maps of perfusion with the heart divided and scored according to a 20-segment model/5-point scoring system, and the appropriate database was selected for gender and the MPI protocol used. The summed rest score of 1 is almost normal and the summed stress score and summed difference scores of 4 and 5 are mildly abnormal. The study was interpreted as probably normal with a breast artifact. Six months later, the patient did not complain of further cardiac symptoms.

Discussion

This case illustrates a common semiquantitative analysis of perfusion that can be performed visually and is provided automatically by most commercially available software. A pixel-based analysis can provide semiquantitative analysis regarding the extent and severity of the defect. SPECT circumferential profile analysis can be performed in a similar way as circumferential profiles of planar images. For each equally spaced radius from the center of the myocardium, the hottest pixel is located along that radius. The data are expressed as a percent of the hottest pixel in the curve, providing only relative perfusion counts. These data can be plotted as polar maps and compared with normal databases. Polar maps or bulls-eyes are graphic displays of sets of circumferential profiles of the short-axis slices. Normal databases vary according to the radiopharmaceutical and protocol used as well as with the gender of the patients. Various software packages are commercially available for quantitative analysis of perfusion SPECT images and have been validated. The most commonly used are the Cequal developed both at Emory University and Cedars-Sinai Medical Center,[50] ECTtoolbox developed at Emory University,[51] and the QGS/QPS developed at Cedars-Sinai Medical Center.[52] Other available software include 4D-MSPECT from University of Michigan,[53] Multidim from Stanford University,[54] and Yale CQ.[55]

The images should be interpreted with reference to the coronary anatomy. A popular method allowing quantification of perfusion abnormalities in relationship to disease likelihood, prognosis, and viability is the segmental analysis using a scoring system to grade the degree of perfusion for each segment of the heart. Current recommendation of the ASNC is division of the heart in 17 segments, adding one apical segment to the 16 segments model typically used for echocardiography (Figures C3-7B and C3-7C).[13]

However, a large number of studies have been published using the Cedars-Sinai 20-segment model, 5-point scoring: It includes 6 segments per slice, distal, midventricular and basal, and two apical segments. Each segment is assigned a perfusion score between 0 and 4, 0 being normal and 4 denoting no perfusion. With the 20-segment model, a summed score of 1 to 3 indicates an equivocally abnormal study, a score of 4 to 7 a mildly abnormal study, a score of 8 to 12 a moderately abnormal study, and a score >13 a severely abnormal study. In currently available software, these scores are generated from an analysis of segmental intensity and its standard deviation from that of normal databases.

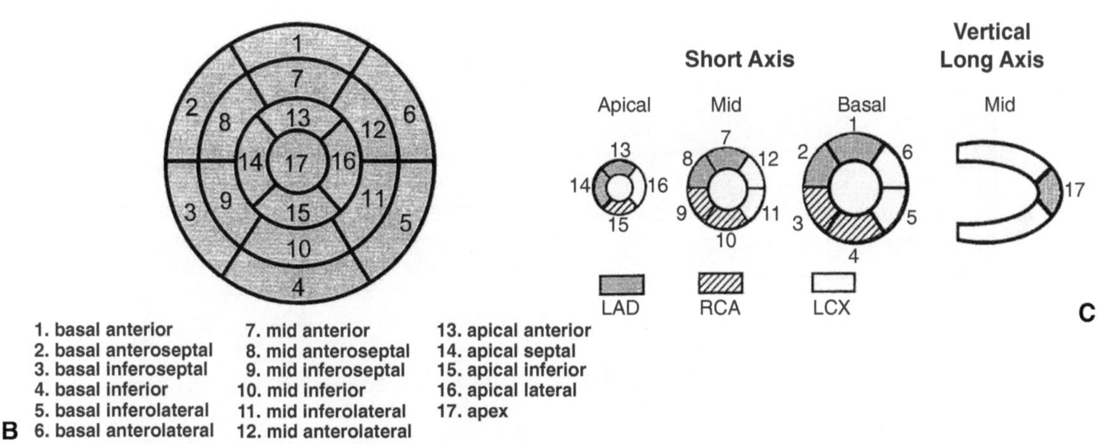

FIGURE C3-7. (B and C) (B and C, from Cerqueira, Weissman, Dilsizian, et al. [13], by permission of *J Nucl Cardiol.*)

These scores must be corrected when an artifact is suspected, whether it is from motion, attenuation, or other sources. The summed stress score is compared with the summed rest score to generate a summed difference score.

Interpretation

Mildly abnormal segmental analysis and perfusion scores probably due to breast attenuation artifact.

Case 3.8

History

A 49-year-old man with a large body habitus and a history of peripheral vascular disease was admitted with unstable angina. A coronary angiogram revealed a 40% stenosis of the LAD, 50% stenosis of the RCA, 90% stenosis of an OM, and normal ventriculographic result. Because of his large body habitus, he was referred for a rest/dipyridamole stress ^{13}N-ammonia PET study displayed in Figure C3-8A. The images were corrected for attenuation using transmission maps acquired with a ring source of ^{68}Ge.

Findings

Despite the large body habitus of the patient, the quality of the images is good and without attenuation artifacts. The stress ^{13}N-ammonia PET images demonstrate moderately decreased uptake in the anterior and lateral wall of the myocardium and the corresponding resting images are normal, indicating ischemia in the territory perfused by the OM with 90% stenosis. The patient underwent successful angioplasty of the OM. A rest/stress ^{13}N-ammonia study was repeated 2 months later and is displayed in Figure C3-8B. The previous defect has now resolved, and there is homoge-

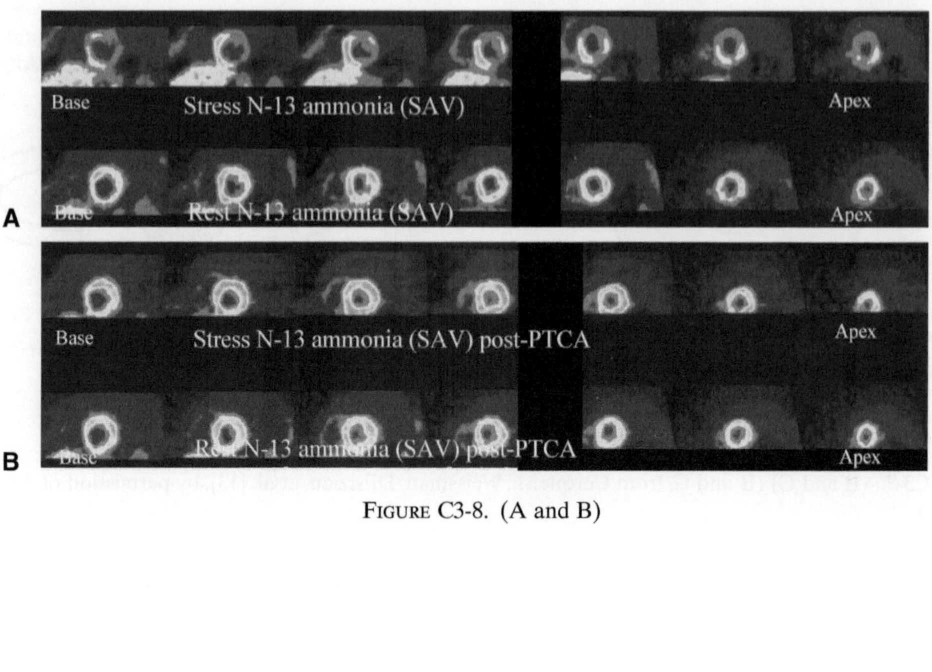

FIGURE C3-8. (A and B)

nous distribution of ^{13}N-ammonia on both rest and stress images (Figure C3-8B).

Discussion

Both ^{82}Rb and ^{13}N-ammonia are positron emitters that accumulate in the myocardium proportional to MBF but require dedicated positron tomographs for imaging. ^{13}N-ammonia requires a cyclotron for its production and has a half-life of 10 minutes, requiring a timely production related to the time of administration. It is rapidly cleared from the blood pool and diffuses intracellularly proportionally to MBF. Its retention depends on its metabolic incorporation into glutamine, thus cellular viability. The imaging protocol for rest/stress ^{13}N-ammonia is depicted in Figure C3-8C.

For ^{13}N-ammonia, the transmission images can be acquired immediately before or after the emission images if the attenuation software can adequately correct for residual emission activity. For the resting study, gated emission images are acquired 1.5 to 3.0 minutes after 10 to 20 mCi of ^{13}N-ammonia is administered intravenously. The images are usually acquired for 5 to 15 minutes. The stress study can be performed using the same protocol during pharmacological stress after a 1-hour waiting period to allow for decay of the resting ^{13}N-ammonia dose. To measure absolute myocardial perfusion rate, the arterial input function can be derived from a region of interest placed in the LV cavity. The dose of ^{13}N-ammonia needs to be infused over 30 seconds and dynamic images need to be acquired with varying frame durations for 4 minutes starting at the time of infusion of ^{13}N-ammonia.[56] Various kinetic models have been developed and validated to measure absolute MBF but are not practical in the clinical setting and are beyond the scope of this chapter.

^{82}Rb is a potassium analog. Unlike ^{13}N-ammonia, it can be eluted from a ^{82}Strontium generator, making it more easily available than ^{13}N-ammonia, which requires a cyclotron onsite. Although ^{82}Rb PET cardiac imaging is reimbursed by third-party payers, the generator (CardioGen-82, Bracco Diagnostics, Inc., Geneva) is expensive and must be replaced monthly, limiting the use of ^{82}Rb PET imaging to large centers that have the volume of referrals to justify the cost. The half-life of ^{82}Rb is 75 seconds, resulting in relative low count-rate images. A theoretical limit in resolution of the ^{82}Rb (compared with ^{13}N) images occurs because the energy of the positrons emitted is higher than that of ^{13}N and the distance traversed by ^{82}Rb positrons is longer than that of ^{13}N before the annihilation process. These two factors together explain the lower quality of ^{82}Rb images compared with ^{13}N-ammonia.

Because of the short half-life, rest/stress studies can rapidly be performed sequentially. Pharmacological stress is usually performed

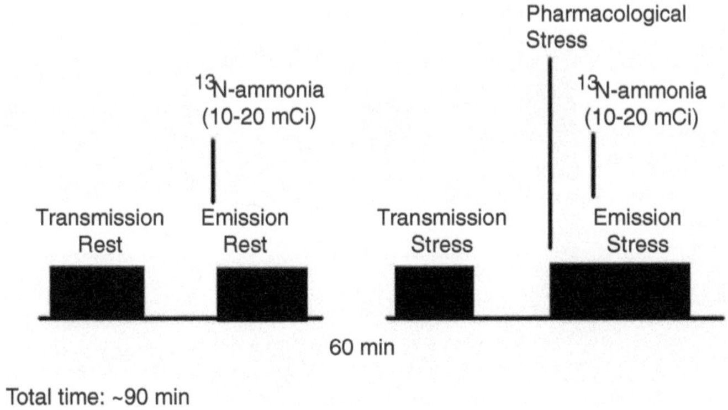

FIGURE C3-8. (C)

with vasodilators with the patient positioned in the gantry of the PET system to start acquisition of the images promptly. The imaging protocol for rest/stress ^{82}Rb study is described in Figure C3-8D and a normal rest/dipyridamole study is displayed in Figure C3-8E.

After positioning the patient in the gantry of the PET system, a scout scan can be performed after administration of a low dose of ^{82}Rb (10 to 20 mCi) to ensure correct positioning of the heart in the field of view, estimate the blood pool clearance time, and select the optimal injection-to-imaging delay time. A transmission scan can then be acquired for 2 to 4 minutes using a ^{68}Ge transmission source or integrated CT x-ray source. The resting study should be performed first to reduce the impact of residual stress effects. The dose administered depends on the type of PET system (bismuth germanate oxide [BGO], lutetium oxiorthosilicate oxide [LSO], or gadolinium oxyorthosilicate [GSO] crystals) and imaging mode (2-D imaging mode requires a higher dose than 3-D). Typically in the 2-D imaging mode with a BGO PET system, 30 to 40 mCi of ^{82}Rb is administered intravenously, and the images are acquired starting at 70 to 90 seconds after administration for patients with an LVEF >50% and 90 to 130 seconds after administration for patients with an LVEF <50%. The emission images are usually acquired for 5 minutes and can be ECG gated. The same sequence of image (transmission and emission) acquisition is performed during vasodilator pharmacological stress and an identical dose of ^{82}Rb. The total rest/stress study time is approximately 45 minutes provided that rest and stress images are corrected for attenuation and gated (see Guidelines references 57–58).

Advantages of PET over SPECT perfusion radiopharmaceuticals are (1) more efficient

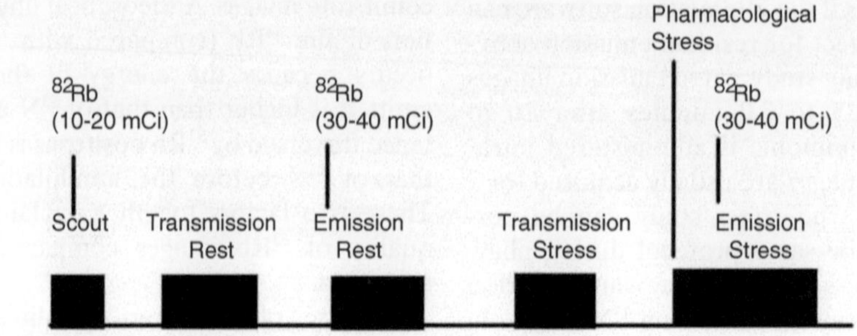

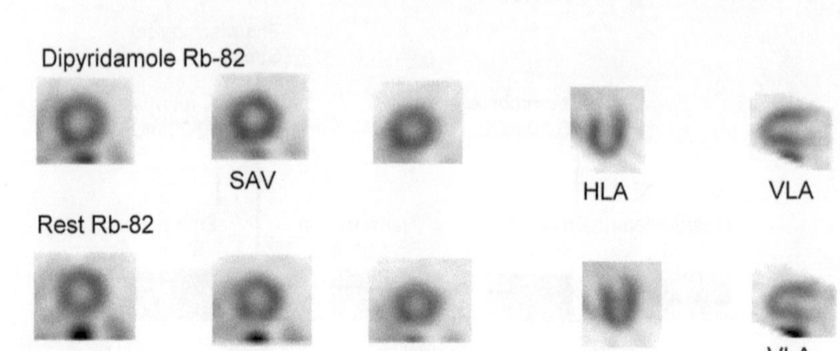

FIGURE C3-8. (D and E) (E, courtesy of J. L. Urbain, Cleveland Clinic Foundation, Cleveland, OH.)

rest/stress protocols because of the shorter half-lives; (2) lower radiation exposure, approximately ten times less than with ^{99m}Tc-labeled radiopharmaceuticals; and (3) higher resolution and superior attenuation correction (particularly important in women and obese patients). The sensitivity for detecting ischemia using PET perfusion scintigraphy is in the 95% range, with a very high normalcy rate in patients without CAD.

^{13}N-ammonia also allows quantitative measurement of coronary blood flow (CBF) and coronary blood flow reserve (CBFR) using compartmental modeling and kinetic analysis. The possibility of evaluation of absolute MBF and CBFR using vasodilators also offers a means of investigating endothelial function and vascular smooth muscle relaxation and detecting early atherosclerosis. Quantitative measurement of MBF with PET is dependent on accurate attenuation correction and lack of motion of the patient during the scanning period, as well as careful calibration of the imaging system.

Patients for whom PET perfusion radiopharmaceuticals are preferable to SPECT are (1) patients with suspected balanced three-vessel disease, (2) patients with suspected small vessel disease (e.g., hypertension, diabetes, heart transplants), and (3) patients in whom significant attenuation artifacts are anticipated.

Interpretation

Lateral wall ischemia in the territory of an obtuse marginal artery demonstrated with rest/stress ^{13}N-ammonia in a patient with a large body habitus.

Case 3.9

History

A 65-year-old man was referred for myocardial perfusion imaging because of an episode of bigeminy seen on a preoperative ECG. He underwent a resting ^{201}Tl/exercise ^{99m}Tc-MIBI gated SPECT study. He exercised 13 minutes on a standard Bruce protocol reaching 100% of his maximum predicted HR without chest pain or ECG changes. His SPECT images are displayed in Figure C3-9.

Findings

The stress images do not display the normal pattern of uptake of an MPI study. The myocardial walls cannot be identified as typically doughnut shaped on the short-axis view or U-shaped in the vertical long-axis views. Instead, the images display blood pool activity in the LV, RV, and great vessels. The resting images show normal perfusion except for mild decreased uptake in the inferior wall that may be related to adjacent activity in the abdomen (see Case 3.10 for additional discussion).

On the anterior planar projection image from the stress study, blood pool activity is visualized in the heart, and there is marked gastric uptake, indicating that free ^{99m}Tc-pertechnetate was administered to the patient instead of ^{99m}Tc-MIBI.

Discussion

The most commonly used radionuclide is ^{99m}Tc because it is readily available from a generator, and has the most suitable physical properties for imaging. When eluted from the generator, ^{99m}Tc is present as heptavalent (+7) pertechnetate (TcO_4^-). Reduced pertechnetate (usually valence +4) combines with a wide variety of chelating agents. Most of the currently used pharmaceuticals are available in kit forms as a lyophilized powder containing the pharmaceutical and a stannous compound as the reducing agent in appropriate proportions. Labeling is performed by simple addition of the ^{99m}Tc-pertechnetate from the eluate of the generator. Rigorous quality control of the radiopharma-

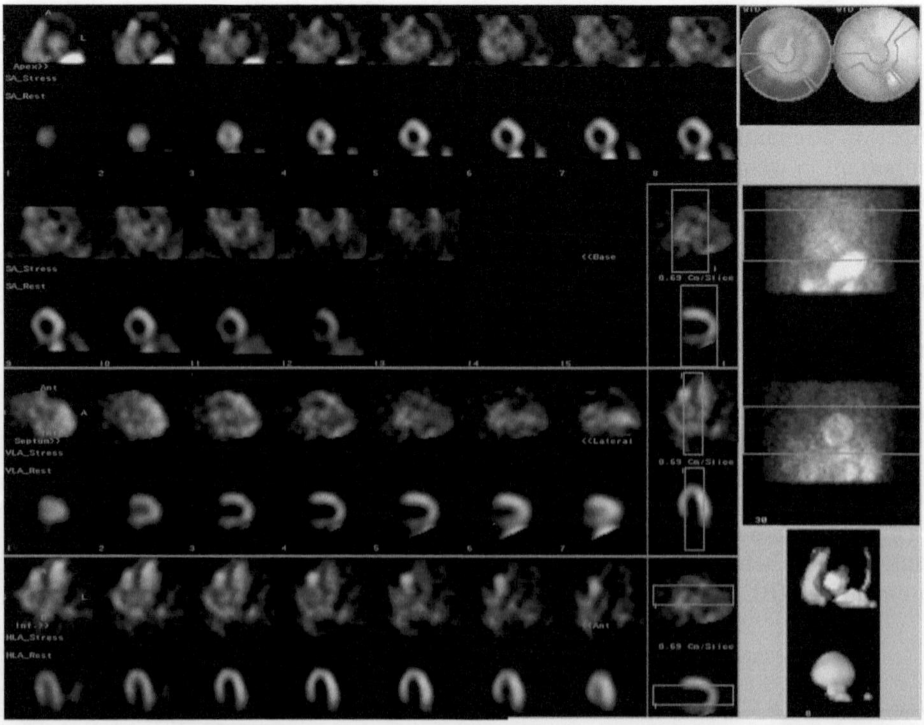

FIGURE C3-9.

ceuticals is performed by radiopharmacies to ensure chemical and radiochemical purity before administration to the patient. Chemical purity is the fraction of the radiopharmaceutical in the desired chemical form, labeled or not (e.g., alumina is a chemical impurity in ^{99m}Tc). Radiochemical purity is the fraction of radionuclide present in the desired chemical form (e.g., free ^{99m}Tc-pertechnetate contaminating ^{99m}Tc-labeled radiopharmaceuticals). Paper chromatography is the most commonly used procedure to analyze ^{99m}Tc-labeled radiopharmaceuticals and to separate the desired labeled pharmaceutical from free ^{99m}Tc and hydrolyzed ^{99m}Tc. Quality control of radiopharmaceuticals also includes pH and ionic strength, particulate matter, toxicity, sterility, and pyrogenicity.[59]

When a radiopharmaceutical is contaminated with free ^{99m}Tc-pertechnetate or if ^{99m}Tc-pertechnetate is accidentally administered to a patient instead of the intended ^{99m}Tc-labeled agent, the typical distribution of ^{99m}Tc-pertechnetate is seen on the images. The biological distribution of ^{99m}Tc-pertechnetate is similar to that of iodide; pertechnetate concentrates in the thyroid, mucous glands of the gastric mucosa (as seen on the anterior planar projection of this patient), and the choroid plexus. In plasma, pertechnetate is loosely bound to proteins and the plasma clearance is slow. Therefore blood pool activity is usually seen on the images. It is excreted renally, so kidneys and bladder activity are also usually seen.

Interpretation

Free ^{99m}Tc-pertechnetate was administered for the stress portion of the study. Similar findings would have been seen in the event of faulty binding of ^{99m}Tc to MIBI or tetrofosmin with resultant high levels of circulating free ^{99m}Tc-pertechnetate.

Case 3.10

History

A 43-year-old woman with hypertension and tobacco use presented with atypical chest pain. She underwent a 1-day, low-dose rest/high-dose adenosine ^{99m}Tc-tetrofosmin gated SPECT study. She was unable to exercise due to severe leg pain related to sciatica. During adenosine infusion, she denied chest pain, and there were no ECG changes suggestive of ischemia. The SPECT images are displayed in Figures C3-10A (supine), C3-10B (prone), and C3–10C (gated study).

Findings

Both the stress and resting SPECT images are abnormal. On the images obtained in the supine position (Figure C3-10A), there is a fixed defect in the anteroseptal wall. However, this defect resolves with prone imaging (Figure C3-10B) and is therefore probably artifactual. There is also a defect in the inferior wall, seen on both the supine and prone images, which appears partially reversible on the rest images in the inferobasal segment. There is prominent gastrointestinal activity adjacent to the inferior wall on all sets of images complicating the interpretation as presented in the following discussion. The gated images (Figure C3-10C) demonstrates a dilated heart with an EDV of 134 ml and an ESV of 70 ml. The LVEF is 47%, and inferobasal hypokinesis is seen. The study was interpreted as worrisome for inferobasal ischemia, although the adjacent gastrointestinal activity could induce artifactual defects in the inferior wall.

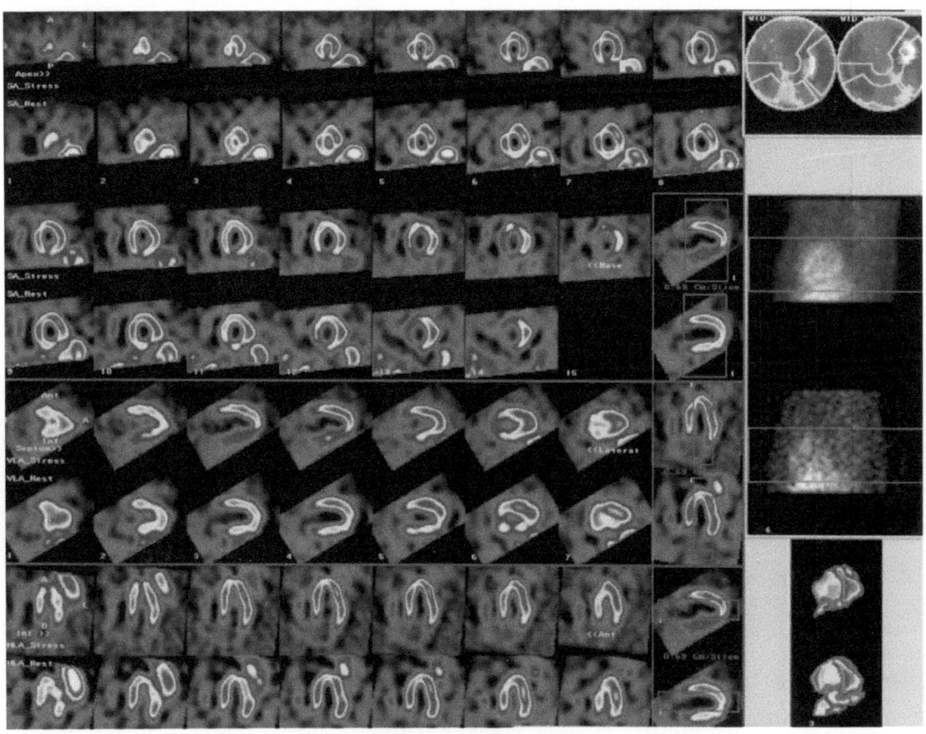

A

FIGURE C3-10. (A)

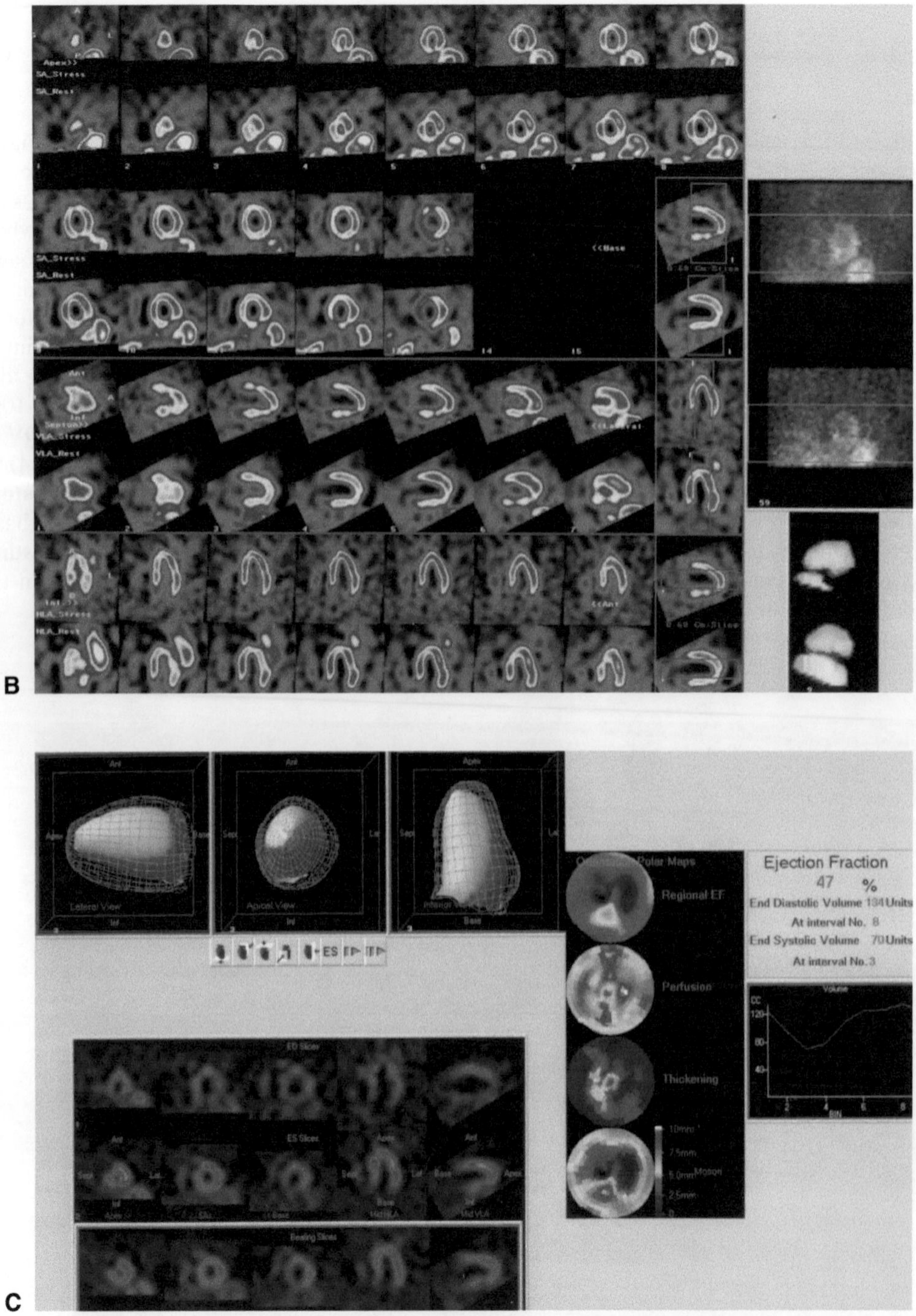

FIGURE C3-10. (B and C)

The patient underwent coronary angiography revealing widely patent coronary arteries. The contrast ventriculogram demonstrated normal wall motion with an LVEF of 52%.

Discussion

^{99m}Tc-labeled radiopharmaceuticals are excreted by the hepatobiliary system, so prominent hepatic uptake or uptake in a loop of bowel adjacent to the inferior wall of the myocardium is not uncommon. If the degree of uptake adjacent to the heart is above that of the myocardium itself, normalization of the SPECT of images may be a problem as discussed in Case 13.3. The interpreting physician must make sure that the SPECT images are displayed correctly so that the maximum color intensity is assigned to the maximum counts in the heart and not to a source of extracardiac uptake.

In addition, a focus of high uptake adjacent to the myocardium can create artifacts by several mechanisms: (1) by overestimation of inferior wall uptake due to scattered activity from the liver or bowel; (2) by underestimation of anterior wall uptake due to artifactual high gastrointestinal uptake overlying the inferior wall; and (3) by underestimation of inferior wall uptake due to oversubtraction of counts from the inferior wall adjacent to the liver or bowel during image processing, as was probably the case in this patient.

The hepatic or gastrointestinal activity is less of a problem with ^{201}Tl imaging, which is predominantly excreted by the kidneys. When using ^{99m}Tc-labeled agents, gastrointestinal uptake is seen more commonly in patients undergoing pharmacologic vasodilator stress and may be minimized by increasing the interval time between tracer injection and image acquisition and/or by adding low-level exercise to vasodilator stress. As discussed in Case 4.8, physical exercise induces vasoconstriction of the splanchnic vessels and diminishes gastrointestinal uptake. Ingestion of fatty food or milk does not significantly increase hepatic clearance but does promote gallbladder contraction, which can sometimes result in more artifact by increasing activity in the bowel. Filling the stomach with food and/or liquids after injection but before imaging can serve to displace interfering bowel activity inferiorly away from the LV. Prone imaging, by increasing the separation of the inferior wall from the abdominal contents, can be used to ameliorate the interference of gastrointestinal activity.

Interpretation

Artifactual perfusion defect in the inferior wall due to adjacent gastrointestinal uptake commonly seen with ^{99m}Tc-perfusion agents.

References

1. Leppo JA, Meerdink DJ. Comparison of the myocardial uptake of a technetium-labeled isonitrile analogue and thallium. *Circ Res.* 1989;65:632–639.
2. Okada RD, Glover D, Gaffney T, et al. Myocardial kinetics of technetium-99m-hexakis-2-methoxy-2-methylpropyl-isonitrile. *Circulation.* 1988;77:491–498.
3. Glover DK, Ruiz M, Yang JY, et al. Myocardial ^{99m}Tc tetrofosmin uptake during adenosine-induced vasodilation as a function of coronary stenosis severity: comparison with ^{201}Tl and regional myocardial blood flow. *Circulation.* 1997;96:2332–2338.
4. Glover DK, Ruiz M, Edwards NC, et al. Comparison between ^{201}Tl and ^{99m}Tc sestamibi uptake during adenosine-induced vasodilation as a function of coronary stenosis severity. *Circulation.* 1995;91:813–820.
5. Wackers FJ, Berman DS, Maddahi J, et al. Technetium-99m hexakis-2-methoxyisobutyl isonitrile: human biodistribution, dosimetry, safety, and preliminary comparison to thallium-201 for myocardial perfusion imaging. *J Nucl Med.* 1989; 30:301–311.
6. Berman DS, Hachamovitch R, Kiat H, et al. Incremental value of prognostic testing in patients with known or suspected heart disease: a basis for optimal utilization of exercise technetium-99m sestamibi myocardial perfusion single-photon emission computed tomography. *J Am Coll Cardiol.* 1995;26:639–647.
7. Kelley JD, Forster AM, Higley B, et al. Technetium 99m-tetrofosmin a new radiopharmaceu-

tical for myocardial perfusion imaging. *J Nucl Med.* 1993;34:222–227.
8. Johnson III G, Alton IL, Nguyen KN, et al. Clearance of ^{99m}Tc N-NOET in normal, ischemic-reperfused, and membrane-disrupted myocardium. *J Nucl Cardiol.* 1996;3:42–54.
9. Rumsey WL, Kuczynski B, Patel B, et al. SPECT imaging of ischemic myocardium using a technetium-99m-nitroimidazole ligand. *J Nucl Med.* 1995;36:1445–1450.
10. Ghezzi C, Fagret D, Arvieux CC, et al. Myocardial kinetics of TcN-NOET: a neutral lipophilic complex tracer of regional myocardial blood flow. *J Nucl Med.* 1995;36:1069–1077.
11. Vanzetto G, Calnon DA, Ruiz M, et al. Myocardial uptake and redistribution of ^{99m}Tc-N-NOET in dogs with either sustained coronary low flow or transient coronary occlusion: comparison with ^{201}Tl and myocardial blood flow. *Circulation.* 1997;96:2325–2331.
12. Nunn A, Linder K, Strauss HW. Nitroimidazoles and imaging hypoxia. *Eur J Nucl Med.* 1995; 22;265–280.
13. Cerqueira MD, Weissman NJ, Dilsizian V, et al. Standardized myocardial segmentation and nomenclature for tomographic imaging of the heart: a statement for healthcare professionals from the cardiac imaging committee of the council on clinical cardiology of the American Heart Association. *J Nucl Cardiol.* 2002;105:539–542.
14. Updated guidelines for nuclear cardiology procedures. *J Nucl Cardiol.* 2001;8:G5–G58.
15. Santana CA, Garcia EV, Folks R. Comparison between ECTb and QGS for assessment of left ventricular function from gated myocardial perfusion SPECT. *J Nucl Cardiol.* 2002;9:285–293.
16. Cellular pathology I: cell injury and cell death. In Cotran RS, Kumar V, Collins T (eds). *Robins Pathologic Basis of Disease*, 6th ed. Philadelphia: Saunders;1999:8.
17. Narula J, Baliga RR. What's in a name? Would that which we call death by any other name be less tragic? *Ann Thorac Surg.* 2001;72: 1454–1456.
18. Itoh G, Tamura J, Suzuki M, et al. DNA fragmentation of human infracted myocardial cells demonstrated by the nick end labeling method and DNA agarose gel electrophoresis. *Am J Pathol.* 1995;146:1325–1331.
19. Strauss HW, Narula J, Blankenberg FD. Radioimaging to identify myocardial death and probably injury. *Lancet.* 2000;356:180–181.
20. Narula J, Baret BL. Noninvasive detection of cell death: From tracking epitaphs to counting coffins. *J Nucl Cardiol.* 2002;9:554–560.
21. Narula J, Petrov A, Pak KY, et al. Very early non-invasive detection of acute experimental non-reperfused myocardial infarction with ^{99m}Tc-labeled glucarate. *Circulation.* 1997;95: 1577–1584.
22. Khaw BA, Nakazawa A, O'Donnell SM, et al. Avidity of technetium 99m glucarate for the necrotic myocardium: in vivo and in vitro assessment. *J Nucl Cardiol.* 1997;4:283–290.
23. Mariani G, Villa G, Rossettin PF, et al. Detection of acute myocardial infarction by ^{99m}Tc-labeled D-glucaric acid imaging in patients with chest pain. *J Nucl Med.* 1999;40:1832–1839.
24. Hofstra L, Liem IH, Dumont EA, et al. Visualization of cell death in vivo in patients with acute myocardial infarction. *Lancet.* 2000;356:209–212.
25. Vriens PW, Blankenberg FG, Stoot JH, et al. The use of ^{99m}Tc annexin V for in vivo imaging of apoptosis during cardiac allograft rejection. *J Cardiovasc Surg.* 1998;116:844–853.
26. Narula J, Acio ER, Narula N, et al. Annexin-V imaging for noninvasive detection of cardiac allograft rejection. *Nat Med.* 2001;7:1347–1352.
27. Green AM, Steinmutz ND. Monitoring apoptosis in real time. *Cancer J.* 2002;8:82–92.
28. Kang PM, Izumo S. Apoptosis and heart failure: a critical review of the literature. *Circ Res.* 2000; 86:1107–1113.
29. Mann DL. Mechanism and models in heart failure: a combinatorial approach. *Circulation.* 1999;100:999–1008.
30. Patel A, Iskandrian AE. MIBG imaging. *J Nucl Cardiol.* 2002;9:75–94.
31. Henderson EB, Kahn JK, Corbet JR, et al. Abnormal ^{123}I metaiodobenzylguanidine myocardial washout and distribution may reflect myocardial adrenergic derangement in patients with congestive cardiomyopathy. *Circulation.* 1988;78:1192–1199.
32. Nakajima K, Taki J, Tonami N, et al. Decreased ^{123}I MIBG uptake and increased clearance in various cardiac diseases. *J Nucl Med Comm.* 1994;15:317–323.
33. Inamura Y, Ando H, Mitsuoka W, et al. Iodine 123 metaiodobenzylguanidine images reflect intense myocardial adrenergic nervous activity in congestive heart failure independently of underlying cause. *J Am Coll Cardiol.* 1995;26: 1594–1599.
34. Simula S, Vanninen E, Viitanen L, et al. Cardiac adrenergic innervation is affected in asymptomatic subjects with very early stage of coronary artery disease. *J Nucl Med.* 2002;43:1–7.

35. Merlet P, Valette H, Dubois-Rande JL, et al. Prognostic value of cardiac metaiodobenzylguanidine imaging in patients with heart failure. *J Nucl Med.* 1992;33:471–477.
36. Merlet P, Benvenuti C, Moyse D, et al. Prognostic value of MIBG imaging in idiopathic dilated cardiomyopathy. *J Nucl Med.* 1999;40:917–923.
37. Nakata T, Miyamoto K, Doi A, et al. Cardiac death prediction and impaired sympathic innervation assessed by MIBG in patients with failing and nonfailing heart. *J Nucl Cardiol.* 1998;5:579–590.
38. Brown KA. Prognostic value of thallium 201 myocardial perfusion imaging: a diagnostic tool comes of age. *Circulation.* 1991;83:363–381.
39. Staniloff HM, Forrester JS, Berman DS, Swan HJ. Prediction of death, myocardial infarction, and worsening chest pain using thallium scintigraphy and exercise electrocardiography. *J Nucl Med.* 1986,27:1842–1848.
40. Weich HF, Strauss HW, Pitt B. The extraction of ^{201}Tl by the myocardium. *Circulation.* 1977;56:188–192.
41. Krahwinkel W, Herzog H, Feinendegen LE. Pharmacokinetics of thallium-201 in normal individuals after routine myocardial scintigraphy. *J Nucl Med.* 1988;29:1582–1586.
42. Dilsizian V, Smeltzer WR, Freedman NMT, et al. Thallium reinjection after stress-redistribution imaging: does 24H delayed imaging following reinjection enhance detection of viable myocardium? *Circulation.* 1991;83:1247–1255.
43. Brown KA, Atland E, Rowen M. Prognostic value of normal technetium 99m sestamibi cardiac imaging. *J Nucl Med.* 1994;35:554–557.
44. Gibson PB, Demus D, Hudson W, Johnson LL. Low event rate for stress-only perfusion imaging in patients evaluated for chest pain. *J Am Coll Cardiol.* 2002;39:999–1004.
45. Beanlands RS, Dawood F, Wen WH, et al. Are kinetics of technetium-99m methoxyisobutyl isonitril affected by cell metabolism and viability? *Circulation.* 1990;82:1802–1814.
46. Younes A, Songadale JA, Maublant J, et al. Mechanism of uptake of technetium-tetrofosmin: uptake into isolated adult ventricular myocytes and subcellular localization. *J Nucl Cardiol.* 1995;2:317–326.
47. Heo J, Powers J, Iskadrian AE. Exercise-rest same-day SPECT sestamibi imaging to detect coronary artery disease. *J Nucl Med.* 1997;38:200–203.
48. Bushberg JT, Leidholdt EM. Radiation protection. In Sandler MP, Coleman RE, Patton JA, Wackers FJ, Gottschalk A (eds.) *Diagnostic Nuclear Medicine*, 4th ed. Philadelphia: Lippincott Williams & Wilkins; 2003:133–164.
49. Rubow S, Klopper J, Wasserman H, et al. The excretion of radiopharmaceuticals in human breast milk: additional data and dosimetry. *Eur J Nucl Med.* 1994;21:144–153.
50. Van Train KF, Garcia EV, Maddahi J, et al. Multicenter trial validation for quantitative analysis of same day rest-stress technetium-99m-sestamibi myocardial tomograms. *J Nucl Med.* 1994;4:609–618.
51. Faber TL, Cooke CD, Folks RD, et al. Left ventricular function and perfusion from gated SPECT perfusion images: an integrated method. *J Nucl Med.* 1999;40:650–659.
52. Germano G, Kavanagh PB, Waechter P, et al. A new algorithm for the quantitation of myocardial perfusion SPECT. I. technical principles and reproducibility. *J Nucl Med.* 2000;41:712–719.
53. Ficaro EP, Kritzman JN, Corbett JR. Development and clinical validation of normal ^{99m}Tc sestamibi database: comparison of 3D-MSPECT to Cequal. *J Nucl Med.* 1999;5:125P.
54. Goris ML, Thompson C, Malone LJ, Franken PR. Modelling the integration of myocardial regional perfusion and function. *Nucl Med Commun.* 1994;15:9–20.
55. Kirac S, Wackers FJ, Liu YH. Validation of the Yale circumferential quantification method using ^{201}Tl and ^{99m}Tc: a phantom study. *J Nucl Med.* 2000;41:1436–1441.
56. Hutchins GD, Schwaiger M, Rosenpire KC, et al. Noninvasive quantification of regional blood flow in the human heart using ^{13}N ammonia and dynamic positron emission tomography imaging. *J Am Coll Cardiol.* 1990;15:1032–1042.
57. Bacharach SL, Bax JJ, Case J, et al. PET myocardial glucose metabolism and perfusion imaging: Part 1-Guidelines for data acquisition and patient preparation. *J Nucl Cardiol.* 2003;10(5):543–556.
58. Schelbert HR, Beanlands R, Bengel F, et al. PET myocardial perfusion and glucose metabolism imaging: Part 2-Guidelines for interpretation and reporting. *J Nucl Cardiol.* 2003;10(5):557–571.
59. Delbeke D, Clanton J. Radiopharmaceuticals. In Sandler MP, Patton JA, Shaff MI, Powers TA, Partain CL (eds). *Correlative Imaging.* Baltimore: Williams & Wilkins; 1989:63–92.

4
Stress Modalities to Evaluate Myocardial Perfusion

João V. Vitola, Otávio J. Kormann, Arnaldo Laffitte Stier, Jr.,
William Azem Chalela, Luis E. Mastrocolla, and Dominique Delbeke

As discussed in Chapter 1, atherosclerotic lesions appear early in life.[1,2] Considering its high incidence, which only increases with aging,[3] the active search for coronary lesions, in the asymptomatic general population, does not seem reasonable. Lesions will often be found but will not necessarily be affecting myocardial perfusion in a significant way. Preservation of perfusion relates to other factors, including (1) the capacity of coronary vessels to dilate, known as coronary blood flow reserve (CBFR) and (2) the existence of a complex net of collateral vessels at the microcirculatory level. Whether coronary lesions will adversely affect myocardial blood flow (MBF) depends highly on the impact they have on CBFR and the existence or absence of good-quality collateral vessels. Evaluation of MBF, under stress, helps to determine the presence of coronary artery disease (CAD) affecting CBFR. The extent of myocardial ischemia and the degree of left ventricular dysfunction are key variables for determining prognosis that can be evaluated in nuclear cardiology using myocardial perfusion imaging (MPI). To test CBFR in nuclear cardiology, several stress modalities can be applied, including exercise, dipyridamole, adenosine, exercise combined with dipyridamole or adenosine, and dobutamine. Other less frequent forms of stress such as arbutamine, cardiac pacing, mental stress, and the cold pressor test, have also been used. These stress modalities are reviewed in this chapter.

Most Commonly Used Protocols

Physical Exercise

Exercise is the most physiological means of promoting coronary dilatation to test CBFR. It promotes vasodilatation by increasing determinants of myocardial oxygen consumption: heart rate (HR), blood pressure (BP), and myocardial contractility. Coronary lesions causing ischemia are identified on MPI as areas of decreased tracer uptake. Findings on exercise MPI are frequently, but not always, accompanied by ST-segment depression on the electrocardiogram (ECG). Under normal conditions, MBF should increase approximately threefold at peak exercise compared with baseline.

Indications

Physical exercise is the stress modality of choice for patients able to exercise adequately, providing valuable information in addition to the perfusion images (compared with pharmacological stress), such as total exercise duration, ST-segment changes, development of symptoms (chest pain), hemodynamic changes (BP and HR), and arrhythmias. In addition, the quality of early myocardial perfusion images is often better with exercise compared with pharmacological stress, and this is related to less hepatic uptake and less inferior wall artifacts with exercise. Contraindications to exercise are listed in Table 4-1.

TABLE 4-1. Contraindications for Various Types of Stress

Contraindications to all type of stress[#]:
High-risk unstable angina*
Acute myocardial infarction (within 2 days)
Uncontrolled symptomatic heart failure
Uncontrolled arrhythmias causing symptoms or hemodynamic compromise
Unwilling or unable to give informed consent (legislation dependent)

Contraindications to exercise[#]:
Absolute
Symptomatic severe aortic stenosis
Acute pulmonary embolism or pulmonary infarction
Acute myocarditis or pericarditis
Acute aortic dissection

*Relative**[†]
Left main coronary stenosis
Moderate stenotic valvular heart disease
Electrolyte abnormalities
Severe arterial hypertension***
Tachyarrhythmias or bradyarrhythmias
Hypertrophic cardiomyopathy and other forms of outflow tract obstruction
Mental or physical impairment leading to inability to exercise adequately
High-degree atrioventricular block

Contraindications to dipyridamole and adenosine:
Second- or third-degree AV block or sick sinus syndrome
Bronchospastic disease manifested by active wheezing/rhonchi, steroid dependency for asthma/COPD, severely depressed FEV1 (<40% predicted), a history of respiratory failure requiring hospitalization
Hypotension (systolic BP < 90 mm Hg)
Ongoing transient ischemic attack (TIA) or recent cerebrovascular accident (<6 months)
Caffeine intake within the past 12 hours
Theophylline intake within the past 48 hours

Contraindications to dobutamine:
Cardiac arrhythmias, including atrial fibrillation and ventricular tachycardia
Severe aortic stenosis or hypertrophic obstructive cardiomyopathy
Hypotension (SBP < 90 mm Hg) or uncontrolled hypertension (SBP > 200 mm Hg)
Aortic abdominal aneurysm greater than 5 cm is a relative contraindication
Presence of LV thrombus is a relative contraindication
Presence of an implanted ventricular defibrillator
LVEF < 25% is a relative contraindication due to increased risk of ventricular arrhythmia

* ACC/AHA Guidelines for the management of patients with unstable angina/non—ST-segment elevation myocardial infarction.
** Relative contraindications can be superseded if the benefits of exercise outweigh the risks.
*** In the absence of definitive evidence, the committee suggests systolic blood pressure of >200 mm Hg and/or diastolic blood pressure >100 mm Hg. Modified from Fletcher et al.[5]
[#] Adapted from Gibbons RJ. ACC/AHA 2002 Guideline Update for Exercise Testing. www.acc.org

Patient Preparation for Exercise Stress

Anti-ischemic drugs should be withheld: beta-blockers for 5 to 7 days (preferably gradually to prevent a rebound effect), calcium channel blockers for at least 2 days, and nitrates for at least 1 day. It is preferable to give additional instructions to prepare for vasodilator stress as well (such as caffeine diet), in case the patient cannot exercise to target HR and an alternative pharmacologic study should become necessary.

Protocols

The goal of exercise is to stress the patient to the maximum predicted heart rate (MPHR) for his age (220-age = maximum HR). If the patient is unable to reach MPHR, then 85% of the MPHR is an acceptable target. If the increase in HR does not reach at least 85% of MPHR, in the absence of typical angina or clearly positive ECG by ST-segment criteria, then exercise should be stopped, and the patient switched to a pharmacological stress protocol. The American College of Cardiology/American Heart Association (ACC/AHA) 2002 guidelines for exercise testing[4] (modified from Fletcher et al.[5]) describe the indications for terminating exercise testing and are listed in Table 4-2.

The most popular methods to exercise patients use the treadmill test (TMT). Several protocols can be used, all staged with incremental physical effort to progressively increase oxygen consumption. Each stage, lasting 2 to 3 minutes, has a set speed and inclination, depending on the protocol. The physical effort performed is measured in metabolic equivalents (METs), multiples from the baseline oxygen consumption, such as 1 MET equals 3.5 ml/kg/min. Each completed stage corresponds to a certain number of METs achieved. Oxygen consumption (VO_2) can be estimated based on the total exercise time. The maximum VO_2 differs between men and women as described here:

$$VO_2 \text{ max for men: } 2.9 \text{ ml·kg·min}^{-1} \times \text{min} + 8.33 \text{ ml·kg·min}^{-1}$$

For example, a man exercising 10 minutes on the Bruce protocol achieves a VO_2 of $2.9 \times 10 + 8.33 = 37.33$ ml/kg/min.

$$VO_2 \text{ max for women: } 2.74 \text{ ml·kg·min}^{-1} \times \text{min} + 8.03 \text{ ml·kg·min}^{-1}$$

For example, a woman exercising 10 minutes on Bruce protocol achieves a VO_2 of $2.74 \times 10 + 8.03 = 35.43$ ml/kg/min.

In 1990, Stuart and Ellestad[6] surveyed 1,375 exercise laboratories in North America and reported that, of those performing TMT, 65.5% routinely used the Bruce protocol. The Bruce protocol starts at initial speed of 1.7 mph on a 10% inclination and patients progress to their maximum capacity at 3-minute intervals using relatively large unequal (2 to 3 METs) increments in workload at each stage, as shown in Table 4-3. This protocol leads to high workload exercise and is suitable for physically active patients, with progressive increments in both speed and inclination on the treadmill. Once stage 4 is achieved, it is usually necessary to run, occasionally creating artifacts on ECG monitoring and recording. Elderly patients and those with physical limitations do not tolerate this

TABLE 4-2. Indications for Terminating Exercise Testing

Absolute indications
Drop in systolic blood pressure >10 mm Hg from baseline blood pressure despite an increase in workload, when accompanied by other evidence of ischemia
Moderate to severe ischemia
Increasing nervous system symptoms (e.g., ataxia, dizziness, or near-syncope)
Signs of poor perfusion
Technical difficulties in monitoring ECG or systolic blood pressure
Patient's request to stop
Sustained ventricular tachycardia
ST-segment elevation (1.0 mm) in leads without diagnostic Q-waves (other than V1 or aVR)
Relative indications
Drop in systolic blood pressure of (10 mm Hg from baseline blood pressure despite an increase in workload, when accompanied by other evidence of ischemia)
ST or QRS changes such as excessive ST-segment depression (>2 mm of horizontal or downsloping ST-segment depression) or marked axis shift
Arrhythmias other than sustained ventricular tachycardia, including multifocal PVCs, triplets of PVCs, supraventricular tachycardia, heart block, or bradyarrhythmias
Fatigue, shortness of breath, wheezing, leg cramps, or claudication
Development of bundle branch block or IVCD that can not be distinguished from ventricular tachycardia
Increasing chest pain
Hypertensive response*
In the absence of definitive evidence, the committee suggests systolic blood pressure of >250 mm Hg and/or a diastolic blood pressure of >115 mm Hg.

ECG: electrocardiogram; PVCs: premature ventricular contractions; ICD: implantable cardioverter-defribrillator discharge; IVCD: intraventricular conduction delay.
* Modified from Fletcher et al.[5]
Reproduced with permission from Gibbons RJ. ACC/AHA 2002 Guideline Update for Exercise Testing. www.acc.org

protocol well. Another commonly used protocol is called Ellestad, in which there is a progressive increase in workload and the changes occur every 2 minutes instead of every 3 minutes (except for stage 1). The speed increments are higher, but the inclination is fixed at 10% up to stage 4. The Kattus and Naughton protocols are better suited for sedentary and elderly patients, with smaller increments of both speed and inclination every 3 minutes. The workload is milder with Naughton compared with Kattus, with the energy consumption in the first two stages being very small for the Naughton protocol. The first seven stages of the protocols discussed previously are shown in Table 4-3. If the patient can tolerate to exercise at higher workloads, then additional stages (8, 9, etc.) can be added. Another protocol, receiving great attention in the literature, is called the *Ramp protocol*, in which the workload increases constantly and continuously. In this case, the exercise capacity is estimated from a brief history and the treadmill protocol can be adjusted to bring patients to their target in about 8 to 12 minutes.

TABLE 4-3. Details of Main Exercise Protocols Used in Nuclear Cardiology

Stage	Min	MPH	Inclination	VO_2	METS
Bruce Protocol					
1	3	1.7	10%	17.5	5
2	3	2.5	12%	24.5	7
3	3	3.4	14%	35.0	10
4	3	4.2	16%	45.5	13
5	3	5.0	18%	56.0	16
6	3	5.5	20%	66.5	19
7	3	6.0	22%	77	22
Ellestad Protocol					
1	3	1.7	10%	16.1	4.6
2	2	3.0	10%	25.8	7.4
3	2	4.0	10%	33.2	9.5
4	2	5.0	10%	42.3	12.0
5	2	5.0	15%	48.4	13.8
6	2	6.0	15%	57	16.6
7	2	7.0	15%	66	18.8
Kattus Protocol					
1	3	1.5	10%	14.7	4.2
2	3	2.0	10%	18.4	5.2
3	3	2.5	10%	22.0	6.3
4	3	3.0	10%	25.9	7.4
5	3	3.5	10%	29.6	8.4
6	3	4.0	10%	33.2	9.5
7	3	4.0	14%	40.7	11.6
Naughton Protocol					
1	2	1	0.0%	6.0	1.7
2	2	2	0.0%	7.0	2.0
3	2	2	3.5%	10.5	3.0
4	2	2	7.0%	14.0	4.0
5	2	2	10.5%	17.5	5.0
6	2	2	14.0%	21.0	6.0
7	2	2	17.5%	24.5	7.0

Physicians performing the test should judge when the ideal moment to inject the tracer is achieved, being aware that the patient should continue exercising for an additional 1 to 2 minutes after injection. Borg described scales for rating perceived exertion.[7] These scales are useful to monitor the patient's fatigue during exercise and assess the moment of near maximum exertion.

Performance

The sensitivity and specificity of MPI using exercise stress for detection of CAD (>50% stenosis) has been summarized by Berman et al.[8] The weighted average sensitivity and specificity of 25 studies performed between 1990 and 1998 was 87% (1515 of 1739 patients) and 73% (431 of 589 patients), respectively.

Using exercise as stress, exercise scores can be calculated, carrying diagnostic but mainly prognostic value. The Duke treadmill score[9] is commonly used to classify patients in a low-, intermediate-, or high-risk category for coronary event, independently of the scintigraphic findings. The Duke score is helpful in patients with a normal or near normal MPI, when balanced CAD is suspected. Patients with severe balanced CAD usually have a poor exercise capacity, severe ST-segment depression on ECG, and a blunted HR response and/or a blunted response or decrease in BP. Chest pain may or may not be present. MPI should be evaluated in the context of other information, including the clinical presentation, CAD risk factors, and the treadmill results. Hachamovitch et al.[10] evaluated the correlation between the Duke score and MPI findings. Both a normal or mildly abnormal MPI study with a high Duke score and a low Duke score but with a severe perfusion abnormality on MPI, are associated with a very high risk of cardiac events and should receive close attention. The fact that a low Duke score with a severe perfusion abnormality is associated with a high risk of cardiac events illustrates the limited sensitivity of exercise ECG to detect ischemia. In addition, there is a good correlation between a poor exercise capacity and higher mortality.[11] Direct assessment of exercise hemodynamics, especially in patients with heart failure, provides additive independent prognostic information compared with clinical evaluation and radionuclide ventriculography.[12]

Dipyridamole

Pharmacological stress represents approximately 34% of the MPI studies performed in the United States.[13,14] Dipyridamole inhibits the action of an enzyme called adenosine deaminase, responsible for the degradation of endogenously produced adenosine. Dipyridamole also blocks the reuptake of adenosine by cells, which again contributes to elevation of adenosine, causing vasodilatation. Dipyridamole increases MBF approximately three- to fourfold compared with baseline.

Indications

Indications for vasodilator stress are (1) inability to exercise, (2) failure to achieve 85% MPHR in the absence of typical angina or >2mm ST-segment depression, (3) concurrent beta-blockade (or calcium antagonist) therapy (relative indication), and (4) presence of left bundle branch block (LBBB) or pacemaker. Contraindications are listed in Table 4-1.

Patient Preparation for Vasodilator Stress

Theophylline and other xanthines (i.e., pentoxifylline) should be withheld for at least 72 hours and all caffeine and caffeinated beverages and foods for 24 to 48 hours before vasodilator infusion.[15] Special attention should be given to stopping consumption of coffee, tea, chocolate, and soft drinks. Patients taking oral dipyridamole (as antiplatelet therapy) should stop it for 24 to 48 hours before vasodilator infusion. Since caffeine is cleared by the liver, special attention should be taken in patients with hepatic failure, especially those evaluated prior to liver transplant.[16] In these cases, exercise or dobutamine stress should be considered.

Protocol

Some investigators have raised questions about the existence of individuals considered *nonresponders* to a dose of 0.56mg/kg of dipyridamole. These nonresponders would have increments of MBF equal or less than twofold baseline that could potentially result in a false-negative MPI study result.[17] There is some evidence that a higher dose of dipyridamole, 0.84 mg/kg, would increase the hyperemic response in some of these patients.[18,19] Awareness should be increased to the occurrence of severe bronchospasm and higher degree atrioventricular (AV) block, which may occur with low or high dose of dipyridamole, requiring prompt discontinuation of the infusion and treatment.

Side Effects

The safety of dipyridamole has been reviewed in a series of 73,806 patients.[20] Dipyridamole (at a dose of 0.56mg/kg) causes side effects in about 50% of individuals, flushing being the most frequent in 43% of patients, chest pain (nonspecific for ischemia) in 20%, and headache in 12% (Table 4-4).[21] The half-life of dipyridamole is approximately 45 minutes. Patients receiving dipyridamole may experience symptoms after completion of the infusion when patients have already left the laboratory. Administration of aminophylline prevents these occurrences in most patients. Aminophylline is administered at 1.0 to 1.5mg/kg or 25mg/minute slow IV push until symptoms resolve with a maximum dose of 250mg.

Performance

The sensitivity and specificity of dipyridamole stress for detection of CAD (>50%) have been described to be in the same range as those for exercise.[18] However, more recently, there has been some evidence that a normal SPECT study result in patients undergoing vasodilator stress may not have the same negative predictive value as compared with exercise stress.[22]

TABLE 4-4. Side Effects Attributable to Vasodilator Stress Testing

	Adenosine* (n = 9,256)	Dipyridamole** (n = 3,911)	Dobutamine*** (n = 1,076)
Chest pain	35%	20%	39%
Flushing	37%	43%	<1%
Dyspnea	35%	3%	6%
Dizziness	9%	3%	4%
GI discomfort	15%	1%	1%
Headache	14%	12%	7%
Arrhythmia	3%	5%	45%
AV block	8%	0%	0%
ST changes	6%	8%	20%–31%
Any adverse effects	81%	50%	50%–75%

* From reference 26.
** From reference 21.
*** From reference 62.
From Hendel, Jamil, and Glover (118), by permission of *J Nucl Cardiol.*

This fact may be related to the higher prevalence of disease and other comorbidities usually present in a population most commonly referred for vasodilator stress.

Adenosine

Adenosine promotes vasodilatation by activation of vascular A_2 receptors, which has an effect on cyclic AMP, reduces the influx of calcium into the intracellular space, and consequently relaxes smooth muscle cells of the coronary arteries. Adenosine increases MBF approximately four- to fivefold above baseline in myocardium supplied by normal arteries, whereas the MBF increases less in myocardium supplied by diseased arteries. The ischemic territories can be identified on MPI as areas of decreased tracer uptake. Ischemic areas can be identified on MPI by heterogenous tracer distribution, due to a differential capacity of vessels to dilate without causing true myocardial ischemia. True myocardial ischemia may occur with administration of adenosine or dipyridamole, when there is a *coronary steal phenomenon*. The steal phenomenon occurs in patients who have part of their myocardium supplied by collateral vessels due to an occluded or critically stenotic coronary artery.[23] When there is true ischemia, ST-segment shifts may be observed during the test as well as clinical evidence of ischemia with typical angina. Wall motion abnormalities may develop as a result of the steal phenomenon during infusion of vasodilators.[19]

Indications

The indications are the same as for dipyridamole. Contraindications are listed in Table 4-1.

Patient Preparation

The patient preparation is the same as for dipyridamole.

Protocol

Adenosine is infused IV with a pump in a volume of 50 ml of saline at a rate of 140 mcg·kg·min^{-1} over 4 to 6 minutes; the rate can be decreased to 100 mcg·kg·min^{-1} without a loss in sensitivity in the event of significant symptoms. Blood pressure, HR, and ECG are monitored every minute. If heart block progresses or does not resolve, infusion should be terminated. Studies comparing 4 versus 6 minutes infusion of adenosine demonstrated similar sensitivity for detection of CAD, and the 4 minutes of infusion was better tolerated.[24] The radiopharmaceutical is administered intravenously 3 minutes into the adenosine infusion. Blood pressure, HR, and ECG are monitored every minute for 10 to 20 minutes or until the patient's hemodynamic status returns to baseline. The indications for terminating adenosine infusion are the same as for dipyridamole described previously.

Side Effects

Approximately 81% of patients undergoing adenosine infusion have some side effects, flushing being the most frequent and occurring in 37% of patients, which is followed by dyspnea in 35%, and AV block in 8% (Table 4-4). The safety of adenosine stress has been demonstrated in a large prospective study of 9,256 consecutive patients.[25,26]

Adenosine has a very short half-life of less than 10 seconds. This does not necessarily mean that all side effects occurring with adenosine resolve after cessation of infusion. Once the adenosine receptors have been activated, a cascade of events is triggered, and therefore, side effects may be much more prolonged than it could be suggested by the drug's short half-life. The antidote to adenosine is aminophylline, 25 mg/minute slow IV push, until symptoms resolve, with a maximum dose of 250 mg. In view of the brief half-life of adenosine, termination of the infusion is often (but not always) adequate to manage adverse events. If possible, wait 2 to 3 minutes after radiopharmaceutical injection to terminate adenosine infusion and give aminophylline. In case of severe ischemic symptoms, administration of sublingual or intranasal nitroglycerin, 0.4 mg, may be necessary, following aminophylline administration.[27]

Performance

For detection of CAD, the sensitivity and specificity of adenosine stress is in the same range as exercise stress.[28–30] The sensitivity and specificity of MPI using vasodilator stress for detection of CAD (>50% stenosis) has been summarized by Berman et al.[8] The weighted average sensitivity and specificity of 15 studies performed between 1990 and 1998 was 89% (1164 of 1306 patients) and 80% (313 of 390 patients), respectively. As described previously for dipyridamole, there has been some recent evidence that a normal SPECT study, in patients undergoing vasodilator stress, may not have the same negative predictive value, as compared with exercise stress.[22] Ischemic ECG changes with normal SPECT images during vasodilator stress are uncommon, but it may be helpful to identify patients at an increased risk for future cardiac events.[31,32]

Combination of Vasodilator and Low Workload Physical Exercise

As discussed previously, pharmacological alternatives have to be considered in patients with poor exercise tolerance and/or those who are unable to reach at least 85% of MPHR. Protocols combining vasodilators (dipyridamole and adenosine) with exercise have been established in the past several years.[33–35] The vasodilator effect of dipyridamole or adenosine has been described to be greater than that of exercise alone, except in cases of nonresponders. Whether or not exercise can contribute to the identification of these individuals is still under investigation, but there are preliminary data to suggest that.[36,37]

Compared with exercise, which is the most physiological stimulus, dipyridamole or adenosine stimuli alone have several limitations, including low sensitivity of the ECG for ischemia and frequent side effects.[21] These vasodilators induce dilatation of the splanchnic vasculature resulting in a higher concentration of radiopharmaceuticals in the liver and intestinal tract.[38] Exercise promotes a redistribution of blood flow to the skeletal musculature and away from intraabdominal organs such as the liver.[39] These effects result in a higher heart-to-liver activity ratio on images obtained after exercise compared with those obtained after vasodilator infusion alone.[40] Some studies have shown that the addition of low workload exercise help to decrease dipyridamole side effects.[41–44] Other studies, using adenosine, have shown similar effects, reducing side effects,[45] arrhythmias,[46] and decreasing technetium-99m-methoxyisobutylisonitrile (^{99m}Tc-MIBI) concentration to the liver.[46] Besides resulting in better image quality, the images can be also be acquired earlier, after administration of the radiopharmaceutical, in patients undergoing a combined exercise/vasodilator protocol compared with vasodilator alone.[33,47]

Indications for Combined Vasodilator and Exercise Stress

Indications for combined vasodilator and exercise stress are (1) inability to exercise to 85% maximum predicted HR, but able to at least walk, and (2) concurrent use of medications that may limit HR increase.

Patient Preparation for Combined Vasodilator and Exercise Stress

A combination of preparations for each type of stress is described in detail previously in this chapter.

Contraindications for Combined Vasodilator and Exercise Stress

The contraindications are the same as described in detail previously in this chapter, as if each type of stress were done separately. It is important to note that patients with LBBB or pacemaker should undergo vasodilator stress alone to reduce the false-positive rate associated with exercise.[48]

Protocols

Most patients for the combined protocol are exercised at low workload as per patient's abilities, such as the first and second stage of a standard or modified Bruce, or some other light protocol such as Kattus or Naughton described previously (see Table 4-3). If the patient can tolerate it, the workload is increased, but if unable to exercise at a higher level, then exercise should be maintained at a lower level (limited to stage 1 or 2 of the protocols described). With exercise plus dipyridamole, the maximum action of the drug occurs between 6 and 9 minutes into the infusion; therefore, the infusion may start before the exercise (approximately at 3 minutes into the infusion), and the tracer should be injected at 6 to 9 minutes from the start of infusion.[33] With adenosine, the infusion is started at the same time as the exercise protocol and the radiopharmaceutical is administered at 2 to 3 minutes into drug infusion, while the patient continues to exercise to maximum tolerance.[35]

Performance

Significant ST-segment changes during low workload (first 3 minutes of a Bruce protocol) are associated with a higher rate of adverse event (Figure 4-1).[49] Importantly, the magnitude of ST-segment depression at this low workload can stratify patients into different risk categories, with approximately 80% of patients with 3 mm of ST-segment depression having cardiac events within 6 years.

The impact of adjunctive adenosine infusion during exercise MPI has been studied as part of a multicenter trial in which 35 patients were enrolled prospectively and underwent both exercise MPI and exercise MPI with a 4-minute adenosine infusion on a separate day (BEAST trial).[50] The summed stress scores (SSS) and summed difference scores (SDS) were greater in the exercise-plus-adenosine group than the exercise-only group. The study concluded that the combined protocol resulted in a greater amount of myocardial ischemia detected on the SPECT images while allowing for the assessment of functional capacity.

Dobutamine

Dobutamine is an inotropic agent, frequently used in intensive care units to increase cardiac output, blood pressure, and urinary output. Dobutamine has a mild effect on alpha-1 receptors, strong effect on beta-1 receptors, and moderate effect on beta-2 receptors. In the heart, dobutamine activates beta-1 receptors.[51] Dobutamine causes increased HR and myocardial contractility, promoting coronary hyperemia through mechanisms similar to exercise. It is a synthetic sympathetic drug developed in the early 1970s[52] for treatment of severe heart failure.[53] In 1984, its use as a stress agent began, initially for MPI and later for stress echocardiography.[54–56] It is a fast-acting drug with the effect starting approximately 2 minutes into infusion. Drug clearance occurs predominantly

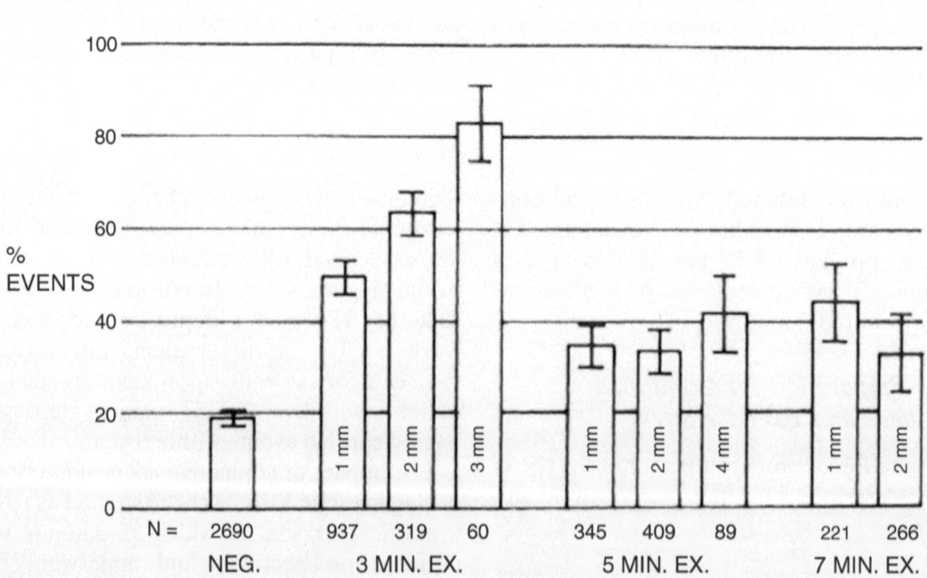

FIGURE 4-1. The incidence of subsequent coronary events (progression of angina, MI, and death) increases with the magnitude of the ST-segment depression only when analyzed at a light workload (3 minutes of exercise = 4 METs; time span 6 years). (Reproduced with permission from Ellestad MH (ed). Predictive implications. In *Stress testing: Principles and Practice.* New York: Oxford University Press; 2003:291.)

by the liver, with a short plasma half-life of approximately 2 minutes.[57,58] Its hemodynamic effects depend highly on the dose infused. At low doses of 5 to 10 mcg/kg/min it activates beta-1 and alpha-1 receptors, which increase myocardial contractility without significant effects on HR. Doses above 10 to 20 mcg/kg/min activate alpha-1 receptors, which increases both the HR and myocardial contractility, resulting in an increase of cardiac output. Doses higher than 30 mcg/kg/min increase significantly the development of ventricular arrhythmias. Dobutamine also causes a reduction of systemic vascular resistance mediated by activation of the beta-2 receptors, which may actually cause the BP to decrease. However, the BP effects of dobutamine are less predictable, but most of the time it will induce a mild increase in BP. The hyperemic effect of dobutamine alone increases MBF approximately twofold above baseline, which is an effect considered lower than that obtained with dipyridamole or adenosine.[59] However, it has been demonstrated that the administration of dobutamine combined with atropine has an hyperemic effect similar to that of dipyridamole.[60]

Indications

In the nuclear laboratory, dobutamine infusion has been mainly indicated to evaluate CAD in patients with COPD who are unable to exercise adequately, as is usually the case in severe COPD. Contraindications for the use of dobutamine are listed in Table 4-1.

Patient Preparation

The patient should be off of beta-blockers for 5 to 7 days, preferably slowly discontinued to prevent rebound effects. Other antianginal medications (calcium channel blockers and nitrates) should also be discontinued as previously discussed in this chapter for exercise testing.

Protocol

The protocol most commonly used for MPI with dobutamine starts with an infusion rate of 10 mcg/kg/min, increasing by an additional dose of 10 mcg/kg/min every 3 minutes, to a maximum dose of 40 mcg/kg/min. Atropine may be used to increase HR, starting at the second stage.[61] Boluses of 0.25 mg of atropine can be given every minute to a maximum dose of 2 mg. Usually, target HR is achieved at the rate of 20 to 30 mcg/kg/min with a small dose of atropine of approximately 0.5 mg. The higher the dobutamine dose given, the higher the incidence of arrhythmias and side effects; the addition of atropine helps to achieve the target HR at lower dobutamine doses. The radiopharmaceutical is injected once the target HR is achieved and the infusion of dobutamine is continued for another minute. ECG and BP are monitored at baseline and every 3 minutes thereafter. Approximately 10% of patients have a nondiagnostic dobutamine-atropine stress test due to failure to reach an adequate hemodynamic response.[62] The interruption criteria are similar to those used for exercise testing, as shown in Table 4-2, with special attention to signs and symptoms of severe ischemia (pain and ST-segment changes) and development of malignant arrhythmias during the infusion.[62–64]

Side Effects

Dobutamine leads to side effects in about 75% of patients, 39% having chest pain that can be treated with sublingual nitroglycerin and 45% having supraventricular tachycardia or ventricular ectopy (Table 4-4).[62] Ventricular tachycardia (VT) occurs in 4% to 5% of patients.[65] Other side effects include headaches (7%), dyspnea (6%), flushing (<1%), nausea, and anxiety, which are usually well tolerated and do not necessitate interruption of the infusion. Symptomatic hypotension occurs rarely and can be treated with infusion of saline. Severe side effects of dobutamine can be reversed by beta-blockers such as esmolol (0.2 mg/kg over 1 minute) or IV bolus of metoprolol (2.5 to 5.0 mg). However, patients undergoing dobutamine infusion often have COPD. Beta-blockers, especially at higher doses, are known to worsen COPD, and should be avoided if possible. When dobutamine induces VT, amiodarone or electric cardioversion may be necessary, especially if hemodynamic instability is present. Despite the relatively high incidence of cardiac arrhythmia with dobutamine, in a study of 3,578 patients reported in the literature, there were no reports of death, MI, or ventricular fibrillation.[66] Safety of dobutamine stress has also been reported in the elderly population[67] and also in heart transplant recipients.[68]

Performance

ST-segment depression on dobutamine ECG has a relatively poor sensitivity, but as with other forms of pharmacologic stress it is highly specific for detection of ischemia. ST-segment elevation in patients without a history of prior MI is strongly associated with severe CAD.[69–71] An analysis of 20 studies demonstrated that the overall sensitivity, specificity, and accuracy of dobutamine MPI to diagnose CAD were 88%, 74%, and 84%, respectively.[70] Parameters such as sensitivity, specificity, and accuracy can vary tremendously in different studies and are highly dependent on multiple factors including the prevalence of CAD in the population, protocols and perfusion agents used, and medications taken by patients at time of testing. Besides, the gold standard used to calculate these variables of MPI is usually the existence of an obstructive lesion, which has its own intrinsic limitations as a predictor of ischemia, which is highly dependent on collateral flow. When ^{99m}Tc-MIBI is used as a tracer, the stress-induced defects appear less pronounced with dobutamine and arbutamine than with other stress methods. This is presumably due to alteration of ^{99m}Tc-MIBI binding to mitochondria secondary to influx of calcium produced by dobutamine.[72,73] However, the literature suggests a good negative predictive value of dobutamine MPI. Normal myocardial perfusion studies with dobutamine are associated with a good prognosis and low cardiac event rate, less than 0.8% per year. Patients with fixed and reversible perfusion defects have a risk of 6.8% and 8.1% for major cardiac events, respectively. If both fixed and reversible cardiac defects are present, the risk is 11.6%.[74,75]

Evaluation of contractile reserve is also possible using gated SPECT ^{99m}Tc-MIBI imaging, in a similar way to echocardiography.[76] The ^{99m}Tc-MIBI images are acquired 1 hour after infusion of the maximum tolerated dose of dobutamine and again during infusion of dobutamine at a low dose. More recently, the administration of nitrate before the rest injection has been combined with low-dose dobutamine infusion during the gated SPECT acquisition to assess both perfusion at rest and at stress, together with contractile reserve, for predicting recovery of regional ventricular function after revascularization.[77,78] This issue is discussed further in Chapter 8.

Less Commonly Used Stress Tests

Arbutamine

Arbutamine is a synthetic catecholamine developed for use as a pharmacological stress agent. It has been approved by the Food and Drug Administration for MPI and echocardiography. This drug is a mixed beta-1 and beta-2 agonist with a mild affinity for alpha-1 receptors.[79] Arbutamine has a chronotropic response similar to that of dobutamine, however with fewer peripheral vasodilating effects. This drug was developed for use in a closed-loop drug delivery system, computerized to constantly monitor the HR response during drug infusion. The device consists of a computer, a single-channel ECG, a noninvasive BP monitor, and IV access. The physician selects the appropriate slope of HR increase for each given patient. The device calculates the dose regimen and adjusts the infusion rate to achieve the expected HR.[59] The most common side effects include tremors (22%), dizziness (11%), headache (11%), paresthesia (7%), arrhythmias (6%), and hypotension (4%).[80]

Performance

The experience with this drug is limited, compared with other forms of stress so widely used today; however, in a comparison of adenosine and arbutamine, a good correlation between both stress modalities was found for classification of stress scores.[81]

Atrial Pacing

Atrial pacing has been used at some institu-tions as an alternative to exercise in the evaluation of CAD. Atrial pacing can be performed through cardiac stimulations from an esophageal access. Zoll.[82] performed the first experimental attempts to stimulate the heart, using ventricular stimulation from the esophagus.

Indications

Transesophageal atrial pacing is an alternative for patients with physical limitations, unable to exercise, and who have contraindications for pharmacological stimulation. This is rare, because patients are usually suitable for one of the forms of stress more commonly used and described previously. Nevertheless, the advantage of pacing involves the possibility of immediate interruption of the stress when severe side effects occur, and a quick return to baseline conditions compared with other forms of stress. Its disadvantage lies in its relative invasiveness, limiting its clinical use. Other indications for atrial pacing, besides stress for MPI and echocardiography, include the evaluation of cardiac arrhythmias, such as sinus and AV node conduction defects.

As for other forms of stress, medications blunting the inotropic and chronotropic response should be discontinued. Contraindications include patients with atrial arrhythmias (fibrillation or flutter), AV block, complex ventricular arrhythmia, recent or complicated MI, uncontrolled hypertension, severe valvular disease, decompensated congestive heart failure (CHF), and esophageal obstruction.

Protocol

The flexible wire with the electrode (size approximately 10F) is placed into the distal esophagus through the nasal cavity. Once the electrode reaches the distal esophagus, it can be repositioned under ECG guidance, and a biphasic P wave is recorded. The increments in induced HR should be gradual, increasing by 10 to 20 bpm. The target HR is 85% of the predicted maximum HR. Augmentation with intravenous atropine may also be used, in a similar manner as for the dobutamine protocol.[83]

Hemodynamic Changes

Compared with other methods (exercise or pharmacological stimulation), atrial stimulation increases HR without much effect on the inotropic response and peripheral vascular resistance. It decreases the systolic volume and the duration of the diastolic period; however, cardiac output is increased secondary to a higher HR. Myocardial contractility may also increase as a consequence of a higher HR, an effect known as *Bowdich-Treppe*.[84] Blood pressure and rate pressure product increases are observed with pacing.[85] Atrial pacing may require a slightly higher HR to induce ischemia compared with dobutamine, probably related to its lower effect on inotropic response and oxygen consumption.[83]

Performance

Lambertz et al.[86] reported a sensitivity and specificity of 67% and 49%, respectively, for ischemic changes on the ECG during atrial pacing, similar to what is seen with exercise ECG. Compared with angiography, the sensitivity of atrial pacing echocardiography varies from 83% to 93% and the specificity from 76% to 100%. These results are comparable with what has been shown for dobutamine echocardiography, which has a sensitivity varying from 72% to 89% and a specificity of 83% to 100%.[87] Atar et al.[84] reported a good concordance between echocardiography and MPI using pacing, with an accuracy of 87%. This concordance was higher in the left anterior descending coronary artery (LAD), and the left circumflex coronary artery (LCX) territories compared with the right coronary artery (RCA).

Mental Stress

The physiological changes induced by mental stress affect mainly the cardiovascular system. These physiological changes are mediated by the autonomic nervous system, especially the sympathetic system. Mental stress is part of a wide group of tests used to evaluate the autonomic system, which also include the tilt test, Valsalva's maneuver, negative pressure applied to lower limbs, and isometric exercises. During mental stress, several tasks are given to the patient, which involve development of an emotional response (challenges, threat, anxiety, and alertness) and induce organic changes mediated by increments of the sympathetic response. Cardiovascular monitoring starts before and continues during and after mental stress is induced.

Acute psychological stress in animals and humans stimulates the central nervous system (CNS), mainly the frontal cortex, which acts on medullary nuclei that have the capacity to modulate the sympathetic activity. This results in an increased peripheral sympathetic discharge,[88,89] and promotes changes preparing the person for a reaction of *escape*, as would happen in the animal model. The hemodynamic changes are many, including increased HR, BP, and cardiac output; splanchnic and cutaneous vasoconstriction; and vasodilatation of vessels to skeletal muscles, partially occurring from activation of the muscular cholinergic system. In the heart, there is a balance between the sympathetic and parasympathetic activity to control the HR, but this increases the vulnerability to some cardiac arrhythmias. Overall, the organic result obtained with an increased peripheral autonomic activation is a reflection of two opposing forces[90]: (1) the signal of alert given by the CNS, which stimulates the sympathetic tone, and (2) activation of the baroreflex, which inhibits the sympathetic tone.[91] Mental stress should only be applied to the appropriate patient population, taking into account the reliability of the responses obtained and the limitations of this form of stress.[92] Mental stress may play a role in the investigation of the relationship between systemic arterial hypertension and cardiovascular disease.[93]

Type A personality is associated with an increased risk (up to threefold) for development of CAD, angina, acute MI, and sudden death.[94] Type A personality is characterized by high level of competition; intense dedication to achieve a high set of objectives; desire for recognition; hostility; involvement with multiple activities; urgency in accomplishing set tasks; intolerance to failure from self and others; impatience; difficulty relaxing; and fast speech, eating, and walking; whereas a type B personality has only a few of these characteristics.

Mental stress testing may induce myocardial ischemia in patients with CAD leading to angina, ECG changes, and cardiac arrhythmias.[95] The increase in oxygen consumption during mental stress may explain ischemic changes, but control by the parasympathetic nervous system is important as well.[96]

As the heart vulnerability to ventricular fibrillation and other cardiac arrhythmias depends on an equilibrium between the sympathetic and the parasympathetic systems, mental stress (and consequently an increased sympathetic activity), may be related to cardiac events such as sudden death.

Mental stress is a valid form of cardiac stress, but has been mainly used to elucidate physiopathological mechanisms of diseases such as CAD and hypertension, as well as the role of emotional stress to induce arrhythmias and sudden death.

Cold Pressor Test

The cold pressor test has been used as a form of cardiovascular stress since 1936.[97] This test can be used to evaluate vascular reactivity of hypertensive patients or those genetically predisposed to hypertension.[97,98] The hemodynamic changes observed during the test are secondary to a global increase in sympathetic activity, resulting in increased plasma catecholamines, arteriolar vasoconstriction, and increased BP.[99]

Indications

Based on these hemodynamic changes, this test has been used to evaluate patients with CAD. Approximately 50% of patients with CAD develop angina when exposed to cold conditions at rest, and a higher percentage of patients when exercise is added.[100,101] (See Case 5.13.)

The exact mechanism of angina associated with cold exposition is not completely known; however, several possible explanations exist for this effect. First, cold leads to increased peripheral vascular resistance and to a higher cardiac workload.[102,103] Second, cold increases the vascular tone of coronary arteries.[104] Third, it is necessary to consider that ischemic response to cold occurs in patients with obstructive CAD, possibly due to an increased sensitivity to catecholamines and/or compromised vasodilator response due to endothelial dysfunction.[105]

Cold pressor test can be used to evaluate vascular reactivity and may be associated with other noninvasive tests, such as echocardiography, MPI, and RVG. This form of stress has also been used with positron emission tomography (PET) and intracoronary US (IVUS), mainly in patients with angina and associated with metabolic disease.[105–109] Other indications for the cold pressor test include the evaluation of LV function in cardiomyopathies, aortic stenosis, and hypertrophic cardiomyopathy with subaortic stenosis.[110] However, this test has been better standardized for the evaluation of CAD and should be considered when there is a limitation for physical exercise and a contraindication for pharmacological stimuli.

Protocol

The test is relatively easy to perform. It consists basically of the immersion of one limb into icy water at 1° to 4°C temperature for a certain period of time. Most of the time the hand is used, for a time varying between 1 and 10 minutes, according to different protocols. The patient should be lying supine during the test. It is recommended that ECG and BP be monitored at baseline, and intermittently during the test and recovery period. Most hemodynamic changes induced by cold occur in the first 15 to 30 seconds, followed by a plateau, persisting for several minutes.

Interruption criteria include intolerance to the test, severe persistent angina, tachycardia (difficult to tolerate), and severe headache.

ECG criteria for positivity are the same as those used for exercise stress.

Hemodynamic responses to cold are the same in patients with or without CAD, consisting of increased systolic and diastolic BP, and a variable HR response that can increase or decrease.[99,111] The BP response is secondary to an increase in vascular resistance and systolic volume. Cardiac output is usually not affected, but changes in ventricular filling do occur and are indirect signs of CAD.[112] A correlation between insulin levels (fasting and after glucose load) and BP response has been observed.[113]

Side Effects

Symptoms that may occur include palpitations (possibly from arrhythmias), chest pain, and headaches from high BP. Chest pain associated with ST depression has a high specificity but low sensitivity for ischemia. Angina has been observed in 12% and ST-segment depression in 15% of patients with CAD.[114–116]

Performance

Cold pressor as a form of stress for MPI has been useful to evaluate myocardial ischemia. The sensitivity depends on disease extent and increases from 40% to 100% in patients with single-vessel compared with three-vessel disease.[117]

New Stress Agents

Selective adenosine A_{2A} receptor agonists have the advantages of fewer side effects than adenosine itself, in particular they do not affect the conduction system.[118] This issue is discussed further in Chapter 18.

Conclusions

In conclusion, various stress methods can be applied during MPI. The optimal stress modality should be individualized for each patient. Ideally, all patients should perform a test with exercise, alone if efficacious, or combined with vasodilators if the exercise capacity is reduced. A purely pharmacologic stress should be used for patients completely unable to exercise or those with LBBB or pacemaker (in these cases, vasodilator stress). Dobutamine is reserved for patients with COPD who do not tolerate exercise. Finally, the choice of the stress modality may vary depending on the population evaluated and particularities of each laboratory, but most of the time the choice of the stress modality is based on the patient's physical condition.

Case Presentations

Case 4.1

History

A 69-year-old man with a history of MI 2 years earlier presented with left arm pain related to exertion. He underwent a TMT showing borderline ST-segment changes and frequent premature ventricular contractions (PVCs) with a period of nonsustained ventricular tachycardia. He was referred for MPI to evaluate risk stratification. In the nuclear laboratory, he underwent TMT using the Bruce protocol and exercised for 9 minutes. His HR increased from 61 to 138 bpm and his BP from 140/80 to 200/100 mmHg. He denied chest pain. His baseline ECG showed right bundle branch block (RBBB). His exercise ECG demonstrated 1.0 to 1.5 mm upsloping ST depression at peak exercise, considered borderline changes for ischemia. During the recovery period, he developed frequent PVCs and a short period of nonsustained ventricular tachycardia. His exercise/rest ^{99m}Tc-MIBI SPECT images are displayed in Figure C4-1A (short-axis views) and C4-1B (horizontal long-axis view).

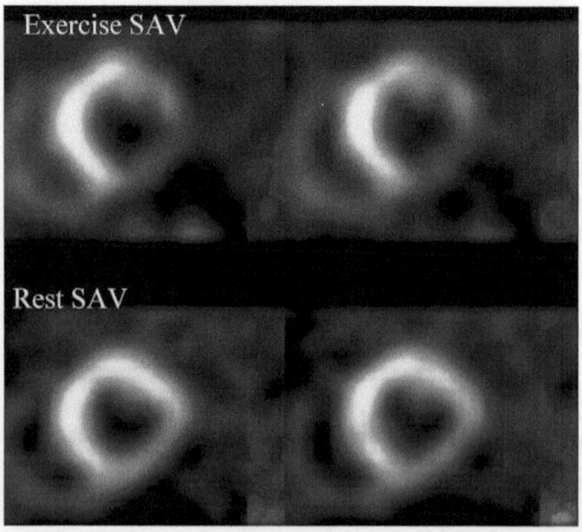

A

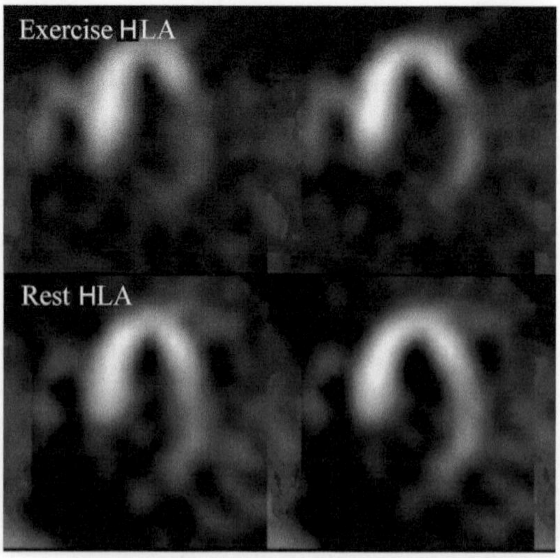

B

FIGURE C4-1. (A and B)

Findings

The stress SPECT images show a large area of moderately decreased uptake, partially reversible at rest and involving the anterolateral and lateral walls. These findings are consistent with ischemia in the territory of a diagonal branch of the LAD and the LCX. In addition, there is a partially reversible defect involving the inferolateral wall compatible with peri-infarct ischemia in this patient with a history of prior MI. The gated images (not shown) demonstrated a moderately dilated left ventricle (LV), a left ventricular ejection fraction (LVEF) of 38%, and moderate hypokinesis of the lateral and inferolateral walls.

Discussion

The SPECT images indicate multivessel CAD, and the patient's anatomy can be predicted by the findings on the SPECT images. Multivessel ischemia, in a patient with a prior MI, places him in a high-risk category for cardiac events. A dilated LV, depressed LVEF, and hypokinesis of the lateral and inferolateral walls are other poor prognostic factors. The severe perfusion abnormalities on the SPECT images are associated with an estimated annual event rate (death or new MI) of approximately 8% to 9%, independently of the treadmill findings (Figure C4-1C). Interestingly, the ST-segment depression on the ECG was only borderline but associated with complex ventricular arrhythmia. Ventricular arrhythmia during exercise is not necessarily indicative of ischemia in the absence of ST-segment depression, but is strongly predictive of ischemia when associated with ST-segment changes. In the current case, borderline ST-segment changes in a patient with a high pretest probability and the presence of complex arrhythmias should raise the suspicion of CAD despite the absence of pain or severe ST-segment changes. In the presence of RBBB, the evaluation of the right precordial lead is compromised, which may decrease the sensitivity of the exercise ECG.

Coronary angiography revealed an occluded LAD, a subocclusive diagonal lesion, an occluded left obtuse marginal branch (filling from collaterals), and an occluded RCA (Figure C4-1D), which also fills from collaterals. This scenario, in a patient with depressed LV function, is an indication for myocardial revascularization, with major benefits, as demonstrated by the CASS study.[119] The patient underwent multivessel coronary artery bypass surgery (CABG) with excellent recovery.

Main Teaching Points of Case 4.1

1. A patient with severe CAD does not always present with chest pain. The presentation

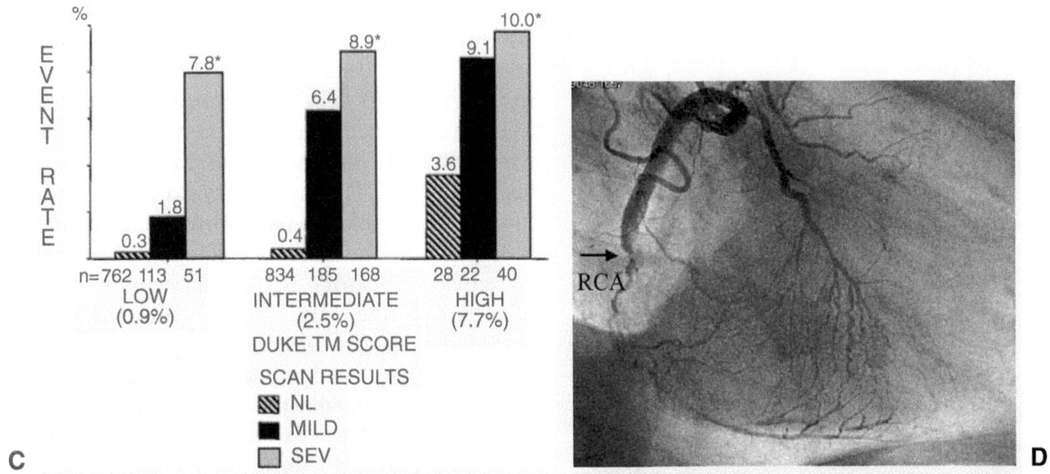

FIGURE C4-1. (C and D) (C, from Hachamovitch, Berman, Kiat, et al. [10], by permission of *Circulation*.)

may be atypical (i.e., arm pain) or silent (no pain at all). Treadmill exercise does not always induce chest pain in patients with severe CAD.

2. A pattern of multivessel disease on MPI is associated with a high risk of cardiac events independent of normal or borderline ST segment changes during exercise.

The presence of RBBB may decrease the sensitivity and specificity of ECG to detect ischemia in the right precordial leads, and this should be taken into account in patients with a high pretest probability for CAD.

3. Multivessel disease indicated by large reversible defects on SPECT imaging and associated with depressed LV function is an indication for myocardial revascularization.

Interpretation

Multivessel disease with indication for surgical revascularization, demonstrated by exercise/rest ^{99m}Tc-MIBI, despite borderline changes on ECG.

Case 4.2

History

An 85-year-old man with CHF and poor exercise tolerance but no risk factors for CAD was referred for MPI using rest/stress ^{99m}Tc-MIBI same day protocol. He complained of occasional exertional chest pain. His resting ECG showed LBBB. He underwent dipyridamole infusion, and the stress/rest SPECT images are displayed in Figure C4-2A.

Findings

A large severe fixed perfusion defect is seen in the inferior wall consistent with a prior MI. In addition, there is mild reversible decreased uptake in the lateral wall extending to the anterolateral region, consistent with myocardial ischemia.

This patient underwent coronary angiography demonstrating critical lesion of the LCX (Figure C4-2B) and an occluded RCA (not shown). He underwent successful stenting of the LCX.

Discussion

The use of vasodilator pharmacological stress rather than exercise was important in this patient because of the presence of LBBB. Conventional exercise stress testing is nondiagnostic in patients with LBBB, because ischemic ST-segment shifts cannot be detected in the presence of LBBB. The Framingham study has

A

B

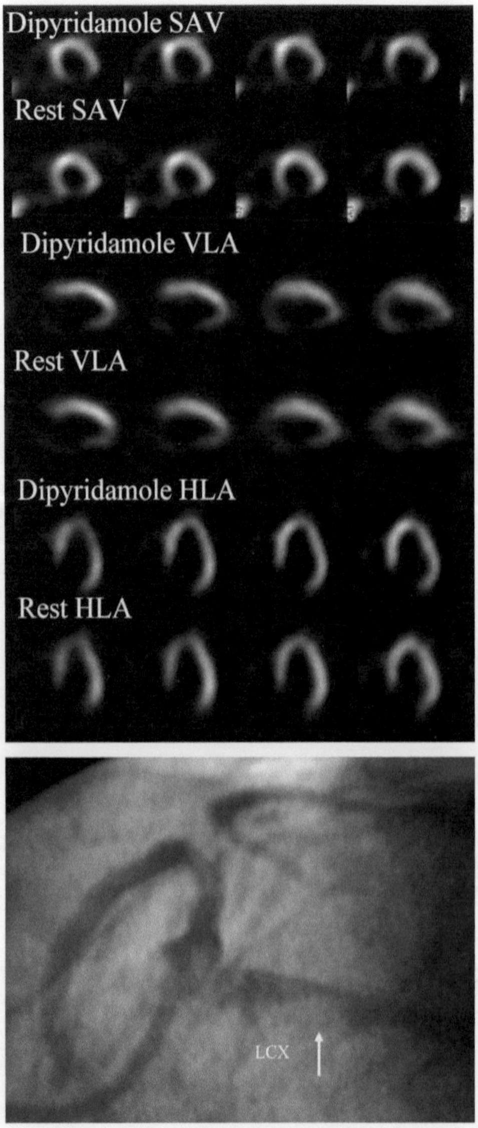

FIGURE C4-2. (A and B)

shown that the occurrence of LBBB in patients with underlying CAD is a strong predictor of mortality,[120] while LBBB in the absence of CAD is associated with a better prognosis.[121] Myocardial perfusion scintigraphy offers a sensitive noninvasive diagnostic technique for the detection of ischemia in patients with abnormal resting ECG including LBBB. Septal wall motion abnormalities occur often in relation to asynchronous contraction of the right and then the left ventricle in patients with LBBB. Exercise may induce perfusion defect involving the anteroseptal and septal region in the absence of significant CAD because the early septal contraction may result in decreased diastolic septal perfusion and result in a reversible septal perfusion defect.[122] The most likely explanation for this finding is delayed perfusion of the septum in LBBB and shortening of diastole when HR increases. Myocardial perfusion occurs in diastole and as the HR increases the diastolic period decreases.[122] As the septum would be the last to be filled in patients with LBBB, a decrease in the diastolic period affects the septum to a greater extent, therefore causing decreased perfusion during exercise. Exercise increases the delay between right and left ventricular activation relative to the duration of systole and would be expected to produce reversible perfusion defects more frequently than dipyridamole or adenosine. Dipyridamole or adenosine increases the HR only slightly, on average approximately 10% of the baseline value, and therefore does not induce artifacts to the same extent as exercise or dobutamine.[123]

Another interesting aspect in this case is that the etiology of CHF was unknown until the ^{99m}Tc-MIBI study was performed. MPI showed evidence of a prior inferior MI, which was silent (there was no history of MI), in addition to ischemia, involving more than one coronary branch. Therefore, CHF is most likely due to ischemic cardiomyopathy. LV function may improve significantly following myocardial revascularization in patients with large areas of ischemic and dysfunctional myocardium, due to hibernation.

Main Teaching Points of Case 4.2

1. Patients with LBBB, as well as those with pacemakers, should be studied using vasodilators stress (dipyridamole or adenosine), which increase the specificity of ischemic findings in the anteroseptal and septal regions. Stress modalities that increase significantly the HR, such as exercise or dobutamine may cause false-positive findings on MPI.

2. Patients with CHF should be thoroughly investigated, attempting to determine its etiol-

ogy. If CHF is a result of ischemic cardiomyopathy, patients can be considered for myocardial revascularization, potentially improving LV function and impacting both morbidity and mortality.

Interpretation

RCA infarct and LCX ischemia demonstrated by dipyridamole ^{99m}Tc-MIBI in a patient with LBBB.

Case 4.3

History

A 58-year-old man with hypertension and hypercholesterolemia was referred for MPI with typical chest pain on exertion. The indication was to determine ischemic burden and cardiac risk. Because of limited exercise capacity, he was stressed with a protocol of dipyridamole combined with low workload exercise. Dipyridamole was infused IV over 4 minutes. Three minutes into the infusion, exercise was started on the treadmill using the Kattus protocol (see Table 4-3). The baseline BP was 130/80 mm Hg and HR was 83 bpm. In the first stage the BP increases to 140/80 but soon drops to 100/60 mmHg as the workload is increased to the second stage (2.0 mph and 10% inclination). His HR did not increase over 100 bpm. The patient started having chest pain, became pale, diaphoretic, and complained of nausea. ^{99m}Tc-MIBI was injected and exercise halted. At this point, the ECG showed a 2-mm downsloping ST-segment depression in V4, V5, V6, DII, and AVF. The patient recovered after administration of 250 mg of aminophylline IV and 0.4 mg of nitroglycerin sublingually. Exercise plus dipyridamole/rest SPECT images are displayed in Figure C4-3.

Findings

The SPECT images demonstrate severe decreased uptake in the inferior wall with stress and partial reversibility at rest. In addition, moderately decreased uptake in the anterolateral, lateral, and inferolateral regions improved at rest. The poststress gated SPECT images revealed akinesia of the inferior wall. These findings are consistent with multi-vessel CAD, with the most critical area being the inferior wall.

Based on these findings, the patient was admitted and referred for coronary angiography showing an occluded RCA (with some collaterals from the left coronary circulation), an 80% proximal LAD lesion, a 90% proximal diagonal lesion, a 90% LCX lesion, and a 90% proximal first marginal. The patient was referred for multivessel CABG.

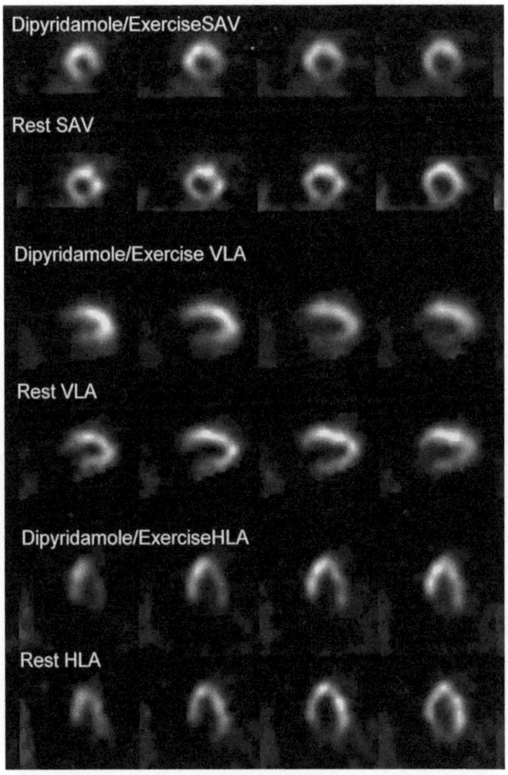

FIGURE C4-3.

Discussion

This patient had a low exercise tolerance but was not unable to do physical stress; therefore, a pharmacological stress combined with low workload exercise was chosen. The Kattus protocol was a good choice for a patient with poor exercise tolerance, compared with Ellestad or Bruce protocol. Combining exercise and vasodilator stress allowed evaluation with MPI at near maximum vasodilatation, from the dipyridamole infusion, and provided hemodynamic information related to the exercise test, all indicative of a poor prognosis: (1) ST-segment depression on low workload,[49] (2) decrease in BP,[124] and (3) blunted HR response to exercise.[125]

Main Teaching Points of Case 4.3

1. Some patients referred for pharmacological stress can perform low-level exercise, and for these patients low workload exercise should be added to vasodilator stimulation.

2. Significant ST-segment depression at low workload exercise is associated with severe CAD and poor prognosis.[49]

3. When exercise is added to dipyridamole, the BP and HR should increase. A drop of BP and a blunted HR response to exercise (if the patient is not taking beta-blockers or calcium antagonists) are indicative of severe CAD.

4. In cases of mild or equivocal findings on scintigraphy, the information provided by the exercise portion of the study, may be helpful in clinical decision making.[126]

Interpretation

Multivessel CAD demonstrated by combined dipyridamole-low workload exercise ^{99m}Tc-MIBI.

Case 4.4

History

A 73-year-old man with a history of hypertension and non-insulin-dependent diabetes for the last 15 years presented with dyspnea on exertion. Four months earlier, he underwent a TMT that was negative for ischemia. Considering the higher incidence of silent ischemia in diabetic patients, he was referred for MPI. Because of his limited exercise tolerance, a protocol of dipyridamole infusion combined with low workload exercise was performed using the Kattus protocol. Dipyridamole infusion preceded the initiation of exercise, as described in Cases 4.3 and 5.6.[33] As sometimes occurs during a combined protocol, the patient exceeded the MPHR at 135 bpm. During exertion he denied chest pain. His resting ECG is shown in Figure C4-4A. His ECG during exercise is shown in Figure C4-4B, and his ECG at recovery (still under effect of dipyridamole) is shown in Figure C4-4C. Aminophylline was given IV and the ECG changes resolved (Figure C4-4D). ^{99m}Tc-MIBI was injected and the stress/rest SPECT images are displayed in Figure C4-4E.

Findings

His resting ECG is unremarkable. His ECG during exercise shows upsloping ST-segment depression. After exercise was interrupted, a repeat ECG clearly shows severe ST-segment elevation from V2 to V6. After administration of aminophylline, the ST changes resolved. The ^{99m}Tc-MIBI SPECT images demonstrate a moderate reversible defect involving the mid and distal anterior wall and septum, extending into the apex. This finding is consistent with a mid LAD lesion, which was confirmed by coronary angiography and intravascular ultrasound (Figures C4-4F and C4-4G). The patient underwent stenting of the LAD with good results confirmed by IVUS (Figure C4-4H).

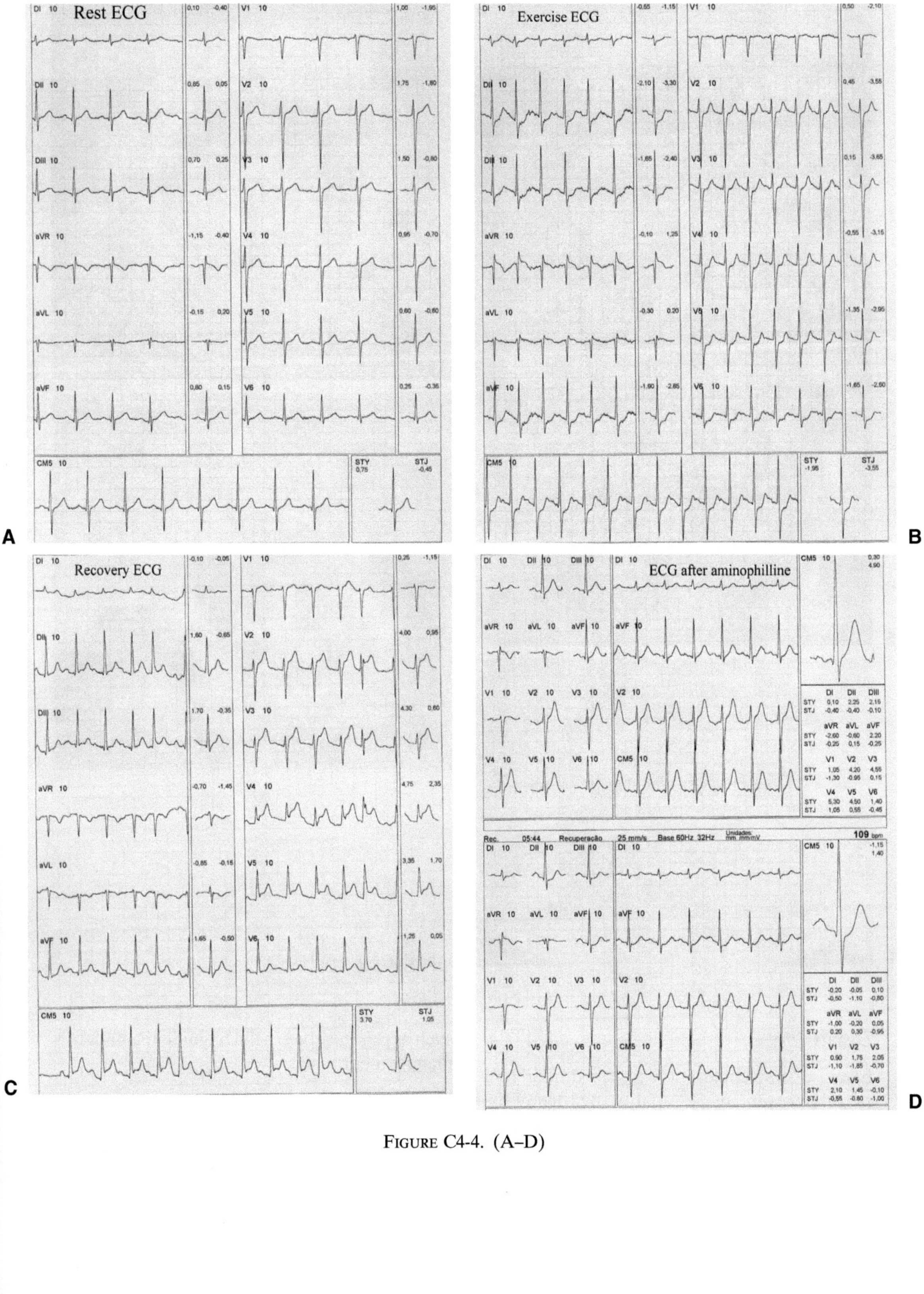

FIGURE C4-4. (A–D)

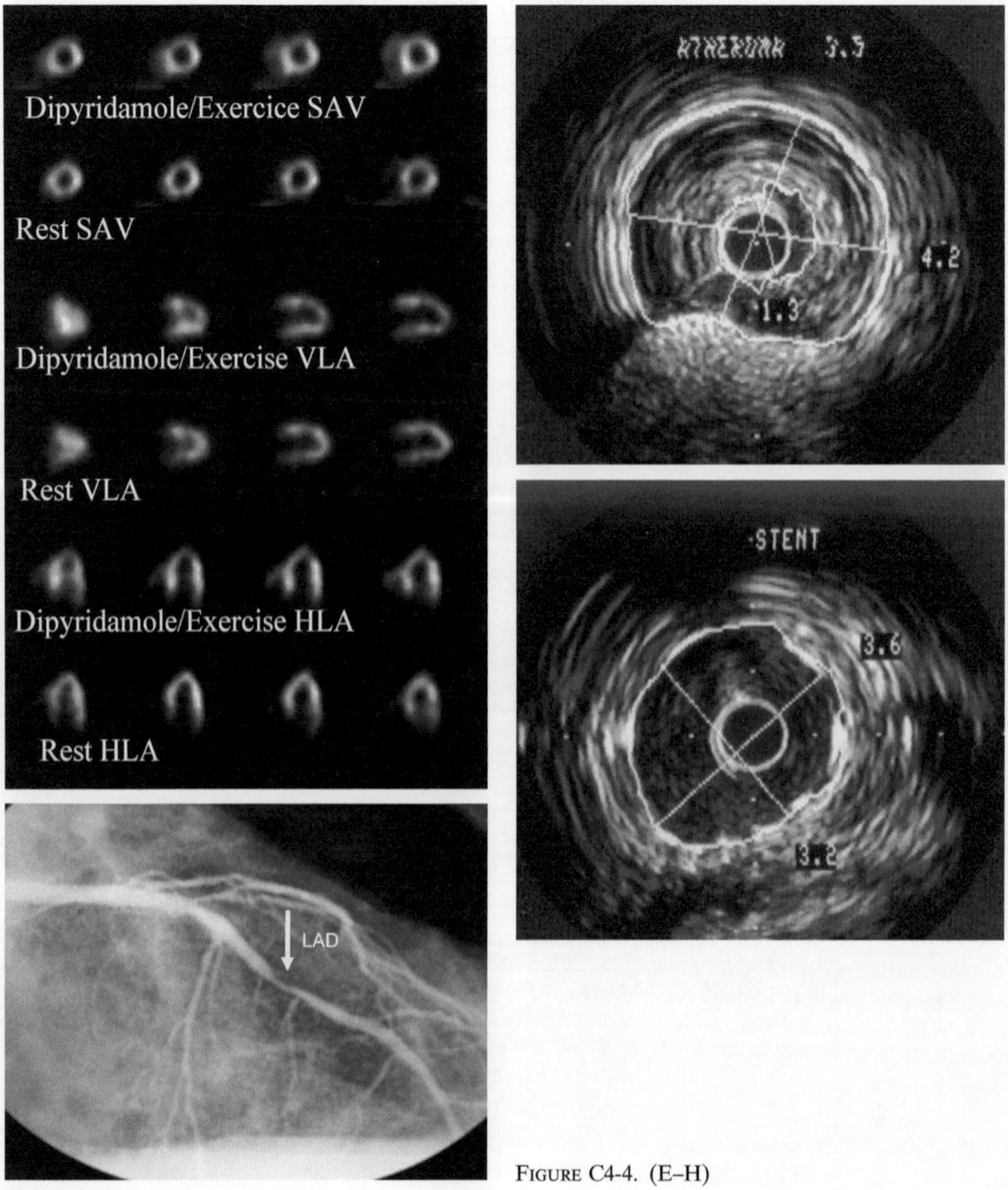

E F G H

FIGURE C4-4. (E–H)

Discussion

Exercise supplementation to vasodilator infusion improves image quality by decreasing splanchnic blood flow and therefore hepatic and intestinal tracer uptake.[33] In addition, exercise provided additional information about the severity of CAD in this patient. When the images are equivocal, additional information such as this may be crucial to guide the patient's management.

Interpretation

LAD ischemia demonstrated by combined dipyridamole-low exercise ^{99m}Tc-MIBI SPECT, causing severe ST-segment elevation reversed by aminophylline administration.

Case 4.5

History

A 53-year-old man with a history of diabetes, hypercholesterolemia, and chronic tobacco use presented with dyspnea on exertion and recent onset of heart failure, but denied any history of angina. Due to the presence of COPD, he underwent dobutamine infusion, to a maximum dose of 30 mcg/kg/min with 1.0 mg of atropine supplementation. His HR increased from 88 to 146 bpm. During the test he complained of chest pain, which resolved 1 minute into recovery. ^{99m}Tc-MIBI was injected at a HR of 146 bpm. The dobutamine/rest ^{99m}Tc-MIBI images are displayed in Figure C4-5A and the ECG during dobutamine infusion is shown in Figure C4-5B.

Findings

The dobutamine stress ECG (Figure C4-5B) demonstrates ST-segment elevation of approximately 2 mm on II, III, and AVF and 1.5 mm in V6. This severe ST-segment change persisted until 6 minutes into recovery. These transient changes are consistent with severe transmural ischemia.

The SPECT images show a large severe reversible perfusion defect involving the entire anteroseptal region and apex and also a moderately reduced reversible defect in the inferoseptal and inferolateral regions. Gated SPECT images (not shown) revealed diffuse LV hypokinesia and an LVEF of 21%.

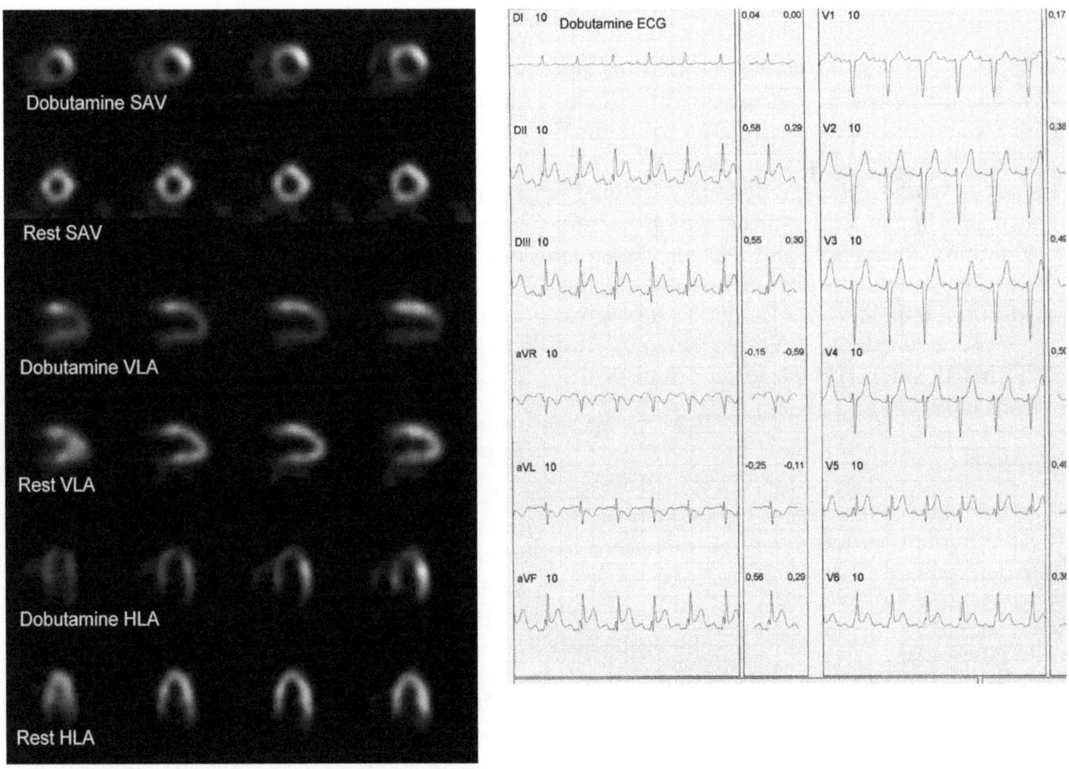

A

B

FIGURE C4-5. (A and B)

Discussion

Dobutamine ECG is relatively poorly sensitive for ischemia but is highly specific.[71] The multi-vessel perfusion defect pattern and depressed LV function indicate multi-vessel CAD. This patient underwent coronary angiography, which revealed severe three-vessel CAD, and surgical revascularization was indicated.

Main Teaching Points of Case 4.5

1. Dobutamine infusion is reserved for patients unable to exercise and who have a contraindication for adenosine or dipyridamole infusion, usually COPD.
2. Dobutamine administration is safe and results in MPI studies with good sensitivity, specificity, and accuracy for establishing the diagnosis and prognosis of CAD.
3. With dobutamine, ECG changes are uncommon, but have high specificity when they occur. ST-segment elevation occurs even less frequently than ST-segment depression but is indicative of severe CAD, causing transmural ischemia.
4. A patient with depressed LV function and evidence of significant 3-vessel disease is in a high-risk category for cardiac events, as demonstrated in the CASS study[119] and should be considered for revascularization.

Interpretation

Extensive 3-vessel disease and ischemic cardiomyopathy demonstrated by dobutamine ^{99m}Tc-MIBI.

Case 4.6

History

A 78-year-old woman with hypertension and hypercholesterolemia presented with significant fatigue and weakness related to minimal exertion but she denied chest pain. She had a history of cardiac bradyarrhythmias and had a pacemaker implanted 1 year before the current evaluation. Considering her old age and risk factors, her attending physician is considering myocardial ischemia with fatigue as a possible "anginal equivalent." A dipyridamole/rest ^{99m}Tc-MIBI study was performed and is displayed in Figure C4-6.

Findings

The rest and stress SPECT images demonstrated normal perfusion.

Discussion

The patient was evaluated using dipyridamole as stimuli for vasodilatation because of her pacemaker. As in LBBB, pacemaker implanted in the right ventricle may lead to an anteroseptal and septal artifact at increased HR during exercise, which was not seen in this case using dipyridamole. Gated SPECT was attempted but synchronization was difficult to obtain due to the wide QRS complex, and it was opted to abort the gating to obtain better quality perfusion images. When gating is suboptimal, leading to significant beat rejection, gating itself may lead to artifacts on the perfusion images; therefore, in these cases, it is better to obtain ungated images. Gating problems are further discussed in Case 13.6.

Main Teaching Point of Case 4.6

1. Patients with pacemakers implanted in the right ventricle should be studied with vasodilators (dipyridamole or adenosine) to avoid artifacts similar to what is seen with LBBB.

Interpretation

Normal dipyridamole/rest ^{99m}Tc-MIBI SPECT is seen in a patient with a pacemaker.

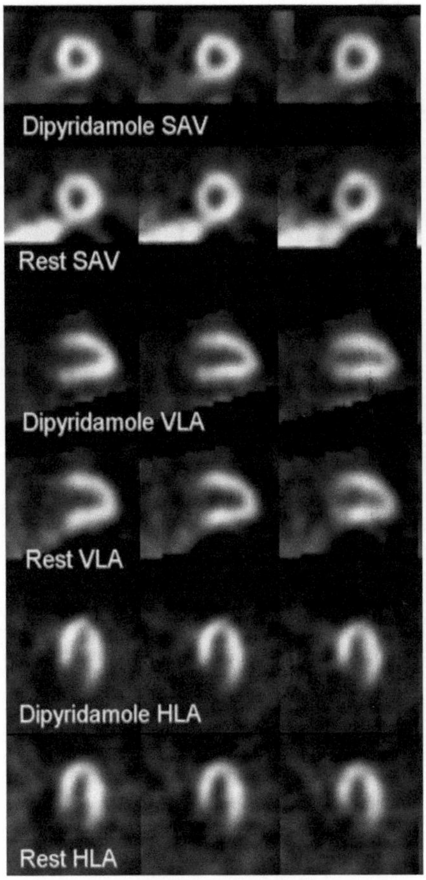

FIGURE C4-6.

Case 4.7

History

A 75-year-old white woman presented with occasional chest pain at rest and severe fatigue on exertion. Her physician was concerned that her symptoms may be related to myocardial ischemia with fatigue as anginal equivalent. She has a past history of hypertension, well controlled with beta-blockers. She also has degenerative joint disease involving the right knee, which limits her exercise capacity and knee surgery was being considered. An adenosine/rest ^{99m}Tc-MIBI study is displayed in Figure C4-7A.

Findings

Adenosine SPECT images demonstrate moderately decreased uptake involving the anterior, lateral, and inferior walls of the myocardium. All these defects resolved on the resting images. During adenosine infusion a short period of complete AV block was observed.

Discussion

The SPECT findings are consistent with multivessel ischemia. The patient underwent

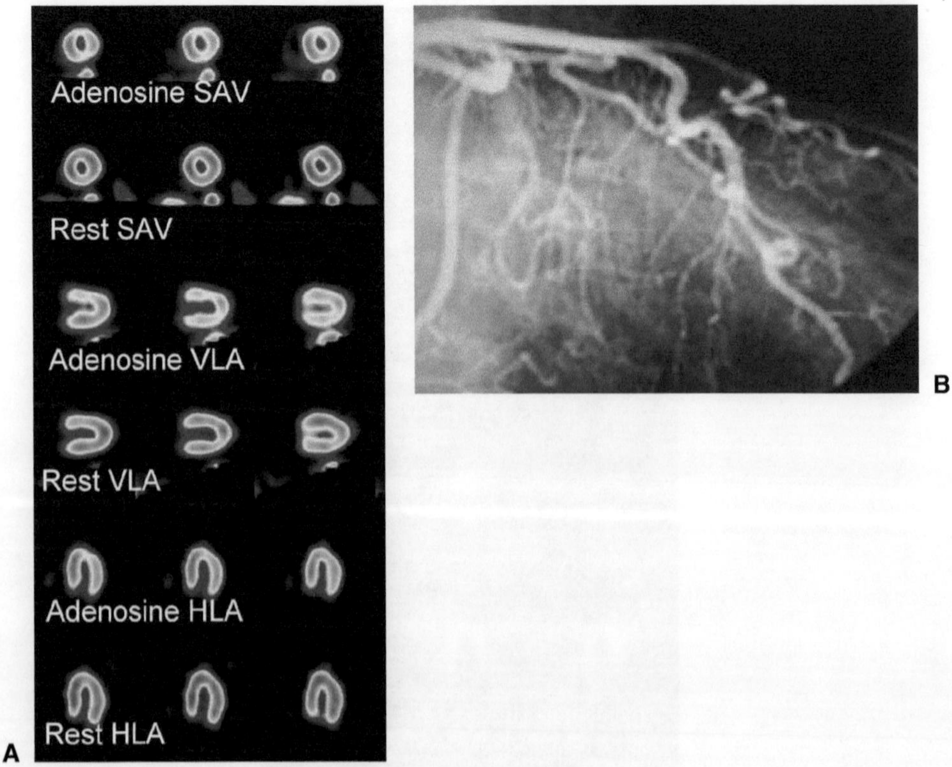

FIGURE C4-7. (A and B)

coronary angiography that demonstrated very tortuous vessels (Figure C4-7B) and slow blood flow, but no obstructive lesions were identified in epicardial vessels. This case was interpreted as significant microvascular disease with probably a severe degree of endothelial dysfunction. The potential role of myocardial perfusion for evaluation of endothelial dysfunction is further discussed in Chapter 17.

Interpretation

Multivessel CAD demonstrated with adenosine ^{99m}Tc-MIBI with no obstruction in epicardial vessels but slow flow and tortuous coronary arteries on angiography suggesting endothelial dysfunction.

Case 4.8

History

Figures C4-8A and C4-8B display an anterior view of the cine-loop display of the stress SPECT images of two different patients who underwent stress/rest MPI for atypical chest pain. How can the differences be explained?

Findings

In Figure C4-8A, there is marked uptake in the liver, whereas in Figure 4-8B, most of the radiopharmaceutical has cleared from the liver and is located in the gallbladder and the bowel.

A 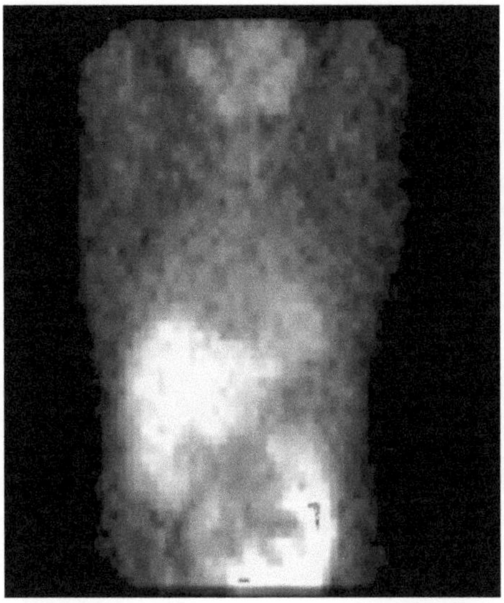

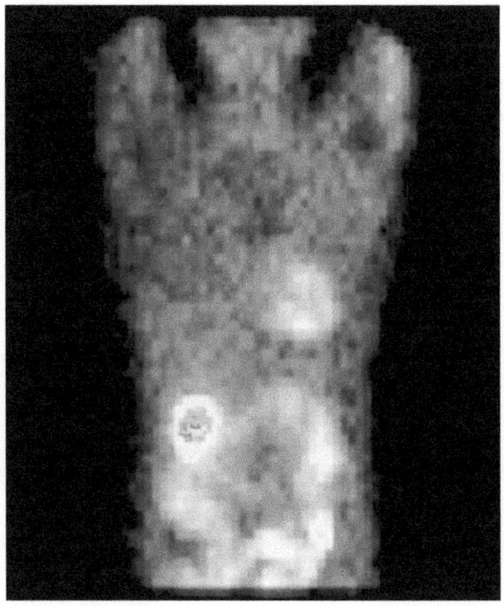 B

FIGURE C4-8. (A and B)

Discussion

Different forms of stress were used in these two patients. The patient in Figure C4-8A was injected with ^{99m}Tc-MIBI during vasodilator (dipyridamole) infusion and the patient in Figure C4-8B during active exercise on the treadmill. In both sets of images, the perfusion radiopharmaceutical was ^{99m}Tc-MIBI. One problem with ^{99m}Tc perfusion radiopharmaceuticals, both MIBI and tetrofosmin, is predominant excretion by the hepatobiliary system, while ^{201}Tl is predominantly excreted by the kidneys. A number of factors influence hepatic uptake of the ^{99m}Tc-perfusion radiopharmaceuticals. The main factors are:

1. Type of radiopharmaceutical: Tetrofosmin clears slightly more rapidly than MIBI.

2. Stress/rest: Dynamic exercise decreases splanchnic blood flow with resultant decrease in gastrointestinal and hepatic uptake. Vasodilator stress with adenosine and dipyridamole results in increased gastrointestinal and hepatic uptake. The addition of submaximal exercise to adenosine or dipyridamole stress tends to decrease hepatic uptake, resulting in improved heart to liver uptake ratio as compared with vasodilator stress alone,[33] allowing acquisition of good quality images earlier after stress than with vasodilator alone.[47]

3. Fasting state: A fatty meal empties the gallbladder but does not affect hepatic clearance of the radiopharmaceutical. In fact, clearance from the gallbladder into the bowel occasionally causes more interference if the activity is located in a bowel loop adjacent to the heart at the time of imaging.

4. Individual variation on hepatic clearance.

The effect of active exercise on regional blood flow has been described by Mitchell and Blomqvist[127] (Figure C4-8C). Physical exercise promotes a significant increase in blood flow to the heart, a major increase in flow to the exercising muscles, and vasoconstriction of the cutaneous and gastrointestinal (hepatic) vasculature. Dipyridamole and adenosine do increase blood flow to the heart but also to the splanchnic circulation, which consequently increases hepatic uptake of the radiopharmaceutical. Post-exercise images can be acquired almost immediately after termination of the exercise and recovery due to the exercise-induced vasoconstriction of splanchnic blood flow. But acquisition of vasodilator stress images must be delayed until hepatic activity has decreased to that less than myocardial

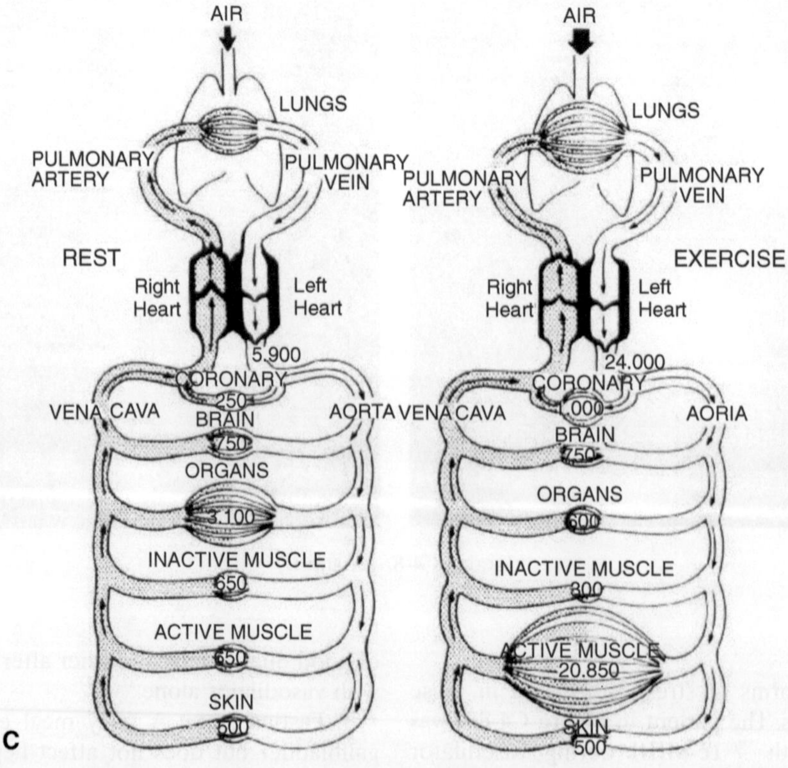

FIGURE C4-8. (C, from Mitchell and Blomqvist [127], by permission of *N Engl J Med.*)

activity. This time period is variable, but 45 to 90 minutes is recommended. Therefore, it is recommended that more time be allowed before imaging after vasodilator stress than exercise to let the radiopharmaceutical clear from the liver and the gastrointestinal tract. Activity in a loop of bowel adjacent to the inferior wall of the heart can create more artifact than hepatic uptake. Therefore, stimulating gallbladder contraction and emptying into the bowel with fatty food or cholecystokinin is not recommended. Ingestion of a full meal and copious liquid after pharmacological stress and before imaging is often helpful, dilating the stomach and displacing any intestinal radioactivity inferiorly away from the heart.[128]

Interpretation

Differential hepatic and gastrointestinal uptake of ^{99m}Tc-MIBI after exercise and dypiridamole stress.

Case 4.9

History

A 50-year-old man with diabetes, hypertension, hypercholesterolemia, and a history of MI 1 year earlier presented with progressive dyspnea. His physician suspected that dyspnea was an anginal equivalent and MPI was performed for risk stratification. Due to his very limited exercise capacity, a pharmacologic study was done using dipyridamole. His resting and dipyridamole ECG are shown in Figures C4-9A and C4-9B. His SPECT dipyridamole/rest ^{99m}Tc-MIBI images are shown in Figure C4-9C.

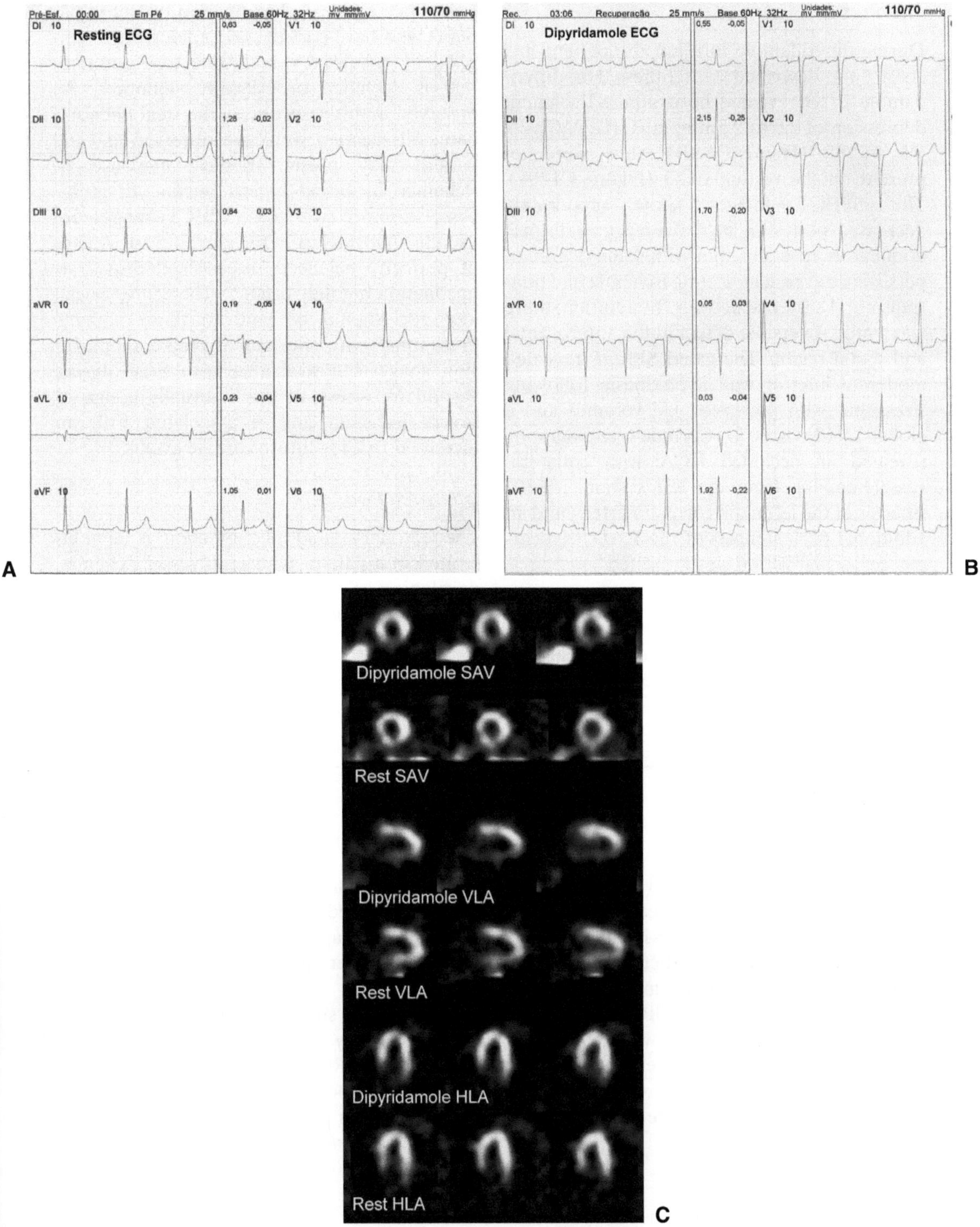

FIGURE C4-9. (A–C)

Findings

During dipyridamole infusion the patient had chest pain, described as tightness. His dipyridamole ECG revealed horizontal ST-segment depression of 2.0 to 2.5mm, in II, III, AVF, V4, V5, and V6 (Figure C4-9B), which were not present on the resting ECG (Figure C4-9A). The SPECT images show moderately decreased perfusion in the inferior wall, predominantly reversible but with some degree of persistence at rest, indicating ischemia and nontransmural scar, respectively. In addition, there was a mild reversible defect in the anteroseptal and septal region. The gated SPECT revealed moderate inferior wall hypokinesia following stress, but with preserved LV volumes and a global LVEF of 60%. Coronary angiography revealed an occluded RCA with collateral vessels coming from the left system, a 65% stenosis of the left main coronary artery, and an additional 60% stenosis of the LAD. Myocardial revascularization was indicated.

Discussion

This case illustrates well the coronary steal phenomenon, which occurs in patients with severe ischemia. The steal phenomenon occurs in patients who have part of their myocardium supplied by collateral vessels, due to a coronary that is occluded or critically stenotic.[129] As observed in this case, during the steal phenomenon, ST-segment shifts are observed and the patient may present clinical evidence of ischemia, including typical angina. In multivessel disease, stress/rest SPECT images are usually abnormal as in the current case. A case of perfectly balanced three-vessel disease is uncommon but may occur.[130] Therefore, special attention should be paid to those patients presenting with normal myocardial perfusion images but with a positive ECG during vasodilator stress, as this is usually a sign of severe ischemia and is associated with an increased risk for future cardiac events.[131,132]

Interpretation

The coronary steal phenomenon is demonstrated in a patient with multivessel ischemia, developing ST-segment depression during dipyridamole infusion.

Case 4.10

History

A 53-year-old woman presented with midsternal chest pain and shortness of breath. The patient had multiple cardiac risk factors including hypertension, tobacco abuse, diabetes, and family history of CAD. The patient underwent a rest/adenosine ^{99m}Tc-tetrofosmin SPECT study for risk stratification. The patient was treated with atenolol and verapamil for her hypertension. The adenosine/rest ^{99m}Tc-tetrofosmin gated SPECT study is shown in Figure C4-10A.

Findings

The study showed homogeneous perfusion throughout the myocardium with no scintigraphic evidence of ischemia or infarction. The LVEF was 36% with global hypokinesis. The patient returned to the hospital before her scheduled next appointment with similar symptoms. Given her quick return and continued symptoms, she was referred for coronary angiography, as shown in Figure C4-10C.

The coronary angiography showed a focal 70% proximal RCA stenosis and 30% mid and distal LAD stenosis. The RCA was stented, and the patient was discharged home. The patient became chest pain free.

Discussion

This patient was treated with atenolol and verapamil for hypertension. These medications

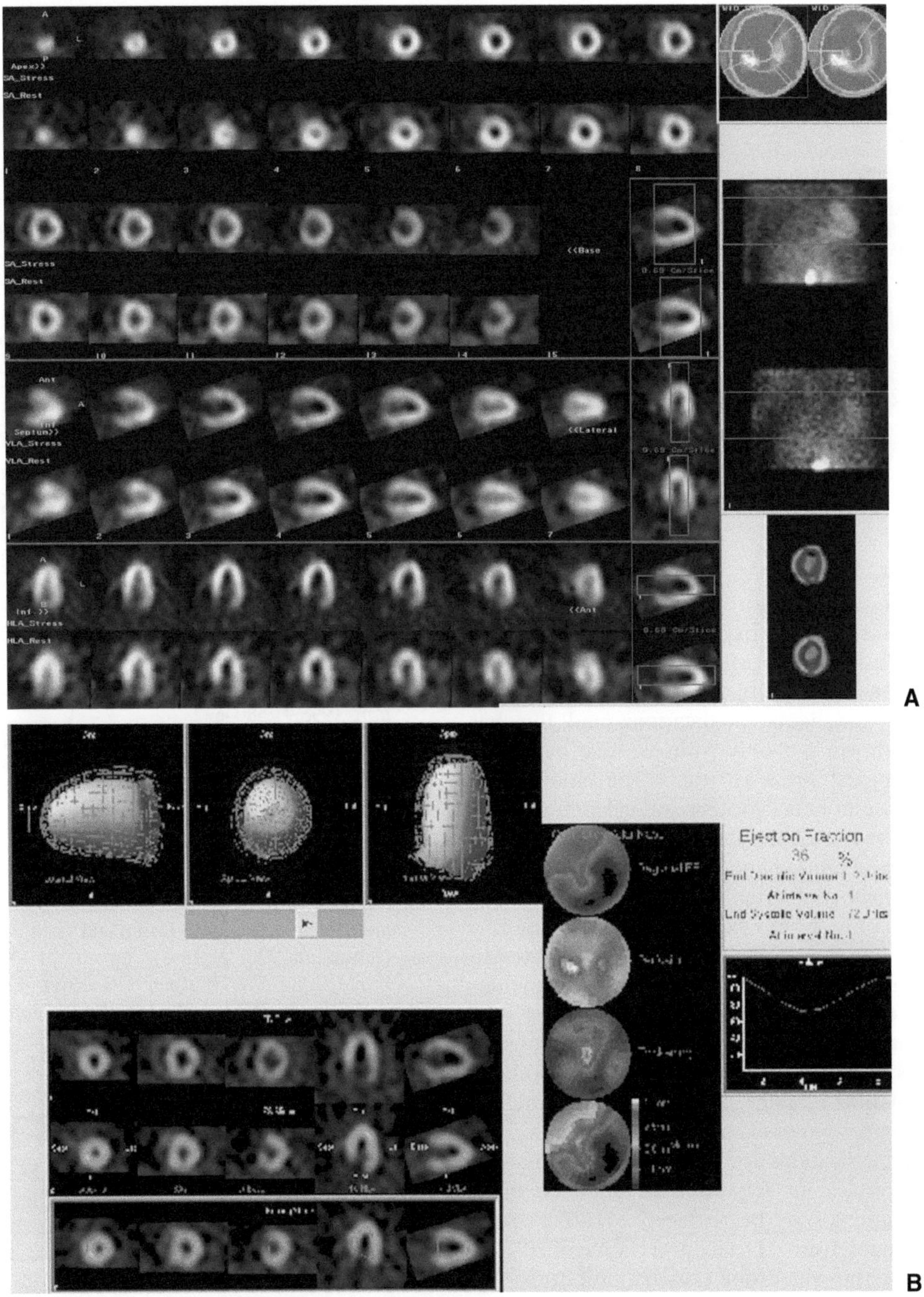

FIGURE C4-10. (A and B)

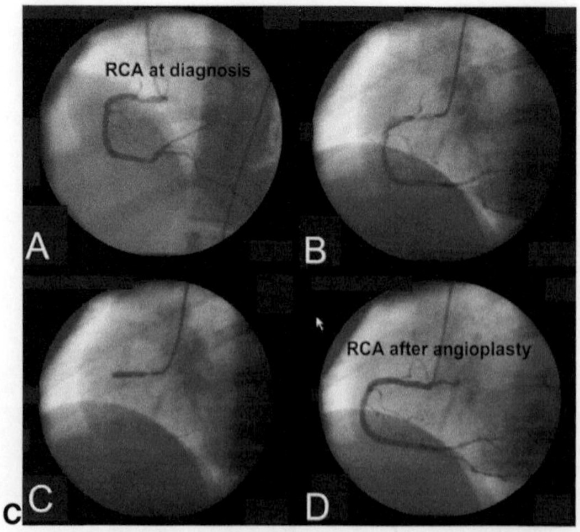

FIGURE C4-10. (C)

were not held before her stress test. Both of these medications have been shown to reduce the sensitivity of rest/stress MPI.[133] The size, number, and severity of defects are lessened by taking antianginal medications, and this has been shown not only with exercise but pharmacological stress as well.[134] The blunted HR response of beta-blockers and calcium channel blockers have been shown to lessen the severity of wall motion abnormalities of dobutamine stress echocardiography.

Certainly when exercise stress is used, a lower hyperemic response can be predicted in the presence of drugs that blunted augmentation of oxygen consumption. However, the mechanism by which these same antianginal drugs interfere with the effects of vasodilator stimulation remains unclear.[134] As a practical approach, patients should discontinue the same medications for pharmacologic stress as for exercise. In hypertensive patients, these medications may be replaced by others such as angiotensin II receptor antagonists or angiotensin-converting enzyme inhibitors.

Interpretation

1. False-negative adenosine ^{99m}Tc-tetrofosmin study performed in a patient on beta-blockers and calcium channel inhibitors.
2. Two-vessel CAD with 70% proximal RCA stenosis was diagnosed, which was amenable to percutaneous coronary intervention.

References

1. Enos WF, Holmes RH, Beyer J. Coronary disease among United States soldiers killed in action in Korea: preliminary report. *JAMA.* 1986;256:2859–2862.
2. McNamara JJ, Molot MA, Stremple JF, Cutting RT. Coronary artery disease in combat casualties in Vietnam. *JAMA.* 1971;216:1185–1187.
3. Tuzcu EM, Kapadia SR, Tutar E, et al. High prevalence of coronary atherosclerosis in asymptomatic teenagers and young adults—evidence from intravascular ultrasound. *Circulation.* 2001;103:2705–2710.
4. Gibbons RJ. ACC/AHA 2002 guidelines update for exercise testing. www.acc.org.
5. Fletcher GF, Balagy G, Froelicher VF, et al. Exercise standards: a statement for healthcare professionals from the American Heart Association writing group—special report. *Circulation.* 1995;91:580–622.
6. Stuart RJ, Ellestad MH. National survey of exercise stress testing facilities. *Chest.* 1980;77:94–97.
7. Borg GA. Psychophysical basis of perceived exertion. *Med Sci Sports Exerc.* 1982;14:377–381.
8. Berman DS, Hayes SW, Germano G. Assessment of myocardial perfusion and viability with technetium-99m perfusion agents. In Depuey EG, Garcia EV, Berman DS (eds). *Cardiac SPECT Imaging.* Philadelphia: Lippincott Williams & Wilkins; 2001:179–210.
9. Mark DB, Hlatky MA, Harrell FE Jr, et al. Exercise treadmill score for predicting prognosis in coronary artery disease. *Ann Intern Med.* 1987;106:793–800.
10. Hachamovitch R, Berman DS, Kiat H, et al. Exercise myocardial perfusion SPECT in patients without known coronary artery disease: incremental prognostic value and use in risk stratification. *Circulation.* 1996; 93(5):905–914.
11. Myers J, Prakash M, Froelicher V, et al. Exercise capacity and mortality among men referred for exercise testing. *N Engl J Med.* 2002; 336(11):793–801.
12. Metra M, Faggiano P, D'Aloi, et al. Use of cardiopulmonary exercise testing with hemo-

dynamic monitoring in the prognostic assessment of ambulatory patients with chronic heart failure. *J Am Coll Cardiol.* 1999;33:943–950.

13. Travin MI, Wexler JP. Pharmacological stress testing. *Semin Nucl Med.* 1999;29:298–318.
14. Cohen MC. A snapshot of nuclear cardiology in the United States. *Am Soc Nucl Cardiol Newsletter.* 1998;5:13.
15. Smits P, Corstens FHM, Aengevaeren WRM, Wackers FJT, Thien T. False negative dipyridamole-thallium-201 myocardial imaging after caffeine ingestion. *J Nucl Med.* 1991;32:1538–1541.
16. Henzlova M, Squire A, Kim-Schuleger L, et al. Screening for coronary artery disease prior to liver transplantation. *J Nucl Cardiol.* 2003; 10(1):S-54.
17. O'Byrne, Rodriguez EA, Maddahi J, et al. Comparison of myocardial washout rate of thallium-201 between rest, dipyridamole with and without aminophylline, and exercise states in normal subjects. *Am J Cardiol.* 1989;64:1022–1028.
18. Wilson RF, White CW. Intracoronary papaverine: an ideal coronary vasodilator for studies of the coronary circulation in conscious humans. *Circulation.* 1986,73:444–451.
19. Picano E, Lattanzi F, Masini M, Distante A, L'Abbate A. High dose dipyridamole echocardiography test in effort angina pectoris. *J Am Coll Cardiol.* 1986;8:848–854.
20. Lette J, Tatum JL, Fraser S, et al. Safety of dipyridamole testing in 73,806 patients: the multicenter dipyridamole safety study. *J Nucl Cardiol.* 1995;2:3–17.
21. Ranhosky A, Kempthorne-Rawson J. The safety of intravenous dipyridamole thallium myocardial perfusion imaging: intravenous dipyridamole thallium imaging study group. *Circulation.* 1990;81:1205–1209.
22. Hachamovitch RJ, Hayes S, Friedman JD, et al. Determinants of risk and its temporal variation in patients with normal stress myocardial perfusion scans—what is the warranty period of a normal scan? *J Am Coll Cardiol.* 2003;41:1329–1340.
23. Feldman RL, Nichols WM, Pepine CJ, Conti CR. Acute effects of intravenous dipyridamole on regional coronary hemodynamics and metabolism. *Circulation.* 1981;64:333–334.
24. Treuth MG, Reyes GA, He ZX, et al. Tolerance and diagnostic accuracy of an abbreviated adenosine infusion for myocardial scintigraphy: a randomized prospective study. *J Nucl Cardiol.* 2001;8:548–554.
25. Abreu A, Mahmarian JJ, Nishimura S, et al. Tolerance and safety of pharmacologic coronary vasodilation with adenosine in association with thallium-201 scintigraphy in patients with coronary artery disease. *J Am Coll Cardiol.* 1991;18: 730–735.
26. Cerqueira MD, Verani MS, Schwaiger M, et al. Safety profile of adenosine stress perfusion imaging: results from the Adenoscan multicenter trial registry. *J Am Coll Cardiol.* 1994;23: 384–390.
27. Johnston DL. Hemodynamic responses and adverse effects associated with adenosine and dipyridamole pharmacologic stress testing: a comparison in 2000 patients. *Mayo Clin Proc.* 1995;70:331–336.
28. Coyne EP, Belvedere DA, Vande-Streek PR, et al. Thallium-201 scintigraphy after intravenous infusion of adenosine compared with exercise thallium testing in the diagnosis of coronary artery disease. *J Am Coll Cardiol.* 1991;17(6): 1289–1294.
29. Verani MS, Mahmarian JJ, Hisxon JB, et al. Diagnosis of coronary artery disease by controlled coronary vasodilation with adenosine and thallium-201 scintigraphy in patients unable to exercise. *Circulation.* 1990;82(1):80–87.
30. O'Keefe JH Jr, Bateman TM, Silvestri R, et al. Safety and diagnostic accuracy of adenosine thallium-201 scintigraphy in patients unable to exercise and those with left bundle branch block. *Am Heart J.* 1992;124(3):614–621.
31. Klodas E, Miller TD, Christian TF, et al. Prognostic significance of ischemic electrocardiographic changes during vasodilator stress testing in patients with normal SPECT images. *J Nucl Cardiol.* 2003;10:4–8.
32. Abbott BG, Afshar M, Berger AK, Wackers FJ. Prognostic significance of ischemic electrocardiographic changes during adenosine infusion in patients with normal myocardial perfusion imaging. *J Nucl Cardiol.* 2003;10:9–16.
33. Vitola JV, Brambatti JC, Caligaris F, et al. Exercise supplementation to dipyridamole prevents hypotension, improves electrocardiogram sensitivity, and increases heart-to liver activity ratio on Tc-99m sestamibi imaging. *J Nucl Cardiol.* 2001;8:652–659.
34. Elliot MD, Holly TA, Leonard SM, Hendel RC. Impact of an abbreviated adenosine protocol

incorporating adjunctive treadmill exercise on adverse effects and image quality in patients undergoing stress myocardial perfusion imaging. *J Nucl Cardiol.* 2000;7:584–589.
35. Samady H, Wackers FJ, Joska TM, et al. Pharmacologic stress perfusion imaging with adenosine: role of simultaneous low-level treadmill exercise. *J Nucl Cardiol.* 2002;9: 188–196.
36. Stein L, Burt R, Oppenheim B, Schauwecker D, Fineberg N. Symptom-limited arm exercise increases detection of ischemia during dipyridamole tomographic thallium stress testing in patients with coronary artery disease. *Am J Cardiol.* 1995;75:568–572.
37. Verzijlbergen JF, Vermeersch PH, Laarman Ascoop CA. Inadequate exercise leads to suboptimal imaging after dipyridamole combined with low-level exercise unmasks ischemia in symptomatic patients with non-diagnostic thallium-201 scans who exercise submaximally. *J Nucl Med.* 1991;32:2071–2078.
38. Taillefer R. Technetium-99m sestamibi myocardial imaging: same day rest-stress studies and dipyridamole. *Am J Cardiol.* 1990;66:80E–84E.
39. Bergman H, Bjorntorp P, Conradson TB, Fahlen M, Stenberg J, Varnauskas E. Enzymatic and circulatory adjustments to physical training in middle aged men. *Eur J Clin Invest.* 1973;3: 414–418.
40. Primeau M, Taillefer R, Essiambre R, Lambert R, Honos G. Technetium 99m sestamibi myocardial perfusion imaging: comparison between treadmill, dipyridamole and transesophageal atrial pacing "stress" tests in normal subjects. *Eur J Nucl Med.* 1991;18:247–251.
41. Casale PN, Guiney TE, Strauss W, Boucher CA. Simultaneous low level treadmill exercise and intravenous dipyridamole stress thallium imaging. *Am J Cardiol.* 1988;62:799–802.
42. Ignaszewski AP, McCormick LX, Heslip PG, McEwan AJ, Humen DP. Safety and clinical utility of combined intravenous dipyridamole/ symptom-limited exercise stress test with thallium-201 imaging in patients with known or suspected coronary artery disease. *J Nucl Med.* 1993;34:2053–2061.
43. Laarman G, Niemeyer MG, Van Der Wall EE, Verzijlbergen FJ, Bruschke AV, Ascoop CA. Dipyridamole thallium testing: noncardiac side effects, cardiac effects, electrocardiographic changes and hemodynamic changes after dipyridamole infusion with or without exercise. *Int J Cardiol.* 1988;20:231–238.
44. Hashimoto A, Palmer EL, Scott JA, Abraham SA, Fischman AJ, Force TL, et al. Complications of exercise and pharmacologic stress tests: differences in younger and elderly patients. *J Nucl Cardiol.* 1999;6:612–619.
45. Thomas GS, Prill NV, Majmundar H, et al. Treadmill exercise during adenosine infusion is safe, results in fewer adverse reactions, and improves myocardial perfusion image quality. *J Nucl Cardiol.* 2000;7(5):439–446.
46. Pennell DJ, Mavrogeni SI, Forbat SM, et al. Adenosine combined with dynamic exercise for myocardial perfusion imaging. *J Am Coll Cardiol.* 1995;25(6):1300–1309.
47. Vitola JV, Ludwig V, Cunha Pereira Neto C, et al. Exercise and dipyridamole combined myocardial scintigraphy allows early evaluation of perfusion and function. *J Nucl Cardiol.* 2003; 10(1)S:87.
48. Ebersole DG, Heironimus J, Toney MO, Billingsley J. Comparison of exercise and adenosine technetium—99m sestamibi myocardial scintigraphy for diagnosis of coronary artery disease in patients with left bundle branch block. *Am J Cardiol.* 1993;71:450–453.
49. Ellestad MH (ed). Predictive implication. In Stress Testing: Principles and Practice. New York University Press; 2003:271–307.
50. Holly TA, Satran A, Bromet DS, et al. The impact of adjunctive adenosine infusion during exercise myocardial perfusion imaging: results of both exercise and adenosine stress test. *J Nucl Cardiol.* 2003;10:291–296.
51. Geleijnse ML, Elhendy A, Fioretii PM, Roelandt JR. Dobutamine stress myocardial perfusion imaging. *J Am Coll Cardiol.* 2000;36(7):2017–2020.
52. Tuttle RR, Mills J. Dobutamine: development of a new catecholamine to selectively increase cardiac contractility. *Circ Res.* 1975;36:185–195.
53. Leier CV, Heban PT, Huss P, et al. Comparative systemic and regional hemodynamic effects of dopamine and dobutamine in patients with cardiomyopathic heart failure. *Circulation.* 1978;58:466–475.
54. Mason JR, Palac RT, Freeman ML, et al. Thallium scintigraphy during dobutamine infusion: non exercise-dependent screening test for coronary disease. *Am Heart J.* 1984;107:481–485.
55. Palac RT, Coombs BJ, Kudenchuk PJ, et al. Two-dimensional echocardiography during dobutamine infusion—comparison with exercise testing in evaluation of coronary disease. *Circulation.* 1984;70 Suppl II:184.

56. Secknus MA, Marwick TH. Evolution of dobutamine echocardiography protocols and indications: safety and side effects in 3001 studies over 5 years. *J Am Coll Cardiol.* 1997;29:1234–1240.
57. Leier CV, Unverferth DV. Drugs five years later: dobutamine. *Ann Intern Med.* 1983;99: 490–496.
58. Kates RE, Leier CV. Dobutamine phamacokinetics in severe heart failure. *Clin Pharmacol Ther.* 1978;24:537–541.
59. Raza JA, Reeves WC, Movahed A. Pharmacological stress agents for evaluation of ischemic heart disease. *Int J Cardiol.* 2001;81(2–3):157–167.
60. Tadamura E, Iida H, Matsumoto K, et al. Comparison of myocardial blood flow during dobutamine-atropine infusion with that after dipyridamole administration in normal men. *J Am Coll Cardiol.* 2001;37:130–136.
61. Cancer B, Karanfil A, Uysal U. Effect of an additional atropine injection during dobutamine infusion for myocardial SPECT. *J Nucl Med Comm.* 1997;18:567–573.
62. Elhendy A, Valkema R, Van Domburg RT, et al. Safety of dobutamine-atropine stress myocardial perfusion scintigraphy. *J Nucl Med.* 1998; 39:1662–1666.
63. Dakik HA, Vempathy H, Verani MS. Tolerance, hemodynamic changes and safety of dobutamine stress perfusion imaging. *J Nucl Cardiol.* 1996;3:410–414.
64. Pennel DJ, Underwood RS, Ell PJ. Safety of dobutamine stress for thallium-201 myocardial perfusion tomography in patients with asthma. *Am J Cardiol.* 1993;71:1346–1350.
65. Picano E, Mathias W, Bigi R, Previtali M. Safety and tolerability of dobutamine-atropine stress echocardiography: a prospective, multicenter study. *Lancet.* 1994;344:1190–1192.
66. Elhendy A, Bax JJ, Poldermans D. Dobutamine stress myocardial perfusion imaging in coronary artery disease. *J Nucl Med.* 2002;43:1634–1646.
67. Elhendy A, van Domburg RT, Bax JJ, et al. Safety, hemodynamic profile, and feasibility of dobutamine stress technetium myocardial perfusion single-photon emission CT imaging for evaluation of coronary artery disease in the elderly. *Chest.* 2000;117:649–656.
68. Elhendy A, van Domburg RT, Vantrimpont P, et al. Impact of heart transplantation on the safety and feasibility of the dobutamine stress test. *J Heart Transplant.* 2001;20:399–406.
69. Gallik DM, Mahmarian JJ, Verani MS. Therapeutic significance of exercise-induced ST-segment elevation in patients without previous myocardial infarction. *Am J Cardiol.* 1993;72:1–7.
70. Elhendy A, Geleijnse ML, Roelandt JR, et al. Evaluation by quantitative 99m-technetium MIBI SPECT and echocardiography of myocardial perfusion and wall motion abnormalities in patients with dobutamine-induced ST-segment elevation. *Am J Cardiol.* 1995;76: 441–448.
71. Maiaresse GH, Marwick TH, Vanoverschelde TL, et al. How accurate is dobutamine stress eletrocardiography for detection of coronary artery disease? *J Am Coll Cardiol.* 1994;24:920–927.
72. Yun JJ, Wu JC, Heller EN, et al. Dobutamine stress has limited value for enhancing flow heterogeneity in the presence of a moderate stenosis when used in conjunction with Tc-99m sestamibi imaging (abstract). *J Am Coll Cardiol.* 1995;25(supp A):217A.
73. Mirta R, Kazuya T, Frank D, et al. Arbutamine stress perfusion imaging in dogs with critical coronary artery stenosis: ^{99m}Tc-sestamibi versus 201-Tl. *J Nucl Med.* 2002;43:664–670.
74. Geleijnse ML, Elhendy A, Domburg RT, et al. Prognostic value of dobutamine-atropine stress technetium-99m sestamibi perfusion scintigraphy in patients with chest pain. *J Am Coll Cardiol.* 1996;28:447–454.
75. Schinkel AF, Elhendy A, van Domburg RT, et al. Prognostic value of dobutamine-atropine stress ^{99m}Tc-tetrafosmin myocardial perfusion SPECT in patients with known or suspected coronary artery disease. *J Nucl Med.* 2002;43: 767–772.
76. Narula J, Dawson MS, Singh BK, et al. Noninvasive characterization of stunned, hibernating, remodelled and nonviable myocardium in ischemic cardiomyopathy. *J Am Coll Cardiol.* 2002;36:1913–1919.
77. Everaert H, Vanhove C, Franken PR. Effects of low-dose dobutamine on left ventricular function in normal subjects as assessed by gated single-photon emission tomography myocardial perfusion studies. *Eur J Nucl Med.* 1999; 26:1298–1303.
78. Leoncini M, Sciagra R, Bellandi F, et al. Low-dose dobutamine nitrate-enhanced technetium 99m sestamibi gated SPECT versus low-dose dobutamine echocardiography for detecting reversible dysfunction in ischemic cardiomyopathy. *J Nucl Cardiol.* 2002;9:402–406.
79. Marwick TH. Arbutamine stress testing with closed loop drug delivery: toward the ideal or

just another pharmacologic stress technique? *J Am Coll Cardiol.* 1995;26:1176–1179.

80. Cohen JL, Chan KL, Jaarsma W, et al. Arbutamine echocardiography: efficacy and safety of a new pharmacologic stress agent to induce myocardial ischemia and detect coronary artery disease. The International Arbutamine Study Group. *J Am Coll Cardiol.* 1995;26:1168–1175.
81. Anagnostopoulos C, Pennell D, Francis J, et al. A comparison of adenosine and arbutamine for myocardial perfusion imaging. *Eur J Nucl Med.* 1998;25:394–400.
82. Zoll PM. Resuscitation of the heart in ventricular standstill by external electrical stimulation. *JAMA.* 1952;247:768–771.
83. Lee CY, Pellikka PA, McCully RB, et al. Nonexercise stress transthoracic echocardiography: transesophageal atrial pacing versus dobutamine stress. *J Am Coll Cardiol.* 1999;33:506–511.
84. Atar S, Cercek B, Nagai T, et al. Transthoracic stress echocardiography with transesophageal atrial pacing for bedside evaluation of inducible myocardial ischemia in patients with new-onset chest pain. *Am J Cardiol.* 2000;86:12–16.
85. Rainbird AJ, Pellikka PA, Stussy VL. et al. A rapid stress-testing protocol for the detection of coronary artery disease. *J Am Coll Cardiol.* 2000;36:1659–1663.
86. Lambertz H, Kreis A, Trumper H, et al. Simultaneous transesophageal atrial pacing and transesophageal two-dimensional echocardiography: a new method of stress echocardiography. *J Am Coll Cardiol.* 1990;16:1143–1153.
87. Gimenez VML. Ecocardiografia de Estresse. In Souza AGMR, Mansur A *SOCESP Cardiologia*,—1ª ed. Vol. 2, Cap 20. São Paulo, Brazil: Atheneu; 1996:173
88. Herd JA. Cardiovascular response to stress. *Physiological Reviews.* 1991;71:305–330.
89. Manuck SB, Kaplan JR, Adams MR, Clarkson TB. Effects of stress and the sympathetic nervous system on coronary atherosclerosis in the cynomolgus macaque. *Am Heart J.* 1988; 116:328–333.
90. Hjemdahl P, Fagius J, Freyschuss U, Wallin BG, Daleskog M, Bohlin G, Perski A. Muscle sympathetic activity and norephinephrine release during mental challenge in humans. *Am J Physiol.* 1989;257:E654–664.
91. Anderson EA, Sinkey CA, Mark A. Mental stress increases sympathetic nerve activity during sustained baroreceptor stimulation in humans. *Hypertension.* 1991;17(suppl III): III43–III49.
92. Linden W. What do arithmetic stress tests measure? Protocol variations and cardiovascular response. *Psychophysiology.* 1991;28(1): 91–102.
93. Cincipirini PM. Cognitive stress and cardiovascular reactivity. I—Relationship to hypertension. *Am Heart J.* 1986;112:1044–1050.
94. Cinciprini PM. Cognitive stress and cardiovascular reactivity II—Relationship to atherosclerosis, arrhythmias and cognitive control. *Am Heart J.* 1986;112:1051–1065.
95. Specchia G, Servi E, Falcone C, Gavazzi A, Angoli L, Bramici E, Ardissimo D, Mussini A. Mental arithmetic stress testing in patients with coronary artery disease. *Am Heart J.* 1984;108: 56–63.
96. Grossman P, Watkins LL, Wilhelm FH, Manolakis D, Lown B. Cardiac vagal control and dynamic responses to psychological stress among patients with coronary artery disease. *Am J Cardiol.* 1996;78:1424–1427.
97. Hines EABG. The cold pressure test for measuring the reactibility of the blood pressure: data concerning 571 normal and hypertensive subjects. *Am Heart J.* 1936;11:1–9.
98. McIlhany ML, Shaffer JW, Hines EA. The heritability of blood pressure: an investigation of 200 pairs of twins using the cold pressor test. *Johns Hopkins Med J.* 1975;136:57–64.
99. Stratton JR, Halter JB, Hallstrom AP, Caldwell JH, Ritchie JL. Comparative plasma catecholamine and hemodynamic responses to handgrip, cold pressor and supine bicycle exercise testing in normal subjects. *J Am Coll Cardiol.* 1983;2:93–104.
100. Backman C, Holm S, Linderholm H. Reaction to cold of patients with coronary insufficiency. *Ups J Med Sci.* 1979;84:181–187.
101. Lassvik C, Areskog NH. Effects of various environmental temperatures on effort angina. *Ups J Med Sci.* 1979;84:173–180.
102. Neill WA, Duncan DA, Kloster F, Mahler DJ. Response of coronary circulation to cutaneous cold. *Am J Med.* 1974;56:471–476.
103. Epstein SE, Stampfer M, Beiser GD, Goldstein RE, Braunwald E. Effects of a reduction in environmental temperature on the circulatory response to exercise in man. Implications concerning angina pectoris. *N Engl J Med.* 1969; 280:7–11.
104. Mudge GH, Grossman W, Mills RM, Lesch M, Braunwald E. Reflex increase in coronary vas-

cular resistance in patients with ischemic heart disease. *N Engl J Med.* 1976;295:1333–1337.

105. Nabel EG, Ganz P, Gordon JB, Alexander RW, Selwyn AP. Dilation of normal and constriction of atherosclerotic coronary arteries caused by the cold pressor test. *Circulation.* 1988;77:43–52.
106. Meeder JG, Peels HO, Blanksma PK, et al. Comparison between positron emission tomography myocardial perfusion imaging and intracoronary doppler flow velocity measurements at rest and during cold pressor testing in angiographically normal coronary arteries in patients with one-vessel coronary artery disease. *Am J Cardiol.* 1996;78:526–531.
107. Meeder JG, Blanksma PK, van der Wall EE, et al. Coronary vasomotion in patients with syndrome X: evaluation with positron emission tomography and parametric myocardial perfusion imaging. *Eur J Nucl Med.* 1997;24:530–537.
108. Vita JA, Treasure CB, Yeung AC, et al. Patients with evidence of coronary endothelial dysfunction as assessed by acetylcholine infusion demonstrate marked increase in sensitivity to constrictor effects of catecholamines. *Circulation.* 1992;85:1390–1397.
109. Zeiher AM, Drexler H, Wollschlager H, Just H. Modulation of coronary vasomotor tone in humans. Progressive endothelial dysfunction with different early stages of coronary atherosclerosis. *Circulation.* 1991;83:391–401.
110. Gould L. Cold pressor test in aortic stenosis and idiopathic hypertrophic subaortic stenosis. Preliminary report. *Am J Cardiol.* 1969;23:38–42.
111. Wasserman AG, Reiss L, Katz RJ, et al. Insensitivity of the cold pressor stimulation test for the diagnosis of coronary artery disease. *Circulation.* 1983;67:1189–1193.
112. Seneviratne BI, Linton I, Wilkinson R, Rowe W, Spice M. Cold pressor test in diagnosis of coronary artery disease: echophonocardiographic method. *BMJ.* 1983;286:1924–1926.
113. Ferrara LA, Mancini M, De Simone GD, et al. Responses of serum insulin and blood pressure to cold and handgrip in obese patients. *Int J Cardiol.* 1991;32:353–359.
114. Verani MS, Zacca NM, DeBauche TL, Miller RR, Chahine RA. Comparison of cold pressor and exercise radionuclide angiocardiography in coronary artery disease. *J Nucl Med.* 1982;23: 770–776.
115. Rootwelt K, Erikssen J, Nitter-Hauge S, Thaulow E. Detection of coronary artery disease with gated cardiac blood-pool scintigraphy: comparison of cold pressor test and dynamic exercise. *Clin Physiol.* 1982;2:459–465.
116. Vojacek J, Hannan WJ, Muir AL. Ventricular response to dynamic exercise and the cold pressor test. *Eur Heart J.* 1982;3:212–222.
117. Ahmad M, Dubiel JP, Haibach H. Cold pressor thallium-201 myocardial scintigraphy in the diagnosis of coronary artery disease. *Am J Cardiol.* 1982;50:1253–1257.
118. Hendel RC, Jamil T, Glover DK. Pharmacologic stress testing: new methods and new agents. *J Nucl Cardiol.* 2003;10:197–204.
119. Coronary artery surgery study (CASS): A randomized trial of coronary bypass surgery. Survival data. *Circulation.* 1983;68:939–950.
120. Schneider JF, Thomas HE Jr, Sorlie P, et al. Comparative features of newly acquired left and right bundle branch block in the general population: The Framingham study. *Am J Cardiol.* 1981;47:931–940.
121. Fahy GJ, Pinski SL, Miller DP, et al. Natural history of isolated bundle branch block. *Am J Cardiol.* 1996;77:1185–1190.
122. Hirzel HO, Senn M, Nuesch K, et al. Thallium-201 scintigraphy in complete left bundle branch block. *Am J Cardiol.* 1984;53:764–769.
123. Burns RJ, Galligan L, Wright L, et al. Improved specificity of myocardial thallium 201 single photon emission computed tomography in patients with left bundle branch block by dipyridamole. *Am J Cardiol.* 1991;68:504–508
124. Hammermeister KE, DeRouen TA, Dodge HT, et al. Prognostic and predictive value of exertional hypotension in suspected coronary heart disease. *Am J Cardiol.* 1983;51:1261–1266.
125. Sandvik L, Erikssen J, Ellestad M, et al. Heart rate increase and maximal heart rate during exercise as predictors of cardiovascular mortality: a 16 year follow-up of 1960 healthy men. *Coron Artery Dis.* 1995;6:667–679.
126. Simons M, Parker JA, Udelson JE, Gervino EV. The role of clinical data in interpretation of perfusion images. *J Nucl Med.* 1994;35:740–741.
127. Mitchell JH, Blomqvist G. Maximal oxygen uptake. *N Engl J Med.* 1971 6;284(18):1018–1022.
128. Boz A, Gungor F, Karayalcin B, Yildiz A. The effects of solid food in prevention of intestinal activity in ^{99m}Tc tetrofosmin myocardial perfusion scintigraphy. *J Nucl Cardiol.* 2003;10: 161–167.
129. Feldman RL, Nichols WM, Pepine CJ, Conti CR. Acute effects of intravenous dipyridamole

on regional coronary hemodynamics and metabolism. *Circulation.* 1981;64:333–334.

130. Gould KL, Hamilton GW, Lipscomb K, Ritchie JL, Kennedy W. Method for assessing stress induced regional malperfusion during coronary arteriography. *Am J Cardiol.* 1974;34:557–564.
131. Klodas E, Miller TD, Christian TF, et al. Prognostic significance of ischemic electrocardiographic changes during vasodilator stress testing in patients with normal SPECT images. *J Nucl Cardiol.* 2003;10:4–8.
132. Abbott BG, Afshar M, Berger AK, Wackers FJ. Prognostic significance of ischemic electrocardiographic changes during adenosine infusion in patients with normal myocardial perfusion imaging. *J Nucl Cardiol.* 2003;10: 9–16.
133. Riou LM, Ruiz M, Rieger JM, et al. Influence of propanolol, enalaprilat, verapamil, and caffeine on adenosine A(2A)-receptor-mediated coronary vasodilation. *J Am Coll Cardiol.* 2002; 40:1687–1694.
134. Sharir T, Rabinowitz B, Livschitz S, et al. Underestimation of extent and severity of coronary artery disease by dipyridamole stress thallium-201 single photon emission computed tomographic myocardial perfusion imaging in patients taking antianginal drugs. *J Am Coll Cardiol.* 1998;31:1540–1546.

5 Myocardial Perfusion Imaging: Detection of Coronary Artery Disease and Miscellaneous Clinical Applications

João V. Vitola, Dominique Delbeke, C. Andrew Smith,
Carlos Cunha Pereira Neto, William H. Martin, and M. Reza Habibian

Several options exist for investigating myocardial ischemia, including exercise testing, stress echocardiography, nuclear perfusion imaging, and coronary angiography. Nuclear perfusion imaging is one of the most sensitive and specific methods for the noninvasive evaluation of myocardial ischemia. The standard criteria to define ischemia on rest/stress MPI is the presence of a stress-induced perfusion defect that reverses on the resting study. Other findings on MPI, associated with extensive coronary artery disease (CAD), include transient ischemic dilatation of the left ventricle (TID) and increased poststress pulmonary accumulation of the perfusion radiopharmaceuticals. (See Case 5.5.)

Numerous reports in the literature demonstrate the high sensitivity and specificity of MPI using various perfusion radiopharmaceuticals and stress protocols, which were summarized in Chapters 3 and 4.[1,2] However, a wide range of performance is reported. This wide range is certainly related to some extent to different radiopharmaceuticals, stress modalities, acquisition and processing protocols, and data analysis, but also, and more importantly, to the referral biases and limitations of coronary angiography (percentage threshold of coronary stenosis) accepted as standard of reference to define significant CAD and ischemia. Limitations of coronary angiography have been well documented in several studies.[3–14] It is becoming more and more evident that a functional component related to endothelial dysfunction plays an important role in ischemia identified on MPI. Intravascular ultrasound (IVUS) may be a better standard than angiography to define significant CAD. (See Case 5.11.)

The average sensitivity and specificity for detection of hemodynamically significant coronary artery stenosis for exercise qualitative ^{201}Tl SPECT are 89% and 76%, respectively.[15–17] The single photon emission tomography (SPECT) technique allows better localization of vascular territories than planar imaging. In 1994, the American Medical Association mandated a Diagnostic and Therapeutic Technology Assessment (DATTA) review of SPECT myocardial imaging (MPI).[18] This extensive review of the literature concluded that for planar imaging the sensitivities and specificities ranged from 67% to 96% and 40% to 100%, respectively, and for SPECT imaging from 83% to 98% and 53% to 100%. A review of quantitative analysis of ^{201}Tl SPECT has shown an overall sensitivity and specificity of 90% and 70%, respectively.[19] The low specificity may be attributed to attenuation artifacts. In addition, because the specificity suffers from post-bias referral to angiography, the normalcy rate may be a more accurate parameter than specificity. The normalcy rate of quantitative ^{201}Tl SPECT averages 89% in the studies previously cited. There is a high degree of concordance between ^{201}Tl and ^{99m}Tc-MIBI regarding sensitivity, specificity, and normalcy rate.[20,21] A relatively recent study of 235 patients showed a sensitivity of 95%, a specificity of 76%, and a normalcy rate of 93% using angiography criteria of >50% stenosis as standard of reference (considering the limitations of such a standard as discussed previously).[22] Poststress gated SPECT with ^{99m}Tc-perfusion radiopharmaceuticals increases the sensitivity for detection of multivessel disease, provides the LVEF known to be a powerful prognostic factor,[23] and may allow identification of postischemic stunning.[24]

Regarding positron emission tomography (PET), a high accuracy of ^{82}Rb and ^{13}N-ammonia myocardial perfusion images for the detection of CAD has been demonstrated in the first study including a large population of patients with a sensitivity and specificity close to 90%.[25] More recently, a joint task force of the American College of Cardiology (ACC), the American Heart Association (AHA), and the Society of Nuclear Medicine (SNM)[26] has reviewed the literature and reported a sensitivity of 87% to 97% and a specificity of 78% to 100% for PET compared with a sensitivity of 89% and a specificity of 76% for SPECT.[27–34] An advantage of perfusion PET may be a higher specificity than ^{201}Tl, probably due to attenuation correction with PET that is certainly an advantage for patients with large body habitus.[35] Another advantage is the possibility of absolute quantitative measurement of coronary blood flow and blood flow reserve that is further discussed in Chapter 17.

This chapter discusses general applications of MPI for detection of CAD, whereas more specific applications are discussed in Chapters 10, 11, and 12. There is more and more evidence that discordance between stress MPI and coronary angiography criteria results from interobserver variability in interpreting studies, threshold to define significant CAD on angiography, and referral bias. In addition, the presence of ischemia is also related to the pattern of coronary stenoses (including the length and stenoses in series), the presence of collateral vessels, and functional components related to endothelial dysfunction, which can be evaluated by MPI, establishing this technique as a standard on its own.

Case Presentations

Case 5.1

History

A 55-year-old man with a family history of CAD presented with atypical chest pain within the last month. He underwent a rest/exercise ^{99m}Tc-MIBI study. He had a poor exercise tolerance and during exercise, he dropped his blood pressure (BP) slightly. His resting ECG was normal, the exercise ECG is shown in Figure C5-1A, and the exercise/rest SPECT images are displayed in Figure C5-1B.

Findings

The exercise ECG demonstrated widespread ST-segment depression consistent with ischemia. SPECT images reveal a large severe reversible perfusion defect in the anterior wall and apex indicative of a proximal left anterior descending (LAD) coronary artery stenosis. The poststress LVEF, left ventricular end-diastolic volume (LVEDV), and end-systolic volume (LVESV) were 50%, 77 ml, and 38 ml, respectively.

On coronary angiography (Figure C5-1C), the left main coronary artery was occluded and the left circumflex coronary artery (LCX) territory was perfused via collaterals from the right coronary artery (RCA). The ventriculogram was normal.

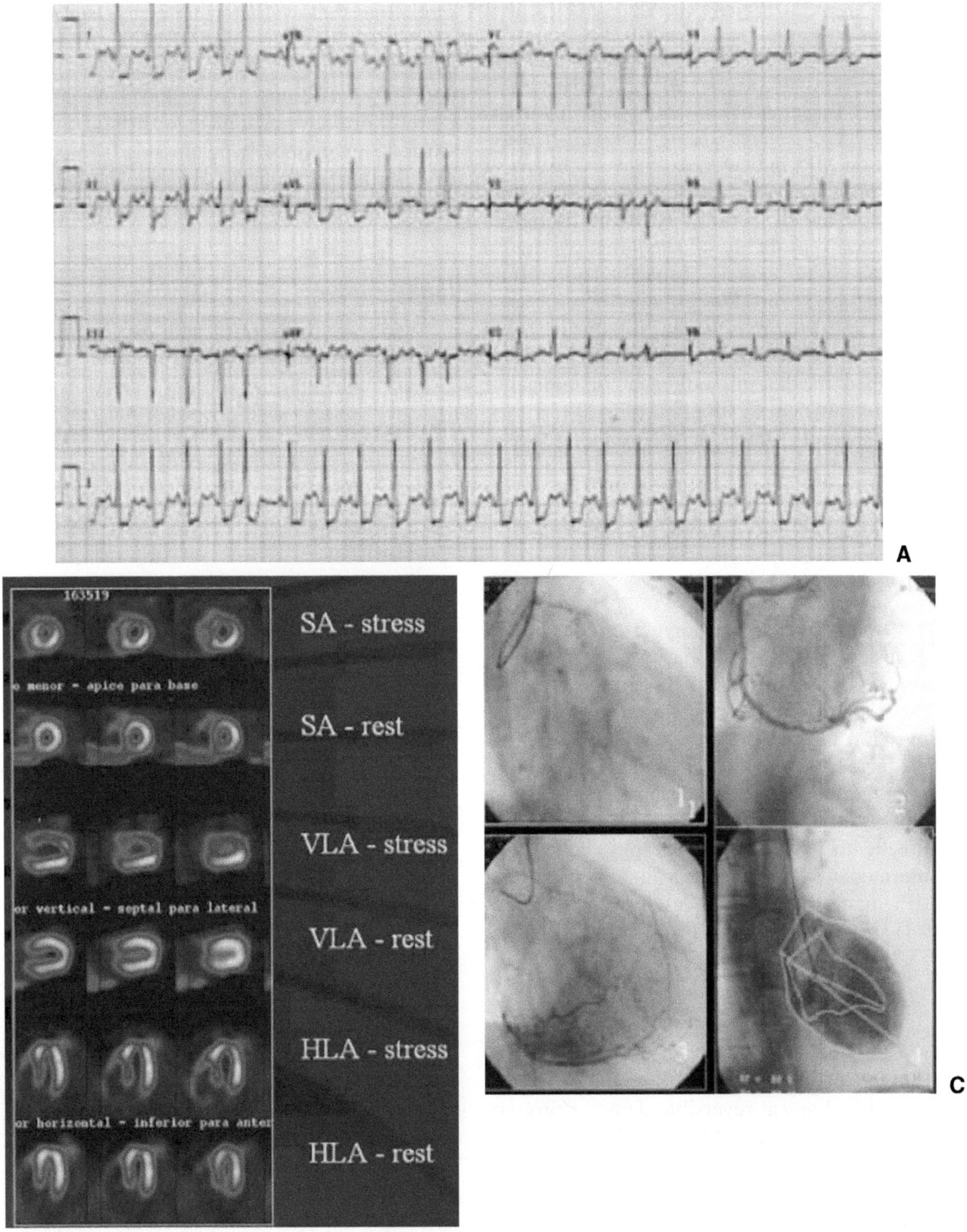

FIGURE C5-1. (A–C, courtesy of Dr. Luiz E. Mastrocolla, from Fleury Laboratories, Sao Paulo, Brazil.)

Discussion

In this patient, poor exercise tolerance, a paradoxical decrease in BP with exercise, widespread ST-segment depression with exercise, and a large severe stress-induced perfusion defect on MPI indicated extensive ischemia of poor prognosis. Despite left main occlusion, collateral vessels from the RCA, perfusing the lateral wall, probably allowed this patient to maintain some exercise capacity and normal LV function at rest. Despite a left main lesion, usually resulting in ischemia in both the LAD and LCX territories, the collateral circulation protected the lateral wall from ischemia but was not sufficient to supply the LAD territory. This is a good example of discordance between modalities that evaluate anatomy versus physiology (angiography versus MPI) and may explain in fact why some patients with certain coronary occlusions may in fact have a completely normally perfused myocardium on MPI. Current guidelines recommended treatment of left main coronary disease with surgical revascularization.

Interpretation

1. Significant drop in BP with exercise indicative of severe ischemia.
2. Left main coronary artery occlusion diagnosed after a severely abnormal rest/stress ^{99m}Tc-MIBI.

Case 5.2

History

A 49-year-old man with hypertension, hypercholesterolemia, and tobacco use presented with a 5-month history of progressive angina. The resting ECG demonstrated new T-waves inversion. Given the typical symptoms, multiple risk factors, and new ECG changes, this patient is at moderate to high risk for CAD. Most patients at high risk for CAD are referred directly to coronary angiography. Patients at intermediate risk are best evaluated with stress MPI first. The patient underwent exercise ^{201}Tl stress-reinjection MPI as shown in Figure C5-2.

Findings

The SPECT images reveal moderate anteroseptal and apical reversible defect. Coronary angiography revealed 80% mid-LAD stenosis distal to the first two diagonals. There was also a muscular bridge present in the distal LAD. The left main coronary artery was angiographically free of disease and the RCA and LCX had 30% to 40% narrowing proximally. The patient underwent successful balloon angioplasty of the mid-LAD. Secondary to a return of similar symptoms, the patient underwent a second exercise stress ^{201}Tl test approximately 5 months after his intervention and that study was normal.

Discussion

This patient had a myocardial bridge in the distal portion of his LAD. Myocardial bridging is an anatomical variation in which a coronary artery takes a course within a segment of the myocardium that compresses the lumen during ventricular systole despite a normal appearance during diastole. Interestingly, myocardial bridging is present in up to 78% of autopsy cases [36,37] and in 0.5% to 16.0% of patients examined by coronary angiography.[38,39] Myocardial bridging most frequently occurs on the LAD. Although most patients are asymptomatic, myocardial bridges may cause ischemia and related complications, including myocardial stunning, infarction, arrhythmia, AV block, transient LV dysfunction, and sudden death.[40] Although, it was believed that the affected coronary is compressed only in systole, IVUS has demonstrated that the vessel narrowing continues even in early diastole, which might account for myocardial ischemia distal to the bridge.[41]

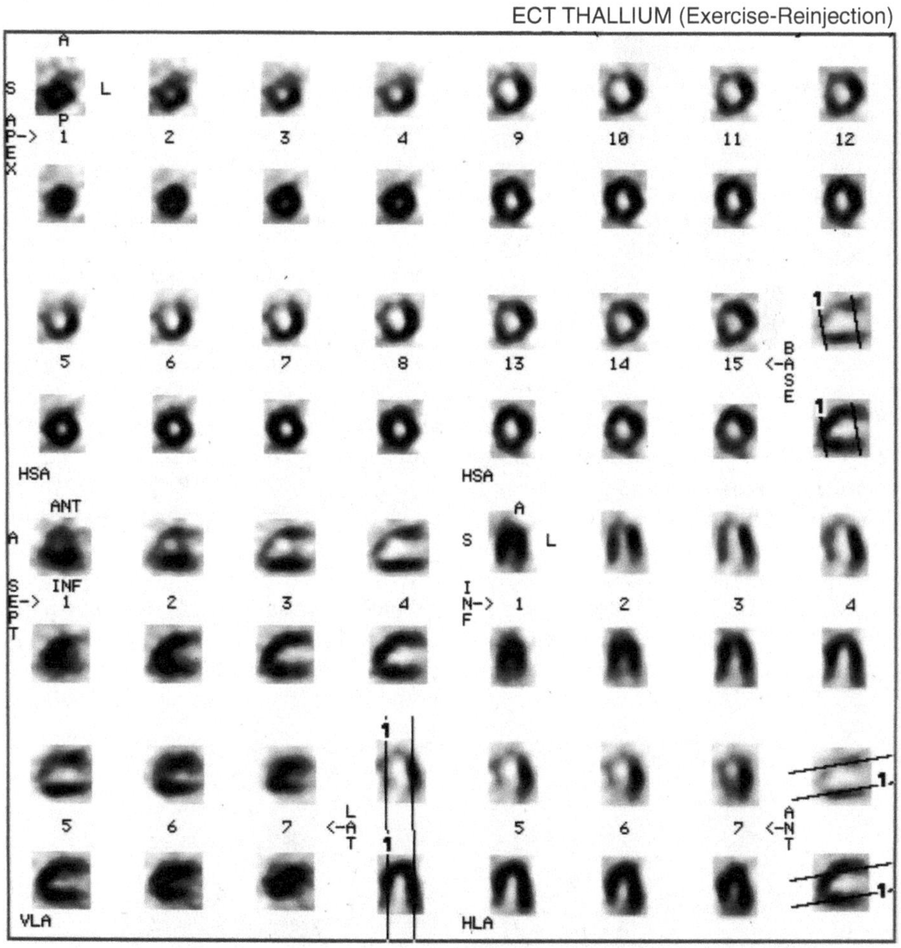

FIGURE C5-2.

Nitroglycerin, administered during angiography, increases the sensitivity for the diagnosis of myocardial bridges compromising blood flow.[42] The proposed mechanisms are an increase in vessel wall compliance and decrease in aortic pressure.

Few studies have reported evaluation of myocardial bridges with MPI. In two small retrospective studies,[43,44] no abnormalities were found with stress ^{201}Tl imaging. However, when myocardial bridges cause ischemia, stress-induced perfusion defects are present on MPI and resolve after the affected artery is bypassed.[45]

In this patient, despite the presence of myocardial bridge, ischemia was most likely due to the mid-LAD stenosis. This is further supported by the normalization of the exercise ^{201}Tl scan 5 months after intervention.

Interpretation

Anteroseptal and apical reversible perfusion defects consistent with myocardial ischemia secondary to severe LAD stenosis.

Distal myocardial bridging of the LAD unlikely to be of hemodynamic significance in this case.

Case 5.3

History

A 53-year-old man with hypertension, hypercholesterolemia, and tobacco use presented with a 4-week history of typical chest pain. The resting ECG revealed left bundle branch block (LBBB). The patient was referred for an exercise/reinjection ^{201}Tl study as shown in Figure C5-3A.

Findings

The SPECT images demonstrated a large severe anteroseptal, septal, and apical perfusion defect that is reversible on the resting images. Considering the presence of LBBB, this study was repeated using pharmacological stress with dipyridamole. The images are shown in Figure C5-3B. Figure C5-3B, using dipyridamole, demonstrated a striking improvement of perfusion in the same areas of severe hypoperfusion previously seen on the exercise study.

Discussion

Reversible defects on exercise myocardial perfusion studies can be artifactual in patients with LBBB.[46–48] These reversible defects are usually located in the anteroseptal or septal region and are HR dependent. Therefore, vasodilator stress, that does not increase the HR to the same extent as exercise, has been recommended as the method of choice to evaluate these patients.[49] The septum's asynchrony with the rest of the LV myocardium causes a decrease in MBF during diastole. This decrease in perfusion is exacerbated at higher HR because the time in diastole is reduced to a greater extent. Some data suggest that extension of the defect to the anterior wall (see Case

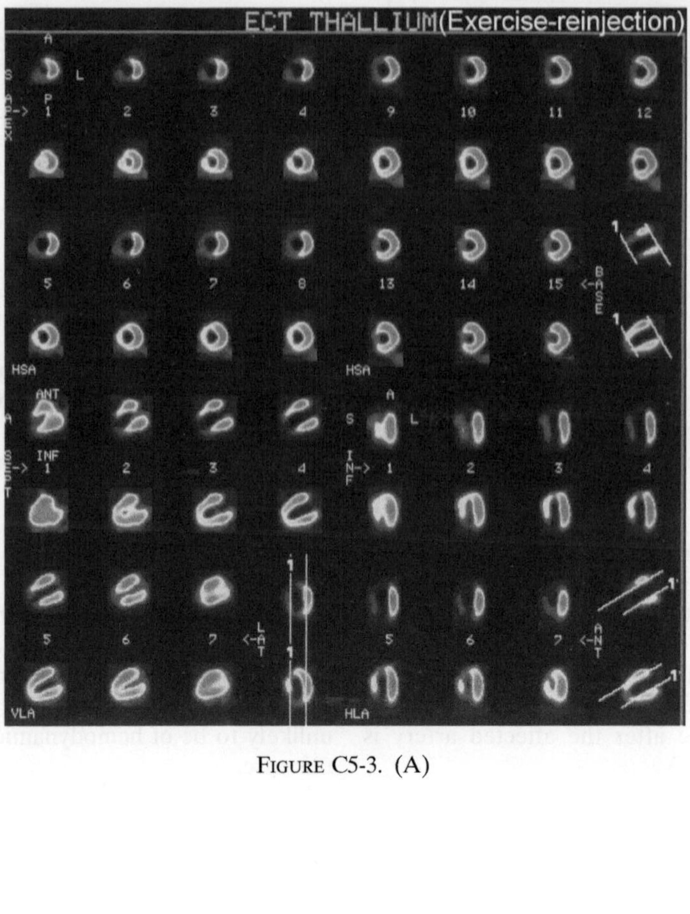

A

FIGURE C5-3. (A)

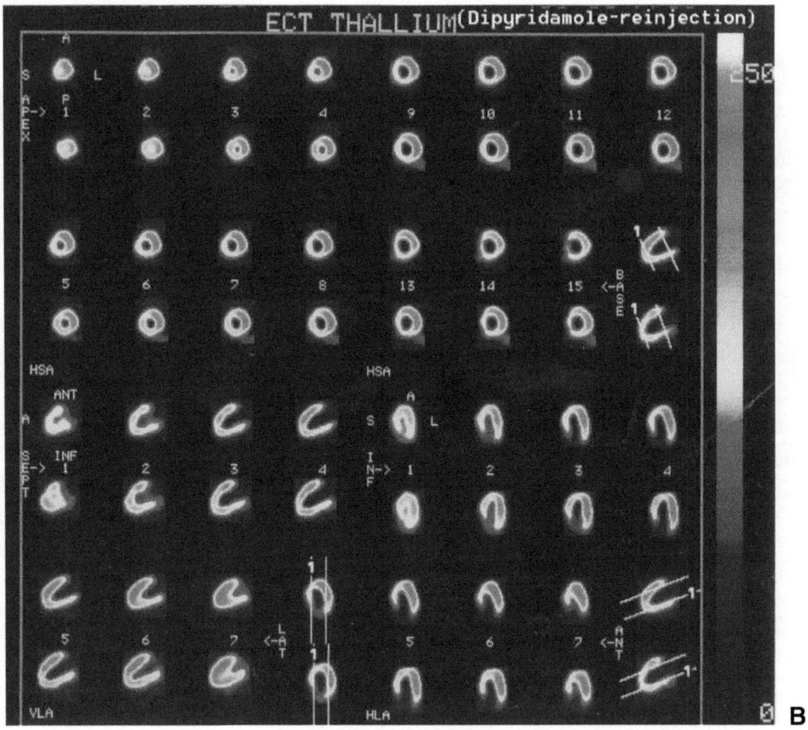

FIGURE C5-3. (B)

5.11) and to the apex may indicate true LAD ischemia and not an artifact.[50]

In this patient, the exercise stress test was followed by a dipyridamole stress test. By using vasodilation as the mode of stress testing in LBBB, diagnostic accuracy is improved, as discussed in Cases 4.2, 5.4, and 13.9. In conclusion, patients with LBBB should be evaluated with vasodilators and not with exercise.

Interpretation

Severe reversible perfusion defect induced by exercise but not dipyridamole in a patient with LBBB.

Case 5.4

History

A 70-year-old woman with hypertension and hyperlipidemia and a strong family history of CAD presented with increasing fatigue over the previous year. She also noted right arm pain that was associated with exertion occurring over the last month. Her baseline ECG showed LBBB. An echocardiogram revealed global hypokinesia, more severe in the anterior wall and an LVEF in the 20% to 30% range. She was referred for a dual isotope rest ^{201}Tl adenosine ^{99m}Tc-MIBI study displayed in Figure C5-4A. She complained of mild chest discomfort during the adenosine infusion but the ECG was nondiagnostic secondary to the LBBB.

A
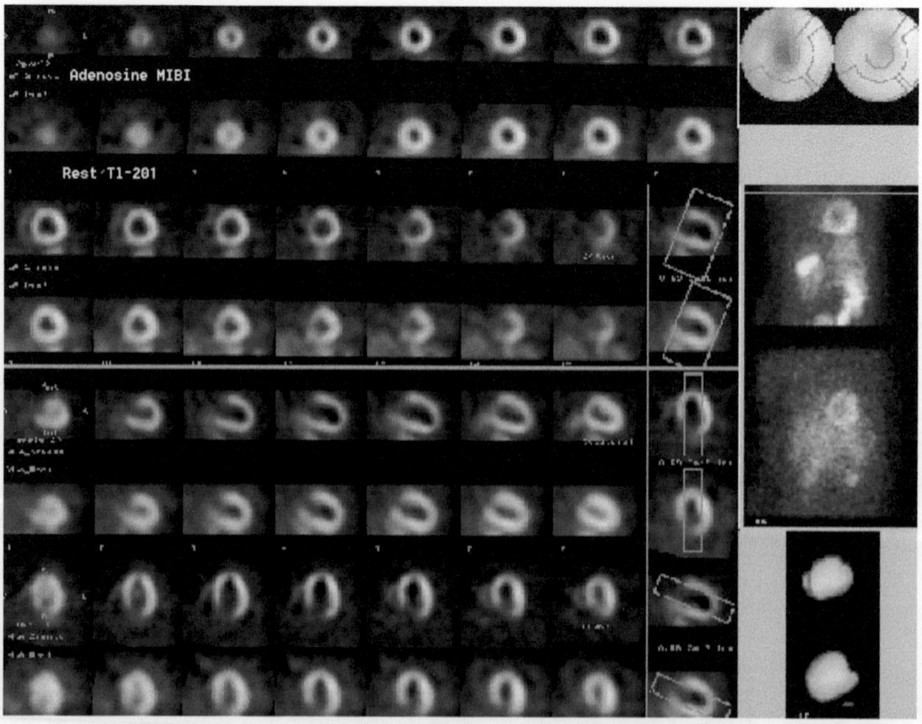

FIGURE C5-4. (A)

Findings

The stress SPECT images demonstrated a moderately large area of moderately decreased uptake in the anterior wall, septum, apex, and the inferoapical segments with substantial reversibility on the resting images. Similar findings were present in images obtained with the patient in the supine and prone positions. In addition, there was mild dilatation of the LV cavity with adenosine compared with rest. The gated images (not shown) revealed an LVEF of 21% with severe hypokinesis of the apex, mid- and distal anterior, and distal inferior walls. The septum was dyskinetic. Coronary angiography (Figure C5-4B) revealed 40% to 50% narrowing

B
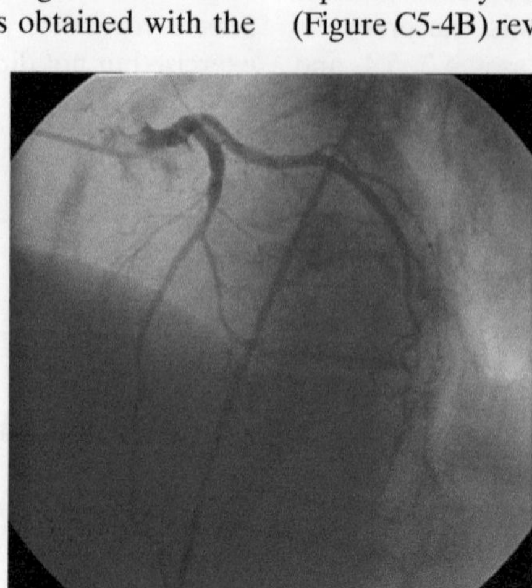

FIGURE C5-4. (B)

of the proximal LAD extending through the distal artery. IVUS was not performed.

Discussion

The results of the adenosine MPI suggest the LAD as the culprit artery for the patient's symptoms. The depressed LV function in this case may be related to both idiopathic cardiomyopathy or ischemic heart disease.

One could argue that the anterior defect is artifactual and due to the underlying LBBB. In this case, the pharmacologic stressor agent was chosen appropriately to lessen the likelihood of this occurring. In patients with LBBB, adenosine and dipyridamole are better pharmacologic choices than dobutamine because they rely on vasodilation rather than increasing the HR. In addition, an artifact due to LBBB is unlikely given the clinical presentation and the large area of ischemic burden identified by adenosine MPI. IVUS, which was not performed here, would be helpful to clarify this issue (see Case 5.11).

This case illustrates the importance of the pattern of perfusion of the epicardial arteries on coronary angiography. Although no high-grade focal stenoses are shown on the study, the distal branches of the LAD are thin and diseased. The ability of the contrast to opacify the distal LAD is less than in the proximal LAD. This suggests that the distal LAD is diffusely diseased with a narrowed lumen that may not be as apparent on angiographic images as a focal stenosis. The diagonal and septal branch vessels of the LAD are also narrowed and short, suggesting diffuse atherosclerotic disease of the distal vessels.

Interpretation

A large area of anterior, septal, apical, and inferoapical ischemia identified by adenosine MPI in a patient with LBBB.

Case 5.5

History

A 75-year-old man with known CAD and aortic stenosis and insufficiency was admitted to the surgery service for a cholecystectomy. Before surgery the patient underwent a preoperative evaluation including a rest ^{201}Tl exercise ^{99m}Tc-tetrofosmin study. The resting ECG showed LV hypertrophy with nonspecific ST-segment and T-wave changes. The patient exercised on a standard Bruce protocol reaching stage II. The exercise was stopped early because of 4 mm ST-segment depression occurring in the left precordial leads (V3–V6). The rest/exercise dual isotope SPECT and gated images are displayed in Figure C5-5A.

Findings

The SPECT images (Figure C5-5A) demonstrated a large partially reversible defect in the inferior wall, extending to the inferoseptal and inferolateral regions, from the base to the apex. The LV cavity viewed on the stress images was dilated compared with the rest images, suggestive of extensive ischemia. The gated images showed an LVEF of 48% with global hypokinesis more pronounced along the inferior wall. Coronary angiography revealed multivessel CAD with a 70% left main stenosis, a 70% stenosis of the mid-LCX, and occlusion of the RCA.

Discussion

The large perfusion defect is likely related to the occluded RCA and possible LCX involvement. Stress-induced LV dilatation and the severe ECG changes occurring early in the stress protocol are both predictors of severe disease. In addition, transient LV dilatation (TID) indicates a poor prognosis.[51–55] The dilatation represents either subendocardial ischemia or true LV cavity dilatation. If there is global subendocardial ischemia on the stress images, the apparent LV dilation is probably due to uptake in a thinner area through the thickness of the myocardium (epicardial region only). It has also been suggested that poststress end-systolic dilation can be due to endocardial postischemic stunning.[56]

A

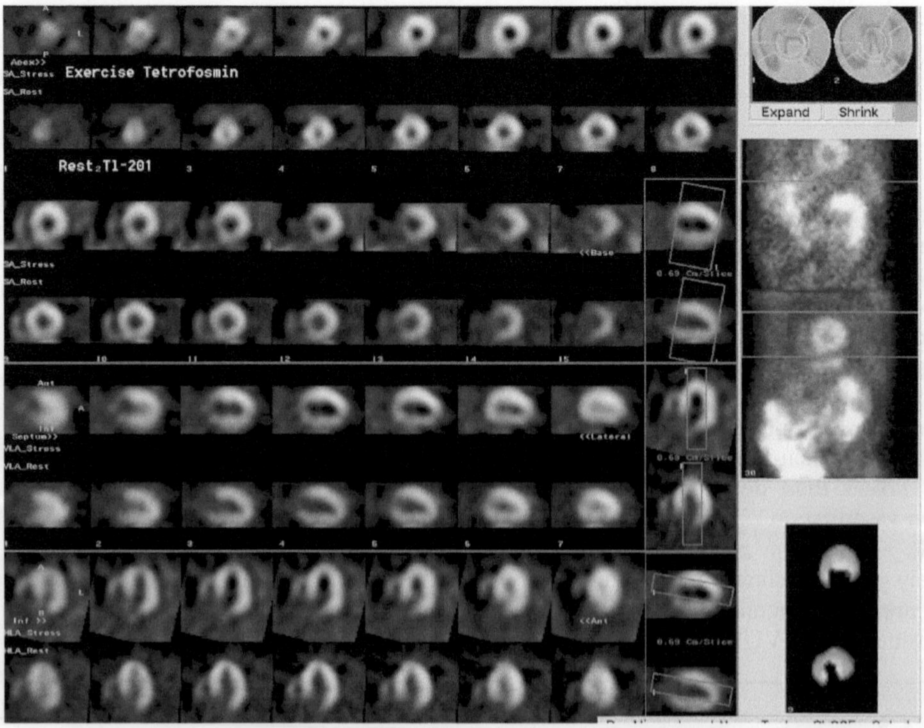

FIGURE C5-5. (A)

Transient ischemic dilation of the LV with stress is a marker of myocardial ischemia and can be determined subjectively or from automatically derived stress and rest ventricular volume measurements. TID must persist post-stress during the actual SPECT acquisition to be detected. It has been first described on ^{201}Tl studies (defined as abnormal when TID ratio >1.12) and has been shown to have a sensitivity of 60% and specificity of 95% for identifying patients with multivessel critical stenoses.[51] The significance of TID after pharmacological stress is similar to that of exercise testing[57] with a similar specificity but lower sensitivity. A study of 110 patients with suspected CAD using dipyridamole ^{201}Tl MPI demonstrated TID more frequently in patients with multivessel disease than those with single-vessel disease and that the sensitivity of TID to identify patients with multivessel disease was 27% and specificity 95%.[58] In addition, ECG changes were observed more frequently in patients with TID.

Normal thresholds for TID ratio can vary slightly according to the type of stress and type of radiopharmaceutical and protocol used (from >1.12 to <1.40).[59] For dual isotope rest ^{201}Tl/exercise ^{99m}Tc-MIBI studies, abnormal TID ratio values correspond to LV endocardial volume ratios greater than 1.20. These criteria identify severe and/or extensive CAD with a sensitivity and specificity of 71% and 95%, respectively.[54] An increased TID ratio has also been associated with a poor prognosis and increased cardiac event rate in a study of 512 patients evaluated with dipyridamole and ^{99m}Tc radiopharmaceuticals.[60]

Another index of severe and extensive CAD is postexercise lung accumulation of ^{201}Tl[61] and ^{99m}Tc-MIBI, thought to be related to significant stress-induced LV dysfunction.[62–65] Increased pulmonary uptake of ^{201}Tl reflects the increased pulmonary capillary wedge pressure that can be caused by CAD but also mitral valve regurgitation or stenosis, decreased LV compliance, and nonischemic cardiomyopathy with LV dysfunction. Although both elevated TID and lung/heart ratio are associated with severe CAD, they have no significant correlation, as demonstrated in a study of 1129 consecutive patients undergoing pharmacological stress with dipyridamole and ^{201}Tl.[63] Increased lung/heart ratio on resting ^{201}Tl images is weakly associated with higher LV end-diastolic pressure and pulmonary wedge pressure and lower LVEF.[64]

Some expressed concern that ^{99m}Tc-perfusion radiopharmaceuticals do not accumulate in the lungs to the same extent as ^{201}Tl does in patients with CAD. However, a phase III multicenter study showed a fair correlation between the two imaging agents when heart/lung ratios of 0.50 and 0.44 were chosen for ^{201}Tl and ^{99m}Tc-tetrofosmin, respectively.[65]

An automatic algorithm assessing lung/heart ratio on exercise ^{99m}Tc-MIBI images correlated well with manually derived values on both ^{99m}Tc-MIBI images and ^{201}Tl images. A lung/heart ratio >0.44 yielded a sensitivity and specificity of 63% and 81%, respectively, for identifying severe and extensive CAD.[65] A study of 149 patients evaluated with exercise ^{201}Tl scintigraphy demonstrated a higher event rate in patients with an L/H ratio >0.5.[66]

An example of a patient with a normal and abnormal L/H ratio is shown in Figures C5-5B and C5-5C, respectively. Both of these patients had a history of anteroseptal MI, presented with atypical chest pain, and were evaluated with a stress/reinjection ^{201}Tl protocol. Both the SPECT images of the first patient displayed in Figure C5-5B and perfusion polar plot of the second patient displayed in Figure C5-5C demonstrated a fixed severe perfusion defect in the apex. However, the L/H ratio was normal at 0.46 (Figure C5-5B) in the first patient who had no cardiac events after a 20 months' follow-up. On the images of the second patient (Figure C5-5C), markedly increased pulmonary uptake

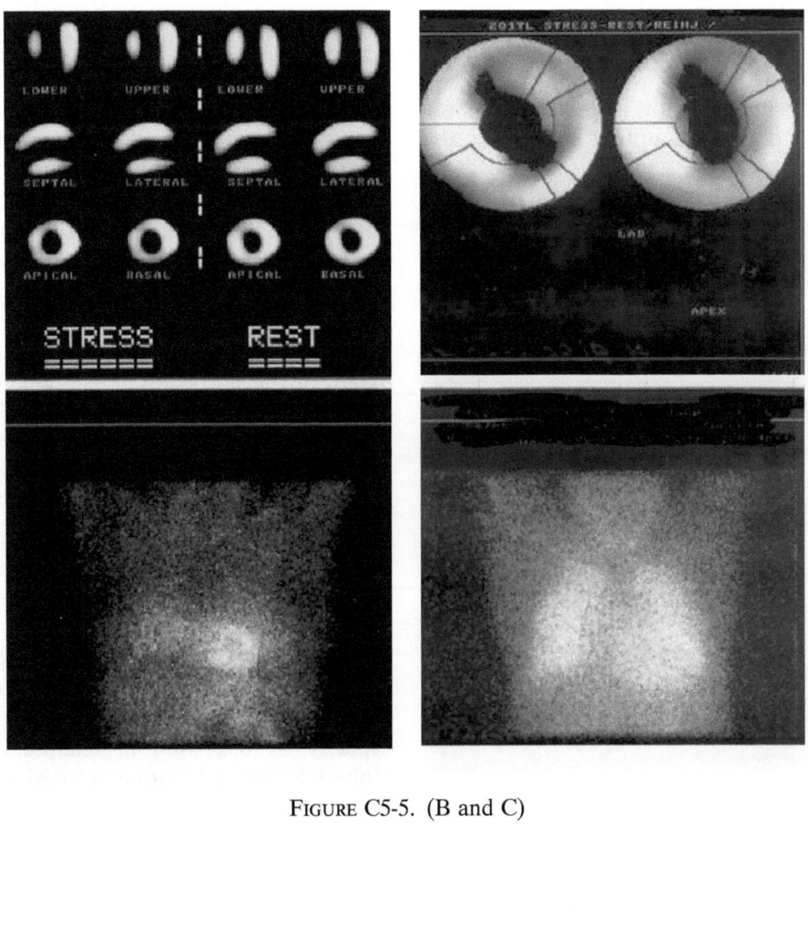

B C

FIGURE C5-5. (B and C)

with an L/H ratio of 0.96 indicated LV dysfunction and multivessel CAD. Coronary angiography proved severe stenosis of all main epicardial arteries, and despite CABG the patient died 6 months later.

Interpretations

1. Severe 3-vessel CAD with left main stenosis.
2. Stress-induced transient ischemic dilatation of the LV cavity.

Case 5.6

History

A 78-year-old man presented with atypical chest pain and was referred for MPI. A combined protocol was performed, adding low workload exercise during dipyridamole infusion. The patient received dipyridamole (0.84 mg/kg) over 4 minutes and also exercised on the Bruce protocol for 3 minutes, starting during the last minute of dipyridamole infusion. The HR achieved was 102 bpm and the exercise ECG was negative for ischemia. The stress/rest SPECT ^{99m}Tc-MIBI images are displayed in Figure C5-6A.

Findings

The SPECT images show an extensive area of severely decreased uptake involving the anteroseptal region, the entire septum and the apex, reversible on the resting images and therefore consistent with ischemia due to a proximal LAD stenosis. There is also evidence of inferior wall ischemia extending to the inferoseptal region, raising the question of single versus multivessel ischemia. The gated images revealed an LVEF of 40% with anterior and septal hypokinesis, indicating possible stress-induced stunning, but hibernation could not be excluded. Coronary angiography revealed 3-vessel disease worse in the LAD and the RCA.

A

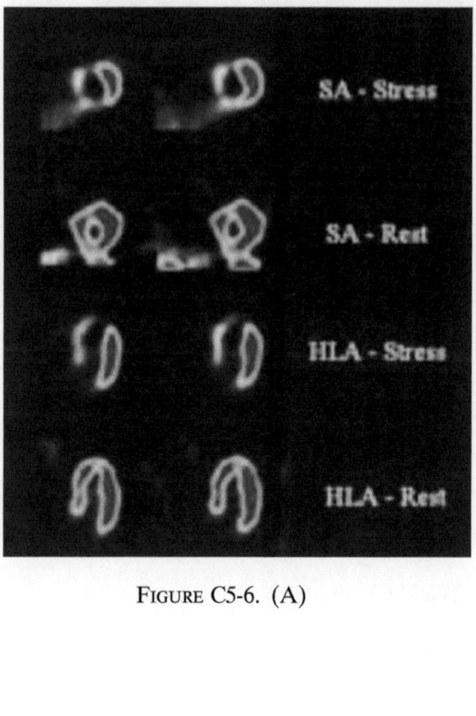

FIGURE C5-6. (A)

Discussion

MPI with SPECT perfusion radiopharmaceuticals demonstrates the relative distribution of perfusion in different coronary territories. In this patient the ischemia in the territory of the LAD with worse coronary blood flow reserve (CBFR) is well demonstrated, but the scan underestimated the ischemia of the less diseased LCX territory. Despite this limitation, stress MPI detects patients with multivessel CAD with high sensitivity (>95%) although the extent of the perfusion defects may be underestimated in some territories. Normal stress MPI in patients with multivessel CAD is rare, unless there is a perfectly balanced disease state. Absolute measurement of MBF such as provided by PET with tracer kinetic analysis and compartmental modeling is necessary to demonstrate noninvasively globally decreased perfusion.

Combination of vasodilator and exercise stress is now well established as the optimal stress modality in patients with limited exercise capacity as discussed in Chapter 4. In the United States, adenosine is used more commonly as a vasodilator stressor with or without

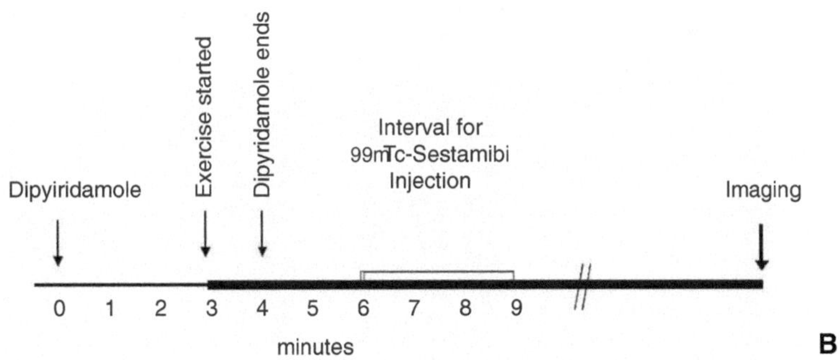

FIGURE C5-6. (B, from Vitola, Brambatti, Caligaris, et al. [67], by permission of *J Nucl Cardiol.*)

combined exercise because of its short half-life limiting the duration of the side effects. However, in many other countries, dipyridamole is still widely used. A protocol combining exercise and dipyridamole is shown in Figure C5-6B.[67]

Another point of discussion is poststress stunning. In a patient with ischemic findings on MPI and decreased LVEF following stress (LVEF of 40% in our patient), stunning may be responsible for LV dysfunction and should be considered as a possibility for this patient. Johnson et al.[68] first demonstrated that post-stress gated ^{99m}Tc-MIBI images do not always represent true LV function at rest, because of stress-induced stunning. Exercise and dipyridamole stress reliably produce segmental wall motion abnormalities in patients with hemodynamically significant CAD. If these wall motion abnormalities persist at the time of SPECT acquisition, they will be detectable on the post-stress gated SPECT display.[69,70] The duration of poststress stunning varies in proportion to the severity and extent of CAD and the stress modality, but may persist for up to 24 hours. Significant post-exercise LV regional dysfunction occurs in the regions of severe ischemia, and the incidence and magnitude of regional stunning are determined by the severity of ischemia. Regional wall motion abnormalities may be more sensitive than global dysfunction for the detection of stunning with gated SPECT studies.[71] Poststress and reversible regional wall motion abnormalities on exercise stress gated ^{99m}Tc SPECT studies are significant predictors of angiographic disease.[72] More recently, transient postischemic stunning has been described on gated ^{201}Tl SPECT studies.[73] If the resting SPECT images are acquired with gating, the resting gated study is usually normal and the resting LVEF is higher.

Interpretations

1. Multivessel CAD demonstrated by combined exercise/dipyridamole ^{99m}Tc-MIBI.
2. Probable poststress stunning.

Case 5.7

History

A 48-year-old man with known CAD, prior inferior MI, and RCA stent underwent MPI to evaluate results of therapy. He was currently asymptomatic. He underwent an exercise ^{201}Tl SPECT exercising to the end of stage II of a standard Bruce protocol. He denied chest pain and had no ECG changes. The stress /3H redistribution ^{201}Tl SPECT images are displayed in Figure C5-7.

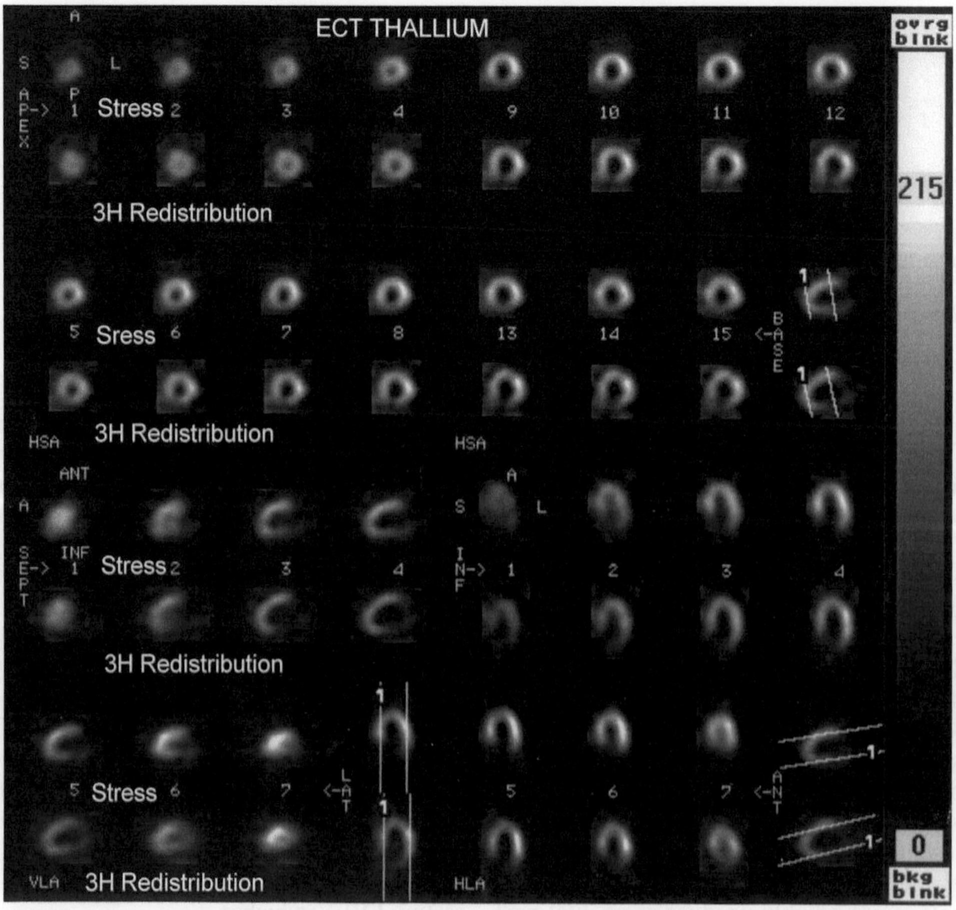

FIGURE C5-7.

Findings

The stress perfusion SPECT images showed mild to moderate decreased ^{201}Tl uptake in the inferior wall (RCA territory). On the rest images the defect in the inferior wall becomes worse and is now graded as moderate to severe. This finding is consistent with a reverse redistribution defect (RRD).

Discussion

RRD is not unusual with ^{201}Tl imaging. The finding is characterized by a defect that is more evident on delayed image as compared with the immediate poststress images. The prevalence of reverse redistribution varies widely[74] from 5% to 9% in patients with chest pain to 75% in patients imaged after thrombolytic therapy in the setting of acute myocardial infarction.[75]

At present, the pathophysiology and clinical significance of this phenomenon are controversial. Reverse redistribution may reflect normal variability in segmental ^{201}Tl clearance in the absence of obstructive CAD. No large series of patients with a low likelihood of CAD have been reported regarding the frequency of RRD and its correlation with significant CAD. However, in the presence of known CAD and recent MI, with or without revascularization, reverse redistribution is common (25% to 75%) and most likely represents viable but abnormal or injured myocardial cells with perfusion sometimes maintained by collateral vessels. There may also be an admixture of viable and nonviable cells. Washout is increased because these cells may not be able to maintain a high intracellular potassium/thallium concentration.[76] When cell integrity has been damaged by previous insult and myocytes are unable to retain thallium, there is RRD in the regions with worse perfusion.[77] In the context of the post-MI patient, who has undergone revascularization (thrombolysis, PTCA, CABG), reverse redistribution probably represents a patent infarct-related artery and salvage of viable myocardium; the prognosis of such patients has not been thoroughly investigated, but preliminary data suggest an improved prognosis as compared with patients with a typical reversible defect. An RRD occurring in a patient with known stable CAD is thought to represent viable and possibly ischemic myocardium in the face of relatively extensive CAD. The prognosis of patients with relatively severe RRDs is similar to patients with typical reversible ^{201}Tl defects. Most of such RRDs resolve after revascularization, and function improves in associated dyssynergic myocardium. Reverse redistribution on reinjection imaging occurs less often but may represent a similar situation. RRD on thallium imaging is identified on rest images; therefore even if the stress ^{201}Tl images are normal, delayed rest images should be obtained. Reverse redistribution may also occur (rarely) with 3 to 4 hour delayed ^{99m}Tc-MIBI imaging, but the clinical significance remains controversial.[78]

Interpretation

Inferior wall reverse redistribution defect on ^{201}Tl imaging, in a patient with history of prior inferior MI and stent the RCA.

Case 5.8

History

A 35-year-old male smoker with a strong family history of CAD presented with a 1-week history of stuttering chest pain radiating to his jaw. He underwent a rest/exercise ^{99m}Tc-tetrofosmin SPECT same day protocol displayed in Figure C5-8A. He exercised for 11 minutes using a standard Bruce protocol with no diagnostic ST-segment changes on ECG or symptoms.

Findings

The stress SPECT images acquired both in the supine and prone position demonstrated a moderate-sized area of mildly diminished uptake along the inferior wall reversible on the resting images. Coronary angiography (Figure C5-8B) showed an interesting congenital anomaly. The patient's RCA had an anomalous take off from the left sinus of Valsalva.

Discussion

The true occurrence of this anomaly is unknown. Total occurrence of congenital anomalies of coronary arteries is still uncommon and occurs in approximately 0.2% to 1.2% of the population.[79] Most of these anomalies are diagnosed within infancy and there is a high mortality without intervention. There are two reported mechanisms of ischemia. The first is the narrowed opening of the RCA as it comes off the aorta. The second is the physical compression of the RCA as it courses between the aorta and the pulmonary trunk. Figure C5-8C is a multislice (16 slices) CT image of another patient to illustrate the course of an anomalous RCA passing between the aorta and the pulmonary artery.

An increased risk of sudden death exists, but in almost all reported cases there have been symptoms of ischemia first. If the opposite coronary anomaly was present in which the left

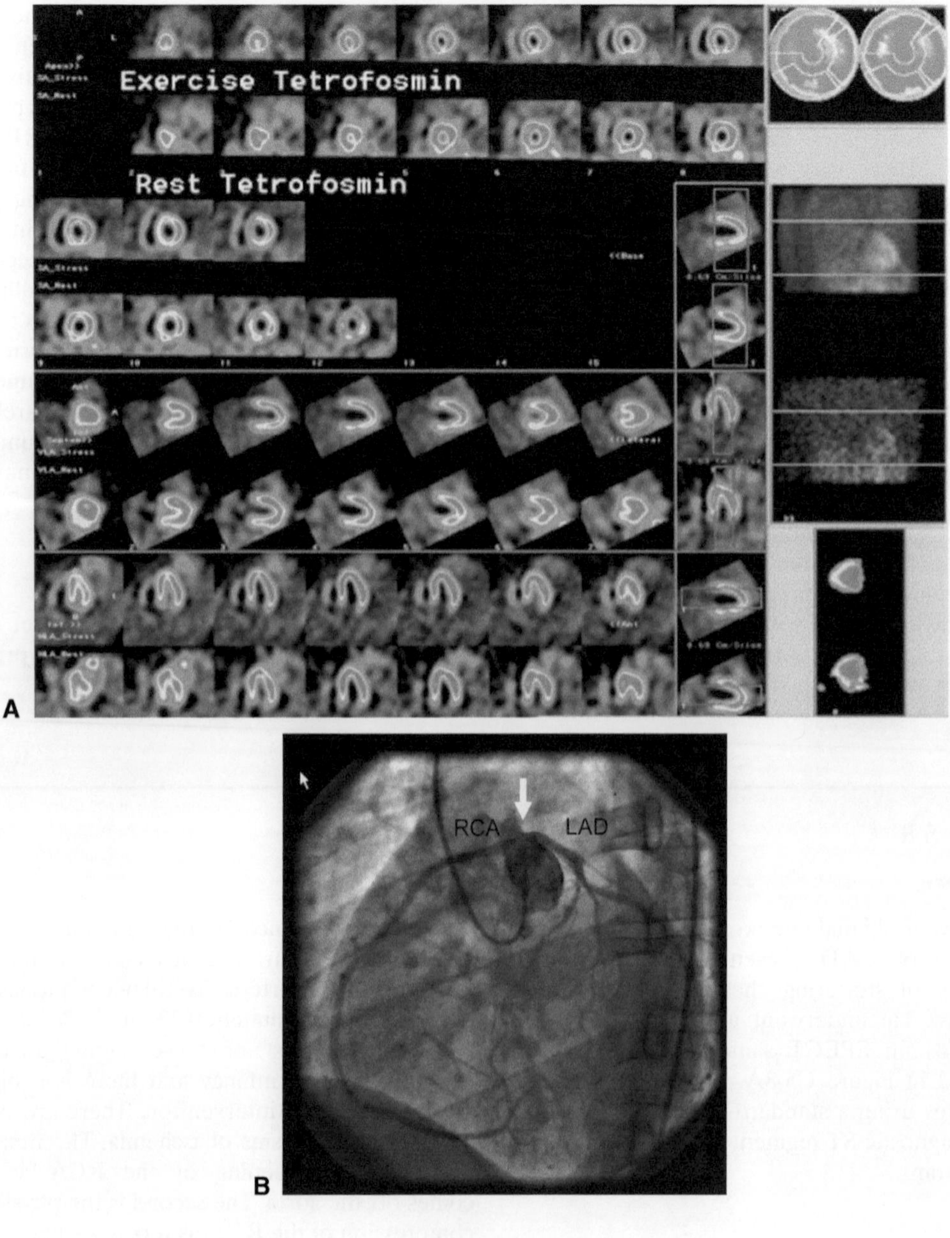

FIGURE C5-8. (A and B)

main artery arises from the right sinus of Valsalva, there is a definite increase in the risk of sudden death even without symptoms.[80] For a patient with this anomaly surgery is indicated regardless of symptoms. In this patient, who presented with typical cardiac symptoms and scintigraphic evidence of ischemia, he would most likely benefit from surgical repair of his anomalous artery.

Interpretation

Anomalous take off of the RCA.

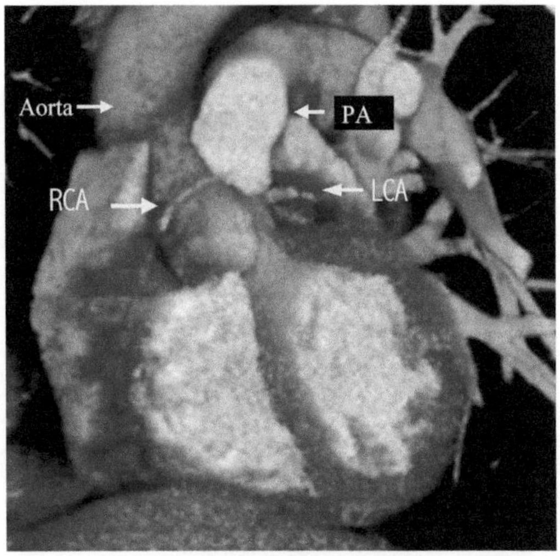

C

FIGURE C5-8. (A–C)

Case 5.9

History

A 13-year-old boy presented with heart failure symptoms at age 11 and was diagnosed with a congenital anomaly of the left coronary artery (anomalous origin of the left coronary artery from the pulmonary artery [ALCAPA]). He underwent surgical repair (Takeuchi procedure) with excellent clinical results. He was referred for a rest/exercise myocardial perfusion study using ^{99m}Tc-MIBI using the same-day protocol displayed in Figure C5-9A. His resting ECG is shown in Figure C5-9B. He exercised 15 minutes using the standard Bruce protocol, had a normal hemodynamic response, normal exercise ECG, and no chest pain on exertion.

Findings

The SPECT images (Figure C5-9A) demonstrated a fixed defect in the distal anterior wall and apex consistent with the presence of scar tissue in the territory of the LAD. The resting ECG (Figure C5-9B) demonstrated anterior R waves consistent with only partial loss of viability in the anterior wall. An early repolarization pattern is seen at rest (ST-segment elevation) in the anterior leads, which is nonspecific, but may be a result from previous MI.

Discussion

From the nuclear cardiology standpoint, an FDG-PET study would be ideal to provide additional information about myocardial viability in the distal anterior wall and apex, but it was not thought to be necessary in this clinical scenario.

This patient's condition (ALCAPA) is rare, with a prevalence of 1/30,000 to 1/300,000 live births, but is the most common clinically important congenital malformation of the coronary circulation.[81] Most cases (90%) present in infancy with severe mortality in the absence of intervention, although there are cases of asymptomatic adult survival. These patients can present with chronic myocardial ischemia that can cause irreversible damage to the myocardium (as demonstrated by SPECT in the current case). The clinical scenario at presentation may vary from heart failure, angina pectoris, syncope while exercising, or sudden death.[82] ALCAPA is characterized by a coro-

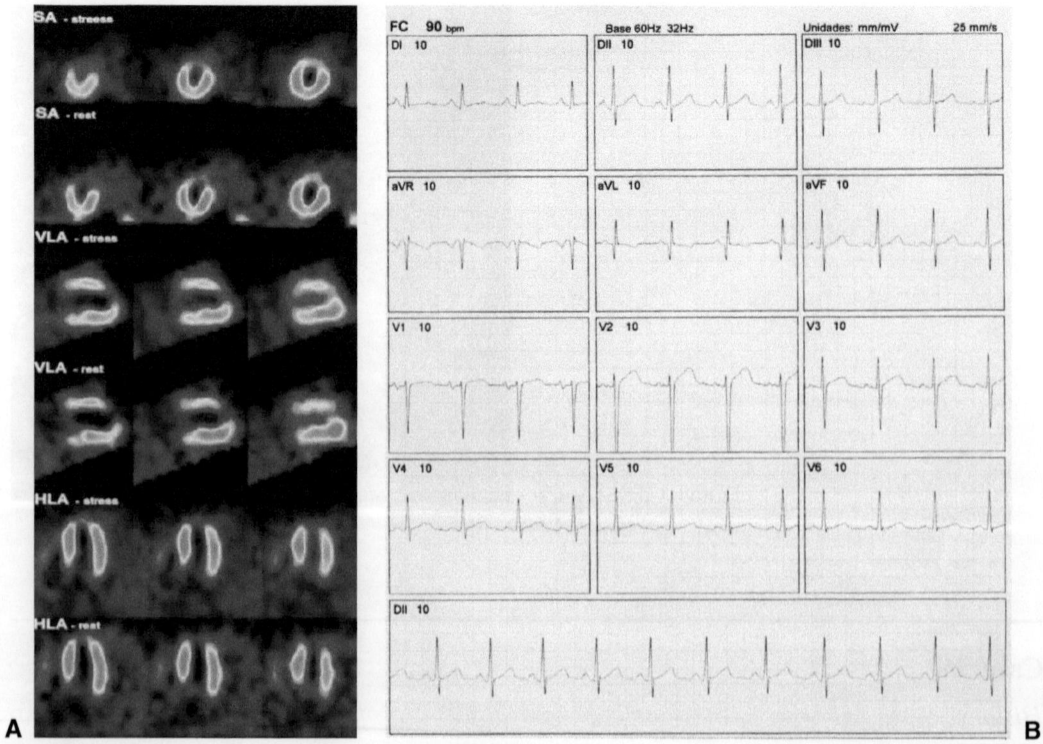

FIGURE C5-9. (A and B)

nary steal that occurs from the RCA through dilated collaterals to the LCA. This condition results in myocardial ischemia with associated MI, papillary muscle dysfunction, and mitral regurgitation. Surgical correction is imperative to reduce irreversible damage to the myocardium. Establishment of a dual coronary artery system is the current goal of the treatment.[81,83–85] Implanting the anomalous coronary artery directly into the ascending aorta is ideal but may not be possible for some unusual anatomic patterns in which the anomalous coronary artery arises in a location remote from the ascending aorta or in which the anomalous coronary artery takes an intramural course between the great arteries. In these situations, other surgical options, such as intrapulmonary baffling (Takeuchi procedure) may be required.[81,85]

The Takeuchi procedure, which was performed in this patient, consists of creating an aortopulmonary window, through which oxygenated blood from the aorta is directed to the coronary artery ostium via a polytetrafluoroethylene tunnel. MPI may be useful to assess surgical results. Some of the complications that may occur include baffle obstruction, baffle leak, and pulmonary artery obstruction.[85] Surgical procedures to achieve physiological correction of the coronary flow abnormalities are effective as long as there is potential for myocardial recovery. However, chronic myocardial ischemia may lead to irreversible damage to the myocardium, especially when the diagnosis is made in adulthood and heart transplantation may be necessary.[82]

Interpretation

Anomalous origin of the left coronary artery.

Case 5.10

History

A 38-year-old white male diabetic patient was referred for MPI because of recent onset of exertional chest pain. He had a history of transposition of the great arteries (TGA) requiring Mustard repair (described in the following Discussion section) at the age of 3 and pulmonic baffle revision (described in the following Discussion section) at age 35 followed by placement of a pacemaker for high-degree AV block. He was referred for a rest/stress adenosine same day ^{99m}Tc-MIBI protocol, displayed in Figure C5-10. No chest pain or significant ECG changes occurred during the adenosine infusion.

Findings

In this patient, the systemic ventricle is located on the right anatomic side. Both the stress and rest SPECT images showed a large fixed defect along the inferior wall and inferoseptal region of the systemic ventricle, with no evidence of reversibility, consistent with nontransmural scar. The gated images (not shown) demonstrated global hypokinesis, and the systemic ventricle ejection fraction was 18%.

Discussion

With TGA, the aorta arises in an anterior position of the anatomical right ventricle (RV) and the pulmonary artery arises from the anatomical left ventricle (LV). Therefore, there is a complete separation between the pulmonary and systemic circulation: the systemic venous blood passes through the right atrium, RV, aorta, and systemic circulation; whereas the pulmonary blood passes through the left atrium, LV and pulmonary artery, and pulmonary circulation. In order for the infant to survive, there must be a communication between these two circuits. In about one third of these patients, associated cardiac defects exist, such as a patent foramen ovale and ductus arteriosus allowing communication between the right and left circulations.[86] In the absence of such associated anomalies, as

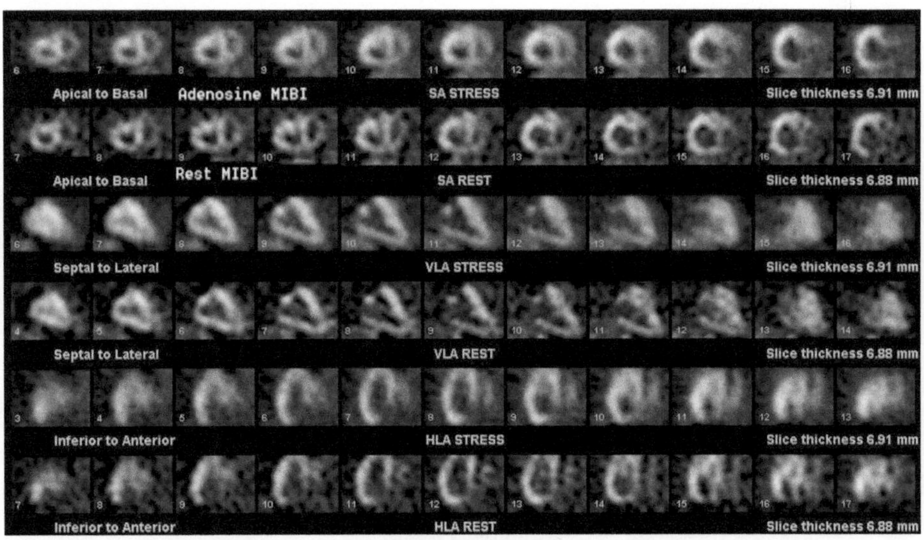

FIGURE C5-10.

was the case in this patient, two surgical procedures have been proposed for patients with TGA. The Mustard repair or *atrial switch* in which the atrial septum is excised, and then a baffle within the atria is reconstructed to direct the systemic blood flow across the mitral valve into the LV and the pulmonary flow across the tricuspid valve into the RV. Thus, the physiologic circulation is restored, although the anatomic RV continued to function as the systemic ventricle, leading to hypertrophy of the anatomical RV as seen on MPI (Figure C5-10). The atrial switch operation has been replaced by arterial switch [86–88] in which the pulmonary artery and ascending aorta are switched, so the pulmonary artery is arising from the RV and the aorta arising from the LV.

The perfusion abnormalities seen in patients with TGA can be explained by the fact that the systemic ventricle (anatomic RV) is supplied by the RCA. This system may provide insufficient flow in the presence of considerable myocardial hypertrophy, seen when the RV functions for a long period of time at the systemic pressures.[89–91] Reversible and fixed perfusion defects with concordant wall motion abnormalities occur in the right (systemic) ventricle 10 to 20 years after Mustard repair for TGA. Ischemia and infarction seem to be important factors in the pathogenesis of ventricular failure.

Interpretations

1. Transposition of the great vessels after Mustard and baffle repair with no evidence of ischemia.
2. Infarction of the inferior wall of the systemic ventricle (anatomical RV).
3. Pacemaker for third AV block, a common complication of TGA.

Case 5.11

History

A 73-year-old man without other risk factors for CAD, but with LBBB, presented with frequent episodes of stress-induced retrosternal chest pain starting a month earlier. His baseline ECG demonstrated LBBB. A resting echocardiogram was normal. He underwent a rest/dipyridamole ^{99m}Tc-MIBI SPECT study displayed in Figure C5-11A.

A

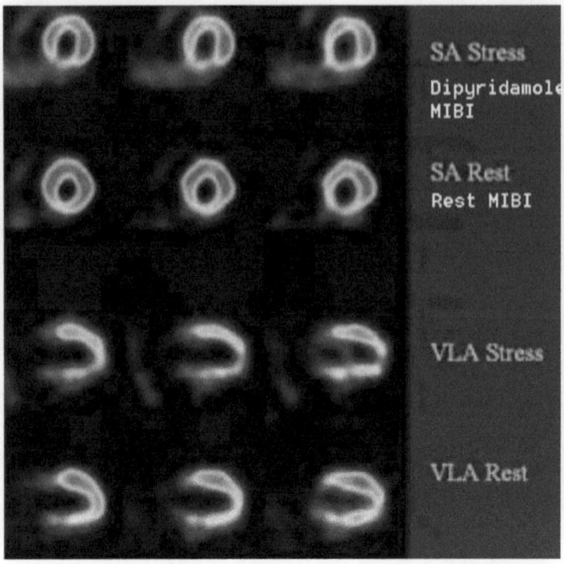

FIGURE C5-11. (A)

FIGURE C5-11. (B)

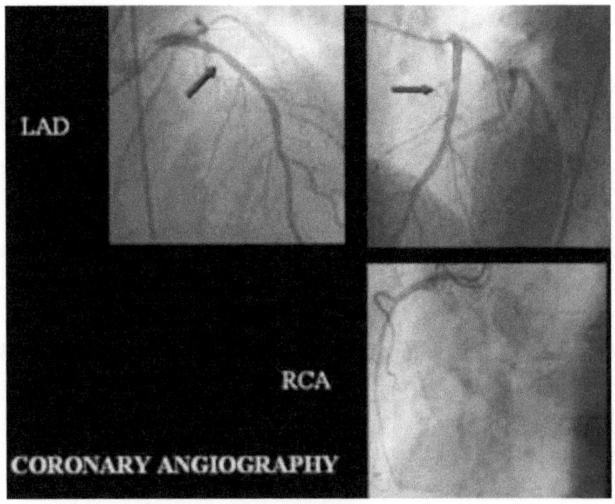

B

Findings

The SPECT images demonstrated mildly reversible decreased uptake in the anterior wall and severe partially reversible decreased uptake in the inferior wall of the myocardium, indicating ischemia in the territories of the LAD and RCA. Coronary angiography (Figure C5-11B) revealed 40% stenosis of the proximal LAD, and the RCA and LCX had mild irregularities.

Discussion

This case is an example of *apparent* discordance between invasive and nuclear imaging results. The typical chest pain of this patient indicates a high pretest probability of ischemia and according to the Bayes theorem, the posttest probability of CAD is high as well (see Figure 1-3). The stress-induced perfusion defects on MPI indicate ischemia in both the LAD and RCA territories. Artifactual perfusion defects in the septum and/or the anteroseptal region should be considered in patients with LBBB but are much less common when the study is performed using vasodilators instead of exercise or dobutamine. In this case, a large portion of the anterior wall is also involved, which favors true ischemia instead of an artifact. An IVUS was performed (Figure C5-11C) and demonstrated that in the region of the LAD

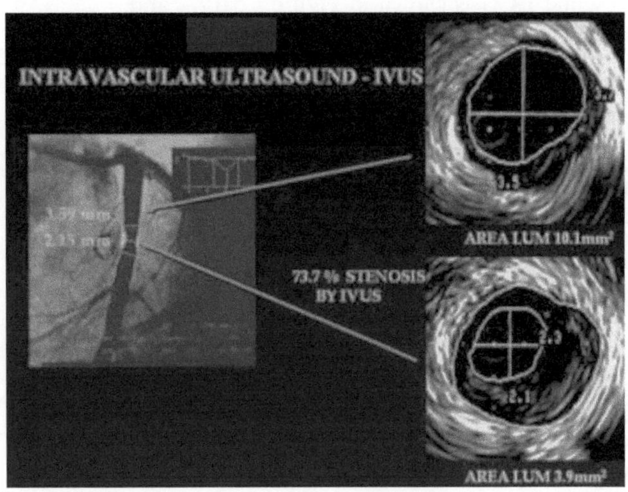

C

FIGURE C5-11. (C, courtesy of Dr. Costantino Costantini, Clinica Cardiologyca Costantini, Curitiba, Brazil.)

lesion, there is severe intimal thickening and luminal narrowing with significant remodeling of the vessel wall. Based on these findings, a stent was placed in the LAD.

The question remaining is whether or not the ischemia in the RCA territory is true or false. Diaphragmatic attenuation may cause artifacts in this area, reducing the specificity of findings in the inferior wall, which is certainly a possibility in this patient. Endothelial dysfunction and microcirculatory abnormalities in the RCA territory are possibilities to be considered and aggressive medical therapy is also indicated for this patient.

Interpretation

Ischemia in the LAD territory demonstrated by rest/dipyridamole ^{99m}Tc-MIBI in a patient with typical chest pain and LBBB and confirmed by IVUS, whereas coronary angiography demonstrated only a 40% stenosis.

Case 5.12

History

A 40-year-old active man, with hypertension and a history of smoking presented with atypical chest pain and progressive fatigue over a 1-month period. He underwent a rest/exercise ^{99m}Tc-MIBI SPECT study. He exercised for three and a half minutes on a standard Bruce protocol and started feeling malaise entering stage II, at which time the radiopharmaceutical was injected. He then experienced an episode of syncope. Early into exercise his BP increased from 120/80 to 150/90 mm Hg and the HR from 95 to 136 bpm. Right after the syncope, his BP was 115/70 mm Hg and the HR 145 bpm. His baseline ECG is shown in Figure C5-12A and the first ECG tracing after his syncope is shown in Figure C5-12B. Complete recovery occurred after 5 minutes and the SPECT images are displayed in Figure C5-12C.

Findings

The baseline ECG demonstrated a right bundle branch block (RBBB) and RV hypertrophy (Figure C5-12A). There were no ST-segment changes or arrhythmia on the ECG obtained immediately after syncope (Figure C5-12B). The SPECT images demonstrated a large RV cavity, thickened RV walls, and a straight septum, suggestive of chronic pulmonary hypertension. There were no reversible perfu-

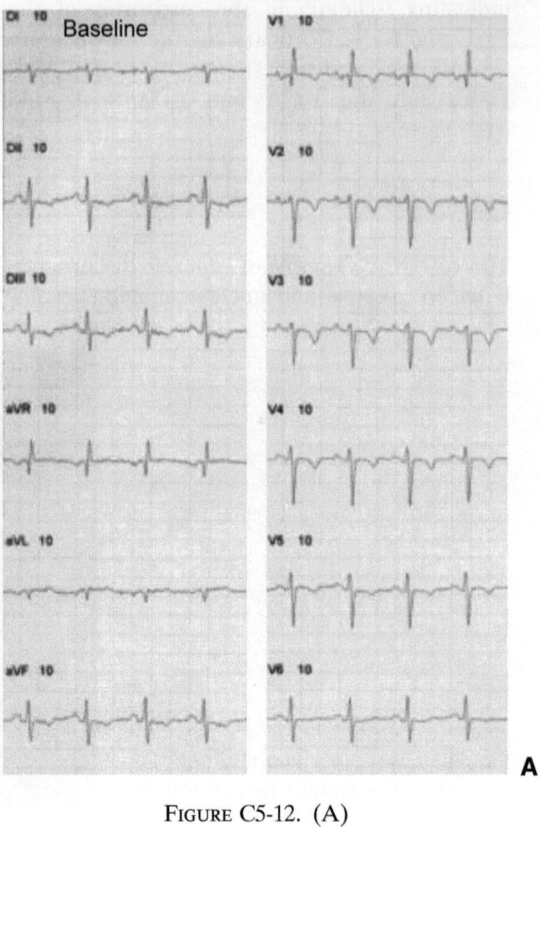

FIGURE C5-12. (A)

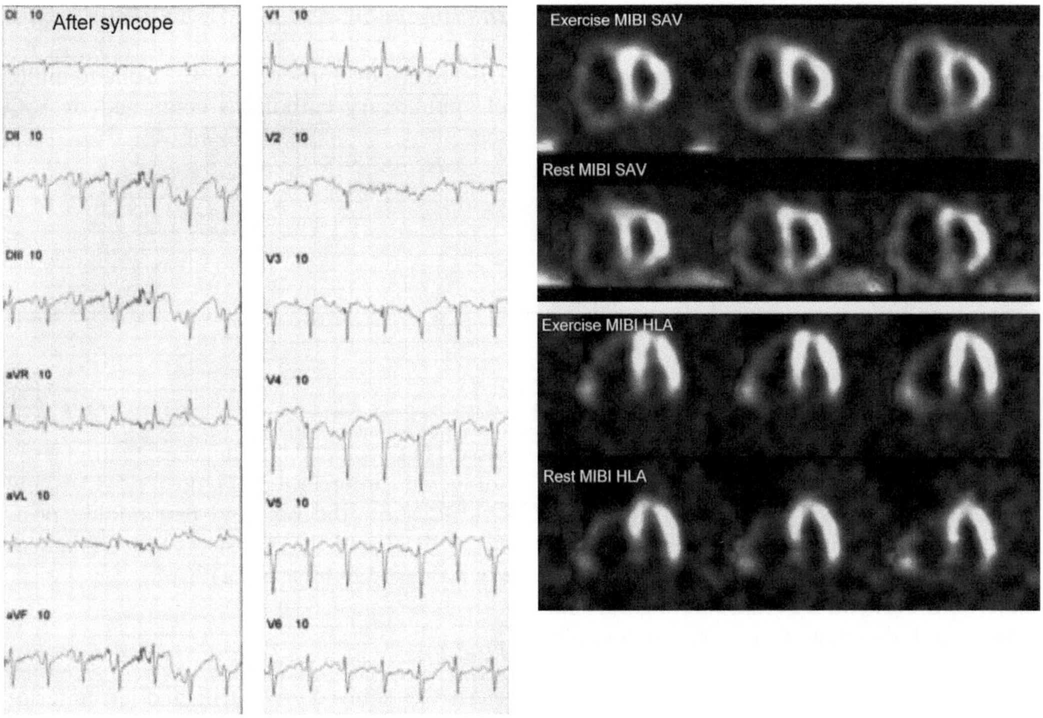

B C

FIGURE C5-12. (B and C)

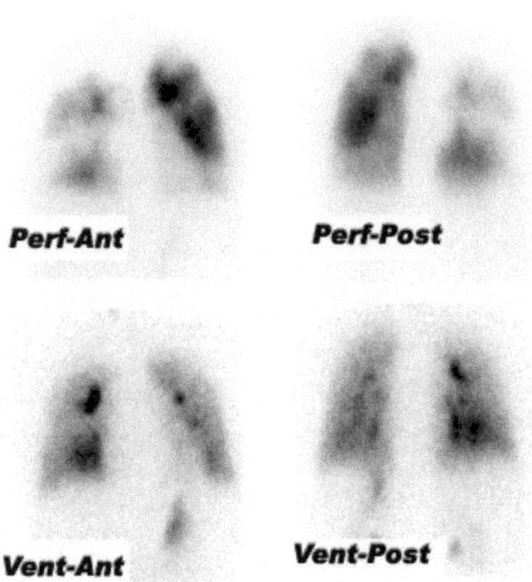

D

FIGURE C5-12. (D)

sion defects to suggest myocardial ischemia. These findings suggest a pulmonary or valvular etiology rather than ischemia, as a cause of syncope. A ventilation/perfusion (V/Q) pulmonary scan was performed (Figure C5-12D), demonstrating large perfusion defects not present on the ventilation images, typical of pulmonary embolism. An echocardiogram revealed a threefold increase in the pulmonary artery pressure and no significant valvular disease.

Discussion

The findings of RBBB and no ST-segment changes on ECG and RV hypertrophy and no reversible perfusion defects on SPECT images suggested chronic pulmonary hypertension rather than ischemia. Chronic pulmonary hypertension was likely due to pulmonary emboli in a patient presenting with atypical chest pain and progressive fatigue. This was confirmed with a V/Q scan. The syncope experienced by the patient while exercising was probably due to an exacerbation of his chronic hypoxemia.

Interpretation

Dilated RV diagnosed by SPECT due to multiple pulmonary embolisms confirmed by V/Q scan.

Case 5.13

History

A 76-year-old man was admitted with chest pain. His past medical history included valve replacement in 1995 to treat severe aortic stenosis and regurgitation, at which time no significant CAD was present. In April 2002 he underwent evaluation because of anginal complaints and dyspnea. Coronary angiography revealed severe aortic regurgitation but only minor irregularities of the coronary arteries, and he underwent a second aortic valve replacement.

After hospital discharge, this patient developed typical anginal complaints both during exercise and at rest during the night. His symptoms were relieved by nitroglycerine. He underwent a rest/exercise ^{99m}Tc-MIBI SPECT study. He exercised 7 minutes on standard Bruce protocol. He developed limiting chest pain, and the study was interrupted. Figures C5-13A and C5-13B show the rest and first minute post-stress ECG, and the rest/stress SPECT images are displayed in Figure C5-13C.

Findings

The ECG showed an RBBB and left anterior hemiblock at rest (Figure C5-13A), but during exercise (Figure C5-13B) there was major ST-segment elevation in leads V3, V4, and V5 (changes in leads V1 and V2 were not taken into consideration due to his RBBB). The SPECT images (Figure C5-13C) demonstrated severely decreased uptake in the apex, anterior, septal, and distal inferior walls, reversible on

A

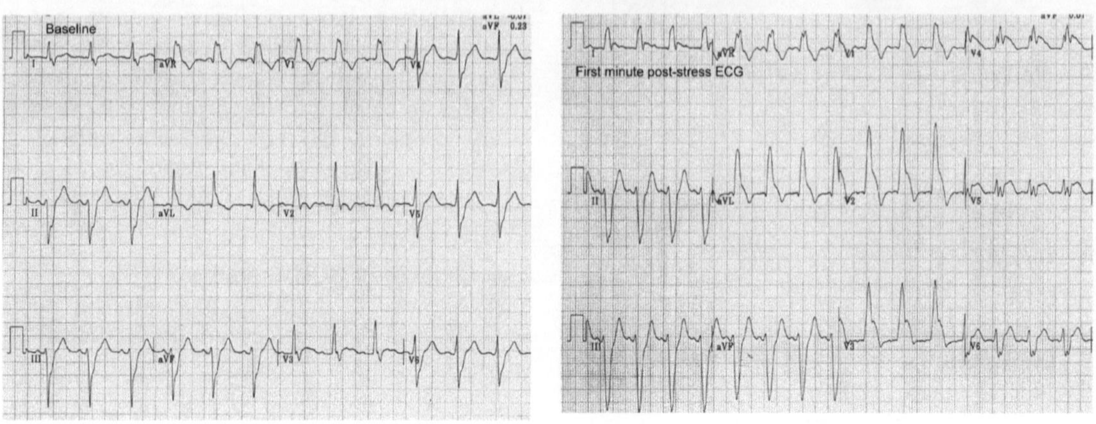

B

FIGURE C5-13. (A and B)

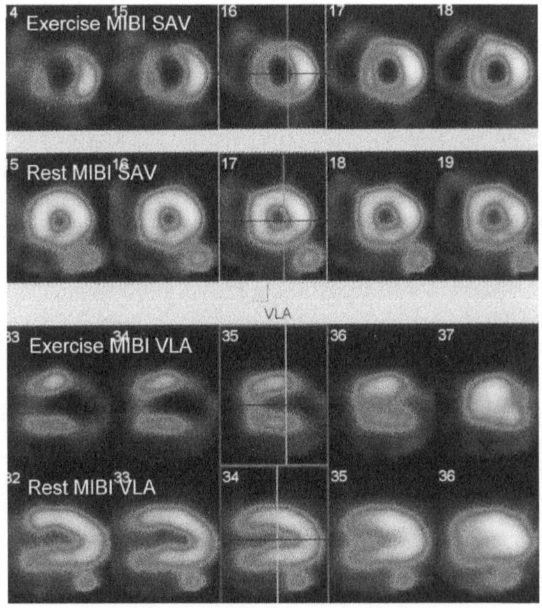

C

FIGURE C5-13. (C, courtesy of Dr. Frans Visser, Amsterdam, The Netherlands.)

the resting images. This indicated extensive and severe ischemia in the LAD territory.

Discussion

Angina due to coronary spasm has been first recognized by Nothnagel in 1867[92] and he proposed the name *angina pectoris vasomotoria*. In 1959, Prinzmetal et al.[93] described the syndrome of *variant angina* characterized by angina at rest and transient ST-segment elevation on ECG. They postulated that the mechanism of chest pain in patients with this finding was due to coronary artery spasm associated with some degree of CAD. The attacks are cyclical in nature and often occur in the morning hours. Ventricular arrhythmias and AV block can occur during the attacks and MI and sudden death are complications.

Approximately 60% of patients with ischemic spasm have definite evidence of underlying CAD, and the other 40% have *normal* or mildly abnormal coronary angiography.[94–96] MacAlpin[94] found that in 90% (62/69) of cases the spasm causing ischemia was precisely superimposed on and limited to the site of a preexisting coronary lesion.

As in this patient, exertional angina coexists in about 50% of patients, and the clinical presentation is sometimes difficult to distinguish from unstable angina. The symptoms of variant angina are relieved by sublingual nitroglycerine within minutes, as was the case in this patient, and should be used promptly. ECG is usually positive for ischemia during chest pain and ambulatory ECG monitoring may be helpful for diagnosis. ST-segment elevation is a hallmark of injury, usually extending all the way from the subendocardium to the subepicardium (transmural ischemia) and is frequently seen with severe spasm. The other aspect is the complaint of nocturnal chest pain. Coronary spasm is known to have a circadian variation, and vessels are more prone to vasoconstriction between 5 and 8 AM (perhaps related to the physiologic catecholamine surge). MPI demonstrated extensive and severe ischemia, in this case in the LAD territory. In a patient with only mild irregularities on coronary angiography, coronary spasm should be seriously considered. IVUS should also be considered to evaluate diffuse intimal thickening, plaque extent, and vascular remodeling.

Provocative testing has been used to make the diagnosis of variant angina when a spontaneous attack cannot be documented. Many stimuli may trigger coronary spasm, including exercise, ergonovine injection, catecholamine release, and exposure to a cold environment.

The cold pressor test and exercise are physiologic stimuli for coronary spasm but with a relatively low sensitivity. Dipyridamole stress appears to induce reversible defects as well as exercise and supports the hypothesis that, in addition to epicardial coronary spasm, dysfunction of the microvasculature is responsible for abnormal coronary perfusion in these patients.[97]

This relationship with cold is very interesting and may explain why those living in countries with cold winters experience coronary spasm more frequently. Approximately 50% of patients with CAD develop angina when exposed to cold conditions at rest. However, a higher percentage develops angina when exercise is added.[98,99] The *cold pressor test*, described in Chapter 4, can be used to evaluate patients suspected of spasm. This test was originally described by Hines and Brown in 1936,[100] and it is still useful today to evaluate vascular reactivity. The other aspect mentioned is the relationship with catecholamine release, especially just before arousal. The cold pressor test increases release of plasma epinephrine by 112%, and an even higher release of 229% is induced by exercise on the treadmill.[101] The pharmacologic agents ergonovine and acetylcholine provoke coronary spasm with a sensitivity of approximately 90%, but a temporary pacemaker should be placed before RCA or dominant left coronary are done because of the high incidence of bradyarrhythmias and conduction disturbances.[102]

Interpretation

Coronary spasm causing severe transmural ischemia detected by rest/exercise ^{99m}Tc-MIBI SPECT.

Case 5.14

History

A 47-year-old man with a history of inferior MI and CABG presented with atypical chest pain. The patient was unable to exercise and underwent a rest/adenosine stress ^{99m}Tc-tetrofosmin same-day protocol study. The gated SPECT images have been analyzed using the Emory Cardiac Toolbox (ECTb)[103] (Figure C5-14A) and QGS/QPS, developed at Cedars-Sinai Medical Center[104] (Figure C5-14B, QPS; and Figure C5-14C, QGS).

Findings

The SPECT images demonstrated a large fixed perfusion in the inferior wall of the myocardium consistent with the known MI. The motion display of the gated images demonstrated inferior wall hypokinesis with both software packages. The LVEF, EDV, and ESV were 42%, 127 ml, and 73 ml by ECTb and 37%, 104 ml, and 66 ml by QGS.

Discussion

Semiquantitative analysis of MPI has been discussed in Chapter 3, especially in Case 3.7. Multiple software packages are commercially available to analyze gated MPIs with different algorithms to identify the epicardial and endocardial borders of the myocardium. Therefore, there are issues regarding normal values and reproducibility of measurements of cardiac volumes between these different software packages. The most distributed software packages to measure LV volumes and EF from gated perfusion tomograms are QGS and ECTb. A study of 246 patients evaluated for CAD and 50 subjects with low likelihood for CAD compared measurements of LVEF, EDV, and ESV obtained using these two software packages. A good linear correlation was found but the LVEF and EDV were significantly lower for QGS than with ECTb.[105] The average values (mean +/− 1 SD) for the 50 patients with low likelihood of CAD are shown in Table 5-1 and are consistent with those published

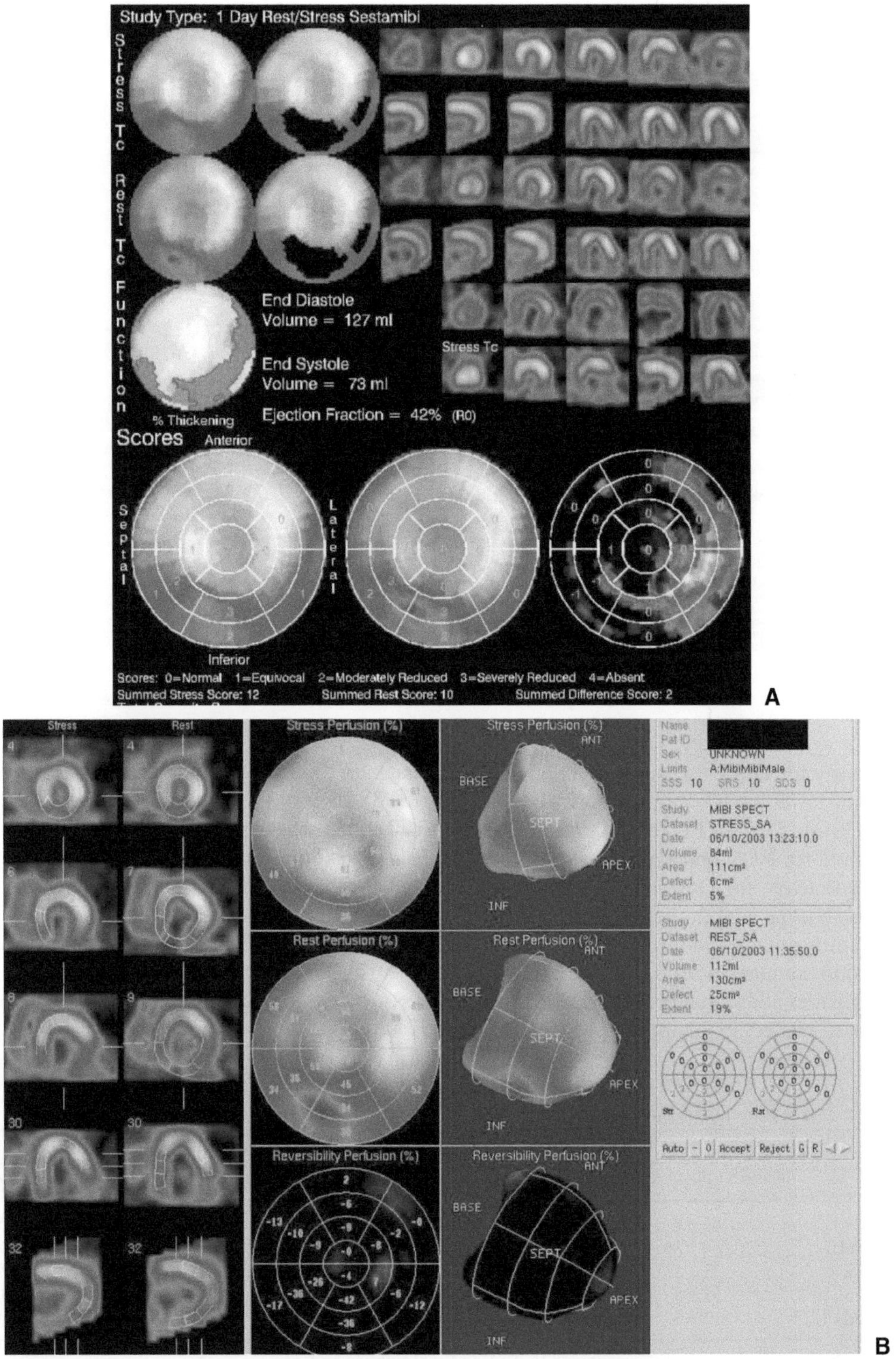

FIGURE C5-14. (A and B)

C
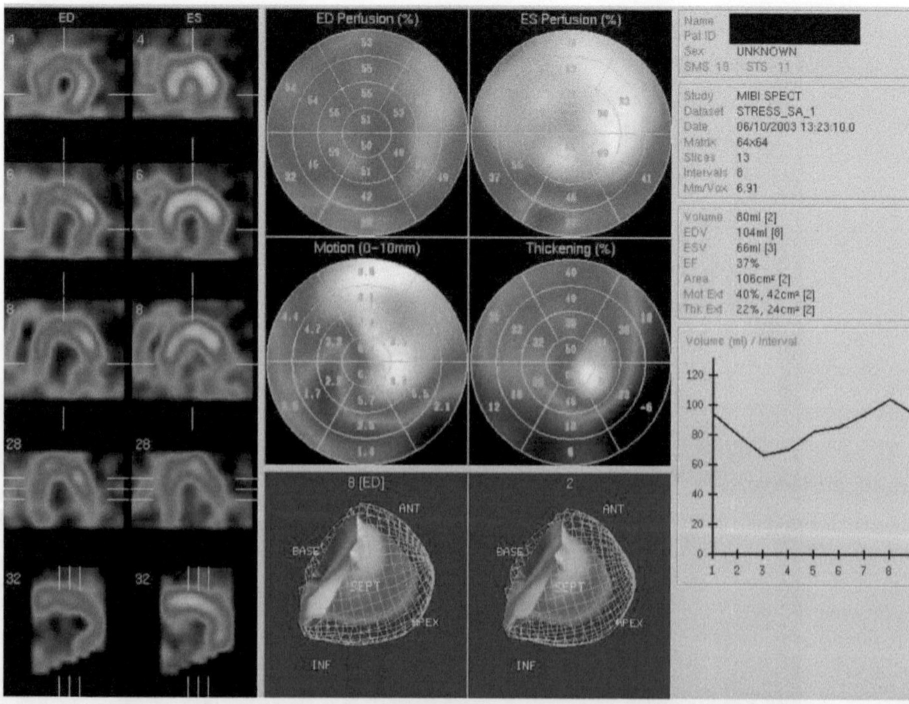

FIGURE C5-14. (C)

previously for QGS.[106] Using a 95% confidence level, the lower limits of normal for LVEF is 44% for QGS and 51% for ECTb, and the upper limits of normal for EDV and ESV are 137 ml and 67 ml, respectively, for QGS and 171 ml and 69 ml for ECTb using an 8 frames/cycle algorithm.

Quantification of the extent and severity of perfusion abnormalities is important as well and provides additional prognostic information that is discussed in Chapter 9. Most software packages provide the summed stress scores (SSS), summed rest scores (SRS), and summed difference scores (SDS) as quantitative indices of perfusion defects by comparison with normal databases for different MPI protocols (see Case 3.7). However, the accuracy of any quantitative index depends on rigorous quality control during acquisition, reconstruction, and processing of the image data as discussed in Chapter 13.

TABLE 5-1. LV Functional Parameters for Subjects at Low Likelihood for CAD

	All		Men		Women	
	QGS	ECTb	QGS	ECTb	QGS	ECTb
EF (%)	62 ± 9	67 ± 8	57 ± 7	63 ± 6	69 ± 8	72 ± 8
EDV (mL)	84 ± 26	105 ± 33	101 ± 20	124 ± 29	63 ± 17	84 ± 24
ESV (mL)	33 ± 17	35 ± 17	44 ± 13	46 ± 14	20 ± 10	24 ± 12
EVD (mL/m^2)	31 ± 8	39 ± 10	35 ± 6	43 ± 9	26 ± 6	34 ± 9
ESV (mL/m^2)	12 ± 5	13 ± 6	15 ± 4	16 ± 5	8 ± 4	10 ± 4

EDV_I, EDV indexed to body surface area; *ESV_I*, ESV indexed to body surface area.

From Nichols, Santana, Folks, et al. (105), by permission of *J Nucl Cardiol.*

TABLE 5-2. Comparative Characterization of Abnormal SPECT Results

	Defect Size		
	Small	Medium	Large
Vascular territories	<1/2	1	2 or 3
SSS[a]	4–8	9–13	>13
Polar maps (% of LV)[b]	<10%	10–20%	>20%
Circumferential profile (% of LV)[c]	<5%	5–10%	>10%

[a] Summed stress score.
[b] Compared with gender-matched normal file and reflects extents only.
[c] Circumferential profiles based on Wachers-Lui-CQ: sum of defects in 36 interpolated slices; compared with normal data files and incorporates both extent and severity.
From Wackers FJT (107) in Sandler, Coleman, Wackers, et al. Diagnostic Nuclear Medicine, by permission of Williams & Wilkins.

In particular, the accuracy of the perfusion scores depends heavily on the accuracy of the oblique axis selection to obtain short-axis myocardial slices perpendicular to the axis of the heart as discussed in Case 13.1 and accurate selection of the apex and base of the heart as discussed in Case 13.2. In addition, the perfusion scores provided by different software packages may differ significantly for the same reason cardiac volumes differ. To our knowledge, there is no published comparison of perfusion indices obtained with different software packages. It is generally recommended to adjust computer quantification of perfusion scores according to visual interpretation of the SPECT images. Table 5-2 provides a comparative categorization of myocardial perfusion abnormalities by commonly used subjective and computer quantification.[107]

For gated SPECT studies, quantification of wall motion and thickening abnormalities is also provided by the commercially available software packages.[108] Reference values for segmental motion (millimeters) and thickening (percent) have been determined for 20 segments in 64 patients with a low likelihood of CAD (<5%) and validated in 201 patients with a likelihood of CAD >5%.[109] In the group of patients with low likelihood of CAD, the average values of motion ranged from 4.8 to 9.5 mm, whereas average thickening ranged from 20% to 69%. In that study, threshold criteria for the detection of motion and thickening abnormalities at individual myocardial segments was expressed as the number of standard deviation (SD) below the mean reference value in each segment and was 2 to 3 SDs below the mean reference value for most segments. The summed motion score (SMS) and summed thickening scores (STS) are the sum of the 20 segment scores (scale of 0 to 5 for motion and 0 to 3 for thickening), as determined for perfusion scores.[110,111] The wide range in normal segmental motion and thickening precludes the definition of a single lower limit of normal.

References

1. Maddahi J, Berman DS. Detection, evaluation and risk stratification of coronary artery disease by thallium-201 myocardial perfusion scintigraphy. In Depuey EG, Garcia EV, Berman DS (eds). *Cardiac SPECT Imaging.* Philadelphia: Lippincott Williams & Wilkins; 2001:155–177.
2. Berman DS, Hayes SW, Germano G. Assessment of myocardial perfusion and viability with technetium-99m perfusion agents. In Depuey EG, Garcia EV, Berman DS (eds). *Cardiac SPECT Imaging.* Philadelphia: Lippincott Williams & Wilkins; 2001:179–210.
3. Detre KM, Wright E, Murphy ML, Takaro T. Observer agreement in evaluating coronary angiograms. *Circulation.* 1975;52:979–986.
4. Zir LM, Miller SW, Dinsmore RE, Gilbert JP, Harthorne JW. Interobserver variability in coronary angiography. *Circulation.* 1976;53: 627–632.
5. DeRouen TA, Murphy JA, Owen W. Variability in the analysis of coronary arteriograms. *Circulation.* 1977;55:324–328.
6. Beauman GJ, Vogel RA. Accuracy of individual and panel interpretations of coronary arteriograms: implications for clinical decisions. *J Am Coll Cardiol.* 1990;16:108–113.
7. Fleming RM, Kirkeeide RL, Smalling RW, Gould KL. Patterns in visual interpretation of coronary arteriograms as detected by quantitative coronary arteriography. *J Am Coll Cardiol.* 1991;18:945–951.
8. Nissen SE. Shortcomings of coronary angiography and their implications in clinical practice. *Cleve Clin J Med.* 1999;66:479–485.

9. Topol EJ, Nissen SE. Our preoccupation with coronary luminology. The dissociation between clinical and angiographic findings in ischemic heart disease. *Circulation.* 1995;92:2333–2342.
10. Ellestad MH. The time has come to reexamine the gold standard when evaluating noninvasive testing. *Am J Cardiol.* 2001;87:100–101.
11. Verna E, Ceriani L, Giovanella L, Binanghi G, Garancini S. "False-positive" myocardial perfusion scintigraphy findings in patients with angiographically normal coronary arteries: insights from intravascular sonography studies. *J Nucl Med.* 2000;41:1935–1940.
12. Kjaer A, Meyer C, Nielsen FS, Parving HH, Hesse B. Dipyridamole, cold pressor test, and demonstration of endothelial dysfunction: a PET study of myocardial perfusion in diabetes. *J Nucl Med.* 2003;44:19–23.
13. Tiatti P, Gragasso G, Monit LD, Setola E, Lucotti P, Fermo I, Paroni R, Galluccio E, Pozza G, Chierchia S, Margonato A. Acute intravenous L-arginine infusion decreases endothelin-1 levels and improves endothelial function in patients with angina pectoris and normal coronary arteriograms: correlation with asymmetric dimethylarginine levels. *Circulation.* 2003;107:429–436.
14. Cox ID, Clague JR, Bagger JP, Ward DE, Kaski JC. Endothelial dysfunction, subangiographic atheroma, and unstable symptoms in patients with chest pain and normal coronary arteriograms. *Clin Cardiol.* 2000;23:645–652.
15. Zaret BL, Wackers FJT, Soufer R. Nuclear Cardiology. In Braunwald E (ed). *Heart Disease.* Philadelphia: Saunders; 1992:276–311.
16. Gerson MC, Thomas SR, Van Heertum RL. Tomographic myocardial perfusion imaging. In Gerson MC (ed). *Cardiac Nuclear Medicine.* New York: McGraw Hill; 1991:25–52.
17. Mahmarian JJ, Verani MS. Exercise thallium-201 perfusion scintigraphy in the assessment of coronary artery disease. *Am J Cardiol.* 1991; 67:2D–11D.
18. Henkin RE, Kalousdian S, Kikkawa RM, et al. Diagnostic and therapeutic technology assessment (DATTA), myocardial perfusion imaging, utilizing single-photon emission-computed tomography (SPECT). *Washington Manual of Therapeutic Technology.* Washington DC, 1994:2850.
19. Mahmarian JJ, Verani MS. Exercise thallium-201 perfusion scintigraphy in the assessment of coronary artery disease. *Am J Cardiol.* 1991; 67:2D–11D.
20. Maddahi J, Kiat H, Friedman JD, et al. Technetium-99m-sestamibi myocardial perfusion imaging for evaluation of coronary artery disease. In Zaret BL, Beller GA (eds). *Nuclear Cardiology: State of the Art and Future Directions.* S. Louis: Mosby; 1993:191–200.
21. Verani MS. Thallium-201 and technetium-99m perfusion agents: Where we are in 1992. In Zaret BL, Beller GA (eds). *Nuclear Cardiology: State of the Art and Future Directions.* St. Louis: Mosby; 1993:191–200.
22. Azzarelli S, Galassi AR, Foti R, et al. Accuracy of 99m-tetrofosmin myocardial tomography in the evaluation of coronary artery disease. *J Nucl Cardiol.* 1999;6:183–189.
23. Sharir T, Germano G, Kang X, et al. Prediction of myocardial infarction versus cardiac death by gated myocardial perfusion SPECT: risk stratification by the amount of stress-induced ischemia and the poststress ejection fraction. *J Nucl Med.* 2001;42:831–837.
24. Sharir T, Bacher-Stier C, Dhar S, et al. Identification of severe and extensive coronary artery disease by postexercise regional wall motion abnormalities in ^{99m}Tc sestamibi gated single-photon emission computed tomography. *Am J Cardiol.* 2000;86:1171–1175.
25. Demer LL, Gould KL, Goldstein RA, et al. Assessment of coronary artery disease severity by positron emission tomography: comparison with quantitative arteriography in 193 patients. *Circulation.* 1989;79:825–835.
26. Guidelines for the American College of Cardiology/American Heart Association task force on assessment of diagnostic and therapeutic cardiovascular procedures (Committee on Radionuclide Imaging), developed in collaboration with the American Society of Nuclear Cardiology. *J Am Coll Cardiol.* 1995;25:521–547.
27. Shelbert HR, Wisenberg G, Phelps ME, et al. Noninvasive assessment of coronary stenoses by myocardial imaging during pharmacologic coronary vasodilation. Detection of coronary artery disease in human beings with intravenous ^{13}N ammonia and positron emission tomography. *Am J Cardiol.* 1982;49:1197–1207.
28. Gould KL, Goldstein RA, Mullani NA, et al. Noninvasive assessment of coronary stenoses by myocardial perfusion imaging during pharmacologic coronary vasodilation. Clinical feasibility of positron cardiac imaging without a cyclotron using generator-produced rubidium-82. *J Am Coll Cardiol.* 1986;7:775–789.

29. Goldstein RA, Kirkeeide KL, Smalling RW, et al. Changes in myocardial perfusion reserve after PTCA: noninvasive assessment with positron tomography. *J Nucl Med.* 1987;28: 1262–1267.
30. Demer LL, Gould KL, Goldstein RA, Kirkeeide RL. Noninvasive assessment of coronary collaterals in man by PET perfusion imaging. *J Nucl Med.* 1990;31:259–270.
31. Demer LL, Gould KL, Goldstein RA, et al. Assessment of coronary artery disease severity by positron emission tomography: Comparison with quantitative arteriography in 193 patients. *Circulation.* 1989;79:825–835.
32. Go RT, Marvick TH, MacIntyre WJ, et al. A prospective comparison of rubidium-82 PET and thallium-201 SPECT myocardial perfusion imaging utilizing a single dipyridamole stress in the diagnosis of coronary artery disease. *J Nucl Med.* 1990;31:1899–1905.
33. Stewart RE, Schwaiger M, Molina E, et al. Comparison of rubidium-82 positron emission tomography and thallium-201 SPECT imaging for detection of coronary artery disease. *Am J Cardiol.* 1991;67:1303–1310.
34. Grover-McKay M, Ratib O, Schwaiger M, et al. Detection of coronary artery disease with positron emission tomography and rubidium-82. *Am Heart J.* 1992;123:646–652.
35. Stewart RE, Schwaiger M, Molina E, et al. Comparison of rubidium-82 positron emission tomography and thallium-201 SPECT imaging for detection of coronary artery disease. *Am J Cardiol.* 1991;67:1303–1310.
36. Bezzera AJ, Prates JC, Didio LJ. Incidence and clinical significance of bridges of myocardium over the coronary arteries and their branches. *Surg Radiol Anat.* 1987;9:273–280.
37. Ferreira AG Jr, Trotter SE, Konig B Jr, et al. Myocardial bridges: morphological and functional aspects. *Br Heart J.* 1991;66:364–367.
38. Noble J, Bourassa MG, Petitclerc R, et al. Myocardial bridging and milking effect on the left descending coronary artery: normal variant or obstruction. *Am J Cardiol.* 1976;37:993–999.
39. Kramer JR, Kitazume H, Proudfit WL, et al. Clinical significance of isolated coronary bridges: benign and frequent condition involving the left descending coronary artery. *Am Heart J.* 1982;103:283–288.
40. Tortoledo F. Stented bridge: another golden gate for the interventional cardiologist. *Cathet Cardiovasc Interv.* 2002;56:64–65.
41. Ge J, Erber R, Ruprecht HJ, et al. Comparison of intravascular ultrasound and angiography in the assessment of myocardial bridging. *Circulation.* 1994;89:1725–1732.
42. Erbel R, Treese N, Alken G, et al. Provocation of myocardial bridging in patients with normal coronary arteries by nitroglycerin and orciprenalin. *Eur Heart J.* 1985;6(suppl):71.
43. Ahmad M, Merry SL, Haibach H. Evidence of impaired myocardial perfusion and abnormal left ventricular function during exercise in patients with isolated systolic narrowings of the LAD artery. *Am J Cardiol.* 1981;48: 832–836.
44. Greenspan M, Iskadrian AS, Catherwood E, et al. Myocardial bridging of the LAD artery: Evaluation using exercise thallium-201 myocardial scintigraphy. *Cathet Cardiovasc Diagn.* 1980;6:173–180.
45. Berry JF, von Mering GO, Schmalfuss C, et al. Systolic compression of the left descending coronary artery: a case series, review of the literature, and therapeutic options including stenting. *Cathet Cardiovasc Interv.* 2002;56:58–63.
46. Patel R, Bushnell DL, Wagner R, Stumbris R. Frequency of false-positive septal defects on adenosine/^{201}Tl images in patients with LBBB. *Nucl Med Commun.* 1995;16:137–139.
47. Hirzel HO, Senn M, Nuesch K, et al. Thallium 201 scintigraphy in complete LBBB. *Am J Cardiol.* 1984;53:764–769.
48. DePuey EG, Guertler-Krawczynska E, Robbins WL. Thallium 201 SPECT in coronary artery disease patients with LBBB. *J Nucl Med.* 1988; 29:1479–1485.
49. Larcos G, Brown ML, Gibbons RJ. Role of dipyridamole thallium-201 imaging in patients with LBBB. *Am J Cardiol.* 1991;68:1097–1098.
50. Larcos G, Gibbons RJ, Brown ML. Diagnostic accuracy of exercise thallium-201 single-photon emission computed tomography in patients with left bundle branch block. *Am J Cardiol.* 1991;68:756–760.
51. Weiss AT, Berman DS, Lew AS, et al. Transient ischemic dilatation of the left ventricle on stress thallium-201 scintigraphy: a marker of severe and extensive coronary artery disease. *J Am Coll Cardiol.* 1987;9:752–759.
52. McLaughlin MG. Transient ischemic dilation: A powerful diagnostic and prognostic finding of stress myocardial perfusion imaging. *J Nucl Cardiol.* 2002 Nov–Dec;9(6):663–667.
53. Kinoshita N, Sugihara H, Adachi Y, et al. Assessment of transient left ventricular dilata-

tion on rest and exercise on ^{99m}Tc tetrofosmin myocardial SPECT. *Clin Nucl Med.* 2002; 27:34–39.
54. Mazzanti M, Germano G, Kiat H, et al. Identification of severe and extensive coronary artery disease by automatic measurement of transient ischemic dilatation of the left ventricle in dual-isotope myocardial perfusion SPECT. *J Am Coll Cardiol.* 1996;27(7):1612–1620.
55. Daou D. Identification of extensive coronary artery disease: incremental value of exercise ^{201}Tl SPECT to clinical and stress test variables. *J Nucl Cardiol.* 2002;Mar–Apr;9(2):161–168.
56. Besletti A, Di Leo C, Alessi A, et al. Poststress end-systolic left ventricular dilation: a marker of endocardial post-ischemic stunning. *Nucl Med Commun.* 2001;22:685–698.
57. Chouraqui P, Rodriguez EA, Berman DS, et al. Significance of dipyridamole-induced transient dilatation of the left ventricle during thallium-201 scintigraphy in suspected coronary artery disease. *Am J Cardiol.* 1990;66:689–694.
58. Toyama T, Caner BE, Tamaki N, et al. Transient ischemic dilatation of the left ventricle observed on dipyridamole-stressed thallium-201 scintigraphy. *Kaku Igaku.* 1993;30:605–611.
59. Kristman JN, Ficaro EP, Corbett JR. Post-stress LV dilation: the effect of imaging protocol, gender and attenuation correction. *J Nucl Med.* 2001;42(Suppl):50P.
60. McClellan JR, Travin MI, Herman SD, et al. Prognostic importance of scintigraphic left ventricular cavity dilation during intravenous dipyridamole technetium-99m sestamibi myocardial tomographic imaging in predicting coronary events. *Am J Cardiol.* 1997;79:600–605.
61. Homma S, Kaul S, Boucher CA. Correlates of lung/heart ratio of thallium-201 in coronary artery disease. *J Nucl Med.* 1987;28:1531–1535.
62. Bacher-Stier C, Sharir T, Kavanagh PB, et al. Postexercise lung uptake of ^{99m}Tc-sestamibi determined by a new automatic technique: validation and application in detection of severe and extensive coronary artery disease and reduced left ventricular function. *J Nucl Med.* 2000;41:1190–1197.
63. Hansen CL, Cen P, Sanchez B, Robinson R. Comparison of pulmonary uptake with transient cavity dilation after dipyridamole ^{201}Tl perfusion imaging. *J Nucl Cardiol.* 2002;9:47–51.
64. Sanders GP, Pinto DS, Parker JA, et al. Increased resting ^{201}Tl lung-to-heart ratio is associated with invasively determined measures of left ventricular dysfunction, extent of coronary artery disease, and rest myocardial perfusion abnormalities. *J Nucl Cardiol.* 2003; 10:140–147.
65. Barr SA, Jain D, Wackers FJ, et al. Tetrofosmin Phase III multicenter study group: Are there correlates of increased thallium uptake on planar tetrofosmin perfusion imaging? *Circulation.* 1993;88:Suppl I-582.
66. Kaminek M, Mysliveck M, Skvarilova M, et al. Increased prognostic value of combined myocardial perfusion SPECT imaging and the quantification of lung ^{201}Tl uptake. *Clin Nucl Med.* 2002;27:255–260.
67. Vitola JV, Brambatti JC, Caligaris F, et al. Exercise supplementation to dipyridamole prevents hypotension, improves electrocardiogram sensitivity, and increases heart-to liver activity ratio on ^{99m}Tc sestamibi imaging. *J Nucl Cardiol.* 2001;8:652–659.
68. Johnson LL, Verdesca SA, Aude WY, et al. Postischemic stunning can affect left ventricular ejection fraction and regional wall motion on post-stress gated sestamibi tomograms. *J Am Coll Cardiol.* 1997;30:1641–1648.
69. Paul AK, Hasegawa S, Yoshioka J, et al. Exercise-induced stunning continues for at least one hour: evaluation with quantitative gated single-photon emission tomography. *Eur J Nucl Med.* 1999;26:410–415.
70. Lee DS, Yog DS, Chung JK, et al. Transient prolonged stunning induced by dipyridamole and shown on 1- and 24-hours poststress ^{99m}Tc-MIBI gated SPECT. *J Nucl Med.* 2000;41:27–35.
71. Paul AK, Hasegawa S, Yoshioka J, et al. Characteristics of regional myocardial stunning after exercise in gated myocardial SPECT. *J Nucl Cardiol.* 2002;9:388–394.
72. Emmett L, Iwanochko RM, Freeman MR, et al. Reversible regional wall motion abnormalities on exercise technetium-99m-gated cardiac single photon emission computed tomography predict high-grade angiographic stenoses. *J Am Coll Cardiol.* 2002;39:991–998.
73. Heiba SI, Santiago J, Mirzaitehrane M, et al. Transient postischemic stunning evaluation by stress gated ^{201}Tl SPECT myocardial imaging: Effect on systolic left ventricular function. *J Nucl Cardiol.* 2002;9:482–490.
74. Hecht HS, Hopkins JM, Rose JG, et al. Reverse redistribution: worsening of 201 thallium myocardial images from exercise to redistribution. *Radiology.* 1981;140:177–181.

75. Weiss AT, Maddahi J, Lew AS, et al. Reverse redistribution of ^{201}Thallium: a sign of non-trasmural myocardial infarction with patency of the infarct related coronary artery. *J Am Coll Cardiol.* 1986;7:61–67.
76. Arrighi JA, Soufer R. Reverse redistribution: is it clinically relevant or a washout? *J Nucl Cardiol.* 1998;5:195–201.
77. Silberstein EB, Devries DF, Reverse redistribution phenomenon in thallium-201 stress tests: angiographic correlation and clinical significance. *J Nucl Med.* 1985:26;707–710.
78. Shih WJ, Miller K, Stipp V. Reverse redistribution on dynamic exercise and dipyridamole stress technetium-99m-MIBI myocardial SPECT. *J Nucl Med.* 1995;36:2053–2055.
79. Frescura C, Basso C, Thiene G, et al. Anomalous origin of coronary arteries and risk of sudden death: a study based on an autopsy population of congenital heart disease. *Hum Pathol.* 1998;29:689–695.
80. Roberts WC. Major anomalies of coronary arterial origin seen in adulthood. *Am Heart J.* 1986;111:941–962.
81. Malec E, Zajac A, Mikuta M. Surgical repair or anomalous origin of the coronary artery from the pulmonary artery in children. *Cardiovasc Surg.* 2001;9 (June):292–298.
82. Nair KK, Zisman LS, Lader E, Dimova A, Canver CC. Heart transplant for anomalous origin of left coronary artery from pulmonary artery. *Ann Thorac Surg.* 2003;75:282–285.
83. Pandey R, Ciotti G, Pozzi M. Anomalous origin of the left coronary artery from the pulmonary artery: results of surgical correction in five infants. *Ann Thorac Surg.* 2002;74:1625–1630.
84. Huddleston CB, Balzer DT, Mendelokk EM. Repair of anomalous left main coronary artery arising from the pulmonary artery in infants: long-term impact on the mitral valve. *Ann Thorac Surg.* 2001;71:1985–1989.
85. Ando M, Mee RB, Duncan BW, Drummond-Webb JJ, Seshadri SG, Igor Mesia CI. Creation of a dual-coronary system for anomalous origin of the left coronary artery from the pulmonary artery utilizing the trapdoor flap method. *Eur J Cardiothorac Surg.* 2002 Oct;22:576–581.
86. Brickner ME, Hillis LD, Lange LA. Congenital heart disease in adults. *N Engl J Med.* 2000 Feb;342(5):334–342.
87. Atik E. Transposição das grandes artérias. Avaliação dos resultados e da conduta atual. *Arq Bras Cardiol.* 2000;75(2):91–93.
88. Triedman JK. Arrhythmias in adults with congenital heart disease. *Heart.* 2002;87:383–389.
89. Hornung TS, Bernard EJ, Jaeggi ET, Howman-Giles RB, Celermajer DS, Hawker RE. Myocardial perfusion defects and associated ventricular dysfunction in congenitally corrected transposition of the great arteries. *Heart.* 1998;80:322–326.
90. Lubiszewska B, Gosiewska E, Hoffman P, et al. Myocardial perfusion and function of the systemic right ventricle in patients after atrial switch procedure for complete transposition: long term follow-up. *J Am Coll Cardiol.* 2000; 36:1365–1370.
91. Millane T, Bernard EJ, Jaeggi E, et al. Role of ischemia and infarction in late right ventricular dysfunction after atrial repair of transposition of the great arteries. *J Am Coll Cardiol.* 2000; 35:1661–1668.
92. Nothnagel H. Angina pectoris vasomotoria. *Dtsch Arch Klin Med.* 1867;3:309.
93. Prinzmetal M, et al. Angina pectoris I. The variant form of angina pectoris. *Am J Med.* 1959;27:375.
94. MacAlpin RN. Relation of coronary arterial spasm to the sites of organic stenosis. *Am J Cardiol.* 1980;46:143–153.
95. MacAlpin RN. Correlation of the location of coronary arterial spasm with the lead distribution of ST segment elevation during variant angina. *Am Heart J.* 1980;99:555–564.
96. Bertrand ME, LaBlanche JM, Tilmant PY, et al. Frequency of provoked coronary arterial spasm in 1089 consecutive patients undergoing coronary arteriography. *Circulation.* 1982:65:1299–1306.
97. Fujita H, Yamabe H, Yokoyama M. Dipyridamole-induced reversible thallium-201 defects in patients with vasospastic angina and nearly normal coronary arteries. *Clin Cardiol.* 2000; 23:24–30.
98. Backman C, Holm S, Linderholm H. Reaction to cold of patients with coronary insufficiency. *Ups J Med Sci.* 1979;84:181–187.
99. Lassvik C, Areskog NH. Effects of various environmental temperatures on effort angina. *Ups J Med Sci.* 1979;84:173–180.
100. Hines EA, Brown GE. The cold pressor test for measuring the reactivity of the blood pressure: data concerning 571 normal and hypertensive subjects. *Am Heart J.* 1936;11:1–9.
101. Robertson D, Johnson GA, Robertson RM, et al. Comparative assessment of stimuli that

release neuronal and adrenomedullary catecholamines in man. *Circulation.* 1979;59: 637–643.
102. Diagnosis and management of patients with unstable angina. In Fuster V, Alexander RW, O'Rourke RA (eds). *Hurst's The Heart*, 10th edition. New York: McGraw Hill; 2001:1263–1266.
103. Faber TL, Cooke CD, Folks RD, et al. Left ventricular function and perfusion from gated SPECT perfusion images: an integrated method. *J Nucl Med.* 1999;40:650–659.
104. Germano G, Kavanagh PB, Waechter P, et al. A new algorithm for the quantitation of myocardial perfusion SPECT I technical principles and reproducibility. *J Nucl Med.* 2000;41:712–719.
105. Nichols K, Santana CA, Folks R, et al. Comparison between ECTb and QGS for assessment of left ventricular function from gated myocardial perfusion SPECT. *J Nucl Cardiol.* 2002;9:285–293.
106. Sharir T, Germano G, Kavanah PB, et al. Incremental prognostic value of post-stress left ventricular ejection fraction and volume by gated myocardial perfusion single photon emission tomography. *Circulation.* 1999;100:1445–1550.
107. Wackers JTH. Myocardial perfusion imaging. In Sandler MP, Coleman RD, Wackers JTH, Patton JA, Gottschalk A, Hoffer PB (eds). *Diagnostic Nuclear Medicine,* 4th ed. Baltimore: Williams & Wilkins; 2002:273–317.
108. Germano G, Erel J, Lewin H, et al. Automatic quantitation of regional myocardial wall motion and thickening from gated technetium-99m sestamibi myocardial perfusion single-photon emission computed tomography. *J Am Coll Cardiol.* 1997;30:1360–1367.
109. Sharir T, Berman DS, Waechter PB, et al. Quantitative analysis of regional motion and thickening by gated myocardial perfusion SPECT: Normal heterogeneity and criteria for abnormality. *J Nucl Med.* 2001;42:1630–1638.
110. Germano G, Kavanagh PB, Waechter PB, et al. A new algorithm for the quantitation of myocardial perfusion SPECT. I. theoretical aspects. *J Nucl Med.* 2000;41:712–719.
111. Sharir T, Germano G, Waechter PB, et al. A new algorithm for the quantitation of myocardial perfusion SPECT. II. Validation and diagnostic yield. *J Nucl Med.* 2000;41:720–727.

6 Myocardial Perfusion Imaging in the Emergency Department

Olímpio Ribeiro França Neto, Dominique Delbeke, João V. Vitola, and Jack A. Ziffer

Management of patients presenting to the emergency department (ED) with chest pain suggestive of acute myocardial infarction (AMI) remains a continuing challenge.[1] Emergency department visits for the evaluation of chest pain or other symptoms suggestive of acute coronary syndromes exceed 5 million each year in the United States, and more than 40% of these visits lead to costly hospital admissions.

Of patients presenting to the ED with acute chest pain, a majority have an electrocardiogram (ECG) that is normal or nondiagnostic for acute myocardial ischemia or infarction, and only a minority eventually are diagnosed with an acute coronary syndrome (ACS).[2]

Typically, these patients are admitted to exclude AMI despite a low incidence of ACS. However, missed ACS in patients who are inadvertently sent home from the ED has significant adverse outcomes and associated legal consequences.[3,4]

A low threshold for admission has been traditional. Because of this approach, fewer than 30% of patients admitted with chest pain ultimately are found to have an ACS. To reduce unnecessary admissions, maintain patient safety, and enhance cost-effectiveness, innovative strategies have been applied to the management of patients with chest pain. Many centers have developed chest pain centers, using a wide range of diagnostic strategies to deal with this dilemma.[1]

Radionuclide myocardial perfusion imaging (MPI) can potentially play an important role in this setting, by providing both a safe and efficient means to risk stratify patients with a low-to-moderate likelihood of unstable angina.[5]

The sensitivity of a rest MPI is not the same when patients are injected after cessation of pain, compared with those injected during angina; therefore, an exercise MPI is warranted for patients who are pain free and have no perfusion defects at rest. Serum cardiac markers, particularly troponins, are very specific for the detection of a larger part of the spectrum of ACS in the ED, including patients with minimal myocardial damage and higher risk for short-term death and nonfatal AMI,[6] but the sensitivity for unstable angina requires additional workup strategies to safely discharge these patients.[7]

The ERASE Trial

Myocardial perfusion imaging with ^{99m}Tc-MIBI in the ED reduces the number of unnecessary admissions, without increasing mistaken discharges, according to the results of ERASE (Emergency Room Assessment of ^{99m}Tc-MIBI in the Evaluation of Chest Pain) trial. The ERASE was the first prospective, multicenter, randomized trial to address this issue, and its findings are in agreement with those of previous observational studies. In ERASE, Udelson et al.[8] randomized 2,475 patients with chest pain or other ischemia symptoms to either standard ED evaluation strategies or usual care plus acute resting MPI using ^{99m}Tc-MIBI SPECT. They found that standard ED assessment was as good as standard care plus ^{99m}Tc-MIBI study in terms of appropriately determining that these patients should be hospitalized (80% to 90%). Both strategies were equally effective in identifying these true ACI patients (13%), where ^{99m}Tc-MIBI scanning seemed to have some advantages was in identifying patients without ischemia who did not need to be hospitalized. In the standard care group, 52% of nonischemic patients were unnecessarily hospitalized, compared with 42% of those who underwent a ^{99m}Tc-MIBI scan, meaning a 10% absolute reduction. What also needs to be considered is that this 10% absolute reduction may not translate into cost savings since it is estimated that 11.3 patients would have to undergo imaging to save one admission. This means that the break-even point "... at which the cost of imaging is exceeded by the cost reduction of the unnecessary admissions is $5519 per admission."[9–11]

Flow Chart for Patient and Patient Selection

Patients who present to the ED with acute chest pain are classified according to the probability of ACS (unstable angina or acute MI). They follow different pathways based on their symptoms, signs, and initial ECG. If there is ST-segment elevation, the diagnosis of AMI is made and the patient is admitted to the coronary care unit (CCU). Treatment is either thrombolysis or angioplasty. The ECG and cardiac enzymes are monitored. If no ST-segment elevation is present, but there is ST-segment depression or ischemic T-wave inversion, the patient is assumed to have unstable angina or non-ST-elevation MI and is admitted to the CCU. Treatment is heparin, aspirin, clopidogrel, beta-blockers, nitroglycerin, and (when indicated) a glycoprotein IIb/IIIa receptor inhibitor. The ECG and cardiac enzymes are monitored. Patients with known CAD and typical symptoms, and those with acute signs of impaired left ventricular function also are admitted to the CCU and follow the same pathway.

Those with intermittent chest discomfort and nondiagnostic ECG findings present the greatest diagnostic challenge in any ED. The strategy is to identify those with ACS using resting MPI as part of a protocol or serial ECGs and serum cardiac markers such as troponin T, troponin I, or CK-MB enzymes. If patients are free of symptoms and these tests are normal, they are referred for different modalities of stress tests. Patients with a clear noncardiac chest pain are sent home.[12–14]

Protocols Most Commonly Used

The chest pain pathway system at emergency departments was developed to rapidly identify patients with significant ECG changes (especially persistent ST-segment elevation), while still identifying CAD in low-to-moderate-risk patients with nondiagnostic ECGs. The pathway can be presented as a flowchart (Figure 6-1). As the patient *travels* down the pathway, decisions are made based on these risks and results, until eventually being either admitted to the hospital or discharged home.[15,16] Other algorithms to evaluate patients presenting with ACS have been published.[17,18]

Comparison of MPI with TMT Alone in the Emergency Department

Treadmill exercise testing (TMT) alone has been often recommended and employed in the ED due its low cost and great availability, when compared with other methods.[19,20] TMT is safe when performed in low to intermediate risk and clinically stable patients.[21] Some groups recommend TMT even in the first hour after admission to the ED, in patients with low probability of CAD (even without the results of serum cardiac markers).[22] The specificity in this case is low (in a population of low pre-test probability) but the negative predictive value is very high.[23] Some other studies show a sensitivity and specificity of a positive or inconclusive test for cardiac events of approximately 75%, and the negative predictive value for events >98%.[24,25]

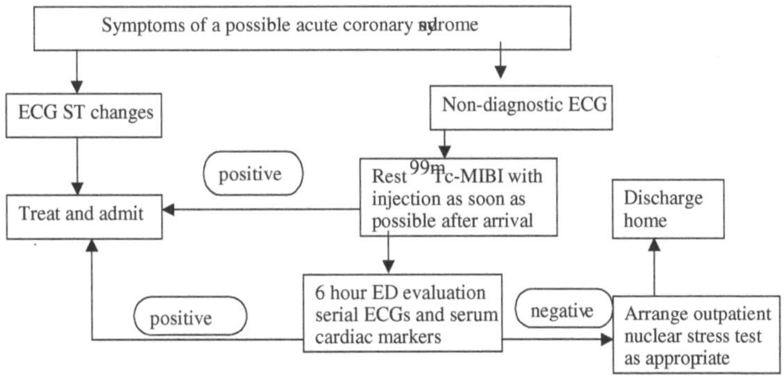

FIGURE 6-1. Pathway for the evaluation of patients with chest pain. (Adapted from Storrow, Gibler, et al. [16], by permission of *Ann Emerg Med.*)

The use of some medications may interfere with the sensitivity of a TMT. Amiodarone, beta blockers, digoxin, or calcium channel antagonists may decrease chronotropic response and, in these cases, the TMT alone may be limited, and other diagnostic options should be considered (e.g., MPI using dypiridamole or adenosine). The indication of a TMT depends on several factors including the patient's ability to perform exercise, the local expertise, and the availability of different testing modalities at different times of the day and different days of the week.[26] Patients who are capable of exercising and have an interpretable ECG (as discussed in Chapter 4) can be evaluated with a simple TMT. Patients who are incapable of exercising or who have an uninterpretable baseline ECG should be considered for pharmacological stress testing.[14,27]

Timing for Serial Enzymes and ECGs

The first 12-lead ECG should be quickly obtained on the patient's arrival to the ED; however, it represents only a *snapshot* of a dynamic process that may be occurring in the heart. Patients with definite or suspected ACS, whose first 12-lead ECG and enzymes are within normal, should be observed carefully for the following hours. A repeat ECG and enzymes should be obtained for 6 to 12 hours after the onset of symptoms.[28] The rise and descent of biochemical cardiac markers may vary and overlap significantly; therefore, it is imperative that physicians incorporate the time from the onset of the patient's symptoms into their assessment of the results of biochemical marker measurements.[29–31] Myoglobin is the earliest marker of myocardial necrosis. Despite being a sensitive marker, it has a low cardiac specificity.

Troponins (Tn), such as TnT and TnI, arise later and are more specific but have a lower sensitivity for the very early detection of myocardial necrosis (e.g., <6h) after the onset of symptoms. This implies that if an early (<6h) troponin test result is negative, a measurement should be repeated 8 to 12 hours after the onset of symptoms. Although the release kinetics of the troponins provide a wider diagnostic window for the diagnosis of MI at a time when creatine kinase CK-MB elevations have returned to normal, the more protracted period of elevation of troponin levels after an MI must be recognized. One possible disadvantage of the use of cardiac-specific troponins is their long (up to 10 to 14 days) persistence in the serum after release.[32]

Myoglobin has greater sensitivity for myocardial necrosis than CK-MB in patients who come to the ED with less than 4 hours of symptoms. The sensitivity is approximately 60% to 80% at presentation and the specificity approximately 80%. False-positive results may occur in patients with seizures, after electrical cardioversion, renal insufficiency, and trauma.

A positive result, 3 to 4 hours after the beginning of symptoms, often indicates AMI with a positive predictive value of >95%. In the same way, a negative result 3 to 4 hours after patient's arrival, decreases the probability of AMI (negative predictive value >90%).[33–36]

CK-MB can be found in cardiac and skeletal muscles and nervous tissues. The sensitivity of CK-MB for MI at presentation is low (30% to 50%) but it increases to 80% to 85% in the first 3 hours, and it reaches 100% in 9 hours (serial CK-MB every 3 to 4 hours). The negative predictive value is 95% in the first 3 hours after admission and patients with intermediate and high probability only reach 100% in 9 to 12 hours. Specificity is 95%. The preferential methodology is CK-MB-mass, which is more specific than CK-MB activity.[37–42]

Serial troponin and early MPI have comparable sensitivities for identifying MI. Perfusion imaging identifies more patients who need revascularization or who have significant CAD, but it has lower specificity for AMI. The two tests can provide complementary information for identifying patients at risk for ACS.[7] Serum troponin T and I are highly specific for acute MI (85% to 95%) but have low sensitivity at presentation. Sensitivity at presentation is 20% to 40%, with a slow increase in the next 12 hours (85% to 99%). The positive predictive value is 75% to 95%, but the negative predictive value at presentation is low (50% to 80%). Troponins remain elevated 7 to 14 days after an MI.[43,44]

Guidelines from the American Society of Nuclear Cardiology

The American Society of Nuclear Cardiology (ASNC) has published a position statement on radionuclide imaging in patients with suspected acute ischemic syndromes in the emergency department or chest pain center.[45] Six studies including a total of 2,113 patients have been performed between 1993 and 1999 and demonstrated a weighted average negative predictive value of 99.2% for detection of ACS with MPI during chest pain. The reliability of the resting scan alone is controversial if the ^{99m}Tc-perfusion agent is administered after chest discomfort resolves. Therefore, it is recommended that the radiopharmaceutical be injected during ongoing chest pain and not more than 2 hours after the symptoms have resolved. Stress testing is recommended to evaluate whether the presence of CAD is a contributor to the symptoms, when ACS is excluded by serial enzymes and ECG plus or minus a rest ^{99m}Tc-MIBI study.

Conclusion

Developing strategies that aggressively identify the patient with ACS can shorten time to therapy and result in improved prognosis in a medical environment where "time is muscle." Furthermore, quickly and safely discharging patients in whom the ACS is not present is necessary. MPI can play a pivotal role in achieving these goals.

Case Presentations

Case 6.1

History

A 43-year-old man with no risk factors presented to the ED with 2 hours of ongoing epigastric pain with a questionable chest component of pain. His ECG and initial laboratory workup were normal. Shortly after presentation, he was injected while symptomatic with 12 mCi of ^{99m}Tc-MIBI, and gated SPECT images were obtained 45 minutes later. The resting ^{99m}Tc-MIBI SPECT and gated images are displayed in Figures C6-1A and C6-1B.

Findings

A very large, severe defect of the lateral wall is seen, continuing to the adjacent anterolateral and inferolateral walls and extending from the base to the apex. The gated images show

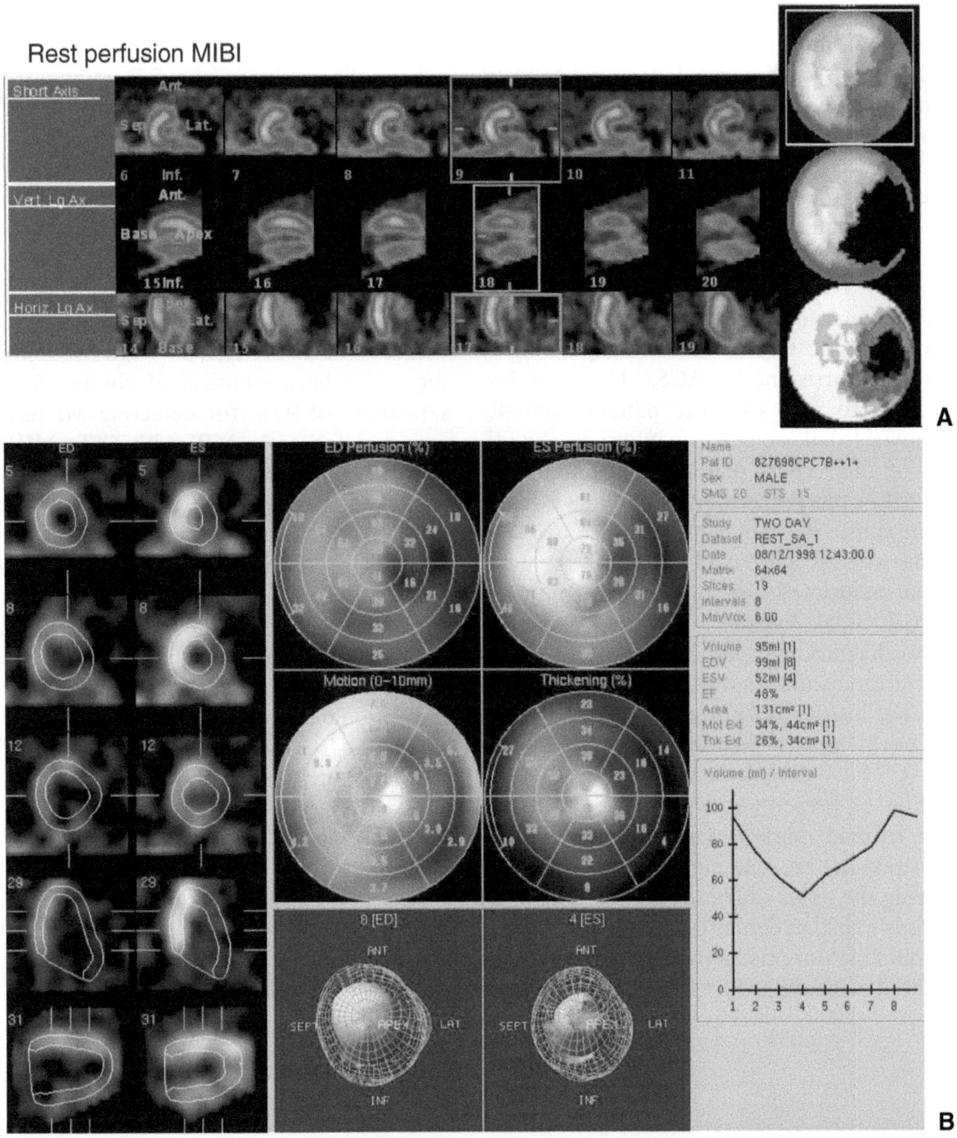

FIGURE C6-1. (A and B)

severely reduced thickening in the region of the defect, with an LV ejection fraction of 48%. These findings are consistent with stunning or necrosis.

The patient was taken emergently to coronary angiography where multivessel CAD was identified, including complete occlusion of his proximal left circumflex coronary artery (LCX). He underwent acute revascularization. Shortly after the completion of his coronary angiography procedure, the patient did develop elevation of serum cardiac markers of necrosis (troponin and CK-MB).

Discussion

Myocardial perfusion imaging identifies high-risk patients and abnormal perfusion before elevation of serum cardiac markers of necrosis,[7] and thus provides for earlier diagnosis in patients with normal or nondiagnostic coronary angiogram results. In this patient, the perfusion defect was in the lateral wall, the area that on conventional ECG has lower sensitivity for detecting the ACS (electrocardiographically silent). The lateral wall is the most common area to identify perfusion defects in patients with an ACS and normal ECGs.

More than 6 million patients per year present to an ED in the United States complaining of chest pain worrisome for ACS.[46] However, less than 20% to 30% of these patients actually have myocardial ischemia or infarct as the etiology of their chest pain. The prevalence of acute MI in this population of patients is 6%.[47] Despite conservative management, 2% to 8% of patients with ACS are inadvertently sent home with an associated risk of death of approximately 10%.[48,49] Various strategies have been used to diagnose MI and ischemia with serial ECG, serum cardiac markers, and echocardiography. The history and physical examination are often not helpful. Fewer than 50% of patients with ACS have diagnostic changes on ECG at the time of presentation to the ED.[50] Early serum cardiac markers (myoglobin, CK-MB, and troponins) become elevated several hours following the onset of chest pain. For example, in a study of 620 patients, the sensitivity of serial troponin I measurements over 8 hours was 92% compared with 39% for the initial measurement.[7] Severe myocardial ischemia or MI produces wall motion abnormalities, and therefore echocardiography in the ED is an attractive option with a high sensitivity (>90%), but poor specificity (<60%).[51]

Patients with nondiagnostic ECGs are a challenge. Wackers et al.[52] demonstrated the ability of ^{201}Tl scintigraphy to detect infarcts within 6 hours of presentation. However, the poor image quality, attenuation artifact, and spontaneous redistribution after injection limits the use of ^{201}Tl in the ED, so ^{99m}Tc-MIBI became the radiopharmaceutical of choice. A similar sensitivity of 92% for detecting MI has been reported for early MPI with ^{99m}Tc-MIBI and serial troponin I measurement.[7] The ERASE trial demonstrated that the addition of acute ^{99m}Tc-MIBI to the standard evaluation for patients presenting with suspected ACS decreased unnecessary hospitalizations among patients without ACS, without reducing appropriate admission for patients with acute ischemia.[8] This particular patient illustrates well the usefulness of acute resting ^{99m}Tc-MIBI when the ECG is nondiagnostic, especially in the LCX territory.

Interpretation

ACS detected by resting ^{99m}Tc-MIBI during chest pain due to occlusion of the LCX, leading to acute revascularization.

Case 6.2

History

A 57-year-old physician experienced atypical chest pain in his office. At presentation to the ED, his laboratory and ECG workup were normal. He was injected while symptomatic with 12 mCi of ^{99m}Tc-MIBI, and gated SPECT images were obtained 1 hour later. The resting ^{99m}Tc-MIBI SPECT and gated images are displayed in Figures C6-2A and C6-2B.

Findings

The images show a moderate sized, mild severity perfusion defect in the lateral wall. Gated images demonstrate normal wall motion (translation) but abnormal thickening during systole. Global measures of LV function and volume were normal, with an LVEF of 54%.

As in Case 6.1, this patient also has abnormal perfusion in the lateral wall, albeit less exten-

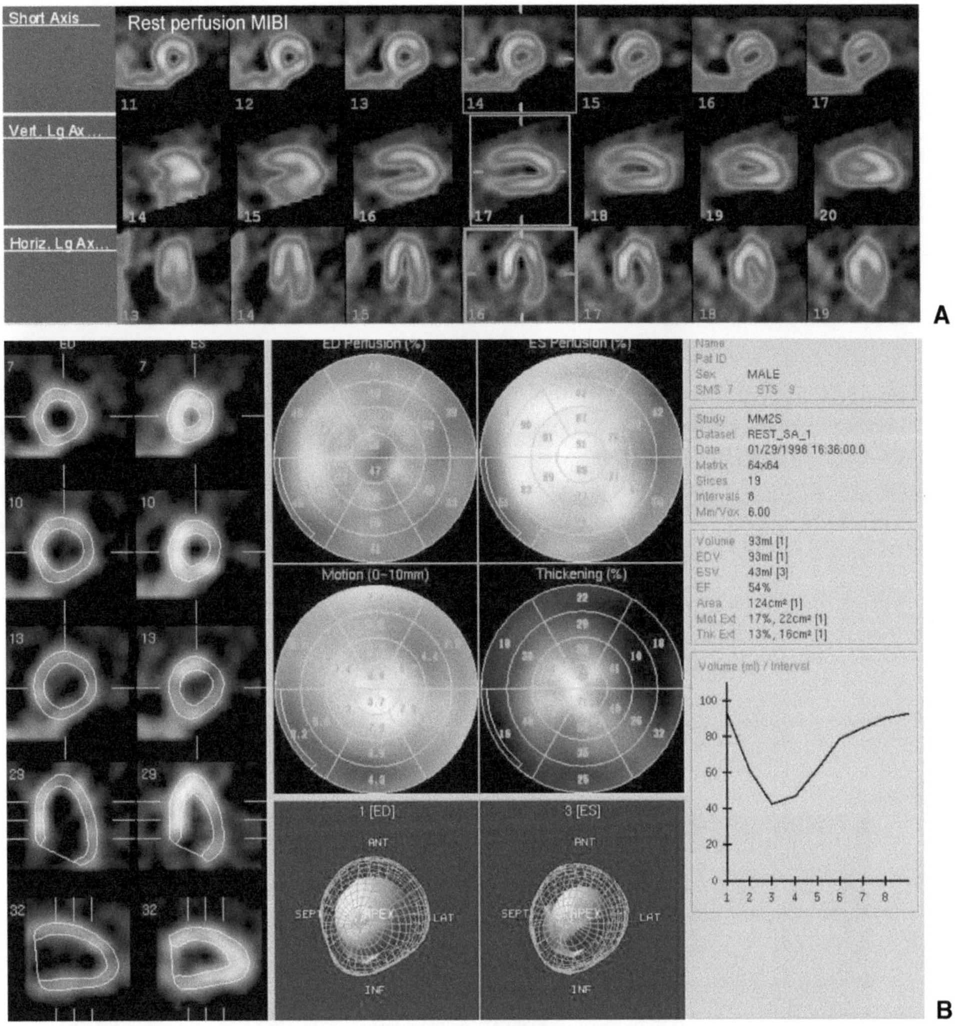

FIGURE C6-2. (A and B)

sively and severely abnormal. He was immediately taken for coronary angiography and a thrombus in his LCX was identified.

Discussion

Detecting abnormal wall thickening, as opposed to wall motion (translation) may provide for a more direct and sensitive method for detecting abnormal function. Importantly, normal function in an area with abnormal perfusion would not necessarily preclude an ACS, because functional images provide data about the characteristics of the LV while the patient is under the camera, whereas perfusion images assess myocardial blood flow at the time of tracer injection, before initial therapy. Nevertheless, abnormal function in the setting of a perfusion defect helps confirm the study result as abnormal.

Interpretation

Resting ^{99m}Tc-MIBI consistent with ACS, involving the lateral wall, with injection during chest pain; finding consistent with the occlusion of an OM found on coronary angiography.

Case 6.3

History

A middle-aged patient presented to the ED with ongoing chest pain and a nondiagnostic ECG. ^{99m}Tc-MIBI (12 mCi) was administered IV during chest pain. The resting gated ^{99m}Tc-MIBI SPECT images are displayed in Figures C6-3A and C6-3B.

Findings

There is moderately decreased uptake in a focal region in the lateral wall and inferolateral region of the LV (Figure C6-3A). The end-diastolic and end-systolic gated images demonstrated hypokinesis in a focal region of the inferolateral wall of the LV. The patient was

A

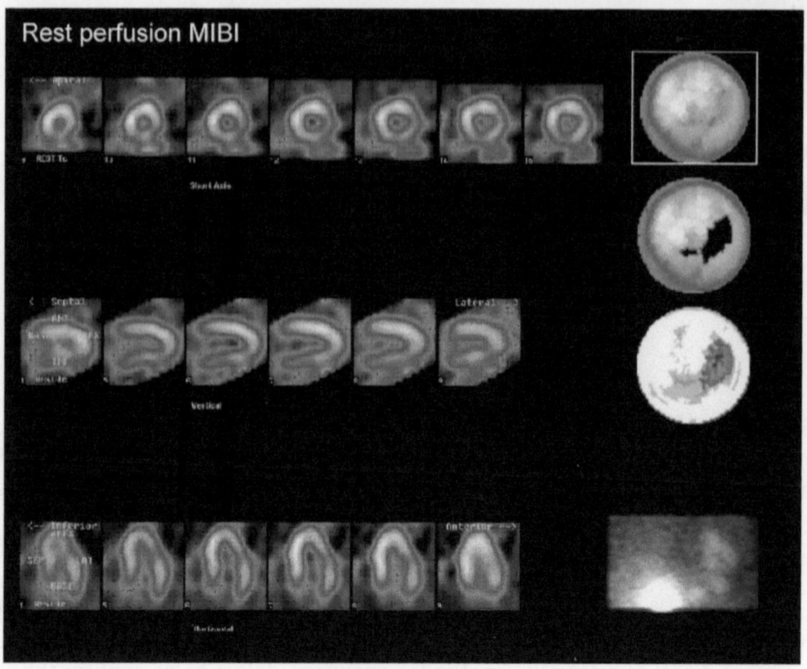

FIGURE C6-3. (A)

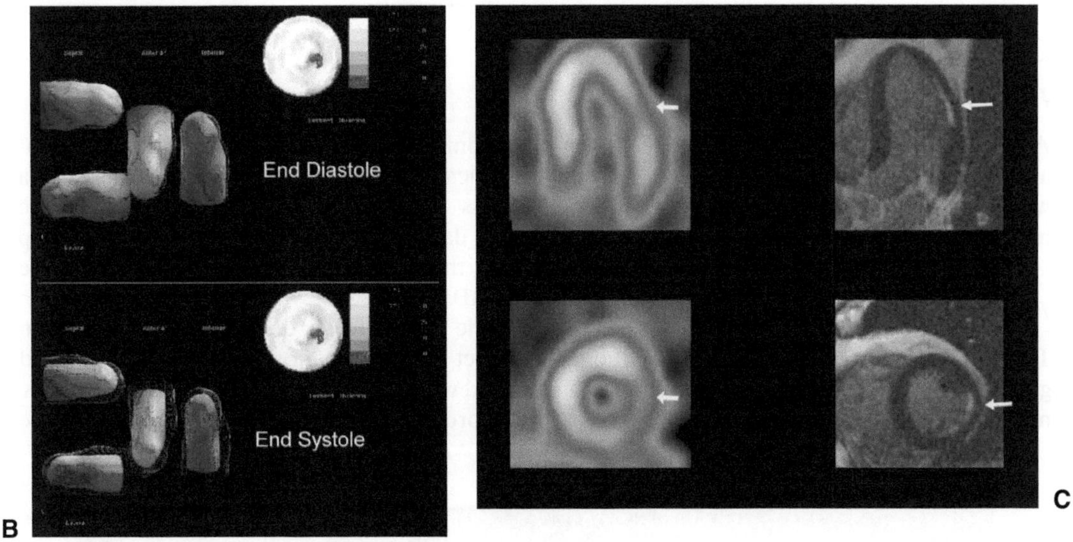

FIGURE C6-3. (B and C)

referred for an MRI with delayed gadolinium (Gd) enhancement demonstrating a focal region of hyperenhancement (arrows, Figure C6-3C) congruent with the perfusion defect on the rest MPI and wall motion abnormality on the gated MPI.

Discussion

The probability of 30-day mortality increases dramatically with the time from symptom onset to treatment. Therefore, early diagnosis of acute MI is critical to decrease mortality. Acute resting MPI provides rapid information. ^{99m}Tc-labeled tracers reflect the condition of the myocardium at the time of administration of the radiopharmaceutical. Images can be obtained as soon as 30 minutes after administration of ^{99m}Tc-labeled tracers or up to 4 hours later because there is no clinically significant redistribution of the radiopharmaceutical. The test can be available 24 hours a day as the radiopharmaceutical is stable for several hours, and the half-life of ^{99m}Tc is 6 hours. The radiopharmaceutical can be administered in the ED during chest pain and again later after the chest pain has resolved documenting a pain-induced defect resolving after the pain has subsided if significant size MI has not occurred.

If gated SPECT images are acquired, as in this case, wall motion abnormalities can be documented and help differentiate a true perfusion defect from an attenuation artifact. Wall motion abnormality can be due to an irreversible injury (MI) or myocardial stunning due to severe ischemia. However, the absence of wall motion abnormality is not helpful since ischemic myocardium may have normal wall motion by the time the image data are acquired. In this patient, a subendocardial MI was documented later with Gd-enhanced MRI. The limitations of acute gated SPECT imaging for evaluation of wall motion abnormalities are similar to those of acute echocardiography.[51]

Interpretation

1. Myocardial infarction diagnosed by rest ^{99m}Tc-MIBI injected during chest pain.
2. Wall motion abnormality on gated SPECT images in the same coronary territory.
3. Delayed-gadolinium enhancement on MRI, documenting a subendocardial MI.

Case 6.4

History

A 38-year-old man presented to the ED 3 hours after resolution of an episode of chest pain. He was administered 3 mCi of ^{201}Tl, and the SPECT images are displayed in Figure C6-4A.

Findings

The study was interpreted as relatively homogenous distribution of the perfusion radiopharmaceutical throughout the myocardium. As the patient was administered the radiopharmaceutical after resolution of chest pain, a stress ^{99m}Tc-MIBI study was performed the next day and the SPECT images were lined-up with the resting study and displayed in Figure C6-4B.

The stress images demonstrated a perfusion defect in the anterior LV wall, septum, and apex, which is reversible on the resting images. A coronary angiogram demonstrated a severe

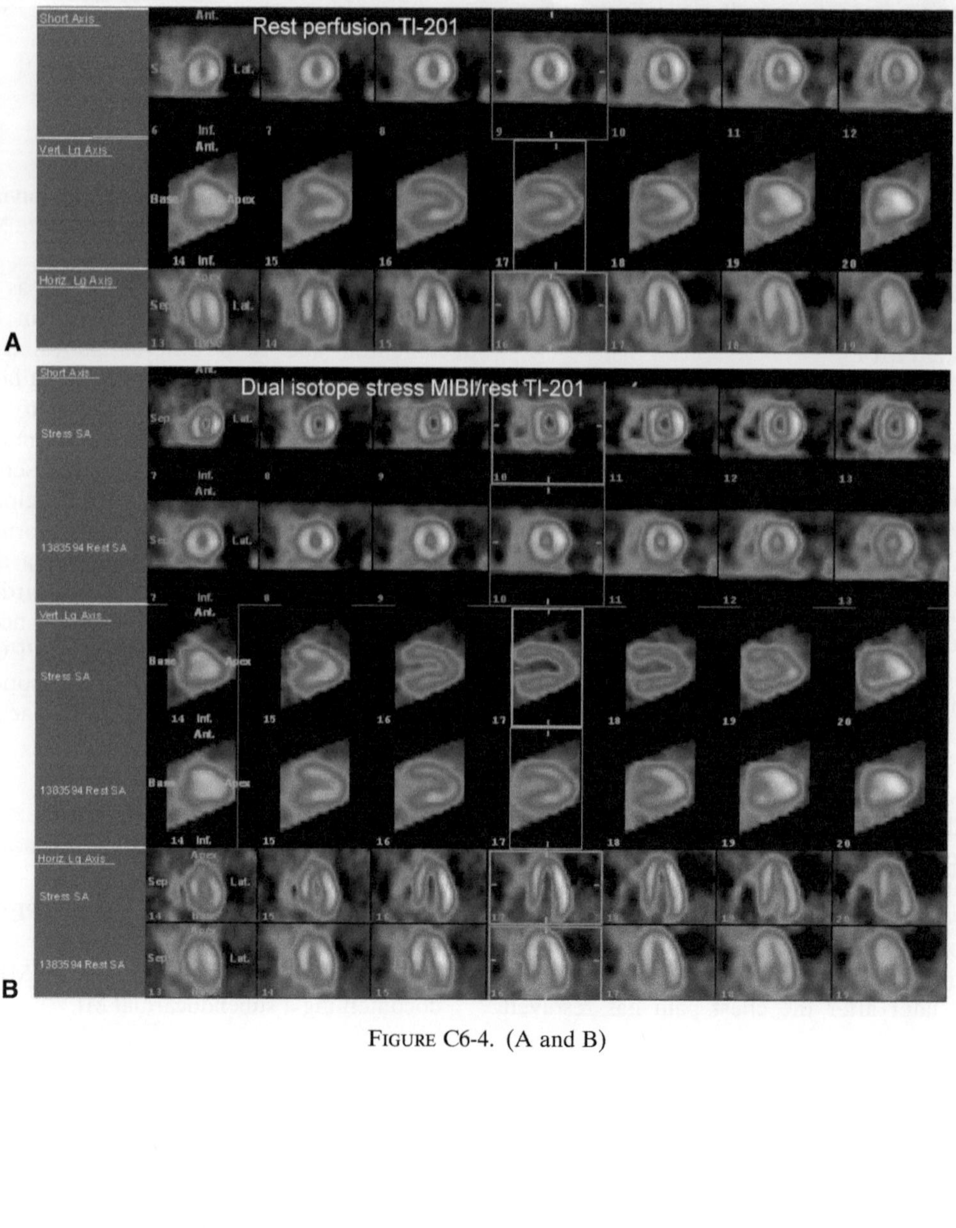

FIGURE C6-4. (A and B)

stenosis of the left anterior descending coronary artery (LAD).

Discussion

Acute rest MPI studies for detection of ACS is becoming an established modality for evaluation of patients presenting to the ED with chest pain and nondiagnostic ECG. When the radiopharmaceutical is administered during chest pain, acute MPI is highly accurate in the diagnosis of ACS as the cause of the patient's chest pain. In a patient with no prior history of MI, the presence of a perfusion defect categorizes the patient as high risk for ACS. Whereas some studies have shown that acute MPIs reveal a defect in most patients injected several hours after resolution of their symptoms,[53] other studies indicate that these defects may normalize rapidly.[54] A recent study investigated this issue in 40 patients undergoing successful coronary angioplasty.[55] Various groups of patients were administered ^{99m}Tc-MIBI during the last balloon inflation (acute MPI), or 15 minutes, 1 hour, 2 hours, 3 hours, 24 hours, or 48 hours later. The sensitivity of the test decreased rapidly when the radiopharmaceutical was administrated after balloon deflation. A defect was seen in all acute MPI, but in only 70% of patients injected at 15 minutes; 37% of patients injected at 1, 2, or 3 hours; and 19% of patients injected at 24 or 48 hours. Therefore, if the resting ^{99m}Tc-MIBI study result is negative, it should be followed by a stress ^{99m}Tc-MIBI study, even with the possibility of using a combination of exercise and vasodilator stress, testing the coronary reserve also in patients receiving beta-blockers in the ED. The stress ^{99m}Tc-MIBI without a rest would be an alternative option to evaluate low-risk patients, giving a quick yet accurate answer.

Interpretation

Normal *pain* SPECT images obtained 2 hours after resolution of chest pain were obtained, but abnormal stress SPECT images demonstrated LAD ischemia confirmed by coronary angiography.

Case 6.5

History

A 44-year-old man presented to the ED with ongoing chest pain. He was administered 25 mCi of ^{99m}Tc-MIBI during chest pain and SPECT myocardial perfusion images were acquired in both the supine and prone position (Figure C6-5).

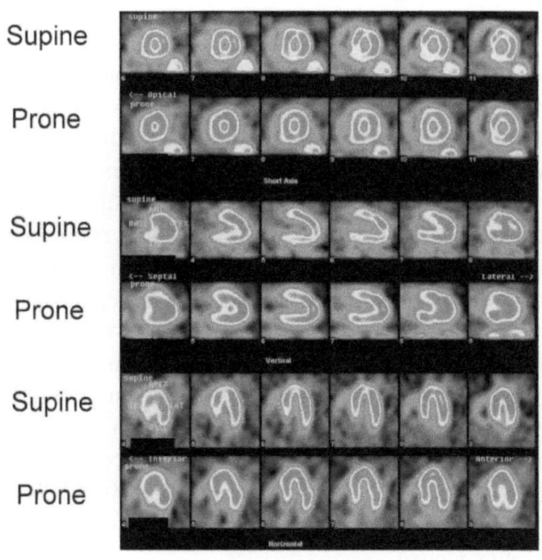

FIGURE C6-5.

Findings

The images demonstrated decreased uptake in the inferior wall with supine imaging that normalizes with prone imaging, allowing interpretation of the study as normal. There is a subtle and small anterior wall defect interpreted as attenuation.

Discussion

Fewer than 30% of patients admitted to the hospital with suspected ACS are found to have infarction or unstable angina, while 2% to 8% of patients with acute MI are inappropriately discharged from the emergency department. Resting MPI is useful to diagnose patients with ACS.[56–60] In addition, studies demonstrated that acute rest MPI reduces the number of admissions and therefore may impact the cost of delivering healthcare.[61,62] Images are usually acquired with gating and the patient in the supine position. As discussed in Case 6.3, a gated acquisition allows evaluation of regional and global wall motion including measurement of the left ventricular ejection fraction (LVEF). In the presence of a perfusion defect, an abnormal wall motion may indicate an MI. If the wall motion is normal, the perfusion abnormality can be related to an attenuation artifact, but normal wall motion does not exclude ischemia.

Prone imaging has been used in rest/stress MPI to further aid in the detection of artifact due to soft tissue attenuation. Supine and prone images of 250 consecutive patients referred from the ED for MPI after administration of ^{99m}Tc-MIBI (25 mCi) during chest pain were reviewed.[63] Supine/prone images were interpreted as abnormal if a defect was seen on both sets of images. Follow-up was performed on the 28 patients who were admitted to the hospital. The addition of prone images doubled the normalcy rate compared with interpretation of supine images only. Among the 28 patients who were admitted, only one patient with a normal resting scan had a proven critical lesion, whereas seven patients with positive scans had proven CAD. It was concluded that the addition of prone imaging doubled the normalcy rate of resting pain MPI, thus avoiding unnecessary admissions to the hospital.

Interpretation

Prone imaging is of value to increase the normalcy rate of resting ^{99m}Tc-MIBI during chest pain.

Case 6.6

History

A 74-year-old man with known CAD and coronary artery bypass grafting (CABG) in the remote past presented to the ED with epigastric pain, starting 2 weeks earlier, at rest, worse after eating spicy food, and worse when lying down after meals. An endoscopy revealed active peptic ulcer disease. Soon after initiation of treatment for peptic ulcer disease, he experienced chest pain and diffuse sweating throughout the night. Two days later in the cardiology office, his ECG showed an RBBB pattern and left axis deviation, but no changes compared with an ECG done 4 years earlier. He was referred for rest/stress MPI with ^{99m}Tc-MIBI SPECT. The resting images are shown in Figure C6-6A.

Findings

The resting images demonstrate severe, large perfusion defects involving the anterior wall, septum, and apex (entire LAD territory) and also the inferior and inferoseptal region (entire right coronary = RCA territory) consistent with multivessel disease. The gated images revealed a dilated left ventricular cavity with an LVEF of 39%.

After interpretation of the resting images, the patient was considered high risk, and the stress component of the study was canceled. On admission, the serum CK-MB levels were slightly elevated but LDH was markedly increased, suggesting that the patient had suffered an acute MI 48 hours earlier at the time of his chest pain. A ^{99m}Tc-pyrophosphate scan

FIGURE C6-6. (A)

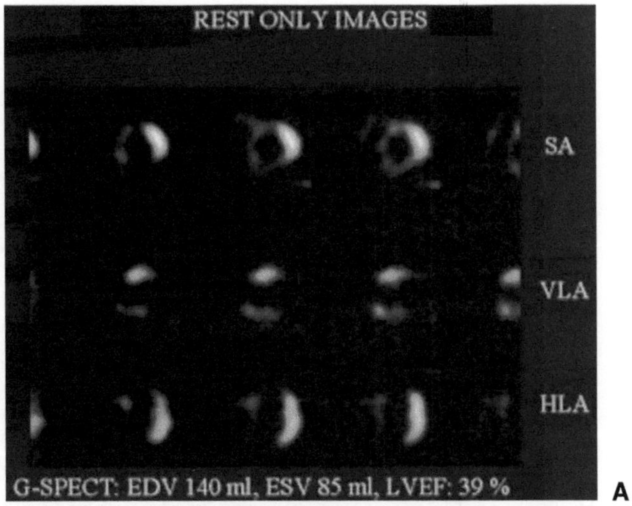

was performed to document the location of his recent MI. SPECT images obtained 2 hours after injection of 20 mCi of ^{99m}Tc-pyrophosphate (Figure C6-6B) revealed intense pyrophosphate uptake, corresponding to the hypoperfused regions on the resting ^{99m}Tc-MIBI images, indicating a large area of recent MI in the territory of the LAD.

The patient underwent coronary arteriography documenting, as expected, an occluded LAD and RCA, occluded graft to the RCA, and a critical stenosis of the graft to the LAD. Based on the pyrophosphate data, indicating that the culprit lesion was in the LAD, a stent was placed in the LAD graft, resulting in dramatic improvement of perfusion and function as shown on Figure C6-6C. If the pyrophosphate images were not available, the culprit lesion could not have been identified, considering that his ECG was not helpful.

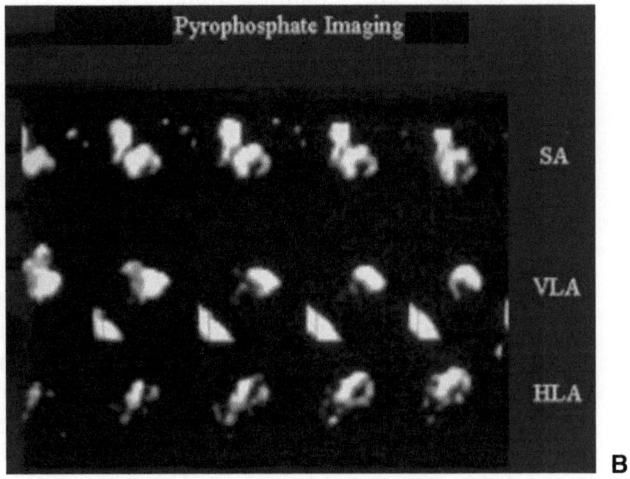

FIGURE C6-6. (B)

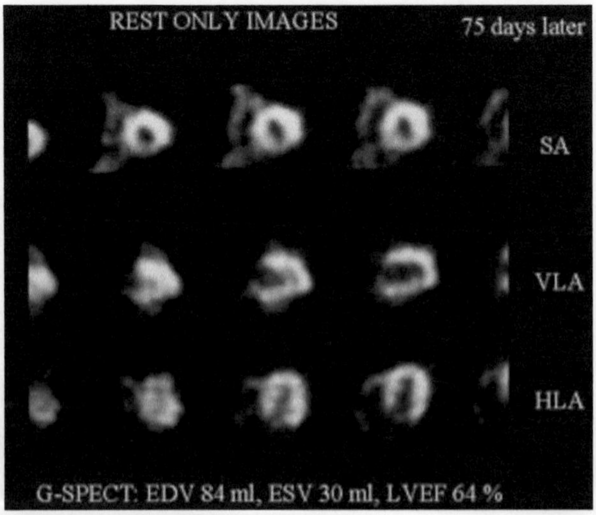

C

FIGURE C6-6. (C)

Discussion

This case is an example of the utility of nuclear imaging in the setting of ACS both with ^{99m}Tc myocardial perfusion radiopharmaceuticals and ^{99m}Tc-pyrophosphate. It illustrates the importance of examining the resting SPECT images before stressing the patient in the clinical setting of high suspicion of a recent MI.

In addition, although ^{99m}Tc-pyrophosphate imaging has limited value for evaluation of patients in the ED as discussed here, it was helpful in this patient to identify the location of MI because multivessel disease was identified on coronary angiography. During severe ischemia there is intracellular deposition of calcium in the mitochondria. ^{99m}Tc-pyrophosphate, initially developed as a bone imaging agent, binds to intracellular calcium in the acutely necrotic myocardium. The maximum uptake occurs at the peri-infarct border where flow is still present but reduced. This may result in a doughnut pattern with absent uptake in the central zone of necrosis where flow is essentially absent. It requires 24 to 48 hours before enough calcium is deposited in the infarct to allow adequate complexing of pyrophosphate to produce a positive image; images may occasionally be positive as early as 12 hours. Activity gradually diminishes over 5 to 7 days but in large infarcts may persist for weeks. Anterior, lateral, and oblique planar views, with or without SPECT, are obtained 2 to 4 hours postinjection. Normally no myocardial activity other than perhaps faint blood pool activity is observed. Physiologic sternal and rib activity are present; costal cartilage calcification or rib metastases can present a diagnostic challenge. Although diagnostic confidence increases as myocardial activity approaches that of ribs and sternum, activity greater than background is considered positive. Diffusely increased myocardial activity is not infrequently observed in patients with large anterior infarctions.

The sensitivity for the detection of small infarcts is relatively low, but in an autopsy series of patients having undergone pyrophosphate scintigraphy, the overall sensitivity for infarction was 89%, the specificity 100%, the positive predictive value 100%, and the negative predictive value 72%.[64] Within the differential diagnosis of a positive scan is myocarditis, pericarditis, persistent blood pool activity, doxorubicin cardiotoxicity, radiation therapy, left ventricular aneurysm, amyloidosis, and acute rejection of a transplanted heart. Due to the time delay necessary to see a positive scan, this modality is not used routinely in the triage of patients with acute chest pain. This technique is most useful in patients with uninterpretable ECG (i.e., LBBB, pacemaker, or MI) but with negative enzymes; or in patients with other confusing factors such as recent trauma, surgery, or cardiopulmonary resuscitation.

Another infarct-avid agent now available is ^{111}In-antimyosin scintigraphy. Antimyosin is a monoclonal murine antibody fragment targeted against human heavy chain myosin; it binds with high specificity to necrotic myocardium. Although uptake of the radiopharmaceutical into damaged myocardial cells occurs immediately after the onset of infarction, imaging must be delayed for 24 to 48 hours to allow blood pool clearance. Using planar imaging, the sensitivity for the detection of transmural infarction is 94% and for nontransmural infarctions is 82%.[65] False-negative results have occurred primarily in patients with inferior/posterior infarctions; SPECT may be helpful in these patients. *False-positive* results have occurred in patients with viral myocarditis and unstable angina without demonstrable infarction. In contrast to pyrophosphate scintigraphy, antimyosin scans may remain positive for as long as 12 months following the clinical event. Thus, the value of a negative scan is more useful in excluding infarction over the prior 6 months than with pyrophosphate.

One limitation of these two imaging modalities available for imaging necrosis, ^{99m}Tc-pyrophosphate and ^{111}In-antimyosin antibodies, is the response time for a disease requiring a quick therapeutic response. Therefore, neither is suitable for use in the ED.

Preliminary studies indicate that ^{99m}Tc-glucarate may be a more suitable radiopharmaceutical because it localizes in the necrotic myocardium within hours after the onset of experimental MI but it is still investigational (see Chapter 3). An additional discussion regarding the beneficial effects of interventional therapy in this patient can be seen in Chapter 10, Case 10.3.

Interpretations

1. Acute anteroseptal MI demonstrated on resting ^{99m}Tc-MIBI.
2. ^{99m}Tc-pyrophosphate imaging helped to identify the culprit lesion, considering that the patient had occlusion of both the LAD and the RCA.

Case 6.7

History

A 70-year-old man with no risk factors for CAD presented with atypical chest pain and recent onset of dyspnea on exertion. The resting ECG and physical examination were normal. The patient was referred for an exercise-only ^{99m}Tc-MIBI SPECT study. The patient exercised for 3 minutes and 48 seconds on a standard Bruce protocol. His peak heart rate (HR) was 140 bpm and blood pressure (BP) 170/100 mmHg. He experienced severe dyspnea during exercise but no chest pain. The exercise ECG was negative for ischemia. The SPECT images are displayed in Figure C6-7A.

Findings

Exercise SPECT images demonstrated homogenous perfusion of the myocardium. However, the right ventricle was slightly prominent, suggesting pulmonary hypertension and in the clinical setting of acute onset of dyspnea and decreased exercise capacity, pulmonary embolism was suspected. The patient was

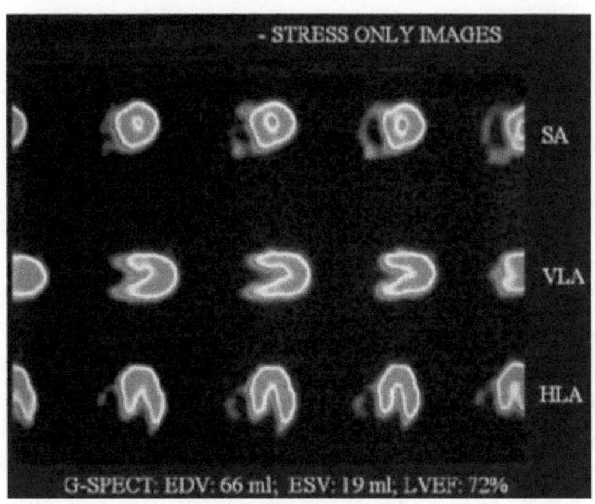

A

FIGURE C6-7. (A)

B
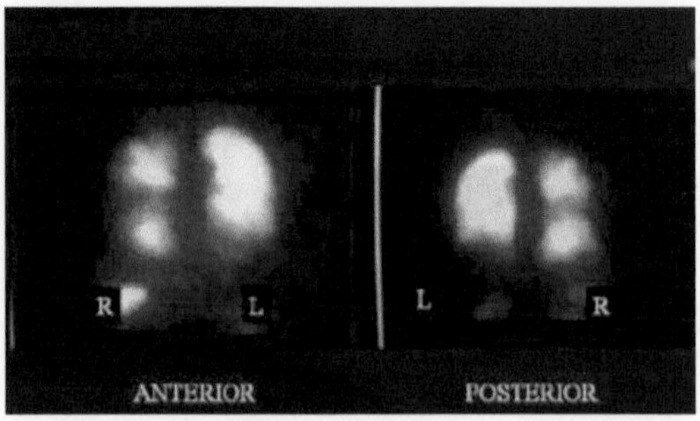

FIGURE C6-7. (B)

referred for a ventilation/perfusion (V/Q) lung scan as shown in Figure C6-7B.

The V/Q scan revealed multiple mismatched perfusion defects bilaterally consistent with pulmonary embolism. Uptake in the myocardium is not visualized on the V/Q scan because a low dose ^{99m}Tc-MIBI was administered for the MPI study and only <4% is retained in the myocardium, whereas 10 mCi ^{99m}Tc-MAA was administered for the pulmonary perfusion scan, with near 100% concentrating in the lungs.

Discussion

Pulmonary embolism is in the differential diagnosis for patients presenting with chest pain and new onset of dyspnea. More than one strategy is available using nuclear imaging in chest pain centers: some use rest myocardial imaging first, some rest followed by stress, and yet some go straight to stress testing associated or not with nuclear imaging as in this case. There is not really only one good strategy since this is a dynamic field in which new information is accumulated every day. The strategies used depend largely on the patient's presentation, what is available at that specific institution, and even the time of day on arrival to the ED. Some institutions are only able to do a treadmill stress test, which is a reasonable option in a low-risk group.[22] However, treadmill testing is suboptimal in patients taking beta-blockers, because of false-negative findings when patients do not reach at least 85% of their predicted maximum exercise capacity (see Chapter 4).

For those having nuclear imaging available in the ED and the chest pain is still ongoing, an injection of ^{99m}Tc-MIBI at rest gives a very high negative predictive value. If the resting ^{99m}Tc-MIBI study result is negative, it should be followed by a stress ^{99m}Tc-MIBI study. The stress ^{99m}Tc-MIBI without a rest would also be a good option in a low-risk patient and would give a quick answer, especially at the end of a working day, as in the case presented.

In this case, the stress MPI study was interpreted as normal, which allowed immediate evaluation with other diagnostic studies, identifying pulmonary embolism as the cause of the patient's symptoms.

Interpretation

Presentation to the ED with atypical chest pain, negative MPI, and positive V/Q scan for pulmonary thromboembolism.

Case 6.8

History

A 63-year-old male, a heavy smoker, with hypercholesterolemia presented with atypical chest discomfort at rest. A resting ECG was performed and is shown in Figure C6-8A. The patient was scheduled for a rest/stress MPI 5 days later. The resting ^{99m}Tc-MIBI images were obtained first and are displayed in Figure C6-8B. The ECG obtained at the time of the resting ^{99m}Tc-MIBI images is shown in Figure C6-8C.

Findings

The ECG performed at the time of the patient's first visit (Figure C6-8A) shows some nonspecific repolarization abnormalities in the lateral leads. The resting ^{99m}Tc-MIBI SPECT

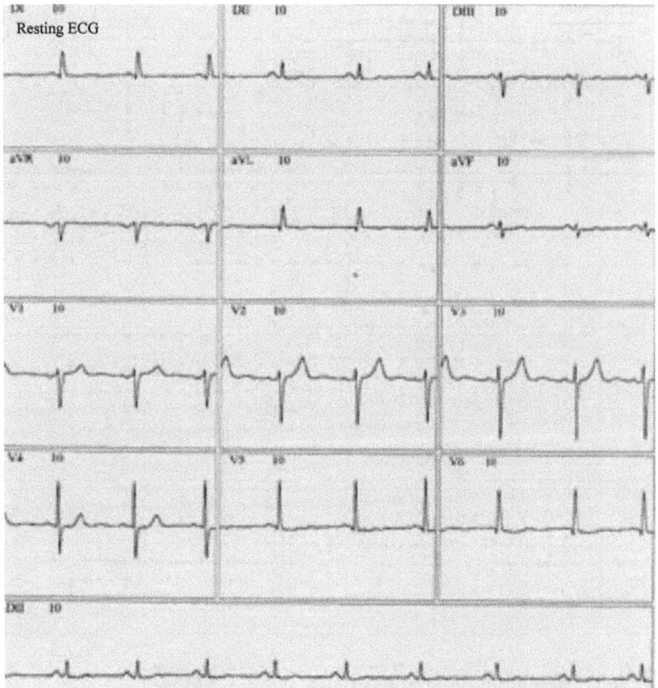

FIGURE C6-8. (A)

images obtained 5 days later demonstrate a large severe inferolateral wall defect (Figure C6-8B), and the ECG at that time (Figure C6-8C) showed evidence of an acute MI in the inferolateral region (ST elevation II, III, AVF, V6).

Discussion

The patient was admitted to the coronary care unit; CK and CK-MB were at the upper limit of normal (a limitation of enzymes on recent events, discussed in the chapter introduction). The patient underwent coronary angiography shown in Figure C6-8D revealing an occluded LCX. He was managed with PTCA and a coronary stent.

ACS (unstable angina or acute MI) has to be considered in patients with complaints of recent onset of chest pain at rest. These patients have to be evaluated immediately to avoid delays in management. This case is a good example of the value of resting ^{99m}Tc-MIBI imaging to diagnose an acute MI. When high-risk patients are scheduled for rest/stress

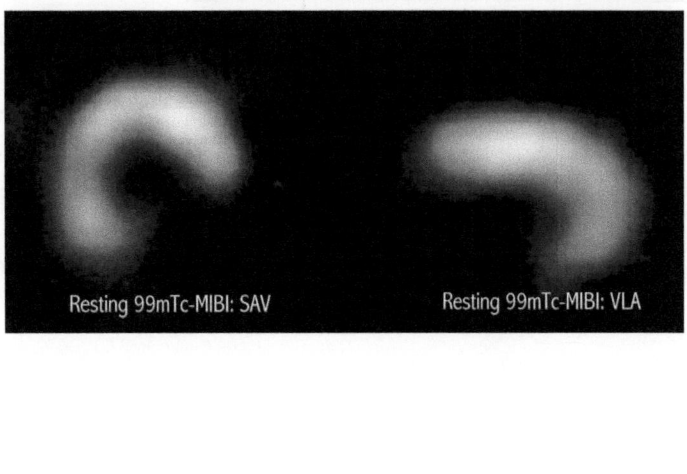

FIGURE C6-8. (B)

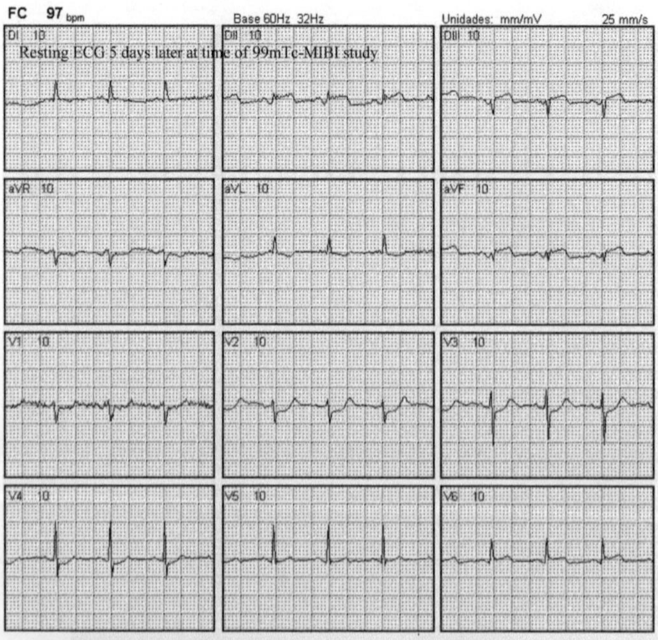

C

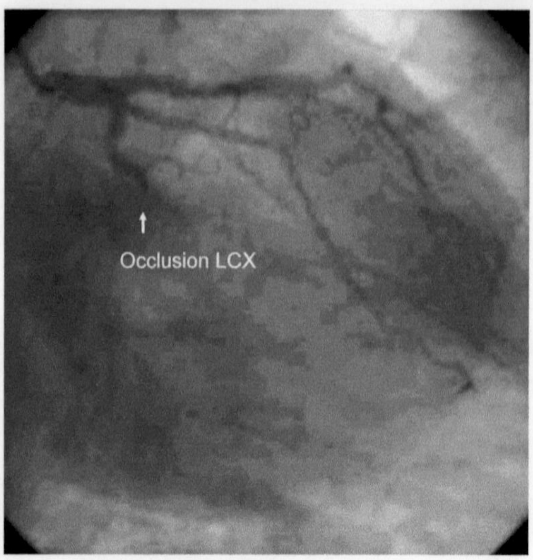

D

FIGURE C6-8. (C and D)

studies, it is imperative that the resting images be reviewed before proceeding to a stress test to avoid stressing a patient with ACS as shown in this case. The strategy applied in this case was evaluated in 2,475 patients in the ERASE trial,[8] as discussed earlier in the introduction to this chapter.

Interpretation

Inferolateral AMI diagnosed by rest MPI in a patient presenting with atypical chest discomfort at rest.

Case 6.9

History

A 62-year-old man with a history of CAD presented to the ED with 2 hours of severe abdominal pain and right chest discomfort. He had undergone CABG 8 years earlier, and MPI 1 year earlier was normal. His ECG and laboratory workup were normal. He was injected while symptomatic with 12.5 mCi of ^{99m}Tc-MIBI. After further clinical assessment, he was thought to have acute cholecystitis, and an ultrasound examination was performed, showing a large gallstone. He was scheduled for emergent laparoscopic cholecystectomy. A request to terminate the nuclear SPECT was made, but the patient was already under the camera. Gated SPECT images were acquired 1 hour after injection, as well as images of his right upper quadrant (RUQ) (Figures C6-9A, C6-9B, and C6-9C).

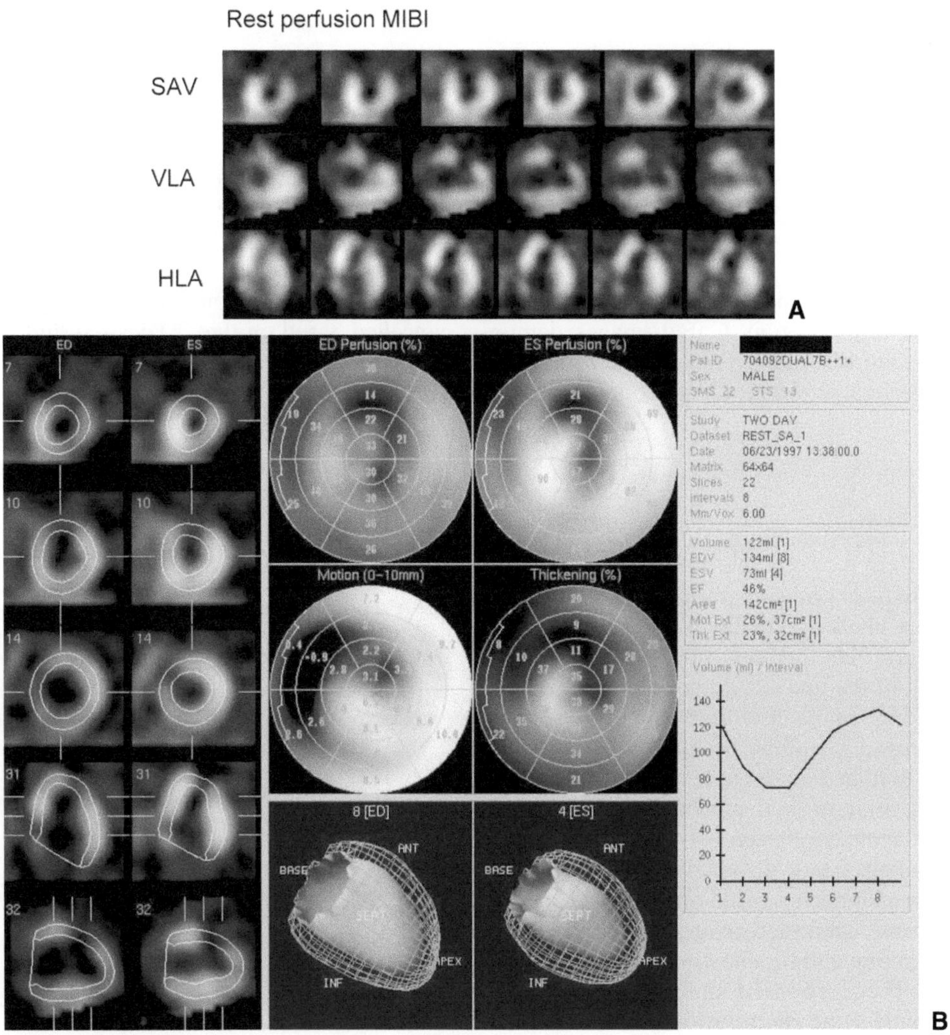

FIGURE C6-9. (A and B)

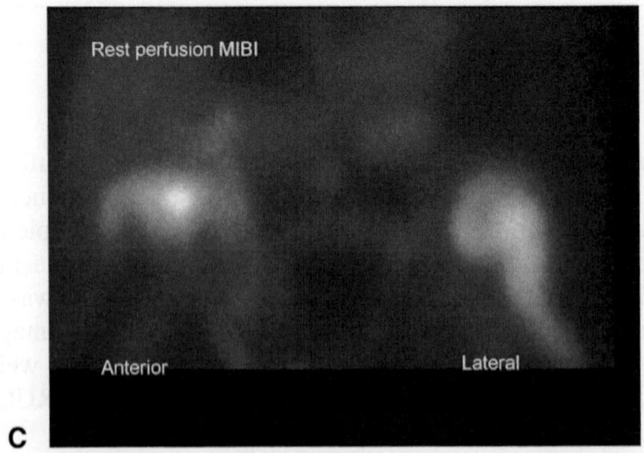

FIGURE C6-9. (C)

Findings

His gallbladder fills with tracer, and there is a large filling defect within the gallbladder compatible with his known gallstone. His SPECT images show two discrete, moderately sized, severe defects, namely in his mid-anterior wall and his basal septum. Gated images demonstrate abnormal thickening in these zones, with a borderline abnormal LV ejection fraction of 46%.

Discussion

His pattern is compatible with a number of possible findings on angiography. His basal septal defect is likely due to disease of the first septal perforator. His mid-anterior wall defect with sparing of the apex could be due to disease of a diagonal, ramus intermedius or obtuse marginal vessel. Given an occlusion of a proximal LAD that had undergone prior CABG, and known prior normal myocardial perfusion, a single acute occlusion of his left anterior descending artery distal to the diagonal and first septal branches could produce this pattern. This was confirmed with urgent coronary angiography, and his cholecystectomy was cancelled. The ^{99m}Tc-MIBI study was also helpful to exclude acute cholecystitis, based on normal filling of his gallbladder.

Interpretations

Myocardial infarction detected by rest ^{99m}Tc-MIBI in a patient with abdominal pain and suspected initially of having acute cholecystitis.

Cholecystectomy, already scheduled, was cancelled based on the ^{99m}Tc-MIBI findings.

References

1. Kirk JD, Diercks DB, Turnipseed SD, Amsterdam EA. Evaluation of chest pain suspicious for coronary syndrome: use of an accelerated diagnostic protocol in a chest pain evaluation unit. *Am J Cardiol.* 2000;85(5A):40B–48B; discussion 49B.
2. Abbott BG, Jain D. Nuclear cardiology in the evaluation of acute chest pain in the emergency department. *Echocardiography.* 2000;17:597–560.
3. Lee TH, Rouan GW, Weisberg MC, et al. Clinical characteristics and natural history of patients with acute myocardial infarction sent home from the emergency room. *Am J Cardiol.* 1987;60:219–224.
4. Pope JH, Aufderheide TP, Ruthazer R, et al. Missed diagnoses of acute cardiac ischemia in the emergency department. *N Engl J Med.* 2000; 342:1163–1170.
5. Abbott BG, Wackers FJ. The role of radionuclide imaging in the triage of patients with chest pain in the emergency department. *Rev Port Cardiol.* 2000;19 Suppl 1:I53–161.

6. Zalenski RJ, Shamsa FH. Diagnostic testing of the emergency department patient with chest pain. *Curr Opin Cardiol.* 1998;13(4):248– 253.
7. Kontos MC, Jesse RL, Anderson FP, Schmidt KL, Ornato JP, Tatum JL. Comparison of myocardial perfusion imaging and cardiac troponin I in patients admitted to the emergency department with chest pain. *Circulation.* 1999; 99(16):2073–2078.
8. Udelson JE, Beshansky JR, Ballin DS, et al. Myocardial perfusion imaging for evaluation and triage of patients with suspected acute cardiac ischemia. A randomized controlled trial. *JAMA.* 2002;288:2693–2700.
9. Rother K. Sestamibi sniffs out false acute cardiac ischemia in the ED. www.theheart.org (cardiology online) 1999;Nov.
10. Wood S. Myocardial scanning for MI improves triage decisions. www.theheart.org (cardiology online); 2002;Dec.
11. Gibbons RJ. Chest pain triage—another step forward. *JAMA.* 2002;288:2745–2746.
12. Ornato JP. Chest pain emergency centers: improving acute myocardial infarction care. *Clin Cardiol.* 1999;22(suppl.8):IV3–IV9.
13. Ornato JP. Critical pathways for triage and treatment of chest pain patients in the emergency department. *Clinician.* 1996;14:53–55.
14. Tatum JL, Jesse RL, Kontos MC, et al. Comprehensive strategy for the evaluation and triage of the chest pain patient. *Ann Emerg Med.* 1997; 29:116–125.
15. Gibler WB, Runyon JP, Levy RC, et al. A rapid diagnostic and treatment center for patients with chest pain in the emergency department. *Ann Emerg Med.* 1995;25:1–8.
16. Storrow AB, Gibler WB, et al. Chest pain centers: diagnosis of acute coronary syndromes. *Ann Emerg Med.* 2000;35:449–461.
17. Christian TF, Clements IP, Gibbons RJ. Noninvasive identification of myocardium at risk in patients with acute myocardial infarction and nondiagnostic electrocardiograms with technetium-99m-Sestamibi. *Circulation.* 1991;83: 1615–1620.
18. Bassan R. Pro-Cardiaco Hospital Diagnostic Algorithm. *Arq Bras Cardiol.* 2002;79(2):196–209.
19. Zalenski RJ, Ting S, et al. A national survey of emergency department chest pain centers in the United States. *Am J Cardiol.* 1998;81:1305–1309.
20. Souza J, Manfroi WC, Polanczyk CA. Teste ergométrico imediato em pacientes com dor torácica na sala de emergência. *Arq Bras Cadiol.* 2002;79:91–96.
21. Lewis WR, Amsterdam EA. Utility and safety of immediate exercise testing of low risk patients admitted to the hospital for suspected acute myocardial infarction. *J Am Coll Cardiol.* 1994; 74:987–990.
22. Amsterdam EA, Kish JD, Diercks DM, et al. Immediate exercise testing to evaluate low-risk patients presenting to the emergency department with chest pain. *J Am Coll Cardiol.* 2002; 40:251–256.
23. Patterson RE, Horowitz SF. Importance of epidemiology and biostatistics in deciding clinical strategies for using diagnostic tests: a simplified approach using examples from coronary artery disease. *J Am Coll Cardiol.* 1989;13:1653–1665.
24. Polanczyk CA, Johnson PA, Hartley LH, et al. Clinical correlates and prognostic significance of early negative exercise tolerance test in patients with acute chest pain seen in the hospital emergency department. *Am J Cardiol.* 1998; 81:288–292.
25. Diercks DB, Gibler WB, Liu T, et al. Identification of patients at risk by graded exercise testing in an emergency department chest pain center. *Am J Cardiol.* 2000;89:289–292.
26. Selker HP, Zalenski RJ, Antman EM, et al. An evaluation of technologies for identifying acute cardiac ischemia in the emergency department: a report from a National Heart Attack Alert Program working group/erratum appears in *Ann Emerg Med.* 1997;29:310/*Ann Emerg Med.* 1997; 29:13–87.
27. Kuntz KM, Fleichmann KE, Hunink MGM, Douglas PS. Cost-effectiveness of diagnostic strategies for patients with chest pain. *Ann Intern Med.* 1999;130:709–718.
28. ACC/AHA Guidelines for the Management of Patients with Unstable Angina and Non-ST-Segment-Elevation Myocardial Infarction. *J Am Coll Card.* 2000;36:970–1062.
29. Wu AH, Apple FS, Gibler WB, Jesse RL, Warshaw MM, Valdes RJ. National Academy of Clinical Biochemistry Standards of Laboratory Practice: recommendations for the use of cardiac markers in coronary artery diseases. *Clin Chem.* 1999;45:1104–1121.
30. Kontos MC, Anderson FP, Hanbury CM, Roberts CS, Miller WG, Jesse RL. Use of the combination of myoglobin and CK-MB mass for the rapid diagnosis of acute myocardial infarction. *Am J Emerg Med.* 1997;15:14–19.
31. Lindahl B, Venge P, Wallentin L. Early diagnosis and exclusion of acute myocardial infarction

using biochemical monitoring. The BIOMACS study group. Biochemical markers of acute coronary syndromes. *Coron Artery Dis.* 1995;6:321–328.
32. Apple FS, Christenson RH, Valdes RJ, et al. Simultaneous rapid measurement of whole blood myoglobin, creatine kinase MB, and cardiac troponin I by the triage cardiac panel for detection of myocardial infarction. *Clin Chem.* 1999;45:199–205.
33. Polanczyk CA, Lee TH, Cook EF, et al. Value of additional two-hour myoglobin for the diagnosis of myocardial infarction in the emergency department. *Am J Cardiol.* 1999;83:525–529.
34. Gibler WB, Gibler CD, Weinshenker E, et al. Myoglobin as an early indicator of acute myocardial infarction. *Ann Emerg Med.* 1987;16:851–856.
35. Brogan G, Friedman S, McCuskey C, et al. Evaluation of a new rapid quantitative immunoassay for serum myoglobin versus CK-MB for ruling out acute myocardial infarction in emergency department. *Ann Emerg Med.* 1994;24:665–671.
36. De Winter RJ, Koster RW, Sturk A, Sanders GT. Value of myoglobin, Troponin T and CK-MB mass in ruling out an acute myocardial infarction in the emergency room. *Circulation.* 1995;92:3401–3407.
37. Christenson RH, Dush SH. Evidence-based approach to practice guides and decision thresholds for cardiac markers. *Scan J Clin Lab Invest.* 1999;230:90–102.
38. Gibler WB, Lewis LM , Erbe RE, et al. Early detection of acute myocardial infarction in patients presenting with chest pain and nondiagnostic ECGs: serial CK-MB sampling in the emergency department. *Ann Emerg Med.* 1990;19:1359–1366.
39. De Winter RJ, Koster RW, van Straalen JP, et al. Critical difference between serial measurements of CKMB mass to detect myocardial damage. *Clin Chem.* 1997;43:338–343.
40. Young GP, Gibler WB, Hedges JR, et al, for the EMCREG II Group. Serial creatine Kinase-MB results are a sensitive indicator of acute myocardial infarction in chest pain patients with nondiagnostic electrocardiograms: The Second Emergency Medicine Cardiac Research Group Study. *Acad Emerg Med.* 1997;4:869–877.
41. Gibler WB, Young GP, Hedges JR, et al. Acute myocardial infarction in chest pain patients with nondiagnostic ECGs: serial CK-MB sampling in the emergency department. *Ann Emerg Med.* 1992;21:504–512.
42. Bassan R, Gamarski R, Pimenta L, et al. Eficácia de uma estratégia diagnóstica para pacientes com dor torácica e sem supradesnível do segmento ST na sala de emergência. *Arq Bras Cardiol.* 2000;74:405–411.
43. Polanczyk CA, Lee TH, Cook EF, et al. Cardiac Troponin I as a predictor of major cardiac events in emergency department patients with acute chest pain. *J Am Coll Cardiol.* 1998;32:8–14.
44. Zimmerman J, Fromm R, Meyer D, et al. Diagnostic marker cooperative study for the diagnosis of myocardial infarction. *Circulation.* 1999;99:1671–1677.
45. Wackers FJT, Brown KA, Heller GV, et al. American Society of Nuclear Cardiology position statement on radionuclide imaging in patients with suspected acute ischemic syndromes in the emergency department or chest pain center. *J Nucl Cardiol.* 2002;9(2):246–250.
46. American Heart Association. *Heart and Stroke Statistical Update.* Dallas: American Heart Association;1998.
47. Heller GV, Stowers SA, Hendel RC, et al. Clinical value of acute rest technetium-99m tetrofosmin in tomographic myocardial perfusion imaging in patients with acute chest pain and nondiagnostic electrocardiograms. *J Am Coll Cardiol.* 1998;31:1011–1017.
48. McCarthy BD, Beshansky JR, Selker HP. Missed diagnoses of acute myocardial infarction in the emergency department. *Ann Emerg Med.* 1993;22:579–582.
49. Lee TH, Rouan GW, Weisberg MC. Clinical characteristics and natural history of patients with acute myocardial infarction sent home from the emergency room. *Am J Cardiol.* 1987;60:219–224.
50. Bilodeau L, Theroux P, Gregoire J, et al. Technetium-99m sestamibi tomography in patients with spontaneous chest pain: correlations with clinical, electrocardiographic and angiographic findings. *J Am Coll Cardiol.* 1991;18:1684–1691.
51. Sabia P, Afrookteh A, Touchstone DA, et al. Value of regional wall motion abnormality in the emergency room diagnosis of acute myocardial infarction: A prospective study using two-dimensional echocardiography. *Circulation.* 1991;84:687–691.
52. Wackers F, Sokole EB, Samson G. Value and limitations of thallium-201 scintigraphy in the acute phase of myocardial infarction. *N Engl J Med.* 1976;295:1–5.
53. Varetto T, Cantalupi D, Altieri A, et al. Emergency room technetium-99m sestamibi imaging

to rule out acute myocardial ischemic events in patients with non-diagnostic electrocardiograms. *J Am Coll Cardiol.* 1993;22:1804–1808.

54. Gallik DM, Obermueller SD, Swarna US, et al. Simultaneous assessment of myocardial perfusion and left ventricular function during transient coronary occlusion. *J Am Coll Cardiol.* 1995;25:1529–1538.
55. Fram DB, Azar RR, Ahlberg AW, et al. Duration of abnormal SPECT myocardial perfusion imaging following resolution of acute ischemia: An angioplasty model. *J Am Coll Cardiol.* 2003; 41:452–459.
56. Kontos MC, Jesse RL, Schmidt KL, Ornato JP, Tatum JL. Value of acute rest sestamibi perfusion imaging for evaluation of patients admitted to the emergency department with chest pain. *J Am Coll Cardiol.* 1997;30:976–982.
57. Weissman IA, Dickinson CZ, Dworkin HJ, O'Neil WW, Juni, JE. Cost-effectiveness of myocardial perfusion imaging with SPECT in the emergency department evaluation of patients with unexplained chest pain. *Radiology.* 1996; 199:353–357.
58. Beller GA. Acute radionuclide perfusion imaging for evaluation of chest pain in the emergency department: need for a large clinical trial. *J Nucl Cardiol.* 1996;3:546–549.
59. Abbott BG, Jain D. Nuclear cardiology in the evaluation of acute chest pain in the emergency department. *Echocardiography.* 2000;17; 597–604.
60. Hilton TC, Thompson RC, Williams HJ, Saylors R, Fulmer H, Stowers SA. Technetium-99m sestamibi myocardial perfusion imaging in the emergency room evaluation of chest pain. *J Am Coll Cardiol.* 1994;23:1016–1022.
61. Knott JC, Baldey AC, Grigg LE, et al. Impact of acute chest pain ^{99m}Tc sestamibi myocardial perfusion imaging on clinical management. *J Nucl Cardiol.* 2002;9:257–262.
62. Heller GV, Stowers SA, Hendel RC, et al. Clinical value of acute rest technetium-99m tetrofosmin tomographic myocardial perfusion imaging in patients with acute chest pain and nondiagnostic electrocardiograms. *J Am Coll Cardiol.* 1998;31:1011–1017.
63. Huntsinger R, Martin WH, Churwell K, Delbeke D. Value of prone myocardial perfusion SPECT imaging (MPI) for patients with chest pain in the emergency department (ED). *J Nucl Cardiol.* 2002;9:S17.
64. Poliner LR, Buja LM, Parkey RW, et al. Clinicopathologic findings in 52 patients studied by technetium-99m stannous pyrophosphate myocardial scintigraphy. *Circulation.* 1979;59: 257–267.
65. Johnson LL, Seldin DW, Becker LC, et al. Antimyosin imaging in acute transmural infarctions: results of a multicenter clinical trial. *J Am Coll Cardiol.* 1989;13:27–35.

7
Evaluation of Cardiac Function

Kenneth J. Nichols, Marvin W. Kronenberg, and Sabahat Bokhari

A plethora of methods now exist for the evaluation of ventricular function. Such methods include radionuclide ventriculography (RVG), contrast ventriculography (CVG), echocardiography, cine-computed tomography (CT), and cardiac magnetic resonance imaging (MRI). For RVG, established methods include first-pass imaging of the left or right ventricles (LV or RV), gated equilibrium imaging, and single photon emission computed tomographic (SPECT) imaging. While all the cardiac imaging methods listed previously may be used to obtain information about ventricular function, an additional advantage of RVG over some methods is its serial repeatability, whether using exercise (planar RVG) or pharmacologic stress.

A combination of visual and calculated data is used to evaluate ventricular performance. For this, electrocardiographic QRS information is matched to the imaging data. The ECG QRS complex is detected by a gating circuit that defines the QRS by a rapid change in voltage per unit time (dV/dt) and produces a gating signal. This signal is shown to the technologist and physician on a monitor and is sent to the imaging system for synchronization with the cardiac cycle. The cardiac cycle may be divided into an arbitrary number of sections, or into 30- to 60-msec sections for as many as are required to span the cycle. For each time frame, a section of computer memory is allocated to allow 64 × 64 or 128 × 128 pixel resolution in byte or word mode. This is determined by the amount of radioactivity injected and the amount of time that is to be allowed for each acquisition. The gating window is set by allowing a period of time before collecting the RVG to estimate the average R-R interval. Then, a tolerance, called the *beat-length window*, is set; this is often 10% of the R-R interval in milliseconds. Extrasystoles are accounted by beat-rejection algorithms. Usually, the premature beat and the next beat are rejected. For enhanced gating, some systems collect each prospective, *good* cardiac cycle data in a preliminary buffer, and then add it to the main buffer if the gating criteria are met. The gating method may be applied to RVG and also to SPECT MPI.

Arrhythmias such as atrial fibrillation produce moderate problems. However, if sufficiently short time frames are collected, systolic function can be accurately assessed, but diastolic time-activity curves may be inaccurate because of beat rejection. Thus, one reasonable strategy for assessing LV systolic performance in patients with atrial fibrillation is to set short time frames and to widen the beat-length window to accept all but very premature beats.

For RVG, established methods include first-pass imaging of the left or right ventricles (LV, RV), gated equilibrium blood pool imaging, and SPECT imaging. For first-pass imaging, it is essential for the linked computer to collect high count rate data accurately as a bolus of radionuclide enters and traverses the central circulation. The physical capacity for extremely rapid analog-to-digital conversion is not usually an issue for equilibrium RVG collection. For the gated equilibrium method, it is clear that the data from a single cardiac cycle would be inadequate to produce a useful image. Thus, the data from many cardiac cycles must be summed to produce enough information to allow visual and quantitative interpretation. For planar RVG, 2 to 8 minutes of data are sufficient to form useful images. For SPECT imaging, 15 to 20 minutes may be required because of the need to acquire approximately 60 planar frames for 180-degree reconstruction.

After the RVG data have been collected, the results are displayed for visual analysis using an endless loop cineangiographic format. Most computer displays allow for four separate ECG-gated images to be viewed simultaneously. These may be of the heart at rest using four different planar projections, or serial views of the heart in two projections, such as anterior and left anterior oblique views, with rest-exercise RVG. Visual analysis allows a general impression of chamber size, wall motion, and the ventricular ejection fraction (EF). The formula to calculate the EF is:

$$EF = [SV/EDV] \times 100\%,$$
$$\text{where } SV = \text{stroke volume and } EDV = \text{end-diastolic}$$

Stroke volume is estimated as EDV—ESV. Regional LV wall motion may be estimated visually using an analysis of extent of the abnormally contracting segments as a fraction or percent of the visually contracting LV and the severity of the abnormality in each LV region. Most systems for studying regional wall motion use 8 or 10 such regions for formal analysis. For planar RVG, these methods are illustrated in the cases to follow.

This chapter emphasizes ECG-gated equilibrium acquisition with the planar method and with SPECT acquisition, the newest scintigraphic method. Intrinsic to each of these methods for evaluation of ventricular function is the use of an intravascular isotopic label. Initially, first-pass studies were acquired using injection of small boluses of ^{99m}Tc, but this procedure was quickly replaced by labeling human serum albumin with this isotope. This, in turn, was replaced by labeling red blood cells (RBCs) themselves, following the chance discovery that RBCs had an affinity for the bone-and infarct-imaging drug, pyrophosphate.[1] Further refinements of the RBC-labeling method have evolved. The original method of pyrophosphate injection followed by injection of ^{99m}Tc (*in vivo* labeling)[2] now competes with a modified *in vivo* method,[3] and an *in vitro* method.[4,5] The latter two methods have the advantage of improved target-to-background ratios, while the former is simpler, with no chance for the accidental injection of another patient's blood.

The following sections discuss planar and then SPECT RVG. For both, validation information is presented, along with physiologic information about the relevant factors that affect ventricular performance related to the specific case.

SPECT RVG

Summary of Biventricular Imaging Techniques

While many imaging techniques successfully image the LV, visual and quantitative assessment of the RV has been more problematic. Presently available techniques for assessing RV function have significant limitations: planar (i.e., nontomographic) RVG studies and echocardiography have limited accuracy and reproducibility, gated first-pass radionuclide angiography (GFP) can be problematic, and CT and cardiac MRI are not widely available and require considerable expertise for RV computations.

Planar RVG RVEF values correlate well with other methods for large groups of patients,[6,7] but may not permit accurate assessment of RVEF in patients in whom the right atrium (RA) and RV outflow tract are markedly abnormal. Planar RVG RVEFs tend to be lower than those from other methods in patients with dilated right cardiac chambers, probably due to inadequate chamber separation of the RV from other chambers, and the difficulty of delineating tricuspid and pulmonary valve planes.[8] Also, planar RVG does not compute volume directly.

The complex, eccentric shape of the RV and its relationship with the infundibulum does not permit the use of conventional 2-dimensional echocardiographic volumetric algorithms based on linear measurements or geometric assumptions. Three-dimensional echocardiography is less affected by distorted chamber anatomy than two-dimensional echocardiography and may be used to reconstruct the RV, but is technically challenging and not widely available. Furthermore, it has not been well validated for RV measurements.

GFP has traditionally been used to measure RVEF and was the measurement technique used in a recent study of sildenafil effects on RVEF in patients with CHF.[9] Although GFP cannot be used to quantify absolute volumes, it is superior to planar RVG for measuring EF because it temporally isolates the RV from other chambers.[10,11] R-wave gating aids these techniques considerably,[12,13] as demonstrated by superior correlations to cine CT obtained with GFP.[14] GFP studies in general have shown better RVEF correlation to cine CT and cardiac MRI than do planar RVG studies.[14,15] However, a problem underlying GFP RVEF accuracy is that it can be difficult to ascertain whether injected tracer is sufficiently well mixed with blood in the RV phase so that constant radioactivity concentration can be assumed for accurate RVEF computations.[16] Thus, GFP requires fortuitous imaging conditions, especially delivery of injected radiotracer at a rate sufficiently slow that the RV phase is seen in more than only one heartbeat, but sufficiently rapid so that there is a distinct time period during which the RV is isolated from the lungs and other chambers.[13] Usually, there are only two to three usable heartbeats during which the RV has sufficient counts, so that it is essential to verify that these are of average duration, and that the patient did not experience an arrhythmia during the RV phase.[17] Otherwise, it becomes impossible to form a composite cinematic representation that is truly representative of RV function.[18] Furthermore, the optimal GFP imaging angle to use to separate the RV from the RA is not known a priori, especially in patients with RV abnormalities, and the tricuspid valve plane is often difficult to define because it translates considerably during contraction.[13,19] Thus, technical problems are the primary impediment to GFP.

Electron beam computerized tomography (EBCT) and MRI are excellent techniques for measuring RV volume and systolic function;[20,21] however, the cost and technical expertise required for these techniques currently limit their widespread clinical application. While RV calculations are difficult for all imaging modalities, cardiac MRI is the most extensively validated method at the present time.[22–24] Investigators have shown excellent correlation between MRI calculations of RV mass versus excised calf hearts,[25] and between MRI measurements of RV volumes when compared to absolute volumes of phantoms of latex and water, and of casts of excised bovine hearts.[26] Recent cardiac MRI technical improvements, including the collection of images of improved signal-to-noise ratio using true-FISP pulse sequences, will undoubtedly facilitate future cardiac MRI RV evaluations.[27]

SPECT RVG provides count-based, 3-dimensional volumetric information. Hence, it is not subject to errors caused by geometric assumptions. Because it is a tomographic technique, unlike planar RVG, it does not have the problem of superimposition of cardiac chambers, thus absolute volumes can be computed; however, SPECT RVG is subject to the traditional limitations of nuclear imaging techniques such as photon-attenuation and partial volume effects. Cardiac MRI values for RVEF and RV size have been found to correlate well with those computed from SPECT RVG data.[28,29] Furthermore, calculations of RV volume are based on robust algorithms that are automatic or semiautomatic.[28,30] Consequently SPECT RVG should prove to be suitable for widespread clinical use.

Until recently, the main focus of SPECT RVG application has been the LV, as evidenced by large multicenter trials for LV assessment by SPECT RVG,[31,32] and the fact that most recent publications regarding cardiac evaluation by SPECT RVG have focused on quantifying the size and function of the LV, not the RV.[30,33,34] These studies have consistently demonstrated that SPECT RVG measurements of LV volume and EF agree closely with corresponding measurements by standard techniques. However, the advantages afforded by SPECT RVG for RV assessment have yet to be fully realized.

SPECT RVG Validated by Physical Phantoms

Recently, SPECT RVG algorithms have been applied to data generated by physical phantoms, consisting of two silicon-rubber chambers driven by two piston pumps simulating crescent-shaped RVs wrapped partway around ellipsoidal LVs.[35] RV and LV true volume and EF ranges were 65 to 275 ml and 55 to 165 ml, and 7% to 49% and 12% to 69%, respectively. Linear correlation coefficients (r) of SPECT RVG observations versus true values for right and LVs were 0.80 and 0.94 for EF and 0.94 and 0.95 for volumes, respectively. Correlations for right and LVs were 0.97 and 0.97 for EF and 0.96 and 0.89 for volumes for interobserver agreement, and 0.97 and 0.98 for EF and 0.96 and 0.90 for volumes, respectively, for interobserver agreement. No trends were detected, though volumes and RVEF were significantly higher than true values.[36]

SPECT RVG Validated by Cardiac MRI

Also recently, SPECT RVG computations have been verified against independent cardiac MRI studies in patients with primary pulmonary hypertension (PPH) and tetralogy of Fallot (TOF).[28] Mean values were not different between SPECT RVG and MRI for RVEF, EDV, or ESV (42 ± 11% versus 41 ± 10%, 135 ± 67 ml versus 139 ± 91 ml, and 87 ± 54 ml versus 85 ± 61 ml, respectively). Significant correlation was found for RVEF, EDV, and ESV ($r = 0.85$, $r = 0.94$, and $r = 0.93$, respectively). No statistically significant trends or biases for RVEF were found, and intraobserver and interobserver comparisons demonstrated good reproducibility. As expected, RV volume was significantly larger, and RVEF significantly lower, for patients with PPH and TOF than were values for individuals at low likelihood for cardiac disease.

SPECT RVG Image Acquisition

As with myocardial perfusion imaging, dual detector gamma cameras can be used efficiently to collect ^{99m}Tc-labeled red blood cell images at 64 projections over a 180-degree circular arc. The 64 × 64 tomograms with a pixel size of 6.4 mm typically are acquired with low-energy high-resolution collimators for 20 to 25 seconds per projection. Total acquisition times of 15 to 20 minutes are typical. Tomograms are acquired with patients at rest, usually at 8 frames per R-R interval, using an R-wave window such that data are collected if R-waves are between 50% and 150% of mean preacquisition HR, as in many myocardial perfusion gated SPECT protocols. It is likely that these imaging parameters will undergo further experimentation, as the use of 16 rather than 8 gating intervals and of beat rejection windows narrower than ±50% will likely result in overall improved SPECT RVG accuracy.[37]

As with all forms of tomographic imaging, careful attention to the quality and integrity of collected data, such as exhibiting no significant patient motion, results in optimal image interpretation and quantitative analyses.[38] Prereconstruction spatial filtering that has been applied successfully to SPECT RVG data have consisted of Butterworth filtering (cutoff = .55 cycles/cm, power = 5.0),[28] or Butterworth (cutoff = 0.6/pixel, pixel size = 0.64 cm, power = 5.0),[30] followed by quantitative ramp x-filtering. Filtered images generally are backprojected to form transaxial slices, which are reoriented into short-axis (SA) sections using manual choices of anterior, inferior, septal, and lateral limits and approximate LV symmetry axes. Reconstruction limiting angles and planes generally are chosen to ensure that the entire RV and LV, as well as portions of the atria and pulmonary artery, are included in the field of view of reoriented images.

SPECT RVG Image Processing

In one form of SPECT RVG processing,[28] midventricular locations are determined automatically by searching for maximum activity in likely RV locations in SA, horizontal long-axis

TABLE 7-1. SPECT RVG Normal Limits for Subjects at Low Likelihood for CAD

	Planar RVG LV	SPECT RVG LV	SPECT RVG RV
EF	67 ± 6%	68 ± 10%	53 ± 8%
EDV		117 ± 39 ml	129 ± 29 ml
ESV		39 ± 25 ml	61 ± 18 ml
N	31	31	31

(HLA), and vertical long-axis (VLA) orientations. The algorithms automatically define SPECT RVG SA regions as corresponding to those contiguous regions that contained counts ≥35% threshold of maximum ED counts over the entire volume. This particular 35% value for the threshold has been used frequently by nuclear medicine investigators in defining endocardial and epicardial surfaces derived from myocardial perfusion or blood pool images.[39] LV and RV EDV are computed from the number of voxels (i.e., 3-D pixels) within these limits, while biventricular EFs and stroke volumes are computed from systolic count changes within these voxels.

In another form of SPECT RVG data processing,[30] the LV is isolated by searching for a *seed point* identified from maximum counts in likely LV 3-D locations, about which endocardial surfaces are determined by pre-curve fit processing, iterative surface fitting, and post-fit filtering. Comparisons of LVEF values computed by this algorithm with planar RVG LVEF have shown high correlation (r = 0.89), with SPECT RVG values 3% higher than planar LVEF values, on average. Automation success rates for this approach have been reported to be on the order of 70% to 85%.[30]

SPECT RVG Quantitative Normal Limits

For the particular algorithms used to compute the RV and LV values of EDV and EF that follow, the following normal limits have been established based on data acquired for male and female patients before beginning chemotherapy for cancer, and for whom there was no evidence of cardiac disease (Table 7-1).

SPECT RVG Tomographic Chamber Visualization

A potentially significant aspect of SPECT RVG data is the ability to view all of the cardiac chambers moving cinematically in all planes simultaneously. The case examples that follow were chosen primarily for their visual impact, to illustrate the range of sizes and shapes of cardiac chambers as revealed by SPECT RVG, across a spectrum of cardiopulmonary diseases.

Case Presentations

Case 7.1

History

A patient with dyspnea was referred for an evaluation of ventricular function. A resting RVG was performed. The technologist varied the gating interval to assess image quality and the effect of frame rate on systolic LV performance. The gating interval was varied to produce 8 and 16 frames per cardiac cycle. The HR was 99 for both studies, and the image quality was the same. Figure C7-1 displays the findings with 8 frames (Figure C7-1A) and 16 frames (Figure C7-1B).

Findings

The time per frame was 76 msec for the 8-frame study (Figure C7-1A) and was 38 msec for the 16-frame study (Figure C7-1B). The LVEF was calculated as 51% in the 8-frame study but was

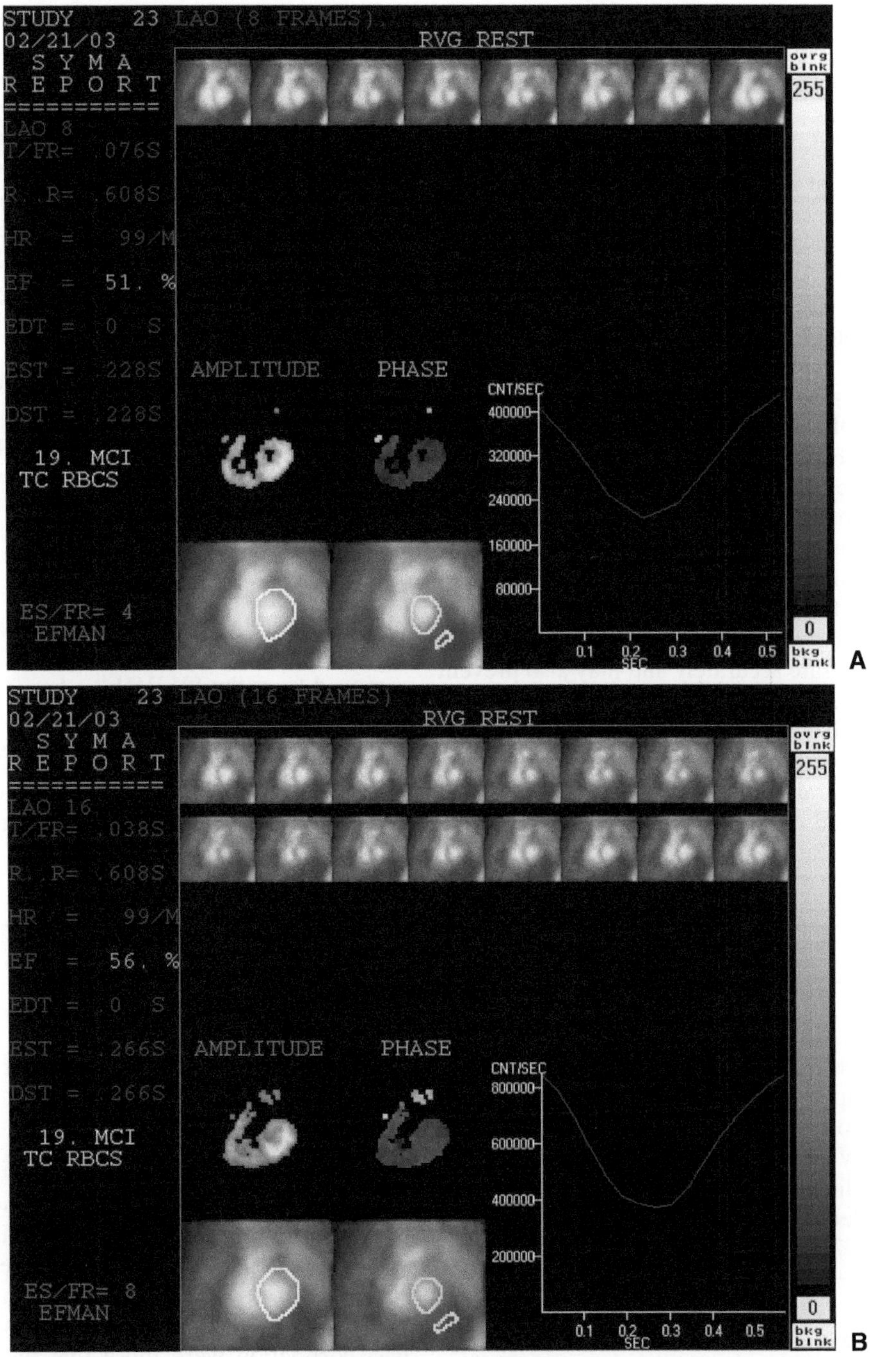

FIGURE C7-1. (A and B)

56% in the 16-frame study. Thus, the importance of an appropriate frame rate for assessing LVEF accurately is clear.

Discussion

This patient had normal cardiac function, and noncardiac causes of dyspnea were likely. This RVG was useful for showing the importance of frame rate for avoiding aliasing, the condition in which the frequency of sampling is inadequate for producing an accurate rendition of the cyclic waveform in question. The sampling frequency of 8 frames per cardiac cycle was inadequate to isolate the ES frame, and thus the LVEF was underestimated. Aliasing occurs most often in patients with normal to high EF and with rapid HR. The frame rate is less important in systole in patients with lower EFs, but an adequate frame rate in diastole is also important, especially if the HR is slow. Loss of diastolic information makes it difficult to assess the filling rate accurately and may also prevent seeing the magnitude of atrial filling as a contributor to LV filling. This is seen in ventricles with poor compliance. One analysis of errors using several methods of gating showed that the method of gating was less important than the frame rate in RVG acquisition.[40]

It should be noted that, by comparison to contrast CVG,[41] dual regions of interest at end-diastole (ED) and end-systole (ES) have been shown to be more accurate[7] for estimating LVEF than a single ROI method, using the ED region with ES activity estimated from the time-activity curve. It should also be noted that the RVG method shows a closer relation to CVG in patients with EFs roughly below 60%.[41,42] Above this level there may be less accuracy in volume estimation by either RVG or CVG.

The placement of the ventricular background region is also an important factor. We systematically analyzed the effects of distance from the LV ROI at end-systole, and the size of the background ROI. There was a 15% variation of background activity between ED and ES when the background region was only 1 pixel removed from the LV ROI, but only an average of 1.2% variation in background activity from ED to ES when the region was 6 pixels removed from the LV ROI.[41]

Interpretation

Normal ventricular function detected more accurately using a greater frame rate for collecting the data to avoid aliasing.

Case 7.2

History

A 65-year-old man was referred for coronary angiography for evaluation of possible CAD. As part of a study, a CVG was performed, followed by obtaining an RVG at rest using the same obliquity at the same time in the catheterization laboratory. The images are displayed in Figure C7-2.

Findings

Figure C7-2 demonstrates the RVG and CVG in the LAO position. The CVG and RVG were traced by outlining the ED and ES frames from the moving CVG and the RVG playback buffer, respectively, without reference to the other study. There was a clear similarity of regional wall motion findings.

Discussion

The RVG accurately reflects CVG findings for regional wall motion. In the previously mentioned study, several methods were examined for expressing the correlation between the findings on RVG and CVG. The methods with the best correlation were those that judged area (or count) reduction using a polar coordinate system with 45-degree ROIs or 90-degree ROIs. In this study, both visually judged and semiautomated border recognition methods showed similarly good results. In the LAO pro-

FIGURE C7-2. (From Steckley, Kronenberg, Born, et al. [43], by permission of *Radiology*.)

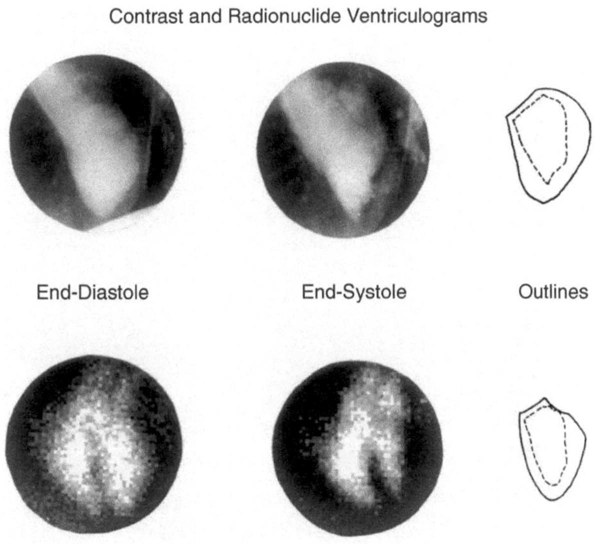

jection, the areas with the best correlation between CVG and RVG were in the regions of the distal interventricular septum, the inferoapical region, and the mid- and distal posterolateral walls in the LAO projection.[43] These r-values ranged from 0.82 to 0.85 using the 45-degree polar coordinate system and a semiautomated system of wall motion analysis. Further, the semiautomated and visual methods of analysis correlated well (r = 0.92 to 0.94 for the polar coordinate systems mentioned previously). In the right anterior oblique (RAO) view, there are similarly good relations between RVG and CVG, except for the inferobasal region of the LV, which is an area of overlap between the LV and the RV.[44]

Interpretation

Good concordance between contrast and radionuclide ventriculographic wall motion estimates.

Case 7.3

History

A 50-year-old man was referred for an exercise perfusion scan to evaluate chest discomfort. A resting perfusion image was collected following injection of 12 mCi ^{99m}Tc-tetrofosmin. Then, the patient exercised on a treadmill using the Bruce protocol. At peak exercise, 25 mCi ^{99m}Tc-tetrofosmin was injected intravenously (IV). Postexercise imaging began 30 minutes later, including ECG gating for evaluation of LV function. During exercise, there was no chest discomfort, and there were no ischemic ECG ST-segment changes. The technologist collected the gated images using both 8 and 16 frames per cardiac cycle. The data collected with 8 frames are displayed in Figure C7-3.

Findings

The images showed normal perfusion, and the gated images showed normal regional and global LV function. The LVEF was 65% using the 8-frame method and was 71% using the 16-frame method. Figure C7-3 demonstrates the findings with the 8-frame method. The reader will note that there is apparently greater activ-

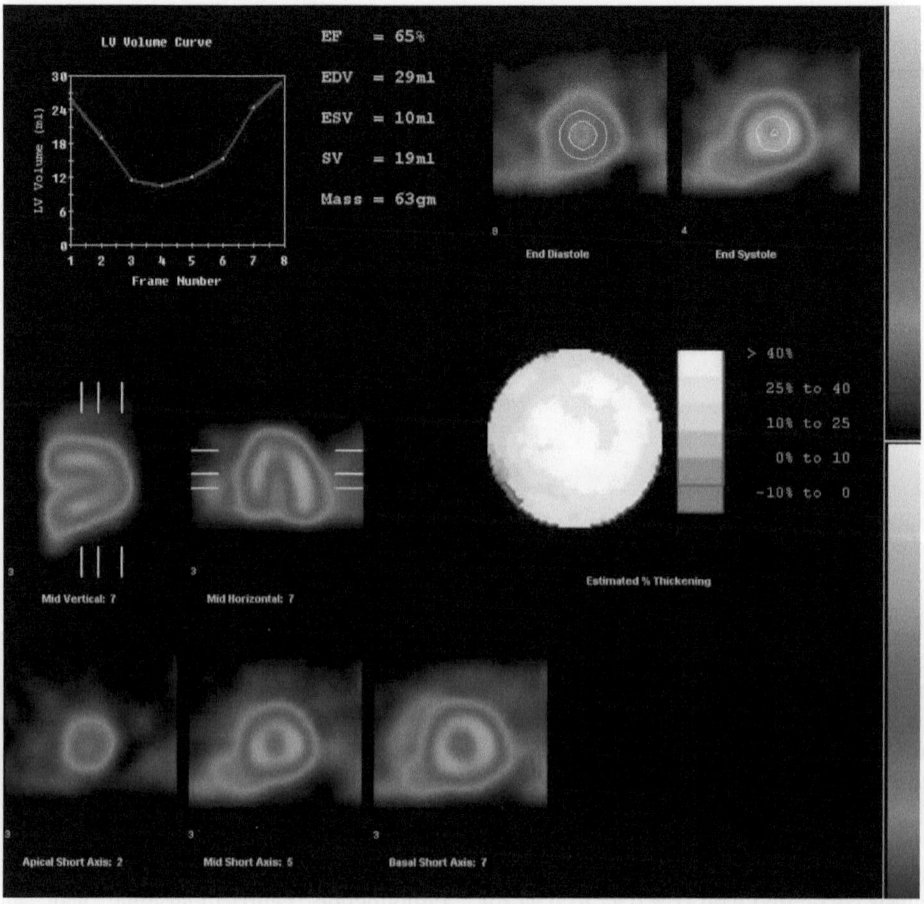

FIGURE C7-3.

ity in frame 8 than in frame 1. This is a common finding and is likely due to delays in sensing the QRS complex and possibly to other electronic delays in the gating circuitry. This then makes frame 1 a collection of data in early systole, while frame 8 shows late diastolic/presystolic activity. The software uses the greatest count activity at end-diastole, regardless of the frame number.

Discussion

This example of gated perfusion imaging demonstrates the same principles as the prior RVG example in terms of sampling frequency. With a regular rhythm, appropriate radioisotopic dosage, and the correct gating, image quality is preserved using the 16-frame collection, and LV global function may be more accurately assessed. Germano et al. found that the LVEF was 3.7% lower with 8 frames than 16 frames per cardiac cycle, although the relation to first-pass RVG EF was excellent with either gating method.[45] The diagnosis of normalcy is enhanced by knowledge of ventricular performance, not just perfusion.

Interpretation

1. Normal ventricular perfusion and performance.
2. More accurate determination of LVEF was obtained with improved sampling frequency.

Case 7.4

History

This 43-year-old man with a history of myocardial infarction (MI) underwent a rest-exercise RVG as part of a study for the detection of myocardial ischemia and evaluation of LV performance. The data are displayed in Figure C7-4.

Findings

At rest, the LVEF was 64% (low limit of normal 50%) (Figure C7-4). There was also a small area of severe hypokinesis in the anterolateral wall, labeled as an abnormally contracting segment (ACS), averaging 19% of the LV perimeter as measured in the combination of LAO and anterior views, with a corresponding regional wall motion score listed. The latter was based on a 5-point rating scale, with 5 equaling hyperkinesis and 0 equaling akinesis or dyskinesis of a segment of the LV. The wall motion abnormality in the mid-anterior wall, but the distal anterior wall and apex contracted normally, suggesting that the infarct-related artery was a diagonal branch of the left anterior descending artery (LAD), rather than the LAD itself. At coronary angiography, this proved to be true, although there was significant 3-vessel CAD warranting coronary artery bypass grafting (CABG). Preoperatively, the patient exercised supine on a bicycle ergometer, and at peak exercise, images were collected for 3 minutes each in the LAO and anterior projections. At peak exercise, the LV dilated, the LVEF decreased, and moderately severe generalized hypokinesis developed. The %ACS increased, and the regional wall motion score decreased.

Three months following CABG, the rest and exercise studies were repeated. Although the LVEF was lower than the preoperative value, the LV size and regional wall motion were similar to the preoperative values. At peak exercise, there was no LV dilation, the LVEF no longer decreased, and wall motion improved in general. The infarct-related %ACS was similar to the resting study.

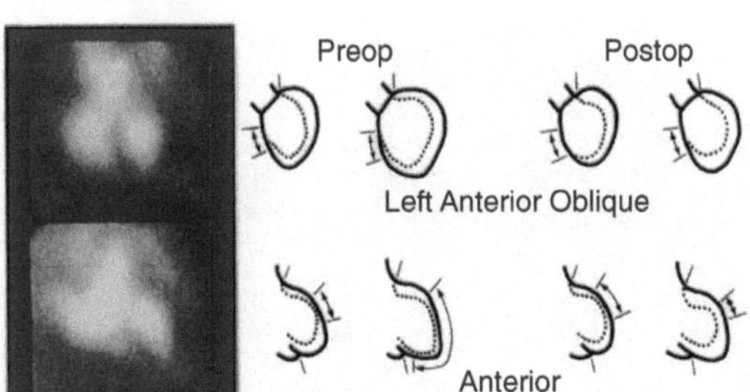

	Preop Rest	Preop Exer	Postop Rest	Postop Exer
EF (%)	64	53	50	54
ACS (%)	19	36	21	13
RWM	31	28	24	37
RPP	7.4	26.6	9.3	27.6

FIGURE C7-4. (From Kronenberg, Pederson, Harston, et al. [48], by permission of *Ann Intern Med.*)

Discussion

This case highlights several features of RVG imaging in ischemic heart disease. First, at rest, a focal wall motion abnormality is a sign of MI, and in several instances, such as this, the infarct-related artery can be defined with some certainty, given a correlative knowledge of coronary anatomy. Second, at peak exercise, there are several ischemic-related findings. As a sign of reduced contractility due to ischemia, the LV dilated diffusely, and the LVEF decreased significantly. Based on reproducibility data, and clinical correlation, the LVEF is considered to change significantly if there is a change of 5 EF units or more. In our laboratory, we obtained 15 serial 2-minute RVGs at rest in a stable patient over a period of 30 minutes. The LVEF varied by ±2 EF units. Thus, a significant change was considered to be 5 EF units (unpublished data), and this is consistent with others' findings.[46]

In addition to the changes in LV size and overall function, there developed a broader area of regional wall motion abnormality, as defined by the %ACS. The regional wall motion score (RWM) did not decline as much as the %ACS increased. The %ACS is a direct measure of an ischemic wall motion abnormality, whereas the RWM score is a summation of abnormal wall motion in the ischemic region and compensatory hyperfunction in nonischemic regions.[47]

The postoperative study showed the effects of improved myocardial perfusion, and the persistent finding of a small area of abnormal wall motion due to the index infarction. The LVEF trended upward, although not strictly by an amount out of the range of reproducibility. Wall motion improved significantly. Compared with the preoperative values, the exercise LVEF was similar to resting LVEF, not improved. The general finding in this study was that, with reperfusion, ischemia was prevented, and the LVEF was preserved, not reduced on exercise.[48] Generally, in cases of stable angina, by revascularization, exercise-induced ischemia is eliminated, and thus, wall motion on exercise remains normal. In contrast, in unstable angina, ischemia and stunning may reduce wall motion at rest, and then, postoperatively, wall motion and EF at rest may actually be improved once the effects of ischemia have resolved.[49]

Interpretation

Chronic ischemic heart disease diagnosed with exercise-induced LV dysfunction and relieved by coronary revascularization.

Case 7.5

History

A 55-year-old man had chest discomfort. As part of a study, he underwent an exercise RVG, and the results were compared with an RVG performed at rest, then during an infusion of the indirect adenosine agonist, dipyridamole. An RVG was performed supine at rest and then with maximal exercise using a bicycle ergometer. Following a rest period, a repeat RVG was performed at rest. Then, dipyridamole was infused to a maximal dose of $0.72\,\text{mg}\cdot\text{kg}\cdot\text{min}^{-1}$ for 6 minutes. Three minutes later, a repeat RVG was obtained. For both studies, LAO and anterior images were obtained, and analysis included LVEF, %ACS, and RWM score. The data are displayed in Figure C7-5.

Findings

During exercise, the systolic blood pressure increased, as expected. The %ACS increased and RWM decreased. During the dipyridamole infusion, the systolic blood pressure changed minimally, but there were similar findings in terms of EF, %ACS, and RWM (Figure C7-5).

Discussion

Many patients do not have the ability to exercise due to orthopedic, vascular, or neurologic problems or general disability. Thus, pharmacologic agents have been employed to demonstrate differences in myocardial perfusion via differences in regional vasodilation distal to significant coronary stenoses.[50,51] In addition to these perfusion defects, using echocardiography, Picano et al. demonstrated inducible

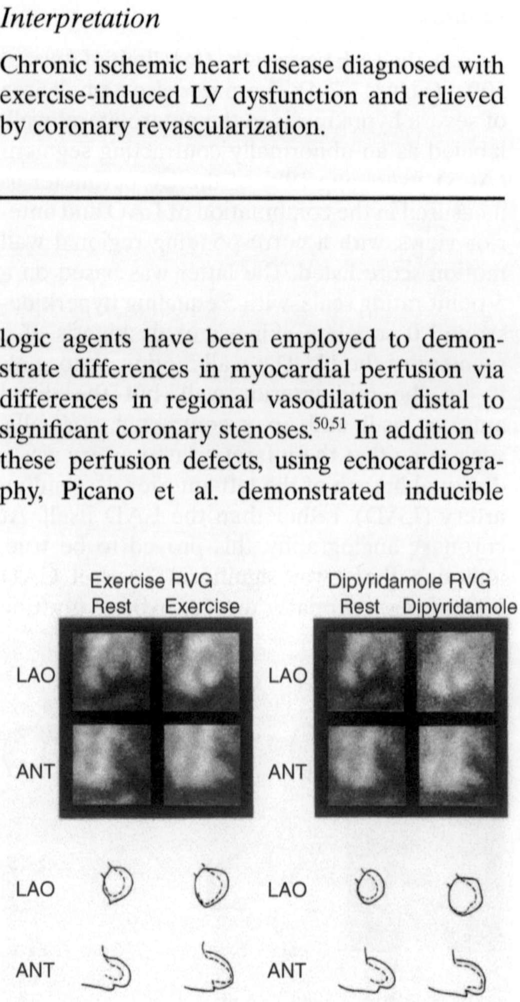

	Rest	Exercise	Rest	Dipyridamole
SBP	160	200	154	130
HR	72	140	76	121
EF	77%	53%	71%	62%
DRWM		-11		-9.5

FIGURE C7-5. (From Cates, Kronenberg, Colins, et al. [54], by permission of *J Am Coll Cardiol.*)

regional wall motion abnormalities following dipyridamole.[52] The standard dose of dipyridamole is $0.56\,mg \cdot kg \cdot min^{-1}$, but Picano et al. also demonstrated that additional regional wall motion abnormalities might be induced by doses of $0.84\,mg \cdot kg \cdot min^{-1}$.[53] The dose chosen for this RVG study was intermediate and successfully demonstrated the ischemic findings noted previously.

While not currently in common use, the dipyridamole RVG method showed that adenosine vasodilation can cause regional myocardial ischemia distal to significant coronary stenoses and expands our knowledge about the physiology of the dipyridamole and adenosine methods. Patients with no significant CAD had an increase in LVEF of 7.9 EF units, whereas patients with CAD had a lack of increase in LVEF as a group, and a tendency to reduction in LVEF with increasing severity of CAD.[54] By receiver operating characteristic (ROC) analysis, the optimal operating point for dipyridamole RVG was a failure to increase the LVEF by 4 or more units; this showed a sensitivity of 65% and specificity of 100% for the detection of CAD of at least 50% in at least one vessel. Thus, dipyridamole RVG showed moderate sensitivity and high specificity for detecting CAD in these patients without prior infarctions. Another possibility to explain these results is that the sensitivity and specificity data reflect closely the actual frequency of ischemic consequences of coronary stenoses, and that some stenoses might, in fact, cause only malperfusion, but not ischemia. A third possibility is that a combination of both may be the actual case. A recent metaanalysis of dipyridamole echocardiography and stress perfusion scintigraphy showed greater sensitivity for the perfusion method, but greater specificity for the dipyridamole echocardiography method in the same patients. However, the difference narrowed when higher doses of dipyridamole were employed.[55]

Interpretation

Myocardial ischemia precipitated by both exercise and dipyridamole in a patient with CAD.

Case 7.6

History

A 76-year-old woman had metastatic breast carcinoma treated with cytoxan and doxorubicin. Subsequently, she developed myelodysplasia and acute myelocytic leukemia. She was treated with thioguanine, cytosine arabinoside, and etoposide. The LV function was monitored with RVG. RVG data before and following therapy are displayed in Figures C7-6A and C7-6B, respectively.

Findings

As shown in Figure C7-6A, the LVEF was 61% before treatment with these three drugs, but following treatment, the LVEF declined to 35% (Figure C7-6B). Chemotherapy was discontinued, and an angiotensin-converting enzyme inhibitor was added for congestive heart failure (CHF). The patient had no evidence of recurrence of the leukemia using maintenance chemotherapy.

Discussion

There has been considerable investigation of anthracycline cardiotoxicity and methods to monitor it. Among others, Alexander et al.[56] reported in 1979 the results of serial RVG in patients receiving doxorubicin. While many patients tolerated the drug well, several showed a progressive decline in LVEF as therapy progressed. Doroshow et al.[57] performed serial studies in mice that demonstrated that those treated with the antioxidant drug, N-acetylcysteine, before receiving doxorubicin, had greater survival than control animals. Thus, it appears that the ability to buffer free radicals in the myocardium affects the ability to tolerate the multiple effects of this class of chemotherapeu-

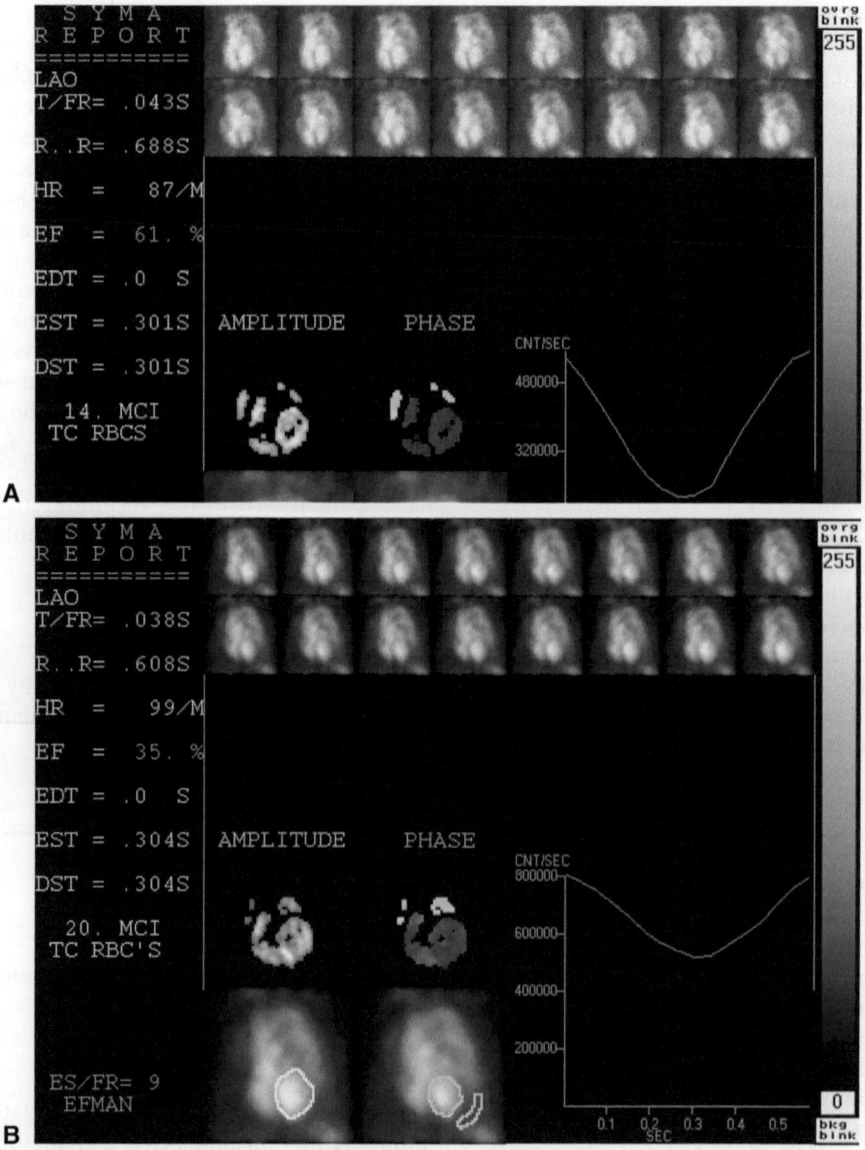

FIGURE C7-6. (A and B)

tic agents. Serial RVG can identify those patients at risk of further LV dysfunction from anthracyline drugs. One recommended method is to monitor patients with clinical risk factors more closely and to evaluate LVEF with RVG in all patients with large cumulative dosages.[58] In our laboratory, we have employed serial LAO images in such patients, rather than a complete, multiple view RVG, for such evaluation. Other imaging methods, such as echocardiography, might be employed in a population of patients; however, RVG affords quantitative, usable data in nearly all patients, as opposed to fewer usable images with echocardiography.

Interpretation

Anthracycline-induced cardiomyopathy.

Case 7.7

History

A 65-year-old woman was enrolled in a study to assess the hypothesis that an arginine vasopressin antagonist causes reverse remodeling of the LV in patients with heart failure. A resting RVG was obtained in the LAO position after labeling the blood using an *in vitro* method. The LV volume was calculated using the method of Links et al.,[59] as shown in Figure C7-7.

Findings

Keeping the same obliquity as during the RVG collection, the center of the LV was identified on a persistence image using a small ^{57}Co marker as a point source of radioactivity. The point source was taped to the skin, and then the camera was rotated to the anterior view. A second static image was acquired. The depth in the chest of the center of the LV from the marker on the skin was identified visually, then counted in pixels and converted to centimeters. In the middle of the RVG collection, a heparinized blood sample had been collected for later use. After the RVG, a 2-ml blood sample was drawn by pipette into a heparinized Petri dish and the sample was counted for 2 minutes (Figure C7-7). A ROI was drawn around the LV at end-diastole. The measured LV activity was then corrected for the known attenuation of ^{99m}Tc activity in water (which is commonly assumed to be the general density of the thoracic structures in general) and by assuming the measured LV activity emanated from a point source at the center of the LV. After a correction for ^{99m}Tc decay, the LV volume was calculated according to the ratio: LV counts/LV volume = Blood sample counts/ Blood sample volume.

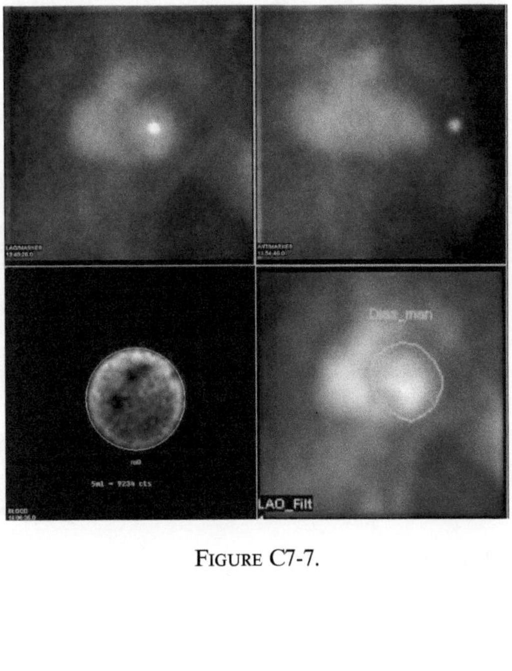

FIGURE C7-7.

Discussion

It is occasionally useful to estimate actual LV or RV volume. This was useful in SOLVD (Studies of Left Ventricular Dysfunction, NHLBI), an evaluation of the effects of an angiotensin-converting enzyme inhibitor (ACE-I), enalapril. In SOLVD,[60] patients were studied before and after randomization to enalapril, or a matched placebo, and mortality and morbidity were assessed. In the Radionuclide Substudy of SOLVD, the mechanism of benefit from ACE-I was investigated. Serial RVGs were obtained at baseline before randomization, and at 3-month intervals until the end of the study. These results demonstrated that enalapril caused a prompt, significant, and persistent reduction in LV volume, termed *reverse remodeling*.[61] This effect was correlated with improved survival in the main population of SOLVD[60] and has also been associated with clinical benefit in patients with heart failure treated with beta-adrenergic blocking drugs.[62] This method is being employed in the present study of the vasopressin antagonist noted previously.

Levy et al.[63] analyzed several methods of volume calculation. In their laboratory, the Links method overestimated LV volume. By contrast, the Links report showed a strong correlation with LV volumes in their own laboratory, with a slope approximating 1 and little residual. Thus, one may legitimately conclude that it is difficult to estimate LV volume with certainty. For all methods of volume estimation, or for imaging in general, consistency is important, and then it is likely that serial comparisons will produce physiologically meaningful results. As discussed in the introduction, SPECT RVG offers a further, improved, accurate method for volume estimation.

Interpretation

1. Dilated LV in a patient with heart failure.
2. LV volume was estimated by depth correction using planar RVG.

Case 7.8

History

A 62-year-old woman diagnosed with breast cancer underwent RVG analysis for cardiac assessment before beginning chemotherapy. The SPECT RVG images are displayed in Figures C7-8A and C7-8B.

Findings

Quantitative results were RVEDV size = 125 ml (normal RVEDV); RVEF = 49% (normal RVEF); LVEDV = 91 ml (normal LVEDV); LVEF = 74% (normal LVEF). Visual examination of regional RV motion, regional LV motion, and of the sizes of LV and RV and the right and left atria all appeared to be normal.

Discussion

Ventricular function often is first evaluated in patients with cancer before the onset of chemotherapy. Many chemotherapeutic agents are known to damage otherwise healthy tissue. Drugs such as doxorubicin,[64,65] used to treat breast cancer, as well as other anthracyclines, have cardiotoxic side effects.[66] Doxorubicin cardiotoxicity is dose-dependent, resulting in myocyte damage culminating in CHF,[67] as illustrated by the example of Case 7.6. Nontomographic (planar) gated scintigraphy of labeled red blood cells (blood pool imaging) has been used for several decades for serial determination of LVEF in patients undergoing chemotherapy.[68] The standard guideline has

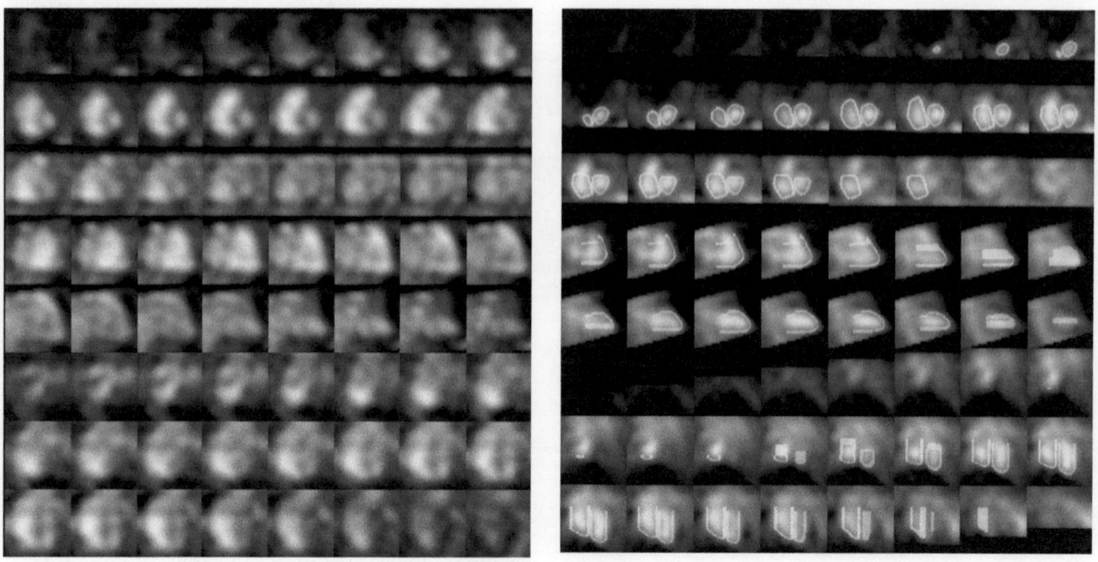

A B

FIGURE C7-8. (A and B)

been to suspend doxorubicin therapy if LVEF decreases below 30%, or if a drop of 10% is observed.[69] Prognosis for patients with LVEF below 30% is poor in general,[70] and for patients with doxorubicin-induced severe CHF, survival is usually less than 2 weeks.[71,72] Therefore, serial imaging of LVEF before, during, and after a course of chemotherapy is often employed. The case study shown here is for a patient with normal cardiac size and function of both RV and LV, to serve as a reference for the subsequent case examples for which RV and/or LV size and/or function are abnormal.

Interpretation

Normal LV and RV by SPECT RVG.

Case 7.9

History

A 52-year-old woman who underwent orthotopic biatrial heart transplantation 15 years earlier was monitored yearly with RVG. The SPECT RVG images are displayed in Figures C7-9A and C7-9B.

Findings

Quantitative results were RVEDV = 296 ml (large RVEDV), but also normal RVEF = 40%; LVEDV = 68 ml (relatively small LVEDV), LVEF = 67% (normal LVEF); RVG LVEF = 79% (high LVEF).

Visual examination of regional RV motion and regional LV motion were normal. Visual examination of RV size appeared mildly enlarged and LV size was normal. The RA size was considered to be enlarged, and the LA size was normal.

A 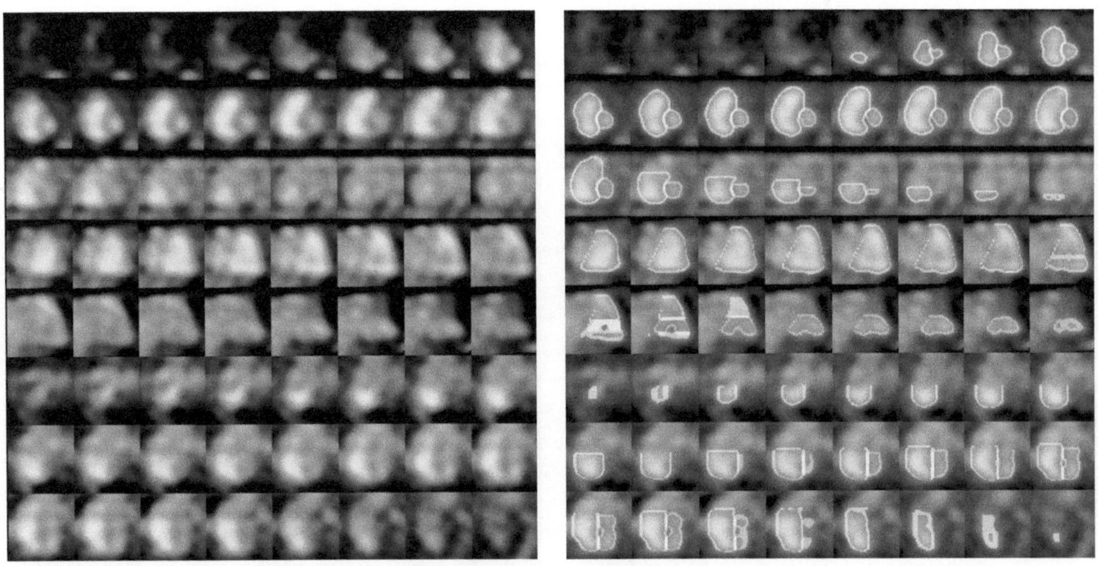 B

FIGURE C7-9. (A and B)

Discussion

After cardiac transplantation patients receive yearly follow-up RVG to evaluate overall function. However, orthotopic biatrial heart transplantation shows an enlarged RA size on RVG. Biatrial transplantation used to be the most common technique, because there was less ischemic time involved, but there was also an increased incidence of atrial arrhythmias due to the size mismatch of atrial remnants. More recently, bicaval cardiac transplantation has been the preferred technique because of a decreased incidence of arrhythmia, need for pacemaker, and risk of mitral or tricuspid regurgitation. In bicaval heart transplantation an enlarged RA size is not seen on RVG.

Interpretation

Biatrial cardiac transplantation; RV dilation, but normal biventricular function.

Case 7.10

History

A 45-year-old woman who underwent orthotopic biatrial cardiac transplantation 10 years earlier was evaluated yearly with RVG. The SPECT RVG images are displayed in Figures C7-10A and C7-10B.

Findings

Quantitative results were RVEDV size = 113 ml (large RVEDV); RVEF = 33% (low RVEF); LVEDV = 88 ml (normal LVEDV); LVEF = 55% (normal LVEF), and RVG LVEF = 67% (normal LVEF).

Visual examination of regional RV motion was reduced. Visual examination of regional LV motion was normal. Visual examination of the RA size was enlarged and LA size was normal.

Discussion

Unlike the patient represented by Case 7.9, the patient shown here has sustained damage to the RV as evidenced by markedly reduced RVEF.

Interpretation

RV dysfunction following orthotopic cardiac transplantation.

A 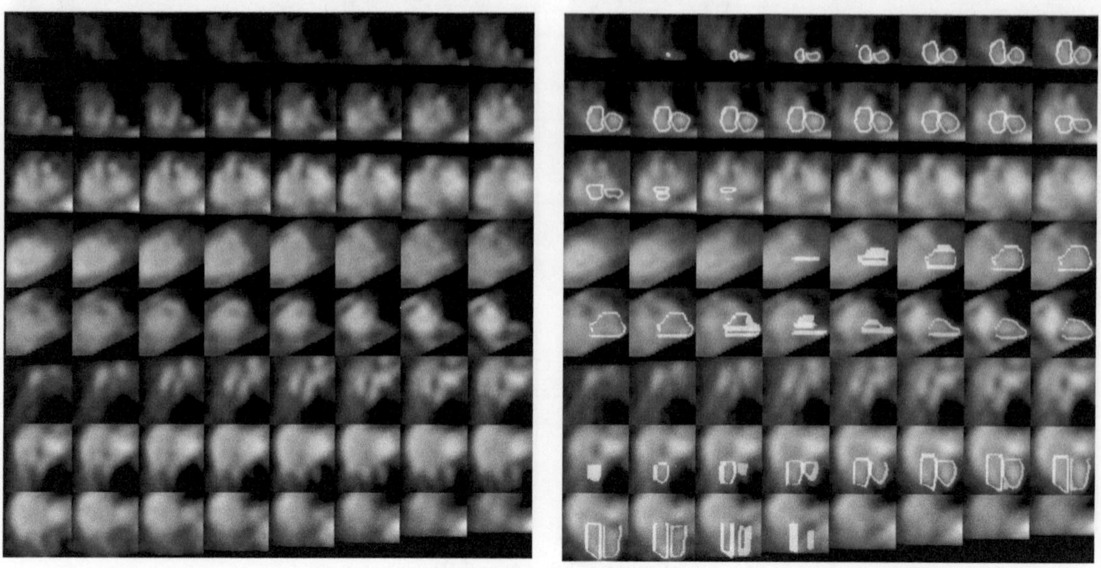 B

FIGURE C7-10. (A and B)

Case 7.11

History

A 54-year-old man with a history of aortic insufficiency and CHF was referred for RVG. Left heart catheterization showed normal coronary arteries. The SPECT RVG images are displayed in Figures C7-11A and C7-11B.

Findings

Quantitative results were RVEDV size = 92 ml (normal RVEDV); RVEF = 46% (normal RVEF); LVEDV = 449 ml (one of the largest recorded LVEDVs); LVEF = 22% (abnormally low LVEF), and RVG LVEF = 22% (abnormally low LVEF).

Visual examination of regional RV motion was normal. Visual examination of regional LV motion showed severe free wall hypokinesis with apical akinesis. The RV size appeared to be normal but the LV size was severely enlarged. RA and LA sizes appeared to be normal.

Discussion

An enlarged LV size, with normal function or global hypokinesis, but normal RV size and function is usually secondary to left-sided valvular regurgitation. However, hypertension or other left-sided heart disorders, such as MI, may be part of the differential diagnosis. In patients who have an enlarged LV with normal EF, a measurement of stroke volume ratio helps in the diagnosis of valvular heart disease. In this case, the LV/RV stroke volume ratio was 2.36, consistent with a severe left-sided regurgitant lesion. Given the normal LA size, the diagnosis of aortic regurgitation is clear because mitral regurgitation would have caused LA enlargement as well as LV dilation.

Interpretation

LV dilation and dysfunction due to chronic aortic regurgitation.

A

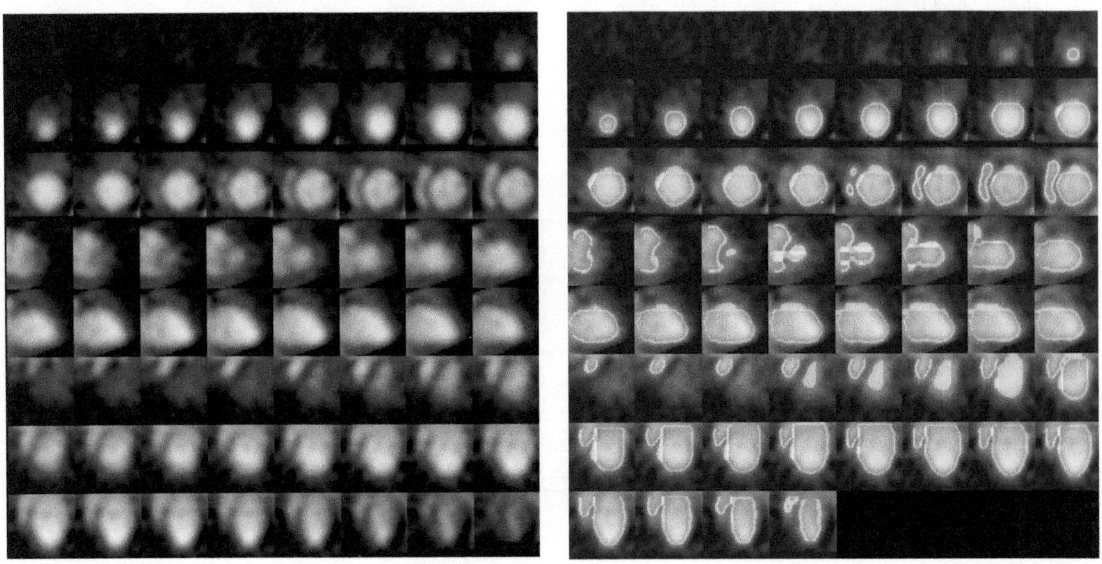

B

FIGURE C7-11. (A and B)

Case 7.12

History

A 29-year-old woman with a history of pulmonary hypertension secondary to atrial septal defect (ASD) (Eisenmenger syndrome) diagnosed 6 years earlier presented with fatigue and shortness of breath and was referred for RVG. Her transthoracic echocardiogram showed a large ASD with right to left shunt. Her right-sided heart catheterization measurements were RA 5mmHg, RV 100/2mmHg, PA 101/40mmHg, pulmonary capillary wedge pressure (PCW) 4mmHg, and PAO_2 saturation 71%. Coronary angiography showed a 60% distal LAD stenosis. The SPECT RVG images are displayed in Figures C7-12A and C7-12B.

Findings

Quantitative results were RVEDV size = 241ml (large RVEDV); RVEF = 25% (low RVEF); LVEDV = 91ml (normal LVEDV); LVEF = 53% (normal LVEF); and RVG LVEF = 63% (normal LVEF).

Visual examination of regional RV motion showed moderate hypokinesis of the free wall and dyskinesis of the RV apex, suggestive of RV apical aneurysm. Visual examination of regional LV motion was normal. RV size was judged to be moderately enlarged and LV size normal. The RA appeared to be enlarged and the LA size was considered to be normal.

Interpretation

Right-sided heart failure due to uncorrected atrial septal defect with pulmonary hypertension (Eisenmenger's syndrome).

A 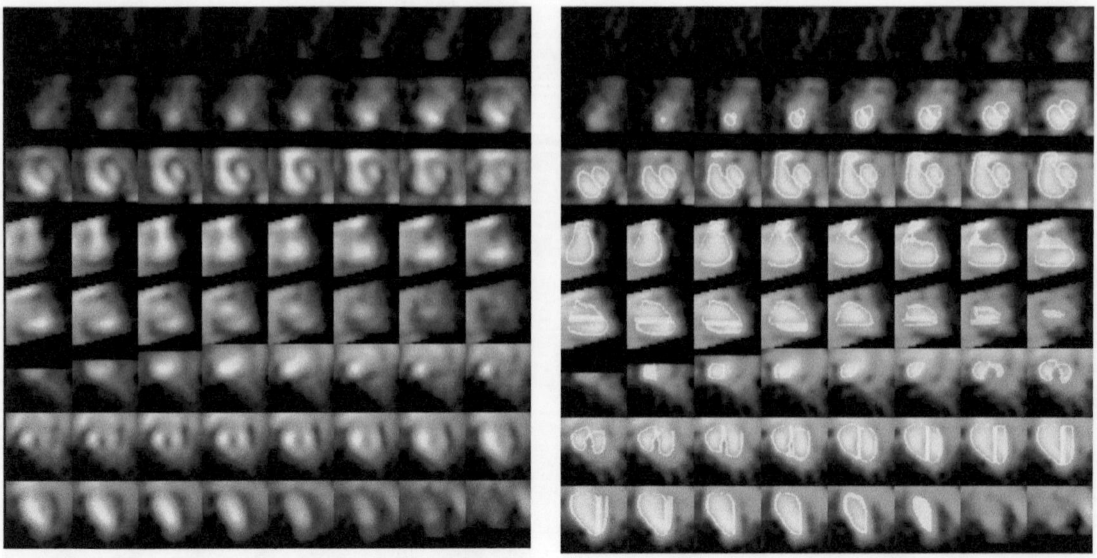 B

FIGURE C7-12. (A and B)

Case 7.13

History

A 63-year-old man with a prior history of anterior wall myocardial infarction and CHF (New York Heart Association Class 3) was referred for RVG. The SPECT RVG images are displayed in Figures C7-13A and C7-13B.

Findings

Quantitative results were RVEDV size = 248 ml (large RVEDV); RVEF = 34% (low RVEF); LVEDV = 127 ml (normal LVEDV); LVEF = 49% (low LVEF); and RVG LVEF = 44% (low LVEF).

Visual examination of regional RV motion showed mild global hypokinesis. Visual examination of regional LV motion showed anterior wall and septal wall hypokinesis and apical dyskinesis. The RV size was judged to be enlarged, and LV size was considered to be mildly enlarged. Visual examination of RA size and LA size were normal.

Discussion

Although both LV and RV are abnormal in this patient, patients with ischemic cardiomyopathy generally have LV regional wall motion abnormality with normal RV motion. They also have LV enlargement and normal RV size. However, patients with dilated cardiomyopathy have RV and LV global hypokinesis and four-chamber enlargement.

Interpretation

Ischemic heart disease with evidence of prior anterior myocardial infarction and LV and RV dysfunction.

A 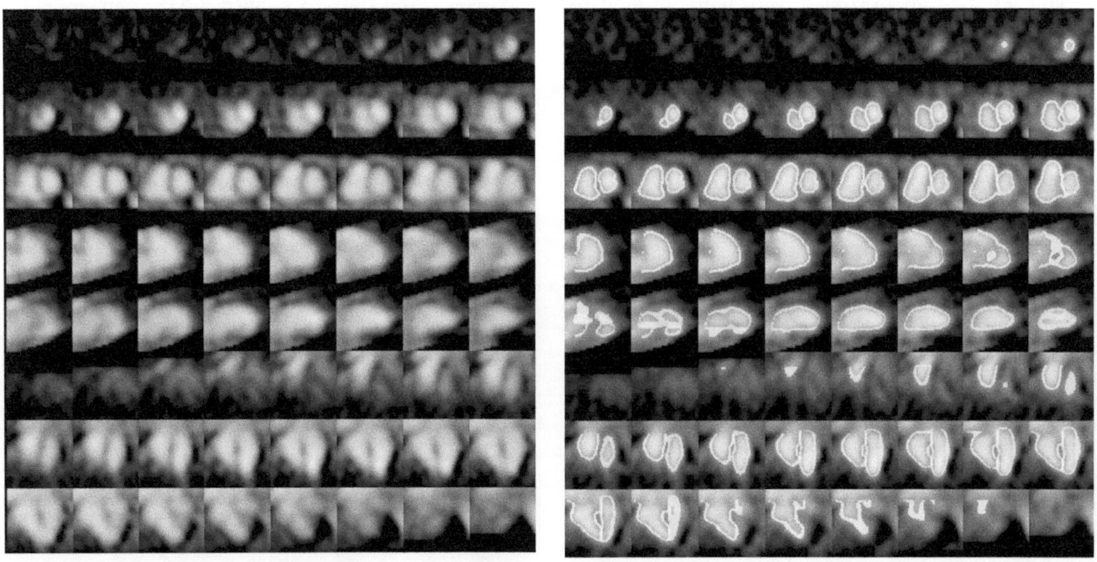 B

FIGURE C7-13. (A and B)

Case 7.14

History

A 53-year-old man with dilated cardiomyopathy presented with progressively worsening shortness of breath over the previous 6 months and was referred for RVG. His coronary angiography showed normal coronary arteries, and right-sided heart catheterization measurements were RA 20mmHg, RV 36/13mmHg, PA 30/17mmHg, PCW 19mmHg, and PAO_2 saturation 35%. The SPECT RVG images are displayed in Figures C7-14A and C7-14B.

Findings

Quantitative results were RVEDV size = 330ml (large RVEDV); RVEF = 15% (low RVEF); LVEDV = 286ml (large LVEDV); LVEF = 24% (low LVEF); and RVG LVEF = 23% (low LVEF).

Visual examination of regional RV motion showed free wall and apical severe hypokinesis. Visual examination of regional LV motion also showed free wall and apical severe hypokinesis. The RV size and LV size both were judged to be moderately enlarged. Visual examination of RA size and LA size indicated that both also were enlarged.

Discussion

Note that, unlike Case 7.13, here both LVEF and RVEF are reduced, and both RVEDV and LVEDV are abnormally increased. One reason for interest in RV size and contractility, per se, is in the study of CHF. CHF is a leading cause of morbidity and mortality in the United States, and currently is the most frequent reason for hospitalization. Epidemiological studies of the role of deteriorating RV function in the progression of CHF have been difficult to conduct due to the difficulty in obtaining RV information, which may have complicated the management of CHF and contributed to poor CHF prognosis.[73] Recently it has become more appreciated that assessment of RV status is important for accurate prognosis.[74–81] Direct RV observations may prove to be important because some patients with CHF can have

A 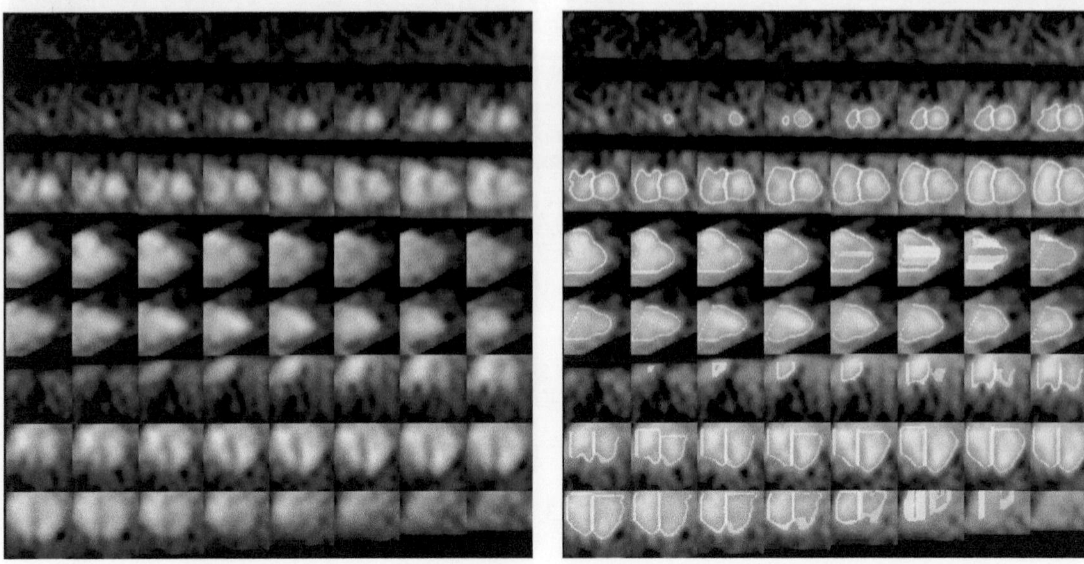 B

FIGURE C7-14. (A and B)

occult RV dysfunction and yet have normal pulmonary artery pressure.[81,82] Also, some studies have shown that RVEF, not LVEF, is a major determinant of functional capacity in patients with CHF,[77,83] suggesting that it may be possible to enhance functional capacity by improving RV function. Treatments of CHF with venodilators that *unload* the RV have been found to improve functional capacity;[84] recently, administration of sildenafil has been shown to produce simultaneous improvement in exercise capacity accompanied by increased RVEF.[9] Therefore, it is plausible that monitoring baseline and time-changes of RV size and contractility could play a role in evaluating efficacy of new pharmaceuticals to treat CHF, and in assessing the degree to which an individual patient responds favorably to a given drug.

Interpretation

Idiopathic dilated cardiomyopathy with 4-chamber dilation and biventricular dysfunction was diagnosed.

Case 7.15

History

A 57-year-old woman with a history of pulmonary hypertension secondary to pulmonary fibrosis presented with shortness of breath and pedal edema that had been progressively worsening over the last 2 years. Chest CT showed diffuse fibrosis and emphysematous changes. Coronary angiography showed normal coronary arteries. Right-sided heart catheterization measurements were RA 9 mmHg, RV 62/0 mmHg, PA 61/27 mmHg, PCW 4 mmHg and PAO_2 saturation 48%. She was referred for an SPECT RVG as displayed in Figures C7-15A and C7-15B.

A 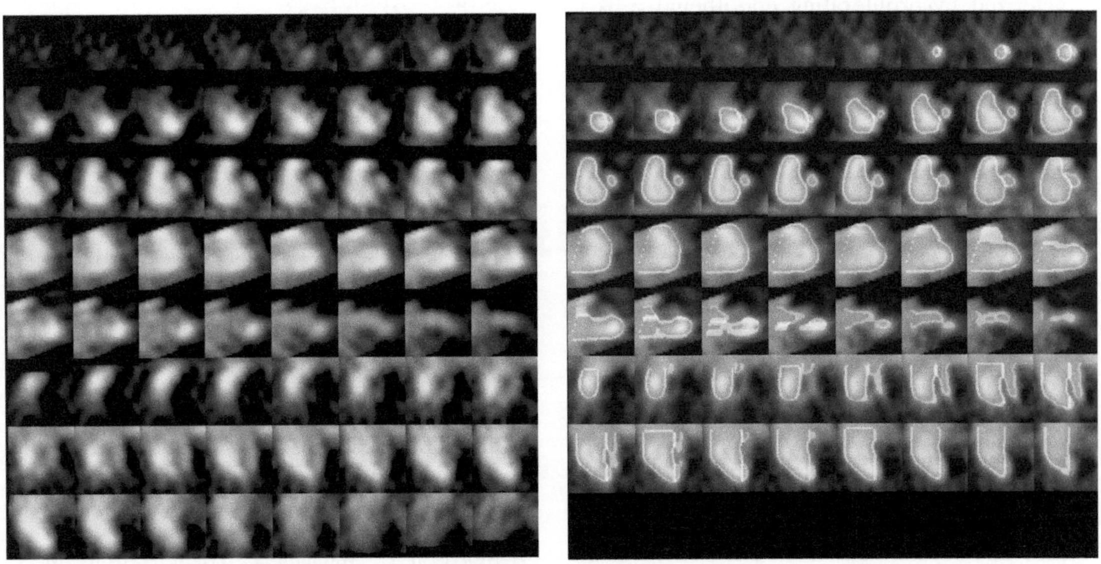 B

FIGURE C7-15. (A and B)

Findings

Quantitative results were RVEDV size = 452 ml (one of the largest recorded RVEDV values); RVEF = 20% (low RVEF); LVEDV = 36 ml (small LVEDV); LVEF = 58% (normal LVEF); and planar RVG LVEF = 67%.

Visual examination of regional RV motion showed severe free wall and apical hypokinesis. Visual examination of regional LV motion was normal. Visual examination of the RA size is enlarged and LA size is normal.

Discussion

RVG is performed in patients with pulmonary hypertension for the diagnosis and monitoring of treatment efficacy. In patients with pulmonary hypertension there is usually RV size enlargement and RV free wall and apical hypokinesis. It is also possible to evaluate septal wall motion. A flattening of the septum is seen in mild to moderate pulmonary hypertension and bowing of the septal wall into the LV cavity occurs in moderate to severe pulmonary hypertension.

Gated blood pool SPECT imaging may well come to play a role in monitoring patients with primary pulmonary hypertension (PPH). PPH is a devastating, terminal disorder,[85] characterized by proliferating endothelial cells in pulmonary arterioles,[86] leading to progressive pulmonary artery hypertension, RV failure and death.[87] An unknown *injury* or triggering mechanism is hypothesized to activate the disease in subjects predisposed to develop PPH. Underlying factors include genetic abnormalities,[88] such as mutations of the bone morphogenic protein receptor-II gene.[89] However, not all patients diagnosed with PPH have this *PPH1* gene, and the actual *triggers* of PPH are not known at this time. Less rare are cases associated with appetite-suppressing drugs such as fenfluramine-phentermine.[90]

Some striking manifestations of PPH are greatly enlarged and/or distorted structures of the right heart, reflecting long-term remodeling processes. Specifics of observed RV abnormalities vary substantially from one patient to the next. The RV and RA can be enlarged, and the pulmonary outflow tract (leading to the PA), can be substantially dilated. RVEF can be markedly reduced. Pronounced RV enlargement can compress the LV, affecting LV function. In the end stage of RV deterioration, patients with PPH generally succumb to right-sided heart failure. One of the intriguing aspects of epoprostenol is the cellular remodeling that appears to take place in the pulmonary vasculature and right heart with drug therapy.[91] Several cardiac MRI and echocardiographic studies documented that for individuals with PPH who respond well to epoprostenol, RV function improves.[92–95]

Interpretation

Primary pulmonary hypertension with severe RV dysfunction.

References

1. Stokely EM, Parkey RW, Bonte FJ, Graham KD, Stone MJ, Willerson JT. Gated blood pool imaging following ^{99m}Tc stannous pyrophosphate imaging. *Radiology.* 1976;120:433–434.
2. Pavel DG, Zimmer AM, Patterson VN. In vivo labeling of red blood cells with ^{99m}Tc: a new approach to blood pool visualization. *J Nucl Med.* 1977;18:303–308.
3. Callahan RJ, Froehlich JW, McKusick KW, Leppo J, Strauss HW. A modified method for the in vivo labeling of red cells with ^{99m}Tc: concise communication. *J Nucl Med.* 1983;24:98–103.
4. Srivastava SC, Straub RF. Blood cell labeling with ^{99m}Tc: progress and perspectives. *Semin Nucl Med.* 1990;20:41–51.
5. Patrick ST, Glowniak JV, Turner FE, Robbins MS, Wolfangel RG. Comparison of in vitro RBC labeling with the UltraTag RBC kit versus in vivo labeling. *J Nucl Med.* 1991;32:242–244.
6. Maddahi J, Berman DS, Matsuoka DT, et al. A new technique for assessing right ventricular ejection fraction using rapid multiple-gated equilibrium cardiac blood pool scintigraphy: description, validation and findings in chronic coronary artery disease. *Circulation.* 1979;60:581–589.
7. Morrison D, Marshall J, Wright A, Kaly M, Henry R. An improved method of right ventric-

ular gated equilibrium blood pool radionuclide ventriculography. *Chest.* 1982;82:607–614.
8. Schulman DS. Assessment of the right ventricle with radionuclide techniques. *J Nucl Cardiol.* 1996;3:253–264.
9. Lachmann JS, Semigran MJ. Sildenafil improves hemodynamic and exercise tolerance in patients with advanced heart failure. *Circulation.* 2002; 106(II):469.
10. Harolds JA, Bowen RD, Powers TA. Right-ventricular function as assessed by two radionuclide techniques: concise communication. *J Nucl Med.* 1981;22:113–115.
11. Morrison DA, Turgeon J, Kotler J, Henry R. Gated first pass radionuclide ventriculography: methods, validation, and application. *Clin Nucl Med.* 1984;9:506–511.
12. Nichols K, DePuey EG, Rozanski A. First-pass radionuclide angiocardiography with single-crystal gamma cameras. *J Nucl Cardiol.* 1997;4: 61–73.
13. Berger HJ, Matthay RA, Loke J, Marshall RC, Gottschalk A, Zaret BL. Assessment of cardiac performance with quantitative radionuclide angiocardiography: Right ventricular ejection fraction with reference to findings in chronic obstructive pulmonary disease. *Am J Cardiol.* 1978;41:897–905.
14. Rezai K, Weiss R, Stanford W, Preslar J, Marcus M, Kirchner P. Relative accuracy of three scintigraphic methods for determination of right ventricular ejection fraction: a correlative study with ultrafast computed tomography. *J Nucl Med.* 1991;32:429–435.
15. Johnson LL, Lawson MA, Blackwell GG, Tauxe EL, Russel K, Dell'Italia LJ. Optimizing the method to calculate right ventricular ejection fraction from first-pass data acquired with a multicrystal camera. *J Nucl Cardiol.* 1995;2:372–379.
16. Maltz DL, Treves S. Quantitative radionuclide angiocardiography: determination of Qp:Qs in children. *Circulation.* 1973;47:1049–1056.
17. Harolds JA, Grove RB, Bowen RD, Powers TA. Right ventricular function as assessed by two radionuclide techniques. *J Nucl Med.* 1981;22: 113–115.
18. Nichols K, DePuey EG, Gooneratne N, Salensky H, Friedman M, Cochoff S. First-pass ventricular ejection fraction using a single-crystal nuclear camera. *J Nucl Med.* 1994;35:1292–1300.
19. Ham HR, Franken PR, Georges B, Delcourt E, Guillaume M, Piepsz A. Evaluation of the accuracy of steady state krypton-81m method for calculating right ventricular ejection fraction. *J Nucl Med.* 1986;27:593–601.
20. Heusch A, Koch JA, Krogmann ON, Korbmacher B, Bourgeois M. Volumetric analysis of the right and left ventricle in a porcine heart model: comparison of three-dimensional echocardiography, magnetic resonance imaging and angiocardiography. *Eur J Ultrasound.* 1999;9: 245–255.
21. Jauhiainen T, Jarvinen VM, Hekali PE, Poutanen VP, Penttila A, Kupari M. MR gradient echo volumetric analysis of human cardiac casts: focus of the right ventricle. *J Comp Assist Tomogr.* 1998;22:899–903.
22. Markewicz W, Sechtem U, Higgins CB. Evaluation of the right ventricle by magnetic resonance imaging. *Am Heart J.* 1987;113:8–15.
23. Sechtem U, Pflugfelder PW, Gould RG, Cassidy MM, Higgins CB. Measurement of right and left ventricular volumes in healthy individuals with cine MR imaging. *Radiology.* 1987;163:697–702.
24. Boxt LM, Katz J. Magnetic resonance imaging for quantitation of right ventricular volume in patients with pulmonary hypertension. *J Thorac Imaging.* 1993;8:92–97.
25. Katz J, Whang J, Boxt LM, Barst RJ. Estimation of right ventricular mass in normal subjects and in patients with primary pulmonary hypertension by magnetic resonance imaging. *J Am Coll Cardiol.* 1993;21(6):1475–1481.
26. Boxt LM, Katz J, Kalb T, Czegledy FP, Barst RJ. Direct quantitation of right and left ventricular values with nuclear magnetic resonance imaging and in patients with primary pulmonary hypertension. *J Am Coll Cardiol.* 1992;19(7):1508–1515.
27. Carr JC, Simonetti O, Bundy J, Li D, Pereles S, Finn JP. Cine MR angiography of the heart with segmented true fast imaging with steady-state precession. *Radiology.* 2001;219(3):828–834.
28. Nichols K, Saouaf R, Ababneh AA, et al. Validation of SPECT equilibrium radionuclide angiographic right ventricular parameters by cardiac MRI. *J Nucl Cardiol.* 2002;9:153–160.
29. Chin BB, Bloomgarden DC, Xia W, et al. Right and left ventricular volume and ejection fraction by tomographic gated blood-pool scintigraphy. *J Nucl Med.* 1997;38:942–948.
30. Van Kriekinge SD, Berman DS, Germano G. Automatic quantification of left ventricular ejection fraction from gated blood pool SPECT. *J Nucl Cardiol.* 1999;6:498–506.

31. Groch MW, Belzberg AS, DePuey EG, et al. Evaluation of ventricular performance using gated blood pool SPECT: A multicenter study [abstract]. *J Nucl Med.* 2000;41:5P.
32. Groch MW, DePuey EG, Belzberg AS, et al. Assessment of left ventricular performance by gated blood pool SPECT: A multicenter study [abstract]. *Circulation.* 2000;102(18):II–725.
33. Bartlett ML, Srinivasan G, Barker WC, Kitsiou AN, Dilsizian V, Bacharach SL. Left ventricular ejection fraction: Comparison of results from planar and SPECT gated blood-pool studies. *J Nucl Med.* 1996;37:1795–1799.
34. Groch MW, Marshall RC, Erwin WD, Schippers DJ, Barnett CA, Leidholdt EM. Quantitative gated blood pool SPECT for the assessment of coronary artery disease at rest. *J Nucl Cardiol.* 1998;5:567–573.
35. De Bondt P, Vandenberghe S, De Sutter J, et al. Comparison of different algorithms for the calculation of left ventricular ejection fraction from planar radionuclide ventriculography studies: A dynamic phantom study [abstract]. *J Nucl Med.* 2001;42:162P.
36. De Bondt P, Nichols K, Vandenberghe S, et al. Validation of gated blood-pool SPECT cardiac measurements tested using a biventricular dynamic physical phantom. *J Nucl Med.* 2003;44:967–972.
37. Germano G, Berman DS. The right stuff. *J Nucl Cardiol.* 2002;9:226–228.
38. DePuey EG. Artifacts in SPECT myocardial perfusion imaging. In DePuey EG, Garcia EV, Berman DS (eds). *Cardiac SPECT Imaging.* New York: Lippincott Williams & Wilkins; 2001: 231–262.
39. Nichols K, DePuey EG, Rozanski A. Automation of gated tomographic left ventricular ejection fraction. *J Nucl Cardiol.* 1996;3:475–482.
40. Juni JE, Chen CC. Effects of gating modes on the analysis of left ventricular function in the presence of heart rate variation. *J Nucl Med.* 1988;29:1272–1278.
41. Kronenberg MW, O'Connor JL, Higgins SB, Pederson RW, Friesinger GC. Analysis of variables affecting calculation of left ventricular ejection fraction using a new technique for border definition. *Proceedings of Computers in Cardiology.* New York: Institute of Electrical and Electronic Engineers, Inc. 1981:107–112.
42. Okada RD, Kirshenbaum HD, Kushner FG, et al. Observer variance in the qualitative evaluation of left ventricular wall motion and the quantification of left ventricular ejection fraction using rest and exercise multigated blood pool imaging. *Circulation.* 1980;61:128–136.
43. Steckley RA, Kronenberg MW, Born ML, et al. Radionuclide ventriculography: Evaluation of automated and visual regional wall motion analysis. *Radiology.* 1982;142:179–185.
44. Jengo JA, Mena I, Blaufuss A, Criley JM. Evaluation of left ventricular function (ejection fraction and segmental wall motion) by single pass radioisotope angiography. *Circulation.* 1978;57:326–332.
45. Germano G, Kiat H, Kavanaugh PB, et al. Automatic quantification of ejection fraction from gated myocardial perfusion SPECT. *J Nucl Med.* 1995;36:2138–2147.
46. Hecht HS, Josephson MA, Hopkins JM, Singh BN. Reproducibility of equilibrium radionuclide ventriculography in patients with coronary artery disease: response of left ventricular ejection fraction and regional wall motion to supine bicycle exercise. *Am Heart J.* 1982;104:567–574.
47. Kerber RE, Marcus ML, Wilson R, Ehrhardt J, Abboud FM. Effects of acute coronary occlusion on the motion and perfusion of the normal and ischemic interventricular septum. An experimental echocardiographic study. *Circulation.* 1976;54:928–935.
48. Kronenberg MW, Pederson RW, Harston WE, Born ML, Bender HW Jr., Friesinger GC. Left ventricular performance after coronary-artery bypass surgery: Prediction of functional benefit. *Ann Intern Med.* 1983;99:305–313.
49. Hamby RL, Tabrah F, Aintablian A, Hartstein ML, Wisfoff BG. Left ventricular hemodynamics and contractile pattern after aortocoronary bypass surgery: factors affecting reversibility of abnormal left ventricular function. *Am Heart J.* 1974;88:149–159.
50. Gould KL, Westcott RJ, Albro PC, Hamilton JW. Noninvasive assessment of coronary stenosis by myocardial imaging during pharmacologic coronary vasodilation. II. Clinical methodology and feasibility. *Am J Cardiol.* 1978;41:279–287.
51. Boucher CA, Brewster DC, Darling C, Okada RD, Strauss HW, Pohost GM. Determination of cardiac risk by dipyridamole-thallium imaging before peripheral vascular surgery. *N Engl J Med.* 1985;312:389–394.
52. Picano E, Distante A, Masini M, Morales MA, Lattanzi F, L'Abbate A. Dipyridamole-echocardiography test in effort angina pectoris. *Am J Cardiol.* 1985;56:452–456.
53. Picano E, Lattanzi F, Masini M, Distante A, L'Abbate A. High dose dipyridamole echocar-

diography test in effort angina pectoris. *J Am Coll Cardiol.* 1986;8:848–854.

54. Cates CU, Kronenberg MW, Colins HW, Sandler MP. Dipyridamole radionuclide ventriculography: A test with high specificity for severe coronary artery disease. *J Am Coll Cardiol.* 1989; 13:841–851.
55. Imran MB, Palinkas A, Picano E. Head-to-head comparison of dipyridamole echocardiography and stress perfusion scintigraphy for the detection of coronary artery disease: a meta-analysis. Comparison between stress echo and scintigraphy. *Int J Cardiovasc Imaging.* 2003;19:23–28.
56. Alexander J, Dainiak N, Berger HJ, et al. Serial assessment of doxorubicin cardiotoxicity with quantitative radionuclide angiocardiography. *N Engl J Med.* 1979;300:278–283.
57. Doroshow JH, Locker GY, Ifrim I, Myers CE. Prevention of doxorubicin cardiac toxicity in the mouse by N-acetylcysteine. *J Clin Invest.* 1981;68:1053–1064.
58. Steinberg JS, Wasserman AG. Radionuclide ventriculography for the evaluation and prevention of doxorubicin cardiotoxicity. *Clin Ther.* 1985;7: 660–667.
59. Links JM, Becker LC, Shindledecker JG, et al. Measurement of absolute left ventricular volume from gated blood pool studies. *Circulation.* 1982;65:82–91.
60. SOLVD Investigators. Effect of enalapril on survival in patients with reduced left ventricular ejection fractions and congestive heart failure. *N Engl J Med.* 1991;325:293–302.
61. Konstam MA, Rousseau MF, Kronenberg MW, et al. Effects of the angiotensin converting enzyme inhibitor, enalapril, on the long-term progression of left ventricular dysfunction in patients with heart failure. *Circulation.* 1992;86: 431–438.
62. Bristow MR. Mechanistic and clinical rationales for using beta-blockers in heart failure. *J Card Fail.* 2000;6(Suppl 1):8–14.
63. Levy WC, Cerqueira MD, Matsuoka DT, Harp GD, Sheehan FH, Stratton JR. Four radionuclide methods for left ventricular volume determination: comparison of a manual and an automated technique. *J Nucl Med.* 1992;33:763–770.
64. Feenstra J, Grobbee DE, Remme WJ, Stricker BH. Drug-induced heart failure. *J Am Coll Cardiol.* 1999;33(5):1152–1162.
65. Rhoden W, Hasleton P, Brooks N. Anthracyclines and the heart. *Br Heart J.* 1993;70:499–502.
66. Ferraresi V, Milella M, Vaccaro A, et al. Toxicity and activity of docetaxel in anthracycline-pretreated breast cancer patients: a phase II study. *Am J Clin Oncol.* 2000;23(2):132–139.
67. Wakasugi S, Fischman AJ, Babich JW, et al. Myocardial substrate utilization and left ventricular function of doxorubicin cardiomyopathy. *J Nucl Med.* 1993;34:1529–1535.
68. Ganz WI, Sridhar KS, Ganz SS, Gonzalez R, Chakko S, Serafini A. Review of tests for monitoring doxorubicin-induced cardiomyopathy. *Oncology.* 1996;53(6):461–470.
69. Schwartz RG, McKenzie WB, Alexander J, et al. Congestive heart failure and left ventricular dysfunction complicating doxorubicin therapy. Seven-year experience using serial radionuclide angiography. *Am J Med.* 1987;82:1109–1118.
70. Cohn JN, Johnson GR, Shabetai R, et al. Ejection fraction, peak exercise oxygen consumption, cardiothoracic ration, ventricular arrhythmias, and plasma norepinephrine as determinants of prognosis in heart failure. The V-HeFT VA Cooperative Studies Group. *Circulation.* 1993; 87:V15–16.
71. Lipshultz SE, Colan SD, Gelber RD, et al. Late cardiac effects of doxorubicin therapy for acute lymphoblastic leukemia in childhood. *N Engl J Med.* 1991;324:808–811.
72. Greene HL, Reich SD, Dalen JE. How to minimize doxorubicin toxicity. *J Cardiovasc Med.* 1982;7:306–310.
73. Mallis GI. Implications of right ventricular dysfunction. *Cardiology Rev.* 2002;19(2):8.
74. Polak JF, Holman BL, Wynne J, Colucci WSL. Right ventricular ejection fraction: An indicator of increased mortality in patients with congestive heart failure associated with coronary artery disease. *J Am Coll Cardiol.* 1983;2:217–224.
75. Di Salvo TG, Mathier M, Semigran MJ, Dec GW. Preserved right ventricular ejection fraction predicts exercise capacity and survival in advanced heart failure. *J Am Coll Cardiol.* 1995;25:1143–1153.
76. Gavazzi A, Berzuini C, Campana C, et al. Value of right ventricular ejection fraction in predicting short-term prognosis of patients with severe chronic heart failure. *J Heart Lung Transplant.* 1997;16:774–785.
77. De Groote P, Millaire A, Foucher-Hossein C, et al. Right ventricular ejection fraction is an independent predictor of survival in patients with moderate heart failure. *J Am Coll Cardiol.* 1998;32:948–954.
78. Karatasakis GT, Karagounis LA, Kalyvas PA, et al. Prognostic significance of echocardiographi-

cally estimated right ventricular shortening in advanced heart failure. *Am J Cardiol.* 1998; 82:329–334.

79. Ghio S, Recusani F, Klersy C, et al. Prognostic usefulness of the tricuspid annular plane systolic excursion in patients with congestive heart failure secondary to idiopathic or ischemic dilated cardiomyopathy. *Am J Cardiol.* 2000; 85:837–842.
80. Forni G, Pozzoli M, Cannizzaro G, et al. Assessment of right ventricular function in patients with congestive heart failure by echocardiographic automated boundary detection. *Am J Cardiol.* 1996;78:1317–1321.
81. Ghio S, Gavazzi A, Campana C, et al. Independent and additive prognostic value of right ventricular systolic function and pulmonary artery pressure in patients with chronic heart failure. *J Am Coll Cardiol.* 2001;37(1):183–188.
82. Ghio S. Prognostic value of right ventricular function in chronic HF. *Cardiology Rev.* 2002; 19(2):9–15.
83. Di Salvo TG, Mathier M, Semigran MJ, Dec GW. Preserved right ventricular ejection fraction predicts exercise capacity and survival in advanced heart failure. *J Am Coll Cardiol.* 1995;25:1143–1153.
84. Gilbert EM, Anderson JL, Deitchman D, et al. Long-term beta-blocker vasodilator therapy improves cardiac function in idiopathic dilated cardiomyopathy: A double-blind, randomized study of bucindolol versus placebo. *Am Med.* 1990;88:223–229.
85. Rubin LJ. Current Concepts: Primary pulmonary hypertension. *N Engl J Med.* 1997;336(2): 111–117.
86. Lee SD, Shroyer KR, Markham NE, Cool CD, Voelkel NF, Tuder RM. Monoclonal endothelial cell proliferation is present in primary but not secondary pulmonary hypertension. *J Clin Invest.* 1998;101:927–934.
87. Wax D, Garofano R, Barst RJ. Effects of long-term infusion of prostacyclin on exercise performance in patients with primary pulmonary hypertension. *Chest.* 2000;116(4):914–920.
88. Barst RJ, Loyd JE. Genetics and immunogenetic aspects of primary pulmonary hypertension. *Chest.* 1998;114(3):231S–236S.
89. Deng Z, Morse JH, Slager SL, et al. Familial primary pulmonary hypertension (gene PPH1) is caused by mutations in the bone morphogenic protein receptor-II gene. *Am J Genet.* 2000; 67:737–744.
90. Abenhaim L, Moride Y, Brenot F, et al. Appetite-suppressant drugs and the risk of primary pulmonary hypertension: International primary pulmonary hypertension study group. *N Engl J Med.* 1996;335:609–616.
91. Fishman AP, Fishman MC, Freeman BA, et al. Mechanisms of proliferative and obliterative vascular diseases. Insights from the pulmonary and systemic circulations. NHLBI Workshop summary. *Am J Respir Crit Care Med.* 1998; 158:670–674.
92. Kramer MR, Valantine HA, Marshall SE, Starnes VA, Theodore J. Recovery of the right ventricle after single-lung transplantation in pulmonary hypertension. *Am J Cardiol.* 1994;73: 494–500.
93. Ritchie M, Waggoner AD, Davila-Roman VG, Barzilai B, Trulock EP, Eisenberg PR. Echocardiographic characterization of the improvement in right ventricular function in patients with severe pulmonary hypertension after single-lung transplantation. *J Am Coll Cardiol.* 1993;22: 1170–1174.
94. Schulman LL, Leibowitz DW, Anandarangam T, et al. Variability of right ventricular functional recovery after lung transplantation. *Transplantation.* 1996;62:622–625.
95. Moulton MJ, Creswell LL, Ungacta FF, Downing SW, Szabo BA, Pasque MK. Magnetic resonance imaging provides evidence for remodeling of the right ventricle after single-lung transplantation for pulmonary hypertension. *Circulation.* 1996; 94:II312–319.

8
Evaluation of Myocardial Viability

Dominique Delbeke, Jeroen J. Bax, William H. Martin, and Martin P. Sandler

Heart failure is becoming a challenging problem in clinical cardiology in terms of the number of affected patients. Approximately 5 million Americans have chronic heart failure (CHF), and 400,000 new cases are diagnosed each year.[1,2] Based on pooled analysis of the 13 multicentered CHF trials published over the past 10 years in the *New England Journal of Medicine*, coronary artery disease (CAD) was the underlying etiology in almost 70% of the 20,000 patients involved in those trials.[1,2] The prognosis of patients with ischemic cardiomyopathy remains poor, despite recent progress in medical therapy. Approximately 35% of the patients have a significant improvement in left ventricular (LV) function post-revascularization with an increase in LV ejection fraction (LVEF) of 5% points or more.[3] Because revascularization procedures are associated with a substantially higher risk in this category of patients,[4] a careful evaluation is mandatory for optimal patient management and risk stratification.

To explain the postoperative improvement in LV function and prognosis, the concept of viability has been proposed. Myocardium that is chronically dysfunctional at rest can still be viable, and patients with viable myocardium have been demonstrated to improve in LV function, heart failure symptoms, and prognosis following revascularization.[5–9] Conversely, patients without viable myocardium do not benefit from revascularization. In addition, preoperative viability testing results in improved perioperative risk stratification,[10] and the presence of viable myocardium in patients with ischemic cardiomyopathy who are treated medically is associated with an extremely high event rate.[11,12]

Hibernating Myocardium

Chronically ischemic myocardium, in which the blood supply is adequate to preserve viability but not to maintain normal cell function, can result in regional dyssynergy (hibernating myocardium).[5,13] Some studies have demonstrated a reduction in resting blood flow in chronic dysfunctional myocardium with improved function post-revascularization, while others indicated that flow reserve (and not resting flow) was impaired and, accordingly, the term *repetitive stunning* was proposed to describe these findings.[14] Revascularization procedures and restoration of normal blood flow to this tissue leads to significant improvement in wall motion and ventricular function in the large majority of patients.

The exact incidence of viable myocardium in patients with chronic ischemic LV dysfunction is not entirely clear. A few studies, however, have focused on this issue (Table 8-1).[15–18] Auerbach and colleagues[16] have evaluated 283 patients with ischemic cardiomyopathy (LVEF 26 ± 8%) with ^{18}F-fluorodeoxyglucose (FDG) positron emission tomography (PET); 156 (55%) patients exhibited some degree of viable tissue. The 3 other studies identified viability in 37% to 57% of the patients studied. Beanlands and colleagues[19] evaluated 67 patients with FDG PET

TABLE 8-1. Prevalence of Viability in Patients with Ischemic Cardiomyopathy

Author	# Pts	LVEF	Viab Technique	Viab Present
Schinkel[15]	83	25 ± 7%	DSE	47 (57%)
Auerbach[16]	283	26 ± 8%	FDG PET	156 (55%)
Fox[17]	27	NA	MPI	10 (37%)
Al-Mohammed[18]	27	19 ± 6%	FDG PET	14 (52%)

DSE: dobutamine stress echocardiography; FDG: ^{18}F-fluorodeoxyglucose; LVEF: left ventricular ejection fraction; MPI: myocardial perfusion imaging; NA: not available; PET: positron emission tomography.
Reproduced with permission from Bax JJ, Delbeke D, Vitola JV, et al. Heart and Lung Transplantation. In Sandler MP, Coleman RD, Wackers JTH, et al. (eds): Diagnostic Nuclear Medicine, 4th ed. Williams & Wilkins, Baltimore, MD, 2002.

in whom therapy was already established. Thus, 11 patients were scheduled for heart transplantation, 38 for revascularization, and 18 for medical treatment. Based on FDG PET findings, therapy was changed in 31 (46%) patients.

Dysfunctional but viable myocardium exhibits different characteristics that form the basis for the different imaging modalities that are currently available for the assessment of myocardial viability (Table 8-2). First, information on contractile function is needed, since assessment of viability is predominantly important in regions with dyskinesia, akinesia, or severe hypokinesia. This information is currently provided noninvasively by echocardiography, radionuclide ventriculography, gated perfusion single photon emission tomography (SPECT), magnetic resonance imaging (MRI), or invasively by contrast ventriculography.

TABLE 8-2. Features Versus Viability Techniques

Feature	Technique
Glucose metabolism	FDG PET/SPECT
Intact cell membrane	^{201}Tl/^{99m}Tc-MIBI and tetrofosmin
Functional mitochondria	^{99m}Tc-tracers
Intact perfusion	^{201}Tl/^{99m}Tc-tracers
Contractile reserve	Dobutamine echo/MRI

MRI: magnetic resonance imaging; PET: positron emission tomography; SPECT: single photon emission computed tomography; FDG: ^{18}F-fluorodeoxyglucose.
Reproduced with permission from Bax JJ, Delbeke D, Vitola JV, et al. Heart and Lung Transplantation. In Sandler MP, Coleman RD, Wackers JTH, et al. (eds): "Diagnostic Nuclear Medicine," 4th ed. Williams & Wilkins, Baltimore, MD, 2002.

Next, information on perfusion is required. With PET imaging a variety of tracers have been used to assess perfusion, including ^{82}Rb, ^{13}N-ammonia, ^{11}C-acetate, and ^{15}O-water. However, these PET perfusion tracers are not widely available because of their short half-lives and/or their cost. Therefore, SPECT tracers are typically used to assess perfusion, i.e., ^{201}Tl and ^{99m}Tc-labeled agents.

Third, cardiac viability is evaluated. The characteristics of cellular viability include cell membrane integrity, intact mitochondria, preserved glucose metabolism, intact resting perfusion, and contractile reserve.[20] Glucose metabolism can be evaluated with ^{18}F-fluorodeoxyglucose (^{18}FDG), fatty acid metabolism with ^{11}C-palmitate, and ^{123}I-beta-methyliodophenyl pentadecanoic acid (BMIPP), and oxidative metabolism with ^{11}C-acetate. Because of its long half-life of 110 minutes, ^{18}FDG is the most practical radiopharmaceutical for clinical studies and ^{18}FDG PET has become the *gold standard* to evaluate myocardial viability. However, a variety of alternative procedures are available for assessing myocardial viability using ^{201}Tl and ^{99m}Tc-labeled agents,[21] as well as dobutamine echocardiography and contrast-enhanced MRI.

Scintigraphy for Evaluation of Viability

^{201}Thallium Imaging

^{201}Tl imaging can be used to assess perfusion/cell membrane integrity.[22] Initial uptake of ^{201}Tl following tracer injection is dependent on regional perfusion, whereas prolonged tracer uptake is dependent on cell membrane integrity and thus myocardial viability. Two main protocols are currently being used for assessment of viability with ^{201}Tl and have been described in Case 3.1: stress-redistribution-reinjection and rest-redistribution. When the clinical question concerns viability only, rest-redistribution provides adequate information.

Stress-Redistribution-Reinjection and Late Redistribution Protocols

Many segments with severe ischemia or hibernating myocardium do not demonstrate reversibility on 4 hours redistribution images following stress.[23] It is well accepted that stress-redistribution ^{201}Tl images underestimate significantly the presence of ischemic but viable myocardium. Late redistribution at 24 hours after stress demonstrates ^{201}Tl redistribution in over 50% of defects that appear to be fixed 3 to 4 hours after stress.[24,25] The positive predictive value of late redistribution is greater than 90% for improvement after revascularization.[24]

Reinjection of ^{201}Tl after the standard 3 to 4 hours redistribution also facilitates uptake of ^{201}Tl in viable regions with fixed defects on stress-redistribution images. The stress-redistribution-reinjection protocol provides information on viability and stress-inducible ischemia combined. Dilsizian et al.[26] determined whether stress-redistribution-reinjection and stress-redistribution imaging provided the same information regarding viability in 100 patients with chronic stable CAD. There was redistribution of ^{201}Tl after reinjection in 49% of fixed defects on stress-redistribution images. For the 20 patients who were studied 3 to 6 months later after angioplasty, 87% of the regions with fixed defects on the redistribution images and identified as viable on the reinjection images improved regional wall motion after angioplasty.[26] All regions with persistent defects on reinjection images before angioplasty had persistent abnormal wall motion after angioplasty. Another study by the same group of investigators compared stress-redistribution ^{201}Tl with reinjection ^{201}Tl and FDG PET in 16 patients.[27] FDG uptake demonstrated viability in 73% of fixed defects on stress-redistribution images. A similar percentage of fixed defects demonstrates viability with reinjection ^{201}Tl images. The severity of the defect is a predictor of viability as well. When irreversible defects were further analyzed according to the severity of the defects in the discordant regions, FDG demonstrated viability in over 80% of the segments with only mild to moderate reduction of ^{201}Tl uptake (50% to 85% normal uptake), whereas FDG uptake was present in only 51% of segments with severe reduction in ^{201}Tl activity. Kitsiou and colleagues[28] have shown that segments with tracer activity ≥50% on the reinjection images are likely to improve in function when superimposed ischemia is present. Thus, the combination of viability and stress-inducible ischemia may allow more accurate prediction of recovery of function post-revascularization.

Another important parameter in the evaluation of myocardial viability is the degree of severity of LV dysfunction. Although ^{201}Tl SPECT using the reinjection protocol yields information regarding regional myocardial viability that is relatively comparable with that provided by FDG PET in patients with severe as well as moderate LV dysfunction, there is discordance in >20% of regions manifesting severe fixed ^{201}Tl defects in patients with severely reduced LV function (LVEF <20%).[29]

Dilsizian et al.[30] have also demonstrated the limited value of 24-hour ^{201}Tl imaging after ^{201}Tl reinjection. In their 50 patients with stable CAD, there were 127 abnormal myocardial regions on the stress images, 55 of which had persistent defects on redistribution images. Forty-five percent of these fixed defects on stress-redistribution images demonstrated improved ^{201}Tl uptake after reinjection. 24-hours ^{201}Tl images after reinjection showed improvement in only 4 of 35 fixed regions involving 6% (3 of 50) of patients.

Rest-Redistribution Protocol

Four patterns in regions with contractile dysfunction can be observed with rest-redistribution ^{201}Tl SPECT: (1) no defect in the dysfunctional region (indicating stunning); (2) initial defect with redistribution (representing hibernating myocardium); (3) initial defect without redistribution with tracer activity on the late images ≥50% (subendocardial necrosis); and (4) initial defect without redistribution with activity on the late images <50% (transmural scar).

Bax et al.[31] have compared the accuracy of rest-4 hour redistribution ^{201}Tl and FDG SPECT in 24 patients to delineate viable myocardium and predict functional recovery after revascularization. FDG SPECT had a sensitivity of 89% and a specificity of 81%, whereas rest-4-hour redistribution ^{201}Tl SPECT had a sensitivity of 67% and a specificity of 77%. However, the difference was not statistically significant.

The available studies with ^{201}Tl rest-redistribution imaging in patients undergoing revascularization have shown an excellent sensitivity to predict improvement of function post-revascularization; however, the specificity has been relatively poor. ^{201}Tl redistribution is a continuum, so the lower specificity is related to the viability criteria that are used.[32] Previous studies have shown that segments with no initial defect (stunned myocardium) or an initial defect with redistribution (hibernation) have a high likelihood of recovery of function. Segments with a fixed defect and activity <50% (transmural scar) will virtually never recover in function. The problem regarding specificity is related to segments with a fixed defect with tracer activity ≥50% (subendocardial scar); these do not frequently improve in function following revascularization and may (at least in part) explain the lower specificity. However, revascularization of these segments may prevent remodeling and be important for long-term prognosis.

The value of 24-hour ^{201}Tl images after resting ^{201}Tl injection-4 hour redistribution has been reported in 30 patients with fixed defects on rest-4 hour redistribution images.[33] Twenty-four-hour redistribution images demonstrated additional redistribution in 30% of the patients. Similar findings were reported by Matsunari et al.,[34] but when a threshold of 60% peak activity was used as an index of myocardial viability, only 3% of the initial ^{201}Tl defects were additionally considered viable by the 24-hour delayed images. In the 14 patients who underwent revascularization, the positive and negative predictive values of the early redistribution images for functional recovery were similar to those obtained by the late images.

^{99m}Tc-Labeled Agents

^{99m}Tc-labeled agents can be used to evaluate perfusion and viability.[35] Most experience has been reported with ^{99m}Tc-MIBI, whereas recent studies have also used ^{99m}Tc-tetrofosmin.[36,37] The uptake and retention of these tracers is dependent on perfusion, cell membrane integrity, and mitochondrial function (membrane potential).

Over the past 15 years, the role of ^{99m}Tc-labeled agents for the assessment of viability has been debated because ^{99m}Tc-MIBI and tetrofosmin do not redistribute significantly over time as ^{201}Tl does. Several studies demonstrated that ^{99m}Tc-MIBI underestimated the presence of viable myocardium as compared with FDG PET, in particular in the inferior wall.[38–41] Several options have been proposed in the literature to improve the detection of viability using ^{99m}Tc-labeled agents. This includes attenuation correction, quantitative evaluation using a different threshold of uptake in the anterior and inferior wall,[42] combining the information of tracer uptake with the functional (wall motion) information when the gated SPECT technique is used,[43] and administration of nitrate before injection of the perfusion radiopharmaceutical.

Nitrate-Enhanced SPECT

Excellent results have been obtained with nitrate-enhanced MIBI SPECT imaging for the detection of viable myocardium.[9,44–47] Nitrates enhance blood flow (and tracer uptake) to myocardial regions that are perfused by severely stenosed arteries. For research purposes, comparison of a resting image and a nitrate-enhanced image have been compared, but for clinical purposes, the best prognostic results may be obtained by comparing post-stress images with nitrate-enhanced resting images. Nitrate can be given sublingually or intravenously (IV). For the IV administration, typically 10 mg of isosorbide dinitrate diluted in 100 ml of isotonic saline solution is infused over 20 minutes to the patient lying supine during electrocardiographic (ECG) and blood pressure (BP) monitoring. The perfusion radiopharmaceutical is administered as soon as the BP drops more than 20 mmHg or 15 minutes after the start of the infusion. Since IV isosorbide is not commercially available in the United States, ^{99m}Tc-MIBI or tetrofosmin can be administered 5 to 10 minutes after sublingual administration of 0.4 to 0.8 mg of nitroglycerin.

The percentage of myocardial segments demonstrating improved uptake on nitrate-enhanced ^{99m}Tc-MIBI images compared with baseline resting ^{99m}Tc-MIBI is in the same range as for the ^{201}Tl rest-redistribution protocol[46] and the ^{201}Tl reinjection images compared with 4-hour redistribution ^{201}Tl images.[48] The optimal criteria for interpretation are further described in Case 8.9.[47]

Nitrate enhancement has been used with resting ^{201}Tl SPECT as well[49] and compared with the rest-4 hour redistribution ^{201}Tl protocol. All the regions identified as viable by the rest-redistribution protocol were identified as viable by the rest-nitrate protocol. Both protocols correctly predicted improvement of regional wall motion after revascularization with a comparable sensitivity (95% and 92%).

Gated SPECT

Evaluation of contractile reserve is also possible using gated SPECT ^{99m}Tc-MIBI imaging.[50] The ^{99m}Tc-MIBI images are acquired 1 hour after infusion of the maximum tolerated dose of dobutamine and again during infusion of dobutamine at a low dose. More recently, the administration of nitrate has been combined with low-dose dobutamine gated SPECT to assess both perfusion and contractile reserve for predicting recovery of regional ventricular function after revascularization.[51,52] For this protocol, dobutamine infusion is started at 5 μcg·kg·min^{-1} for 5 minutes and then increased to 10 μcg·kg·min^{-1} with the patient under ECG and BP monitoring. Gated SPECT imaging is started after 3 minutes of the 10 mcg·kg·min^{-1} dosage, which is maintained until the acquisition is completed. The combined use of low-dose dobutamine nitrate-enhanced ^{99m}Tc-MIBI gated SPECT had a higher predictive accuracy for predicting regional wall motion improvement than low-dose dobutamine echocardiography.[52]

FDG Imaging

Since the 1990s, FDG imaging has been used to assess glucose metabolism.[53] Under normal resting conditions, cardiac metabolism is mainly oxidative with free fatty acids (FFA) and glucose being the major sources of energy. In the presence of ischemia, however, oxidative metabolism of FFAs is decreased and glucose becomes the preferred substrate for the myocardium. Depending on the degree of residual oxygen availability, glucose may predominantly be metabolized anaerobically. The amount of energy produced by anaerobic glycolysis may not be adequate to maintain contractility but sufficient to preserve the cellular integrity. This is one explanation of the situation in dysfunctional but viable myocardium: contraction is severely reduced or absent while glucose utilization and viability are maintained. FDG, an analog of glucose, enters the cells by the same transport mechanism as glucose and is intracellularly phosphorylated by a hexokinase to FDG-6-phosphate (FDG-6-P). Unlike glucose-6-P, FDG-6-P does not enter into further enzymatic pathways and remains trapped in the myocyte proportionally to the glycolytic rate, providing a good tracer for myocardial metabolic imaging.

Patient Preparation

The myocardium can use several substrates for its metabolism, depending on various factors including hormonal status and availability of substrates. Therefore, FDG uptake in the myocardium is highly dependent on the dietary conditions (i.e., plasma levels of FFA, glucose, and insulin). High insulin levels with the resultant suppression of FFA promote FDG myocardial uptake, whereas high FFA levels inhibit FDG uptake.

In the fasting state, the myocardium uses predominantly fatty acids for its metabolism and the myocardial distribution of FDG is often heterogenous. Only 50% of PET myocardial images obtained in fasting patients are interpretable.[54] Therefore, for evaluation of myocardial viability using FDG, the levels of circulating substrates/hormones need to favor utilization of glucose by the myocardium. This is accomplished by loading the patient with glucose.

Several protocols are available to promote cardiac FDG uptake, including (1) oral glucose loading, (2) hyperinsulinemic euglycemic clamping, and (3) the administration of nicotinic acid derivatives. Oral glucose loading is the most frequently used approach, although it results in uninterpretable images in as many as 10% of patients in some studies.[55]

The reference method is the euglycemic hyperinsulinic clamp, a labor-intensive and time-consuming procedure, allowing regulation of metabolic substrates and insulin levels and providing excellent image quality in most patients.[56] Martin et al.[55] have adapted the clamping protocol and described a rather elegant and simpler protocol: a fixed glucose-insulin-potassium (GIK) solution was infused over 30 minutes, followed by FDG injection, which resulted in excellent image quality with 99% of the images being interpretable.

Finally, Knuuti et al.[57] demonstrated that oral administration of a nicotinic acid derivative (acipimox) may be an alternative to clamping. Acipimox inhibits peripheral lipolysis, thus reducing plasma FFA levels, and thus indirectly stimulating cardiac FDG uptake.[58,59] Bax et al.[60] and Kam et al.[61] demonstrated the success of FDG imaging using acipimox in nondiabetic patients. Bax et al.[60] reported the quality of FDG images using different patient preparations; all patients underwent three cardiac FDG studies following oral glucose loading, acipimox administration, or during hyperinsulinemic euglycemic clamping. The image quality was expressed as a myocardium-to-background ratio, being 2.2 ± 0.3 with oral glucose loading ($P < 0.05$ versus acipimox and clamping), 2.9 ± 0.7 with acipimox administration, and 2.8 ± 0.8 with clamping. Visually, the FDG images were superior with clamping and after acipimox administration as compared with oral glucose loading. Kam et al.[61] confirmed good quality of FDG image after acipimox in 50 nondiabetic patients using a dual isotope technique with FDG and ^{99m}Tc-tetrofosmin.

Since acipimox is unavailable in the United States, a 30-minute infusion of a fixed glucose-insulin solution is the most practical yet effective technique for stimulating myocardial FDG uptake in nondiabetic patients.

As diabetes is a disease affecting glucose metabolism, achieving homogenous myocardial glucose metabolism after loading diabetic patients with glucose is a well-known problem. Diabetic patients have been excluded from all the large FDG PET studies. Unfortunately, CAD is a frequent complication of diabetes and sometimes patients are evaluated for CAD before a diagnosis of diabetes has been established. Methods for loading nondiabetic patients with glucose have been modified to optimize myocardial glucose utilization in diabetic patients with variable success.[62–65] The subject of glucose loading is further discussed in Case 8.6.

Protocols for FDG Imaging: FDG PET Versus FDG SPECT

FDG PET

Since FDG is a positron emitter, the optimal systems to image FDG imaging are dedicated positron tomographs operating in the coincidence mode. Over the past 15 years, numerous studies have used FDG PET to evaluate tissue viability in patients with chronic CAD and depressed LV function. The initial work in patients was performed by the UCLA group and demonstrated the existence of matches and mismatches.[66] Subsequently, Brunken et al.[67,68]

demonstrated that 40% of the regions with Q waves on the ECG and severe wall motion abnormalities showed FDG uptake, indicative of residual viability, and that FDG PET was capable of detecting residual viability in over 50% of fixed defects identified by ^{201}Tl stress-redistribution imaging.

FDG SPECT

Driven by the increased demand for FDG PET studies to assess viability, considerable effort has been invested in the development and optimization of ultra-high-energy 511 keV collimators to allow FDG imaging without a PET system.[69–74] The five direct comparisons between FDG PET and FDG SPECT with a total of 113 patients demonstrated excellent agreement for assessment of viability (ranging from 76% to 100%) (Table 8-3).[75–79] The NIH-group studied 28 patients with chronic CAD and a mean LVEF of 33 ± 15%.[79] These patients underwent both FDG PET and FDG SPECT following oral glucose loading. Regional LV function was evaluated by RVG or gated SPECT imaging. When a 50% FDG uptake threshold was used to distinguish between viable and nonviable tissue, both techniques provided comparable information in 920 of 977 segments, yielding an agreement of 94%. When the analysis was restricted to 41 akinetic segments, FDG PET and SPECT yielded concordant information in 80% of segments. The other comparative studies also demonstrated a good agreement between both modalities. However, a comparative study between FDG PET and SPECT in patients undergoing revascularization (with recovery of function post-revascularization as an independent measurement for viability) is still lacking.

FDG Coincidence

More recently, conventional dual-head gamma cameras capable of coincidence imaging have been developed; this approach enhances resolution of the system, but necessitates the use of attenuation correction. Three direct comparisons between FDG PET and gamma camera coincidence imaging have shown suboptimal agreement (Table 8-3)[80–82]; this agreement was even less when attenuation correction was not applied for coincidence imaging. Moreover, the segments with disagreement were located predominantly in the septum and inferior wall, suggesting the influence of attenuation. These studies indicate that accurate attenuation correction is more important with coincidence imaging than SPECT. Further studies, in

TABLE 8-3. Direct Comparative Studies Between FDG PET and FDG SPECT/Gamma Camera Coincidence Imaging

Author	# Pts	LVEF (%)	Pts with MVD (%)	Pts with Previous MI (%)	Agreement (%)
PET vs SPECT					
Burt[75]	20	NA	NA	NA	93
Martin[76]	9	NA	NA	NA	100
Bax[77]	20	39 ± 16	83	100	76
Chen[78]	36	NA	NA	NA	90
Srinivasan[79]	28	33 ± 15	93	64	94
PET vs gamma camera coincidence imaging					
Hasegawa[80]	20	NA	80	100	48
De Sutter[81]	19	44 ± 13	63	100	70
Nowak[82]	21	41 ± 13	80	57	74

LVEF: left ventricular ejection fraction; MI: myocardial infarction; MVD: multivessel disease; NA: not available; pts: patients.

Reproduced with permission from Bax JJ, Delbeke D, Vitola JV, et al. Heart and Lung Transplantation. In Sandler MP, Coleman RD, Wackers JTH, et al. (eds): "Diagnostic Nuclear Medicine," 4th ed. Williams & Wilkins, Baltimore, MD, 2002.

particular with functional follow-up after revascularization, are needed.

Imaging Protocols

The perfusion and FDG data can be acquired sequentially or simultaneously. With PET and gamma camera-based dual-head coincidence imaging, only sequential acquisition is possible. With SPECT imaging both sequential and simultaneous acquisitions are possible.

The initial FDG SPECT studies used ^{201}Tl as a perfusion tracer and were thus acquired sequentially. This approach has been validated extensively over time and has been proven comparable with FDG PET in terms of prediction of improvement of function post-revascularization.[53] The more recent SPECT studies have used a dual-isotope simultaneous acquisition (DISA) protocol that has similar accuracy in predicting functional outcome post-revascularization as FDG PET imaging. Important advantages of the DISA protocol are the reduction in acquisition time and the perfect alignment between the perfusion and FDG data. Moreover, with gated SPECT imaging (performed mainly with ^{99m}Tc-labeled agents), the information on regional contractile function (to identify the dysfunctional regions) can also be provided by SPECT, thus avoiding misalignment between 2-D echocardiography or RVG and SPECT. The interpretation of FDG imaging in isolation, without comparison to a concurrent perfusion study, appears attractive, but the accuracy for predicting functional outcome after revascularization is suboptimal, mainly due to overestimation of functional recovery.[83] In these studies, cutoff criteria for FDG uptake are used to classify dysfunctional segments as viable or nonviable.

Viability Criteria for FDG Imaging

For the data analysis, different approaches have been reported, including absolute quantification requiring dynamic imaging, semiquantitative analysis using static imaging, and visual analysis comparing perfusion and metabolism.

Perfusion-FDG Match and Mismatch

For optimal prediction of functional recovery, integration of perfusion and FDG uptake is needed. Several patterns of myocardial perfusion and FDG uptake can be seen in dysfunctional myocardium (Table 8-4). (1) Based on the concept of *hibernation*, segments with reduced perfusion but preserved FDG uptake (perfusion-FDG mismatch) are classified as viable. Indeed, many studies have indicated that these segments usually improve in function following adequate revascularization.[84–92] (2) In contrast, segments with reduced perfusion and concordantly reduced FDG uptake (perfusion-FDG match) are considered scar tissue and only rarely improve in function following revascularization. (3) Additional studies have demonstrated that dysfunctional segments with near-normal resting perfusion and preserved FDG uptake also frequently improve in function if served by a significantly stenosed vessel. These segments may represent areas of repetitive stunning.[93] The pattern of decreased blood flow with maintained metabolism identifies myocardial segments that have the potential to improve after revascularization. The approach of the combined perfusion-FDG mismatch has been extensively documented as a good predictor of regional wall motion improvement post-revascularization, as well as improvement of heart failure symptoms, exercise capacity, and prognosis (see Outcome after Revascularization, later in this chapter).

TABLE 8-4. Myocardial Perfusion and FDG Uptake Patterns in Dysfunctional Myocardium

	Resting Perfusion	FDG Uptake
Repetitive stunning	Normal	Normal/increased
Hibernation	Reduced	Normal/increased
Transmural scar	Severely reduced	Severely reduced
Nontransmural scar	Mildy reduced	Mildly reduced

Reproduced with permission from Bax JJ, Delbeke D, Vitola JV, et al. Heart and Lung Transplantation. In Sandler MP, Coleman RD, Wackers JTH, et al. (eds): "Diagnostic Nuclear Medicine," 4th ed. Williams & Wilkins, Baltimore, MD, 2002.

Normalized FDG Uptake

Cut-off values of normalized FDG uptake are applied when FDG is used without a perfusion tracer. Most frequently a cutoff value of ≥50% of maximum is used to identify viable myocardium.[94] This approach, however, may not be accurate in the prediction of functional recovery, since segments with severely reduced perfusion may still have increased FDG uptake although less than 50% of normal or maximum. Also, segments with a mild reduction in perfusion and concordantly reduced FDG uptake (but still ≥50% of normal or maximum) are likely to represent areas of subendocardial necrosis and will not improve in function following revascularization; these segments have been referred to as *mild match* in some studies. Indeed, the superiority of combined assessment of perfusion and FDG uptake over the use of FDG alone for prediction of functional outcome has been demonstrated.[95] Finally, if normalized FDG uptake is used, the optimal cut-off value has not been defined adequately. Some studies[94] have used a 50% cut-off value, whereas other studies using ROC-curve analysis showed that the optimal cut-off value for prediction of functional recovery was much higher (85% to 90% of maximum uptake).[96]

Absolute Glucose Utilization

Another option is the use of absolute quantification of regional glucose utilization. Fath-Ordoubadi et al.[97] have used ROC-curve analysis and identified the cut-off value of regional glucose utilization ≥0.25 µmol/min/g as the optimal predictor of improvement of regional LV function post-revascularization. Applying this cut-off value in a subsequent study, a sensitivity of 99% but a specificity of only 33% for predicting improvement of LV function were obtained.[83] Similar to using normalized FDG uptake, the specificity is suboptimal, indicating that many segments defined as viable by quantitative FDG imaging do not improve in function after revascularization. Again, this is most likely caused by nontransmural scars that contain a certain amount of viable nonischemic myocardium, which cannot improve in function with revascularization.

Fatty Acid Analog Metabolic Imaging

During ischemia there is suppression of fatty acid metabolism, so tracers of fatty acid derivatives have the potential for early detection of ischemia, even at rest. ^{11}C-palmitate is a radiolabeled straight fatty acid that is taken up and then cleared by the myocardial cells, allowing evaluation of oxidative metabolism. However, it is labeled with the short-lived positron emitter ^{11}C (half-life = 20 min) and requires the complexity of dynamic PET imaging and compartmental modeling, available only in a research environment and cumbersome to perform clinically.

^{123}I-BMIPP is a radioiodinated branched fatty acid analog that is trapped in the myocardium with little washout, therefore reflecting fatty acid utilization in the myocardium.[98] Clinical applications of ^{123}I-BMIPP include detection of ischemia, as well as evaluation of myocardial infarction (MI) and cardiomyopathy.

^{123}I-BMIPP can identify ischemic myocardium as areas of reduced uptake at rest. A study of 111 patients presenting with acute chest pain compared imaging findings using ^{99m}Tc-tetrofosmin, ^{123}I-BMIPP, and coronary angiography performed within 24 hours of the episode of chest pain.[99] Fourteen percent of patients showed abnormal ^{123}I-BMIPP uptake with normal perfusion at rest, and these patients were the most likely to have severe coronary stenosis or vasospasm on angiography. This is probably related to prolonged impairment of fatty acid utilization that can persist after acute coronary insufficiency has resolved, the equivalent of *metabolic stunning*.

The prognostic significance of a normal ^{123}I-BMIPP study was better than that of rest/stress MPI in a group of 167 patients with angina pectoris but no prior MI.[100] The majority of dysfunctional segments with less ^{123}I-BMIPP uptake than ^{201}Tl (discordant uptake) are often associated with increased FDG uptake indicative of ischemic but viable myocardium likely to improve after revascularization.[101–103] Further studies are necessary to clarify the potential role of ^{123}I-BMIPP imaging compared with ^{201}Tl or FDG for identification of stunned or hibernating myocardium and risk stratification. Although available in Asia since the early 1990s, ^{123}I-BMIPP is still investigational in the United States. This topic is further discussed in Case 18.9.

Scintigraphic Imaging for the Evaluation of Viability: Conclusions

In summary, FDG PET currently represents the gold standard for assessment of myocardial viability. Patient preparation demands pre-injection glucose loading, which can be cumbersome. For accurate interpretation, FDG images must be correlated with perfusion images.

When FDG PET imaging is not available, alternative scintigraphic techniques using FDG-SPECT, ^{201}Tl SPECT (using the stress-reinjection, 24-hour-delayed or rest-redistribution protocols), and nitrate-enhanced ^{99m}Tc MIBI or tetrofosmin gated SPECT provide comparable results.

Evaluation of viability with ^{201}Tl or ^{99m}Tc-agents may be the first choice in diabetic patients and metabolic imaging with FDG appears to be the most sensitive modality for detection of viability in patients with severe LV dysfunction (LVEF <20%).

Dobutamine Stress Echocardiography

Dobutamine stress echocardiography can be used to assess myocardial contractility. Experimental studies have shown that infusions of low-dose dobutamine (5 to 10 mcg·kg·min^{-1}) can increase contractility in dysfunctional but viable myocardium, a phenomenon referred to as *contractile reserve*. Segments without viable myocardium do not exhibit this contractile reserve. Many studies in patients have demonstrated the value of dobutamine stress echocardiography to identify viable myocardium.[104] As discussed in the following section on Prediction of Recovery of Function Post-Revascularization, dobutamine stress echocardiography is highly specific but less sensitive than scintigraphic techniques.

More recently, the protocol has been modified into a low-dose/high-dose protocol. With this protocol, the infusion rate of dobutamine is stepwise, starting at 5 mcg·kg·min^{-1} (and using 5- to 10-mcg increments) until the maximum rate of 40 mcg·kg·min^{-1} is reached; supplemental atropine may be used to achieve target heart rate if necessary. This protocol allows assessment of viability at the lower infusion rate (5–10 mcg·kg·min^{-1}) with evaluation of ischemia at the higher doses. The safety of this protocol in patients with severely depressed LV function was demonstrated by Poldermans et al.[105] in 200 patients with depressed LVEF (<35%), hypotension or cardiac arrhythmias occuring in only 11% and 6% of patients, respectively.

Four patterns in regions with contractile dysfunction can be observed (Table 8-5): (1) bipha-

TABLE 8-5. Different Responses to Dobutamine in Chronic Dysfunctional Myocardium

	WM Response at Low Dose	WM Response at High Dose	Representing
1. Biphasic reponse	Improved	Worsening	Viability, superimposed ischemia
2. Direct worsening	Worsening	Worsening	Critical stenoses
3. Sustained improvement	Improved	Improved	Subendocardial scar with viable tissue
4. No change	No change	No change	(Transmural) scar

WM: wall motion.

Reproduced with permission from Bax JJ, Delbeke D, Vitola JV, et al. Heart and Lung Transplantation. In Sandler MP, Coleman RD, Wackers JTH, et al. (eds): "Diagnostic Nuclear Medicine," 4th ed. Williams & Wilkins, Baltimore, MD, 2002.

sic response (initial improvement followed by worsening of wall motion), (2) worsening (direct deterioration of wall motion without initial improvement), (3) sustained improvement (improvement of wall motion without subsequent deterioration), and (4) no change (no change in wall motion during the entire study). All patterns except pattern 4 (which represents scar tissue) indicate the presence of viable myocardium.

Magnetic Resonance Imaging

Magnetic resonance imaging (MRI) has also been used to detect viability (Table 8-6).[106] This modality is discussed in more depth in Chapter 14 and Case 18.12. The initial studies of myocardial viability used resting MRI focused on the end-diastolic wall thickness (EDWT), systolic wall thickening (SWT), and signal intensity without contrast enhancement. Early observations revealed severely reduced EDWT, reduced/absent SWT, and decreased signal intensity in patients with previous infarction. A comparison of MRI with FDG PET showed that segments without SWT and EDWT <5.5 mm were mainly nonviable on FDG PET imaging.[107] Moreover, segments with EDWT <5.5 mm virtually never showed recovery of function post-revascularization. However, segments with EDWT ≥5.5 mm did not always improve in function post-revascularization, indicating the need for additional testing in segments with EDWT ≥5.5 mm to accurately predict outcome post-revascularization. Subsequently, Baer and coworkers[107] demonstrated that the presence of contractile reserve during low-dose dobutamine MRI in segments with EDWT ≥5.5 mm allowed accurate prediction of outcome post-revascularization.

More recent technical improvements, namely the availability of ultrafast imaging sequences with a significant reduction of imaging time, have initiated several studies that examined the combination of pharmacological stress and MRI for the detection of suspected CAD. The most well-developed stress-MRI technique is wall motion imaging during dobutamine stress. This technique is analogous to stress echocardiography, but MRI has the inherent advantages of better resolution, higher reproducibility, and true long- and short-axis imaging with contiguous parallel slices.[108] However, the clinical impact of MRI for the diagnosis of CAD is still low.

The most recent studies concerning MRI have used contrast agents; Kim et al.[109] have demonstrated the use of gadolinium (Gd)-enhanced MRI for the detection of viability and subsequent prediction of improvement of function in 50 patients with chronic ischemic LV dysfunction. Using this approach, hyperenhanced regions represent scar tissue, and with the high resolution of MRI, it is possible to detect different stages of infarct transmurality. The results showed nicely that the higher the transmurality, as evidenced by hyperenhancement, the lower the likelihood of recovery of function post-revascularization. In contrast, segments without hyperenhancement had a high likelihood of recovery. A more recent study by Klein et al.[110] evaluated the performance of contrast-enhanced MRI compared with PET as the gold standard for detection and quantification of scar tissue in 31 patients. Scar

TABLE 8-6. Parameters Derived from Magnetic Resonance Imaging for the Assessment of Viability

Technique	Parameters	Clinical Relevance
Resting MRI	End-diastolic wall thickness	EDWT <5.5 mm represents scar
	Systolic wall thickening	Absence of SWT represents scar
	Signal intensity (without contrast)	Decreased SI represents scar
Dobutamine MRI	Contractile reserve	Presence of CR represents viability
Contrast MRI	Hyper-enhancement	Enhanced myocardium represents scar

CR: contractile reserve; EDWT: end-diastolic wall thickness; SI: signal intensity; SWT: systolic wall thickening.
Reproduced with permission from Bax JJ, Delbeke D, Vitola JV, et al. Heart and Lung Transplantation. In Sandler MP, Coleman RD, Wackers JTH, et al. (eds): "Diagnostic Nuclear Medicine," 4th ed. Williams & Wilkins, Baltimore, MD, 2002.

tissue on PET was defined by concordantly reduced perfusion and glucose metabolism. The sensitivity and specificity of MRI in identifying patients with matched flow/metabolism defects were 96% and 86%, respectively. When the segments were analyzed, sensitivity and specificity were 100% and 94%. The infarct mass measured on PET and MRI correlated well (r = 0.81). MRI hyperenhancement was a better predictor of scar than end-diastolic and end-systolic wall thickness or thickening. Ongoing investiga-tions will further define the applications of contrast-enhanced MRI.

Prediction of Recovery of Function Post-Revascularization

The presence of viable tissue has been related to a superior outcome post-revascularization.[53] If the extent of viable tissue is large, improvement of LVEF can be anticipated. There are also relations between the presence of viable tissue and improvement of heart failure symptoms and/or exercise capacity post-revascularization. Finally, various retrospective analyses have shown that patients with viable myocardium had an excellent long-term prognosis, whereas patients with viable tissue who did not undergo revascularization had a high event-rate over time.[8,11]

Different end-points have been used against which viability tests have been validated. The most frequently used end-point is prediction of improvement of regional function following revascularization. Recently, an updated meta-analysis was published on the prediction of functional recovery post-revascularization using any one of the aforementioned techniques.[104] Inclusion criteria for this meta-analysis included (1) prospective study, patients with chronic CAD undergoing revascularization; and (2) results should allow assessment of sensitivity/specificity to predict improvement of regional function. A total of 850 studies conducted from 1980 to 2001 were identified; 105 of these encompassing 3034 patients met the inclusion criteria (Table 8-7).[104] The incidence of recovery of regional function varied substantially between all studies (ranging from 16% to 91%), suggesting inclusion of different study populations. Still, when all studies were pooled, a sensitivity of 84% and a specificity of 69% were obtained.

An important discrepancy was noted between the sensitivity/specificity of dobutamine stress echocardiography and nuclear imaging. When the metaanalysis was restricted to 11 studies with 325 patients who underwent both low-dose dobutamine echocardiography and some form of rest nuclear imaging (thus both protocols only focusing on viability without ischemia), nuclear imaging appeared significantly more sensitive in the prediction of functional recovery, whereas dobutamine echocardiography was more specific. A relatively recent study by Bax et al.,[111] including 73 patients with an average LVEF of 32%, compared sequential testing with dobutamine echocardiography and resting-4 hour redistribution ^{201}Tl to predict recovery post-

TABLE 8-7. Pooled Data from Studies Focusing on Prediction of Recovery of Function Post-Revascularization

Technique	# Studies/Pts	Sens (%)	Spec (%)	NPV (%)	PPV (%)
FDG PET	20/598	93	58	86	71
^{201}Tl	33/858	87	55	81	64
^{99m}Tc tracers	20/488	81	66	77	71
Dobutamine echo/MRI 32/1090	81	80	85	77	
Pooled data	105/3034	84	69		

Data based on reference 104.

Reproduced with permission from Bax JJ, Delbeke D, Vitola JV, et al. Heart and Lung Transplantation. In Sandler MP, Coleman RD, Wackers JTH, et al. (eds): "Diagnostic Nuclear Medicine," 4th ed. Williams & Wilkins, Baltimore, MD, 2002.

revascularization. For patients with an intermediate likelihood of viability by dobutamine echocardiography, the addition of ^{201}Tl imaging improved the sensitivity of dobutamine echocardiography from 63% to 78% and the specifity remained unchanged (80%).

Improvement of Regional LV Function

Many studies have employed FDG PET to evaluate tissue viability and predict improvement of function after revascularization. The results of 12 FDG PET studies (with a total of 322 patients) were pooled to determine the value of FDG PET for the prediction of improvement of regional (not global) LV function following revascularization.[9] Pooling of the results yielded a sensitivity of 88% with a specificity of 73% and a negative predictive value of 86% with a positive predictive value of 76%.

Although it is interesting to pool these studies to provide an estimation of the diagnostic accuracy of FDG PET to predict improvement of function, these data should be interpreted with caution because of the lack of standardization of metabolic conditions, protocols, and viability criteria of FDG PET studies to assess myocardial viability.

Improvement of Global LV Function

From a clinical point of view, improvement of global LV function may be more relevant than improvement of regional LV function. The number of studies focusing on improvement of global function post-revascularization is significantly less than those focusing on improvement of regional LV function. A total of 29 studies with 758 patients focused on prediction of improvement of global LV function; these studies were uniform in showing a significant improvement of LVEF in patients with viable myocardium, whereas patients without viable myocardium did not show improvement of global LVEF.[104] The results are summarized in Table 8-8. Importantly, the criteria to classify a patient as viable differed substantially among the different studies. ROC-curve analysis was applied and demonstrated that 25% of the LV being dysfunctional but viable may be the optimal threshold to predict improvement of LVEF post-revascularization.[112]

Improvement of Symptoms

Another end-point used in viability studies, is prediction of improvement in heart failure symptoms and exercise capacity. Heart failure symptoms are difficult to assess; in the clinical setting, the New York Heart Association

TABLE 8-8. Pooled Data from Studies Focusing on Prediction of Improvement of Global LV Function Post-Revascularization

		Patients with Viability		Patient Without Viability	
Technique	# Studies/Pts	LVEF pre	LVEF post	LVEF pre	LVEF post
FDG PET	12/333	37%	47%	39%	40%
^{201}Tl	5/96	30%	38%	29%	31%
^{99m}Tc tracers	4/75	47%	53%	40%	39%
DSE	8/254	35%	43%	35%	36%
Mean	29/758	37%	45%	36%	36%

LVEF pre and post represent LVEF before and after revascularization respectively. DSE: dobutamine stress echocardiography; FDG: F18-fluorodeoxyglucose; LVEF: left ventricular ejection fraction; PET: positron emission tomography; pts: patients. Data based on reference 104.

Reproduced with permission from Bax JJ, Delbeke D, Vitola JV, Poldermans D, et al. Heart and Lung Transplantation. In Sandler MP, Coleman RD, Wackers JTH, et al. (eds): "Diagnostic Nuclear Medicine," 4th ed. Williams & Wilkins, Baltimore, MD, 2002.

TABLE 8-9. Prediction of Heart Failure Symptoms Post-Revascularization in Relation to Presence/Absence Viability

Author	Technique	# Pts	NYHA Pre	NYHA Post
Haas[10]	FDG PET	34	3.0	1.6
Schwarz[116]	FDG PET	32	1.4 ± 1.2	0.1 ± 0.3
Beanlands[115]	FDG PET	18	3.0 ± 0.8	1.6 ± 0.7
Dreyfus[113]	FDG PET	46	3.1 ± 0.3	2.0 ± 0
Bax[112]	FDG SPECT	47	3.4 ± 0.5	1.7 ± 0.8
Marwick[114]	DSE/FDG PET	63	2.6 ± 0.7	1.9 ± 0.7
Bax[3]	DSE	62	3.2 ± 0.7	1.6 ± 0.5
Gunning[117]	^{201}Tl RR	19	2.7 ± 0.6	1.3 ± 0.7

NYHA pre and post represent NYHA before and after revascularization, respectively. DSE: dobutamine stress echocardiography; FDG: F18-fluorodeoxyglucose; NYHA: New York Heart Association classification; PET: positron emission tomography; SPECT: single photon emission computed tomography; ^{201}Tl RR: ^{201}Tl rest-redistribution.

Reproduced with permission from Bax JJ, Delbeke D, Vitola JV, et al. Heart and Lung Transplantation. In Sandler MP, Coleman RD, Wackers JTH, et al. (eds): "Diagnostic Nuclear Medicine," 4th ed. Williams & Wilkins, Baltimore, MD, 2002.

(NYHA) classification is frequently used. Several studies have evaluated NYHA class before and after revascularization in patients evaluated for myocardial viability (Table 8-9).[3,10,112–117] These studies indicate that NYHA class improved significantly in patients with viable myocardium. One study of 36 patients undergoing CABG demonstrated that the magnitude of improvement in heart failure symptoms was directly related to the preoperative extend and magnitute of myocardial viability as assessed by FDG PET imaging.[118]

A more objective measure of functional improvement is exercise capacity. Marwick and colleagues[119] evaluated 23 patients with FDG PET imaging before revascularization and demonstrated that patients with extensive zone of mismatch improved significantly in exercise capacity post-revascularization (from 5.6 ± 2.7 METS to 7.5 ± 1.7 METS). Similar results were reported by DiCarli et al.[118] and Gunning et al.[117]

Viability and Long-Term Prognosis

It has been hypothesized that in patients with ischemic cardiomyopathy the presence of viable tissue protects the patients from perioperative events and that the postoperative improvement of LV function, symptomatology, and exercise capacity may translate into improvement of long-term survival.

The assessment of perioperative risk was addressed by Haas et al.[10] The authors analyzed 76 patients with chronic CAD and depressed LV function; 35 patients underwent surgical revascularization on the basis of clinical presentation and results of coronary angiography only. Another 41 patients underwent preoperative FDG PET, and patients were referred to surgical revascularization on the basis of the extent of viable tissue defined by FDG PET in addition to the clinical and angiographic data. Small areas of viable tissue and large areas of scar tissue were deciding factors against surgery. Accordingly, seven patients were treated medically or underwent heart transplantation and 34 were revascularized. In the patients who did not undergo FDG PET, a higher perioperative event rate was observed, accompanied by a higher short-term (30 days) and long-term (12 months) mortality. Moreover, the patients who did undergo FDG PET needed inotropic support less frequently and had a significantly higher rate of uncomplicated recovery.

Long-term prognosis and survival may be the most ideal end-point in the clinical setting. Several studies are now available that have related viability to long-term prognosis; it should be emphasized, however, that all of these studies were retrospective analyses. Several prognostic studies have been performed employing FDG PET, ^{201}Tl imaging, and dobutamine echocardiography.[3,117,120–135] The pooled data demonstrated a high mortality in all groups, except in the group of patients with viable myocardium who underwent revascularization. As stated before, the main shortcoming of these studies is their retrospective, nonrandomized character. A metaanalysis reviewing studies including 3,088 patients demonstrates a strong association between myocardial viability on noninvasive testing and improved survival in patients with chronic CAD and LV dysfunction who underwent revascularization.[11] Absence of viability was associated with no significant difference in outcomes irrespective of treatment strategy.

These results suggest that residual viability in patients with ischemic cardiomyopathy is an unstable substrate and prone to future events. Following this hypothesis, timely revascularization may be favored. There is mounting evidence that myocardial hibernation represents an adaptation to ischemia that cannot be maintained indefinitely. Biopsy specimens taken from hibernating myocardium during cardiac surgery show structural degeneration characterized by reduced quantities of structural proteins, loss of myofilaments, and disorganization of the cytoskeleton, with varying degrees of fibrosis.[136,137] The severity of morphologic degeneration seems to correlate with the timing and degree of functional recovery after revascularization. Pooled data from 13 studies (947 patients) receiving medical therapy after viability assessment suggest that the relative risk of clinical events in patients with viable myocardium decreases with increasing length of follow-up.[138] Currently two reports have demonstrated the benefit of timely revascularization in patients with viable myocardium on FDG PET. Beanlands et al.[115] evaluated 35 patients with chronic CAD and depressed LVEF; 18 patients underwent early revascularization ($<12 \pm 9$ days) and 17 underwent late revascularization (145 ± 97 days). In the early group, the preoperative mortality was lower, more patients experienced improved LVEF postoperatively, and the event-free survival was higher. Similar findings were reported by Schwarz et al.[116]

Left ventricular (LV) remodeling (increased LV volumes and cavity size) is also a predictor of poor outcome in patients with ischemic cardiomyopathy undergoing coronary artery surgery, as demonstrated in two studies. Louie et al.[139] reported that a preoperative LV end-systolic volume (ESV) of 70ml or greater, assessed by echocardiography, was shown to be a marker of poor outcome post-revascularization. Another study demonstrated that patients with an end-systolic volume index greater than $100\,ml/m^2$ did not have improved regional and global LV function after revascularization and therefore were more likely to suffer from postoperative heart failure and death.[140] In view of the poor outcome of this population with medical treatment or delayed revascularization, an argument can be made to assess these patients early in their course and proceed with revascularization if abundant viability is demonstrated. Otherwise transplantation could be contemplated.

Conclusions

The number of patients with CHF secondary to chronic CAD is rising. Potential therapies include medical treatment, heart transplantation, and revascularization. Revascularization is considered the best option, when feasible and when viable myocardium is present. Different nuclear imaging techniques are available for the detection of viability, using ^{201}Tl-chloride, ^{99m}Tc-labeled tracers, and FDG PET and SPECT. Although FDG PET is currently the most accurate technique for evaluation of myocardial viability, dobutamine stress echocardiography and MRI may also provide alternative options. Scintigraphic techniques are more sensitive, and techniques evaluating contractile reserve such as dobutamine stress echocardiography are more specific. Viability has been related to improvement of regional and global function after revascularization, to improvement in heart failure symptoms and exercise capacity, and to a superior long-term prognosis. Patients with viable myocardium have fewer complications at surgery and have a better long-term survival. In contrast, the patients with viable myocardium who are treated medically experience a very high event-rate and mortality. Thus, viability assessment is an important part of the diagnostic work-up of patients with chronic ischemic LV dysfunction and may help to guide optimal treatment. The American society of Nuclear Cardiology has recently published guidelines for FDG PET imaging.[141,142]

Case Presentations

Case 8.1

History

A 39-year-old woman with CHF and previous MI presented with new onset of chest pain. A rest ^{99m}Tc-MIBI myocardial perfusion study revealed a defect in the anterior, septal, and apical walls in both the supine and prone positions. The gated images demonstrated global hypokinesis and distal anterior, septal and apical dyskinesis, with an LVEF of 28%. The patient was referred for evaluation of myocardial viability. An FDG PET study was performed and compared with the rest ^{99m}Tc-MIBI SPECT perfusion. Before FDG administration, the patient was loaded with glucose using an IV infusion of insulin and dextrose. Both the ^{99m}Tc-MIBI SPECT and the FDG PET images were transferred to the same imaging workstation, oriented and lined up similarly for interpretation (Figure C8-1).

Findings

A large area is seen of severely decreased perfusion and metabolism in the anteroseptal wall and apex with no mismatched defect.

Discussion

The severe matched defect in the LAD distribution indicated that there is a low likelihood (<10%) of seeing improved wall motion after

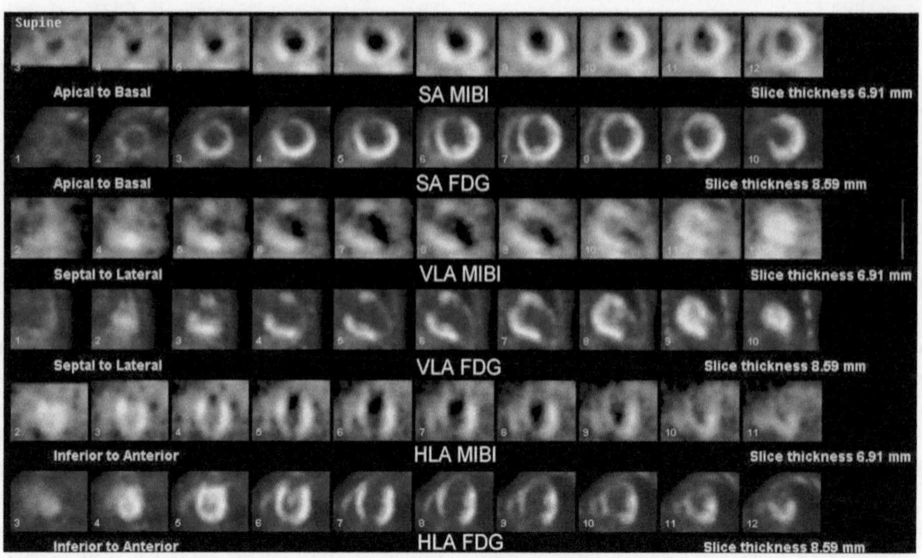

FIGURE C8-1.

revascularization, so she was treated medically. Furthermore, patients without myocardial viability are more likely to experience perioperative morbidity at the time of thoracotomy. Dysfunctional myocardium with severe hypoperfusion at rest may be infarcted or still viable. An extensive literature demonstrates that patients with ischemic but viable myocardium are at high risk for cardiac events if they are not revascularized.[8,11] Revascularization of ischemic/hibernating myocardium will affect improvement in regional function. If the volume of dysfunctional but viable myocardium is >25% of the LV mass, it is probable that the global LVEF will increase by >5% EF units.[112] Infarcted myocardium is hypometabolic by FDG imaging and will not exhibit improved wall motion following revascularization.

Various techniques are available for identification of dysfunctional viable myocardium. Evaluation of glucose metabolism with FDG PET is probably the most sensitive and accurate modality currently available. Several criteria have been developed for assessment of viability using FDG PET, but the most accurate is the comparison of regional perfusion and metabolism.

For comparison with FDG PET images, the best perfusion agents are PET perfusion radiopharmaceuticals because of similar resolution of the images, similar method for attenuation correction, and similar display. ^{13}N-ammonia is a short-lived positron emitter trapped intracellularly as glutamine proportionally to blood flow. Because of the short half-life of ^{13}N-ammonia, a cyclotron adjacent to the PET tomograph is necessary for a timely production just before the time of administration. ^{82}Rb is another positron emitting flow agent that is produced by a commercially available generator and thus can be used without access to a cyclotron. PET perfusion imaging is more sensitive than conventional SPECT imaging for detection of CAD due to the better resolution of the images, accurate soft tissue attenuation correction, and the ability to provide quantitation of coronary blood flow (CBF) and coronary blood flow reserve (CBFR) using kinetic modeling. Furthermore, due to the extremely short half-life of ^{82}Rb (1.3 minutes), a rest/stress protocol can be completed within 60 to 80 minutes, providing a high departmental throughput and convenience to the patient. The sensitivity for the detection of ischemia using perfusion PET is reported to be 95% as compared with 85% to 92% for ^{201}Tl and ^{99m}Tc-MIBI SPECT. In addition, if a matching perfusion defect is demonstrated with ^{13}N-ammonia or ^{82}Rb PET, an FDG PET study can be performed to determine viability.

However perfusion PET radiopharmaceuticals are not currently widely available because of the cost of the generator for ^{82}Rb and the short half-life of ^{13}N-ammonia (T ½ of 10 minutes) preventing distribution. Therefore, many institutions compare FDG PET images with SPECT perfusion images, as was the case for this patient.

When interpreting images obtained with two different imaging systems (SPECT and PET), the interpreter should have in mind the limitations related to the differences in the techniques used. For example in this case, the ^{99m}Tc SPECT perfusion images have a lower resolution than the FDG PET images, so a ^{99m}Tc perfusion defect will appear somewhat smaller than a matched FDG PET defect. The SPECT perfusion images have not been corrected for attenuation while the FDG PET images have. Although the two sets of images could be displayed with the same computer system and color scale, the thickness of the slices has to be a multiple of the original pixel size and could not be adjusted. Therefore, the thickness of the slices is 8.6 mm for the PET images and 6.9 mm for the SPECT images.

Interpretation

Anteroseptal and apical myocardial scarring demonstrated by matched ^{99m}Tc-MIBI SPECT/FDG PET defect.

Case 8.2

History

A 67-year-old man with a known ischemic cardiomyopathy presented to the emergency department (ED) with syncope. Due to the presence of atrial fibrillation with a rapid ventricular response and runs of ventricular tachycardia, he was admitted to the coronary care unit. A coronary angiogram revealed a 75% stenosis of the LAD (Figure C8-2A), 50% stenosis of the LCX, occlusion of the RCA with collateral circulation (Figure C8-2B), and global hypokinesis with an LVEF of 20%. An FDG PET study performed for viability assessment was compared with a resting ^{99m}Tc-MIBI SPECT perfusion study. Before FDG administration, the patient was loaded with glucose using an IV infusion of insulin and dextrose. The ^{99m}Tc-MIBI SPECT and FDG PET images were transferred to the same imaging workstation, oriented and lined up similarly for interpretation (Figure C8-2C).

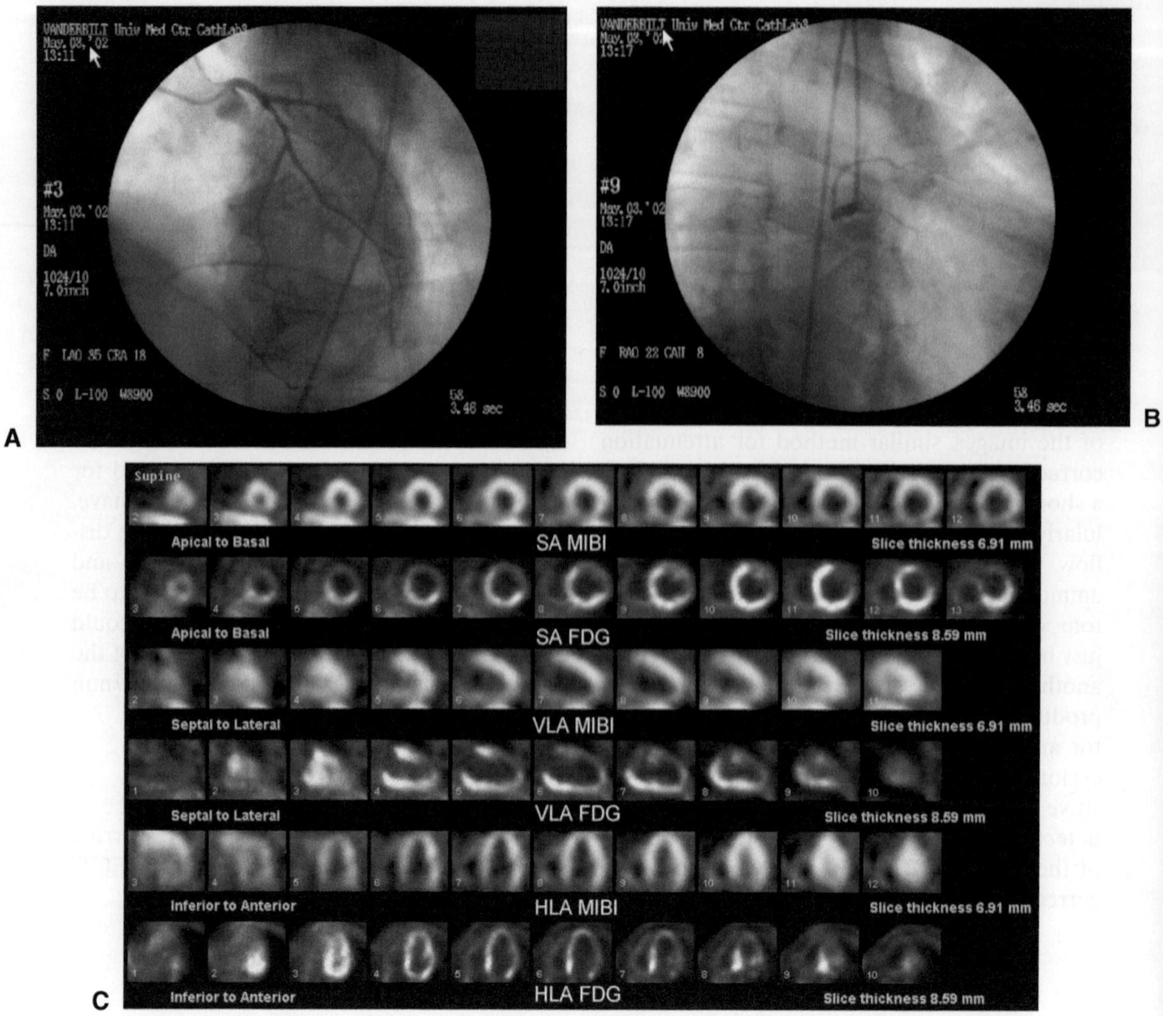

FIGURE C8-2. (A–C)

Findings

The rest ^{99m}Tc-MIBI myocardial perfusion study demonstrated a large severe fixed inferior wall defect in both the supine (Figure C8-2C) and prone (not shown) positions. The gated images (not shown) demonstrated global hypokinesis worse in the anteroseptal region and apex and an LVEF of 23%. The large area of decreased perfusion in the inferior wall of the myocardium demonstrates FDG uptake and therefore is viable. The large region of ischemic but viable myocardium in the inferior wall has an excellent potential for recovery of function post-revascularization. The patient was referred for CABG but refused intervention.

Discussion

The mismatched perfusion/metabolism in the inferior wall indicates injured but viable myocardium that most likely will benefit from revascularization. The interpretation of the FDG images may be somewhat confusing because the highest level of FDG uptake is in the inferoseptal wall that is the region with the least perfusion. Because the images are normalized to the pixel with most activity in the myocardium, the remainder of the myocardium appears hypometabolic compared with the region of ischemic myocardium. If the FDG images were interpreted without perfusion images, the decreased activity along the anterolateral wall could be misinterpreted as an infarct. This example demonstrates the importance of comparing perfusion and metabolic images for accurate interpretation. The pathophysiological mechanism underlying this phenomenon is the inhibition of lipolysis and decreased serum levels of fatty acids during ischemia, shifting the metabolism of the myocardium toward glucose. Therefore, the FDG uptake in ischemic regions may be above the level of uptake in normal myocardium. Anaerobic metabolism with severe ischemia results in supraphysiologic FDG uptake.

This patient is an example of ischemic cardiomyopathy with a large volume of hibernating myocardium. Hibernating myocardium refers to a state of persistently impaired LV dysfunction in the resting basal state attributable to a chronic reduction in CBF. Hibernating myocardium implies that if regional blood flow is restored, myocardial function will improve. Only 25% to 40% of unselected patients with severe CAD and LV dysfunction demonstrate improvement in global LVEF with revascularization. Therefore, the need for assessment of viability is imperative, as substantial gain can be achieved in such patients if revascularization can be accomplished. At present, FDG imaging is considered the most accurate modality for viability determination.

Interpretation

Ischemic but viable myocardium in the inferoseptal wall demonstrated by mismatched resting ^{99m}Tc-MIBI SPECT/FDG PET defects.

Case 8.3

History

A 62-year-old man with multiple risk factors and previous CABG presented with typical angina and elevated circulating troponins. He was diagnosed with an acute MI and underwent a coronary angiogram showing proximal occlusion of all native vessels, a patent internal mammary graft (LIMA) to the LAD and saphenous venous grafts (SVG) to the posterior descending artery (PDA) and obtuse marginal (OM). The SVG graft to the OM was severely stenosed at the anastomosis (Figure C8-3A, LAO view). The patient was referred for evaluation of viability with FDG PET imaging. Before FDG administration, the patient was loaded with glucose using an IV infusion of insulin and dextrose. A resting ^{99m}Tc-MIBI SPECT perfusion study was performed for comparison. Both the ^{99m}Tc-MIBI SPECT and FDG PET

A

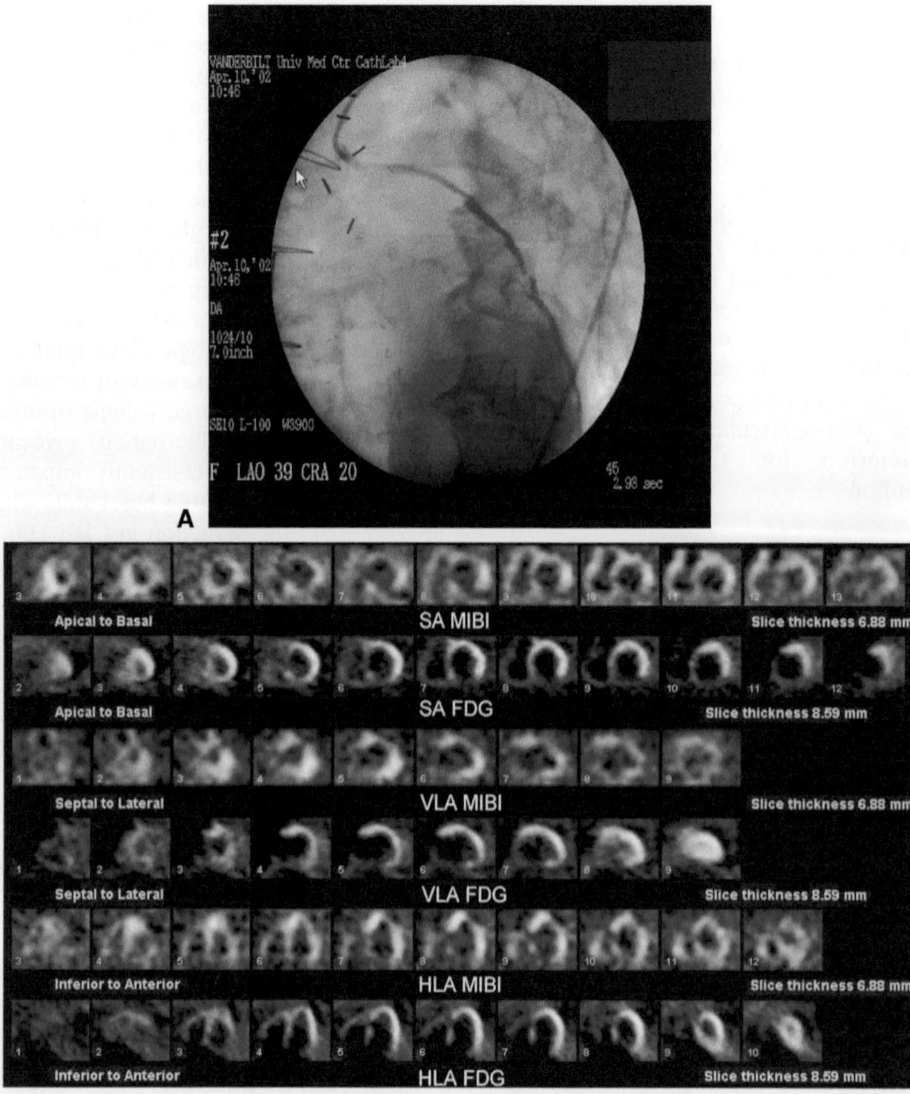

B

FIGURE C8-3. (A and B)

sets of images were transferred to the same imaging workstation, oriented and lined up similarly for interpretation (Figure C8-3B).

Findings

On the resting perfusion images, there is severely decreased uptake in the inferior wall and moderately decreased uptake in the anterior wall, septum, and anterolateral wall. The gated images (not shown) demonstrated biventricular dilatation, global hypokinesis and a severely depressed LVEF of 19%. The FDG images revealed no uptake in the inferior wall consistent with scarring but marked glucose uptake in the anterolateral wall indicating ischemic but viable myocardium that will benefit from revascularization. The region of dysfunctional ischemic but viable myocardium corresponds to the territory perfused by the stenosed SVG graft to the obtuse marginal branch. The patient underwent angioplasty and stenting of the SVG to the obtuse marginal. Three months later, his clinical symptoms and exercise capacity had markedly improved.

Discussion

This is an example of a patient with ischemic but viable myocardium who improved after revascularization. The improvement post-revascularization can be assessed using several criteria including improvement of regional or global LVEF and improvements of symptoms and exercise capacity.

Both Eitzman et al.[120] and DiCarli et al.[118,121] demonstrated a significant improvement of heart failure symptoms following revascularization, most evident in patients with viable tissue on FDG PET. It has been hypothesized that the postoperative improvement of LV function, symptoms, and exercise capacity may translate into improved long-term survival. Several studies have related viability to long-term prognosis; it should be emphasized, however, that these are all retrospective and nonrandomized studies, and that a prospective randomized study is needed to draw definitive conclusions.

Several studies have specifically addressed the long-term prognostic value of FDG PET.[117,121,122,124,126] In these studies, a total of 549 patients were included. The patients were grouped according to treatment (revascularization/medical) and viability status (absent/present). The mean follow-up varied from 12 to 29 months. All studies included hard events (death, infarction), and 4 studies also considered soft events (e.g., late revascularization, unstable angina). The pooled results showed that the highest event-rate (42%) was observed in the "viable patients" who were treated medically. In contrast, the lowest event-rate (9%) was observed in the patients with demonstrable viability who underwent revascularization. The groups of patients without viability also had relatively low event-rates. A study of 93 patients by DiCarli.[138] similarly concluded that patients with low LVEF and evidence of viable myocardium by PET have improved survival and symptoms with CABG compared with medical therapy.

Interpretation

Ischemic but viable myocardium anterolateral wall demonstrated by mismatched resting ^{99m}Tc-MIBI SPECT/FDG PET defects, plus inferior scarring manifested by a matched defect.

Case 8.4

History

A 57-year-old woman with a remote history of CAD and MI is currently asymptomatic. However, a rest/adenosine myocardial perfusion study performed at an outside institution revealed a dilated LV and a large fixed perfusion defect in the mid to distal anterior wall, septum and apex with an LVEF of 26%. A coronary angiogram revealed 90% stenosis of the LAD (Figure C8-4A) and akinesis of the anterior wall, septum, and apex. The patient was referred for evaluation of viability with FDG PET imaging. Before FDG administration, the patient was loaded with glucose using an IV infusion of insulin and dextrose. A resting ^{99m}Tc-MIBI SPECT perfusion study was performed for comparison. Both the ^{99m}Tc-MIBI SPECT and FDG PET images were transferred to the same imaging workstation, oriented, and lined up similarly for interpretation (Figure C8-4B).

Findings

The resting perfusion study demonstrated decreased uptake in the mid to distal anterior wall, septum, and apex both in the supine (Figure C8-4B) and prone (not shown) position, similar to the outside study. The gated study (not shown) revealed global hypokinesis more severe in the distal anterior wall, septum,

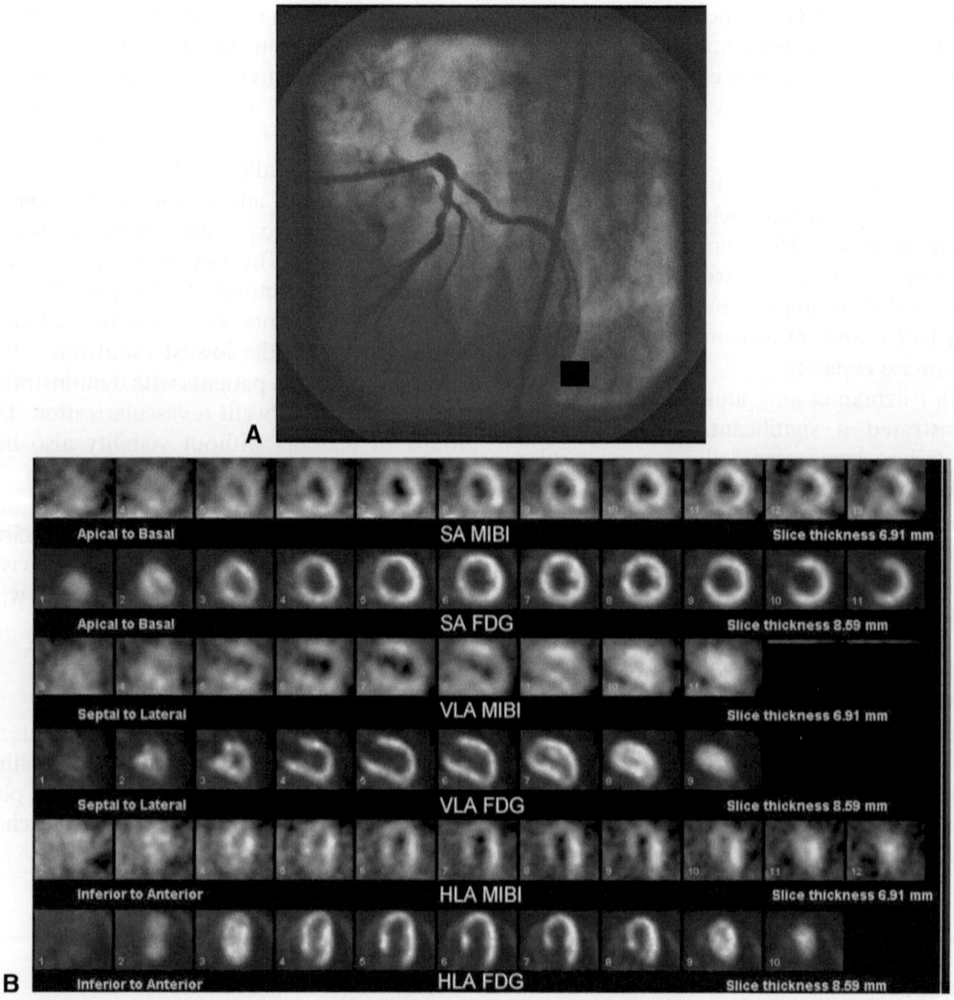

FIGURE C8-4. (A and B)

and apex with an LVEF of 30%. The FDG images revealed glucose metabolism in the distal anterior wall and apex indicating ischemic but viable myocardium that would benefit from revascularization. A stent was placed in the LAD.

Discussion

This is another example of a patient with ischemic but viable myocardium who improved after revascularization. The most objective criteria to document improvement post-revascularization is probably improvement of regional wall motion or global LVEF, although symptomatic improvement and both short- and long-term outcome (MI, death) are most important.

Many studies have employed FDG PET to evaluate tissue viability and predict improvement of regional function after revascularization. The first study, by the UCLA group, involved 17 patients with a depressed LVEF (32 ± 14%) who were scheduled for surgical revascularization.[84] Perfusion was assessed by ^{13}N-ammonia PET, and FDG PET was performed following oral glucose loading. Regional LV function was evaluated before and 3 months after revascularization; 37 segments improved in function post-revascularization, with 35 being classified as viable on PET. Conversely, 30 segments did not improve in function, with 24 classified as nonviable by PET. Thus, the sensitivity and specificity to predict improvement of regional LV function post-revascularization were 95% and 80%, respectively. The results of 12 FDG PET studies (with a total of 322 patients) were pooled to determine the value of FDG PET for the prediction of improvement of regional LV function following revascularization.[9] Pooling of the results yielded a sensitivity of 88% with a specificity of 73% and a negative predictive value of 86% with a positive predictive value of 76%.

Improvement of global LVEF is clinically more relevant than improvement of individual segments, since LVEF is an important prognostic parameter of survival. It is likely that the improvement of LVEF translates to improvement of heart failure symptoms, exercise capacity, and survival. In the study by Tillisch et al.,[84] global LVEF was evaluated before and 3 months after revascularization. The authors demonstrated that a significant improvement in LVEF occurred (from 30 ± 11% to 45 ± 14%) in patients with a substantial volume of viable myocardium as defined by FDG PET. Studies that have evaluated global LVEF before and after revascularization are summarized in Table 8-8. In these studies, the average LVEF improved significantly in patients with viable tissue on FDG PET imaging, ranging from 7% to 18% absolute increase in LVEF. In the patients without viable tissue (included in FDG PET studies), however, the LVEF did not increase significantly, ranging from 4% absolute increase to 12% absolute decrease in LVEF. Moreover, Pagano et al.[143] have shown that a linear relation existed between the extent of viable myocardium and the absolute change in LVEF. Bax et al.[112] demonstrated using ROC analysis that 25% dysfunctional but viable LV may be the optimal threshold to predict improvement of global LVEF after revascularization.

Interpretation

Ischemic but viable myocardium in the distal anterior wall and apex demonstrated by mismatched resting ^{99m}Tc-MIBI SPECT/FDG PET defects.

Case 8.5

History

A 69-year-old woman with a history of CAD, documented MI, and CHF presented with worsening dyspnea on exertion. A rest-24-hour redistribution ^{201}Tl perfusion study revealed severe hypoperfusion of all regions of the myocardium except the lateral wall. The patient was referred for evaluation of viability with FDG PET imaging. Before FDG administration, the patient was loaded with glucose using an IV infusion of insulin and dextrose. Both the 24-hour ^{201}Tl SPECT and the FDG PET images were transferred to the same imaging workstation, oriented, and lined up similarly for interpretation (Figure C8-5A).

Findings

On the 24-hour ^{201}Tl images, the uptake is inhomogenous throughout the myocardium and is decreased in the septum, anterior, and inferior wall of the myocardium. The FDG PET images demonstrated the presence of glucose metabolism in the septum, apex, anterior and inferior wall, indicating ischemic but viable

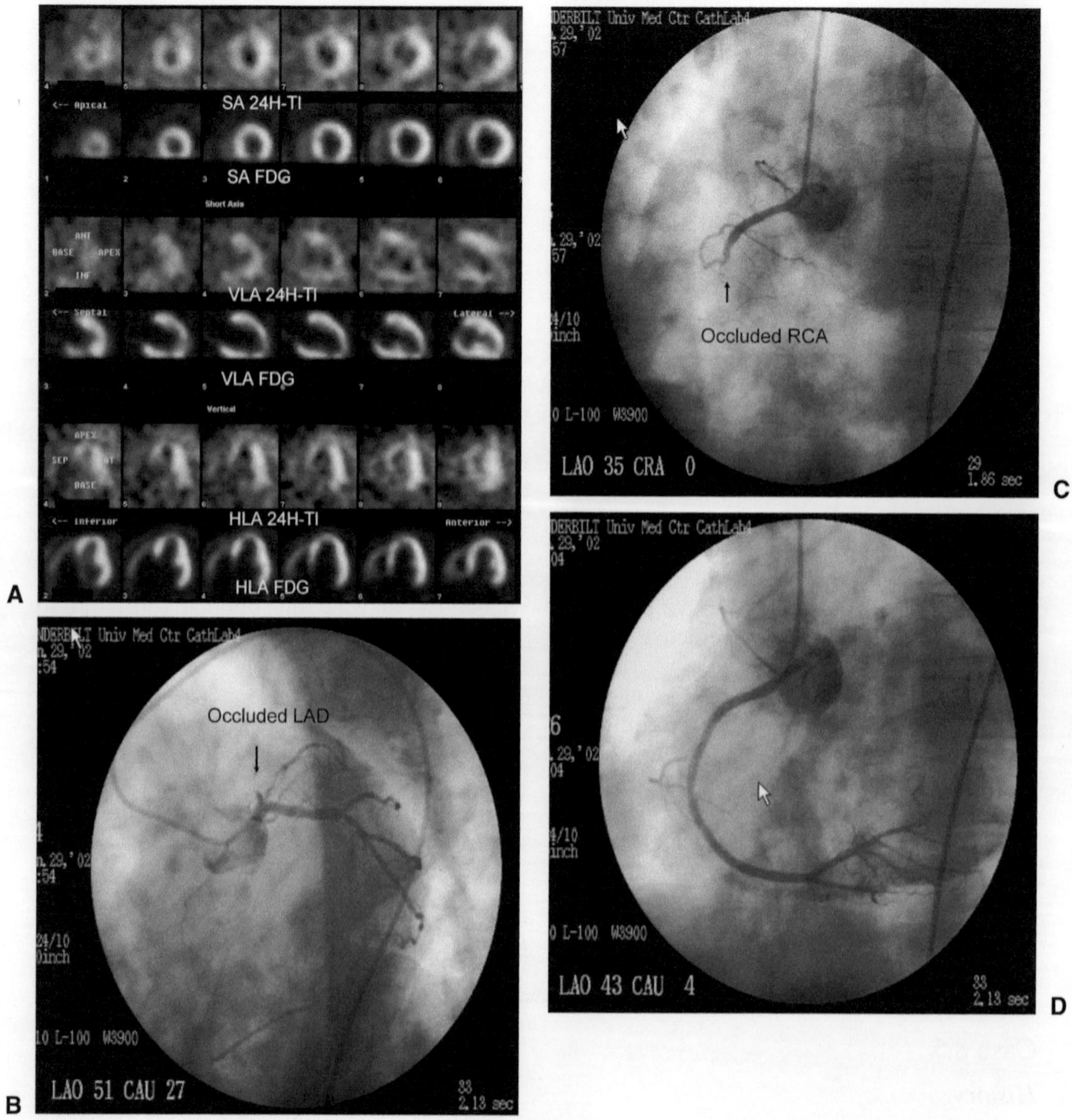

FIGURE C8-5. (A–D)

myocardium, which is likely to improve post-revascularization. A coronary angiogram revealed occlusion of the LAD (Figure C8-5B) and the RCA (Figure C8-5C). In addition, there was a 40% luminal stenosis of the LCX and the ventriculogram revealed LVEF of 20%. Stents were placed in both the LAD and RCA. Figure 8-5D demonstrates good flow through the RCA after the procedure. At her 3-month follow-up visit, her symptoms and exercise tolerance had markedly improved.

Discussion

This case illustrates several aspects of the evaluation of myocardial viability using scintigraphic techniques. The first point is the difference in quality of the 24-hour SPECT ^{201}Tl images compared with FDG PET images. The superior quality of the FDG PET images is related to the better resolution of the PET compared with the SPECT technology, as well as a difference in count rate. Even when the imaging time is increased to acquire 24-hour SPECT ^{201}Tl images, the images are often noisy and this is related to a low count rate, making the interpretation difficult. Another advantage of the PET technology is the routine availability of attenuation correction.

The second point is the value of 24-hour versus 4-hour delayed images after a resting ^{201}Tl injection. The value of routine acquisition of additional images at 24 hours is still debated in the literature.[33,34] In this case, the 24-hour delay to acquire the redistribution images was related to the patient's convenience.

The third point is identification of ischemic viable myocardium with FDG imaging in regions that appear to be of borderline viability on rest-redistribution ^{201}Tl images. Although FDG imaging appears more sensitive and specific than rest-4-hour redistribution ^{201}Tl images for prediction of recovery after revascularization, the difference was not significant in a study of 24 patients.[31] However, the degree of severity of the LV dysfunction is important, FDG imaging can demonstrate viability in fixed defects on stress-reinjection ^{201}Tl SPECT images in patients with an LVEF <20%.[29]

For patients evaluated for stress-induced ischemia with ^{201}Tl, two protocols are commonly used to maximize detection of viability in compromised myocardium: the stress-redistribution-late redistribution and the stress-redistribution-reinjection protocols. Evidence of stress-induced perfusion defects on ^{201}Tl images that redistribute after 4 hours is indicative of ischemic viable myocardium but fixed defects do not necessarily indicate scarring. The identification of viable myocardium is improved by the addition of a third set of images obtained at 24 hours that allows a longer period of redistribution for ^{201}Tl.[30] A prospective study by Yang et al.[25] demonstrated that late redistribution occurs in 53% of the patients with fixed defects on stress-redistribution images. However, fixed defects at 24 hours do not exclude viability, as 37% of segments that remain fixed on both 4 hours and 24 hours images also improve after revascularization.[24] The case of this patient illustrates the limitations of ^{201}Tl to detect myocardial viability, even using the optimal protocol. In addition, the suboptimal count statistics at 24 hours often makes the images difficult to interpret even if the acquisition time is increased.

The concept of reinjection of a booster dose of ^{201}Tl (1.0 to 1.5 mCi) 15 to 30 minutes prior to acquiring the rest redistribution images was introduced in the early 1990s. In a study of 100 patients with 33% of fixed defects after 4-hour redistribution images, Dilsizian et al.[26] demonstrated that there is improvement of ^{201}Tl uptake in 49% of these fixed defects on images obtained after reinjection of 1 mCi of ^{201}Tl. In addition, patients with regions identified as viable improved wall motion after percutaneous transluminal coronary angioplasty (PTCA). ^{201}Tl reinjection protocols have been shown to provide incremental prognostic information compared with clinical, exercise, and stress-redistribution data.[129,130]

Interpretation

Ischemic but viable myocardium anterior wall, septum, apex, and inferior wall demonstrated by mismatched resting 24-hour ^{201}Tl/FDG PET defects.

Case 8.6

History

A 57-year-old diabetic male patient was admitted with CHF and episodes of ventricular tachycardia. He had no symptoms to suggest ischemia. A coronary angiogram revealed occlusion of the RCA, 90% stenosis of the mid-LAD, 90% stenosis of the proximal LCX, global hypokinesis, and an LVEF of 25%. Considering possible revascularization, the patient was referred for evaluation of ischemia and viability using a resting FDG SPECT/stress adenosine ^{99m}Tc-MIBI SPECT dual isotope single acquisition protocol (DISA) (Figure C8-6). Before FDG administration, the patient was loaded with glucose using an IV infusion of insulin and dextrose.

Findings

The ^{99m}Tc-MIBI SPECT perfusion images demonstrated a large severe perfusion defect in the inferior wall and a smaller one in the anteroseptal region. Although the FDG SPECT images are of suboptimal quality due to diabetes, glucose metabolism is quite homogenous throughout the myocardium indicating viability. In addition, there is dilatation of the LV cavity with stress that is frequently seen in multivessel CAD. Considering the amount of viable myocardium found, the patient was referred for CABG.

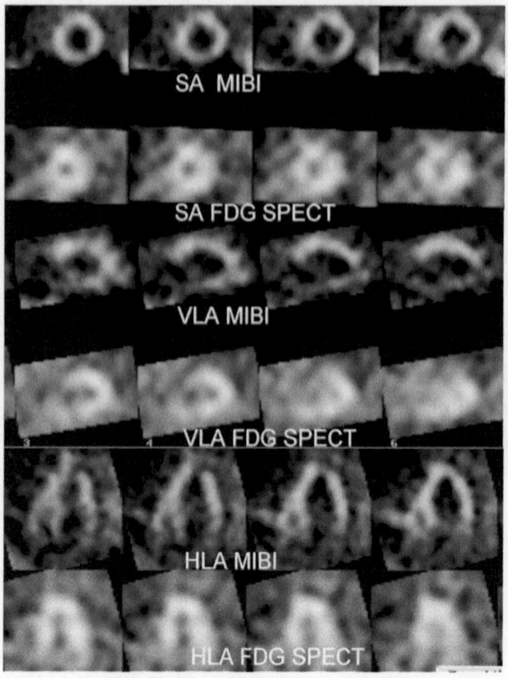

FIGURE C8-6.

Discussion

The perfusion/metabolism mismatches are consistent with ischemia in two vascular territories. This patient is an example of ischemic cardiomyopathy with a large volume of hibernating myocardium demonstrated by FDG SPECT rather than PET. Hibernating myocardium refers to a state of persistently impaired LV dysfunction in the resting basal state that is attributable to a chronic reduction in CBF. Angina may or may not be present, especially considering the presence of diabetes.

The available evidence in the literature on FDG SPECT for prediction of improvement of regional LV function is less extensive than that for PET. One study evaluated 55 patients with severe CAD and depressed LV function (LVEF = 39 ± 14%) with FDG SPECT before revascularization.[9] Data were acquired sequentially: ^{201}Tl SPECT was used to assess resting perfusion and FDG SPECT was performed using hyperinsulinemic euglycemic clamping. Echocardiography was performed before and 3 months after revascularization to assess regional wall motion. Of the 281 segments with abnormal contraction preoperatively, improved function occurred in 94 segments after revascularization, with 80 being viable on FDG SPECT. Conversely, 187 segments did not improve in function, and 141 of these segments were classified as nonviable by FDG SPECT. Accordingly, the sensitivity and specificity to predict improvement of regional LV function post-revascularization were 85% and 75%, which is virtually identical to the pooled data for FDG PET imaging.

Prediction of improvement of global LV function has also been evaluated using FDG SPECT. Forty-seven patients with ischemic cardiomyopathy (LVEF 30 ± 6%) were studied with the sequential SPECT protocol before surgical revascularization.[112] Of interest, most of these patients presented with heart failure symptoms instead of angina pectoris. LVEF was assessed before and 3 to 6 months after revascularization by radionuclide ventriculography. A direct relation between the extent of viable myocardium and the change in LVEF post-revascularization was observed. The patients were subsequently divided into three groups, according to the number of dysfunctional but viable segments on FDG SPECT (using a 13-segment model). Group A consisted of 22 patients without substantial viability (<3 viable segments, mean 1.0 ± 0.8); group B consisted of 17 patients with an intermediate amount of viable tissue (3 to 5 segments, mean 4.1 ± 0.8); and group C consisted of 8 patients with a large amount of viable tissue (>5 segments, mean 7.4 ± 1.4). The largest increase in LVEF was observed in group C (from 30 ± 5% to 44 ± 10%, p = 0.001); 7 of 8 (88%) patients showed a significant increase in LVEF (mean increase 16 ± 6%). Patients in group B showed a moderate increase in LVEF (28 ± 7% to 32 ± 9%, p = 0.002), while patients in group A did not show improvement in LVEF.

The change in heart failure symptoms in relation to preoperative viability was assessed in these same 47 patients.[112] Using FDG SPECT, the patients were divided into three groups, as described previously. Heart failure symptoms were graded before and 3 months after revascularization using the NYHA classification. Importantly, the average NYHA score before revascularization was comparable among the three groups. The largest improvement in NYHA score was again observed in group C (from 3.4 ± 0.5 to 1.7 ± 0.8, p = 0.001). Patients in group B showed a slightly less improvement in NYHA score (from 3.3 ± 0.5 to 2.2 ± 1.0, p = 0.003). Patients in group A showed no improvement in symptoms (3.1 ± 0.5 versus 2.9 ± 0.8, ns).

To date, two centers have reported preliminary prognostic data on FDG SPECT studies. In a large cohort of 135 patients with depressed LV function undergoing FDG SPECT and a follow-up of 28 ± 11 months, Bax et al.[144] demonstrated that the event-rate was highest (60%) in the patients with viable myocardium treated medically, and the lowest event-rate (4%) was observed in the patients with viable myocardium undergoing revascularization. Intermediate event-rates were observed in the patients with nonviable myocardium who were revascularized (16%) or treated medically (9%). Similar findings have been reported by Wijffels et al.[145] Importantly, these data are very similar to the FDG PET data.

When using the DISA ^{99m}Tc-MIBI/FDG SPECT protocol, the FDG is administered at rest after glucose loading. The patient can be stressed after a 30-minute distribution phase of FDG and the ^{99m}Tc-MIBI is administered at peak stress. This protocol allows evaluation of stress-induced ischemia as well as viability in one setting. If the ^{99m}Tc-MIBI is administered at rest at the same time as the FDG, only viability can be assessed.

The metabolic conditions during FDG imaging are extremely important; they determine myocardial FDG uptake and image quality. High insulin levels accompanied by suppressed FFA levels promote FDG uptake, whereas high FFA levels inhibit FDG uptake. Several protocols are available to promote cardiac FDG uptake. Oral glucose loading is the most frequently used approach, although it results in uninterpretable images in approximately 10% of nondiabetic patients,[55] and more commonly in patients with impaired glucose tolerance or diabetes mellitus. The hyperinsulinemic euglycemic clamp allows near-perfect regulation of metabolic substrates and insulin levels, ensuring excellent image quality in virtually all patients.[56] However, the procedure is laborious and time-consuming. A shorter (30 min) and more practical IV glucose/insulin loading procedure has been used with success in nondiabetic patients.[55] Oral administration of a nicotinic acid derivative (acipimox) may be an alternative to clamping; acipimox inhibits peripheral lipolysis, thus reducing plasma free fatty acid levels, and thus indirectly stimulating cardiac FDG uptake.[59] Initial data suggest that good image quality can be obtained using this approach.[60]

As diabetes is a disease affecting glucose metabolism, the fasting—oral glucose loading protocol is most often not effective in diabetic patients.[64] Unfortunately, CAD is a frequent complication of diabetes, and sometimes patients are evaluated for CAD even before a diagnosis of diabetes has been established. The methods used for loading nondiabetic patients with glucose have been modified to optimize myocardial glucose utilization in diabetic patients with variable success.[65] The reference method is the euglycemic hyperinsulinic clamp, a rigorous and time-consuming procedure, allowing regulation of metabolic substrates and insulin levels and providing excellent image quality in most patients, and especially in patients with non-insulin-dependent diabetes mellitus.

Interpretation

Severe multivessel disease with viability in the inferior and anterior walls demonstrated by DISA ^{99m}Tc-MIBI/FDG SPECT study. This information was critical for making a decision regarding revascularization.

Case 8.7

History

A 71-year-old man with ischemic cardiomyopathy, and remote CABG presented with worsening CHF. The patient was evaluated for stress-induced ischemia and myocardial viability using a resting FDG SPECT/ stress adenosine ^{99m}Tc-MIBI DISA SPECT (Figure C8-7). Before FDG administration, the patient was loaded with glucose using an IV infusion of insulin and dextrose. The patient denied chest pain during adenosine infusion, and the ECG showed no diagnostic changes of ischemia.

Findings

The large inferior wall perfusion defect is metabolically inactive as demonstrated by the absence of FDG uptake, representative of myocardial scarring. The remainder of the LV is viable with adequate perfusion at stress. In this case, the matched ^{99m}Tc-MIBI/FDG defect at the inferior wall precluded consideration of RCA bypass grafting since the probability of gaining improved inferior wall motion after revascularization would be less than 10%. The patient was treated medically.

Discussion

Modified SPECT gamma camera systems that accept 511 keV photons for FDG imaging are now commercially available. FDG metabolic SPECT imaging can be combined with ^{99m}Tc-MIBI perfusion imaging to give information regarding perfusion and metabolism using sequential imaging or a DISA protocol. FDG evidence of viability has been reported in as many as 50% of segments with fixed perfusion defects using rest/stress ^{99m}Tc-MIBI protocols (without nitrate) as well as in 40% to 50% of fixed ^{201}Tl defects with stress-redistribution protocols (not reinjection and 24-hour protocols). If a dedicated PET system is unavailable, accurate assessment of viability can be accomplished using a dual-head gamma camera equipped with ultra-high-energy 511-keV collimators.

Interpretation

Inferior wall MI demonstrated by matched ^{99m}Tc-MIBI/FDG SPECT defects.

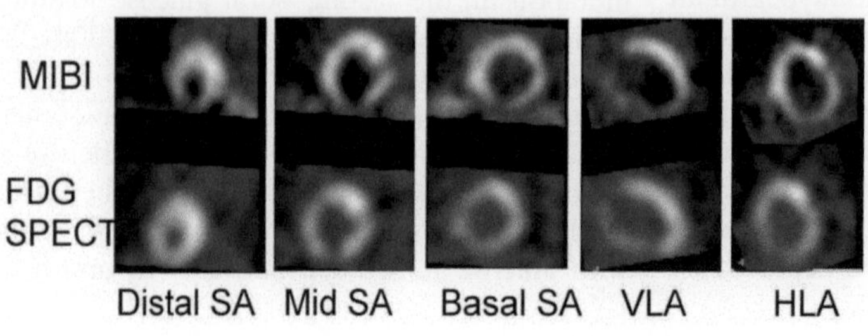

FIGURE C8-7.

Case 8.8

History

A 72-year-old diabetic male patient with known CAD, HTN, and CHF was referred for evaluation of chest pain. An echocardiogram revealed an LVEF of 20%. An FDG PET study was performed and compared with resting ^{99m}Tc-MIBI SPECT perfusion performed the same day. Before FDG administration, the patient was loaded with glucose using an IV infusion of insulin and dextrose. Both the ^{99m}Tc-MIBI SPECT and FDG PET images were transferred to the same imaging workstation, oriented, and lined up similarly for interpretation (Figure C8-8).

Findings

Along the inferior wall there appears to be a mismatched perfusion and metabolic defect in the supine imaging position suggestive of ischemia. In the prone imaging position, the inferior perfusion abnormality is only mild and matches the mild metabolic defect along the inferior wall. There is no anterior wall perfusion abnormality at rest. Gated MIBI SPECT cine images reveal a dilated heart with global hypokinesis and an LVEF of 21%. Coronary angiography revealed a 90% stenosis of the proximal LAD and moderate disease in the LCX and RCA. A PTCA of the LAD was performed successfully.

Discussion

The matched pattern of perfusion and metabolism indicates that there is no evidence of myocardium at risk that is viable in the resting state. Improvement of the inferobasal defect on prone imaging suggests an attenuation artifact from the diaphragm. The partial resolution of the inferobasal defect on MIBI images and complete resolution on FDG images may be explained by attenuation correction of the FDG PET images but not on the ^{99m}Tc-MIBI SPECT images. This may sometimes result in the appearance of a mismatched inferior wall abnormality suggestive of ischemia. Prone imaging or correction for attenuation artifact may be necessary in these instances.

The same problem occurs when comparing ^{99m}Tc-MIBI/FDG SPECT images. One must remember that there is more soft tissue attenuation of the 140-keV ^{99m}Tc photons than there is of the 511-keV ^{18}F photons when imaged with SPECT. A significant problem with cardiac SPECT imaging is the frequent occurrence of artifactual myocardial defects due to photon attenuation by extra-cardiac soft tissues. This problem is magnified with coincidence imaging, making attenuation correction more important for PET than for SPECT. Anteroseptal defects are seen in women as a result of overlying breast tissue in as many as 35% of cases. The relative decrease in inferior wall activity is a frequent occurrence in normal patients of both sexes due to interposition of the diaphragm and subdiaphragmatic fat between the heart and the detector(s). This results in lower specificity for inferior wall defects than for anterior and lateral wall defects.

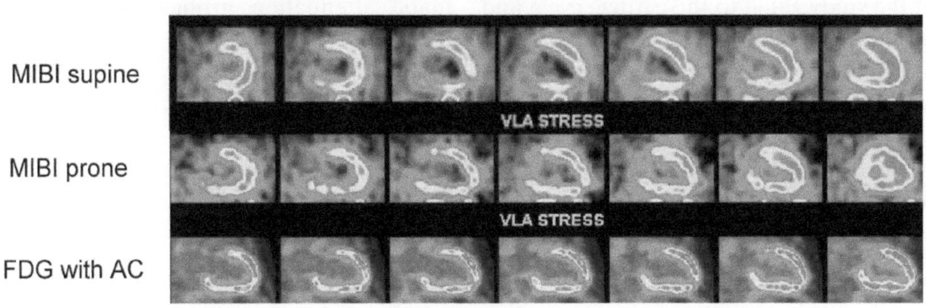

FIGURE C8-8.

Prone imaging may be used as a means of correcting for soft tissue attenuation by altering the position of the soft tissues, breasts, or diaphragm, in relation to the position of the heart. In many cases, the breast attenuation artifact seen with supine imaging improves or resolves with prone imaging because the breast is displaced laterally. Even when it does not resolve, it may be seen to change location, indicative of soft tissue effect. The heart is mobile within the thoracic cavity and swings up and away from the diaphragm when a patient is imaged in the prone position, so that the heart is spatially separated from the diaphragm, causing the inferior wall perfusion defect seen in the supine position to improve significantly or resolve. When using ^{201}Tl, there is a significant improvement in inferior counts in the large majority of patients imaged prone versus supine (striking in approximately 25%), with a resultant improvement in inferior wall specificity of approximately 24%. Because of the higher count rates obtained with ^{99m}Tc-labeled radiopharmaceuticals, soft tissue attenuation artifacts may be a less frequent and less severe problem, but they remain a dilemma more frequently than initial reports indicated. Because of the high 511-keV energy of ^{18}F, attenuation artifacts may not be as severe with FDG SPECT imaging. For that reason, it is strongly recommended that all patients undergoing ^{201}Tl or ^{99m}Tc SPECT and FDG SPECT cardiac imaging be imaged in both the supine and prone positions to decrease erroneous interpretations of reversibility along the inferior wall (or the anterior wall in women).

The high count density seen with ^{99m}Tc-MIBI and ^{99m}Tc-tetrofosmin imaging allows acquisition of the study gated to the cardiac cycle and viewing as a continuous cine display, even with DISA ^{99m}Tc-MIBI/FDG imaging. The cine loop display allows evaluation of LV regional wall motion, segmental systolic wall thickening, and global systolic function. With appropriate software, LVEF can be determined. ECG-gated myocardial perfusion images are useful in determining if matched defects are caused by breast or diaphragmatic attenuation versus true infarct or scar by the presence or absence of corresponding wall motion abnormalities. Regional wall motion can be assessed by subjective evaluation of endocardial excursion, and segmental wall thickening by changes in color intensification from end-diastole to end-systole. Whereas an infarct would be expected to demonstrate impaired wall motion and thickening, a soft tissue attenuation artifact should be associated with normal wall motion and thickening. In a study of 285 patients, gated acquisitions reduced the number of *borderline* results from 31% to 10%.[43] This should result in improved specificity and allows a more accurate measure of viability as well. However, patients with ischemic cardiomyopathy often suffer from severe global hypokinesis and low LVEF, so regional wall motion and wall thickening may be difficult to evaluate.

The severe stenosis of the LAD would probably have been detected with a rest-stress myocardial perfusion scintigraphy, but the patient was considered at too high risk to be stressed at the time.

Interpretation

Artifactual ^{99m}Tc-MIBI/FDG SPECT mismatch in the supine imaging position due to diaphragmatic attenuation artifact demonstrated by prone SPECT imaging.

Case 8.9

History

A 52-year-old man without cardiac risk factors presented with recent signs of heart failure. He underwent an echocardiogram showing global ventricular dysfunction and an LV thrombus. His coronary angiography showed severe lesions of the LAD, LCX, and RCA. He was referred for myocardial perfusion imaging (MPI) using a nitrate-enhanced ^{99m}Tc-MIBI protocol for assessment of myocardial viability. Baseline ^{99m}Tc-MIBI images were compared with images

A

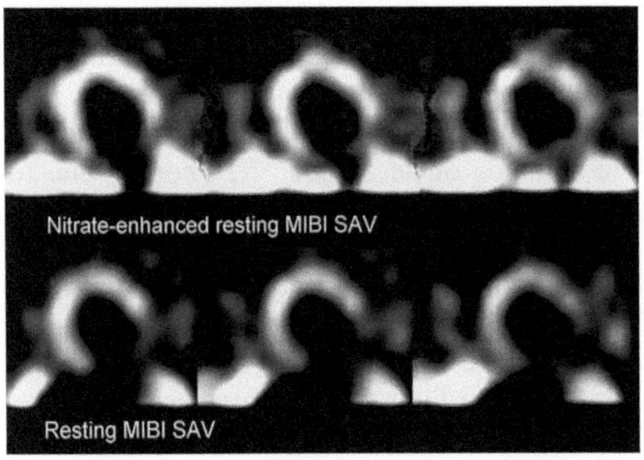

FIGURE C8-9. (A)

obtained when ^{99m}Tc-MIBI was administered 5 minutes following sublingual administration of nitroglycerin (0.4 mg × 2 at 5-minute intervals because there was no significant decrease of the blood pressure after the first dose). The SPECT images without and with nitroglycerine are displayed in Figure C8-9A.

Findings

The images without nitroglycerin showed moderated decreased uptake along the anterior and lateral walls and marked decreased uptake along the inferior wall and apex. After nitroglycerin, there is evidence of viability of the anterior, lateral, and inferolateral walls. No sign of viability exists along the inferior segment or apex. The gated images showed marked global hypokinesis of the LV and a reduced LVEF.

A similar case of another patient is displayed in Figure C8-9B. A 69-year-old man with known CAD and four-vessel CABG presented with typical angina and CHF. The coronary angiogram revealed 90% stenosis of the left main stem and occlusion of all native vessels. The internal mammary graft to the LAD was patent with a 50% stenosis. The SVG to the RCA was patent, but the grafts to a diagonal branch and to the OM were occluded. He was currently maximized on medical therapy including carvedilol, enalapril, simvastatin, diuretics, and aspirin, but remained symptomatic. His echocardiogram at rest revealed an LVEF of 45%. Revascularization was contemplated depending on viability assessment by MPI. The patient underwent a baseline and nitrate-enhanced resting ^{99m}Tc-MIBI SPECT displayed in Figure C8-9B. The baseline ^{99m}Tc-MIBI SPECT images reveal moderately decreased uptake in the anterior, lateral, and inferior walls. Following nitrate administration there is a significant increase in ^{99m}Tc-MIBI uptake in all coronary territories. Based on these findings, the patient was referred for revascularization.

Discussion

Viability detection with ^{99m}Tc-labeled perfusion radiopharmaceuticals has been debated in the literature for years. Early studies suggest that ^{99m}Tc-MIBI underestimates viability compared with other methods such as ^{201}Tl and FDG PET.[38,40] Later studies have demonstrated that the ^{99m}Tc-perfusion radiopharmaceuticals could identify myocardial hibernation when using quantitative SPECT criteria.[41] These agents remain bound intracellularly to the mitochondria of viable myocytes under conditions of myocardial stunning and hibernation, producing severe myocardial asynergy. A further increase in ^{99m}Tc-MIBI, for detection of viable myocardium, was achieved by performing quantitative resting and nitrate-enhanced imaging.[44] The mechanisms by which nitrates increase blood flow to hypoperfused myocardial segments appear to be dilatation of stenotic epicardial vessels and improvement of collateral flow. In addition, the decrease in LV preload and afterload induced by nitrates could improve subendocardial perfusion and therefore

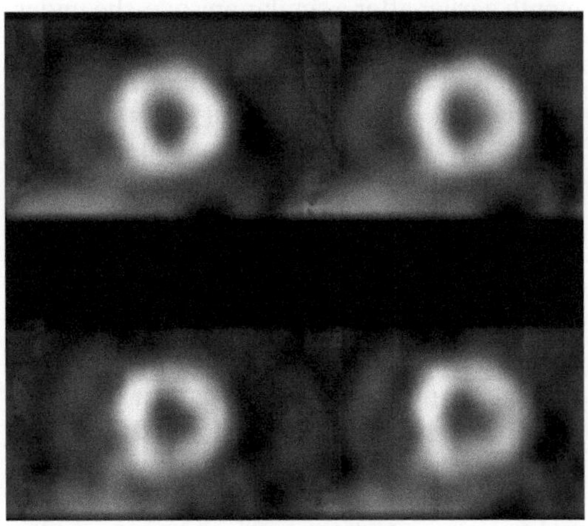

B

FIGURE C8-9. (B)

help to differentiate between hibernating myocardium and subendocardial scar.

Evaluation of the clinical success of coronary revascularization can be performed comparing the global LVEF pre-revascularization and post-revascularization. Sciagra et al.[47] have described a relationship between the extent and severity of ^{99m}Tc-MIBI defects and the post-revascularization changes in LVEF. The relationship was slightly better using nitrate-enhanced images than the resting ones. Typically, the criteria used for detection of viability are resting ^{99m}Tc-MIBI uptake >60% of the average uptake in the segment with the highest activity or nitrate ^{99m}Tc-MIBI uptake >65%. The same group of investigators demonstrated that the best criterion for detecting viability was a combination of the resting and nitrate-enhanced study: a nitrate-induced increase of >10% or nitrate-induced increase <10% but nitrate activity >65%. Using the receiver operating characteristic analysis (ROC) curve, this criterion achieved the best results with a sensitivity of 81% and a specificity of 69% for prediction of improvement of the global LVEF of 5% points.[46]

Gated SPECT allows evaluation of ventricular regional wall motion, segmental systolic wall thickening, and global systolic function. Preserved systolic thickening indicates viability in the instance of decreased ^{99m}Tc counts due to attenuation and not scar. It has been shown that the acquisition of gated SPECT images during low-dose dobutamine infusion allows detection of contractile reserve in asynergic segments with results comparable with low-dose dobutamine echocardiography.[51] More recently, it has been demonstrated that the combined use of low-dose dobutamine nitrate-enhanced ^{99m}Tc-MIBI gated SPECT had a higher predictive accuracy (sensitivity of 77% and 57% and specificity of 88% and 85%, respectively) for predicting regional wall motion improvement than low-dose dobutamine echocardiography.[52]

Interpretation

Ischemic but viable myocardium in the anterolateral wall and infarcted myocardium in the inferior wall demonstrated with resting ^{99m}Tc-MIBI SPECT with and without administration of nitrate.

Case 8.10

History

A 63-year-old female patient presented with a prolonged episode of chest pain at rest. One month earlier after a similar episode, she underwent coronary angiography revealing occlusion of the mid-LAD, but attempted angioplasty was unsuccessful. Her past medical history was significant for a remote right pneumonectomy for tuberculosis. Her resting ECG is shown in Figure C8-10A. During the next few days she had an acute episode of dyspnea and was found to have a pulmonary thromboembolism in the left lung apex (Figure C8-10B). She was referred to the nuclear laboratory for MPI and risk stratification. Due to poor exercise capacity, an adenosine ^{99m}Tc-MIBI SPECT was performed first. The resting study was performed the next day and because of the history of prolonged chest pain and known occlusion of the mid-LAD, sublingual nitroglycerin was administered before administration of the ^{99m}Tc-MIBI dose for better evaluation of viability. The adenosine/nitrate-enhanced resting ^{99m}Tc-MIBI SPECT images are displayed in Figure C8-10C. The acquisition could not be gated because of frequent premature atrial contractions.

Findings

There are no Q waves on the resting ECG to indicate a transmural MI, and although the specificity of absent Q waves is relatively low, this suggests that some myocardium in the LAD territory is still viable despite the occlusion of the mid-LAD. The lung perfusion scan demonstrates evidence of the right pneumonectomy performed for tuberculosis and the heart is shifted to the right. In addition, decreased uptake in the left lung apex is consistent with a

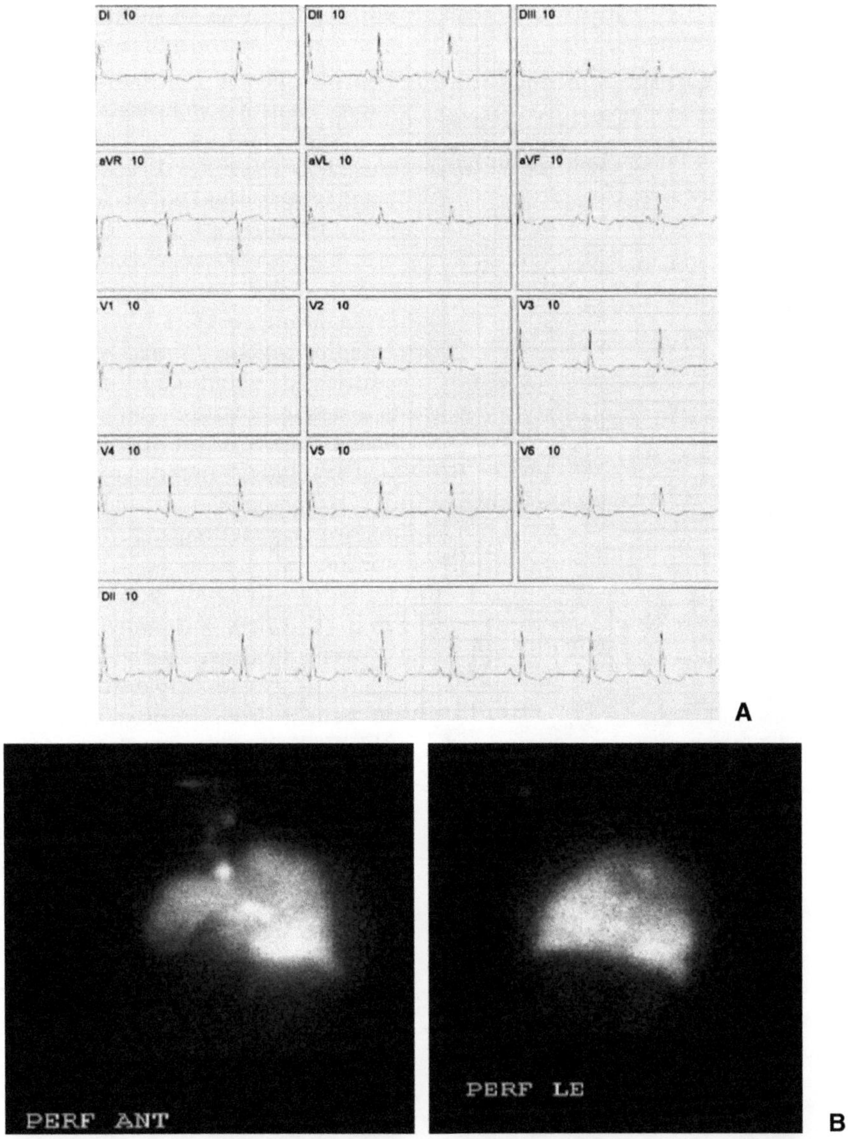

FIGURE C8-10. (A and B)

pulmonary embolism in the setting of an episode of acute dyspnea. The SPECT images demonstrate severe decreased uptake in the anterior wall of the myocardium that is partially reversible on the nitrate-enhanced resting images. This indicates ischemia of the anterior wall associated with an area of scar.

Revascularization should certainly be considered for this patient. In a patient with single-vessel CAD, PTCA is the first choice but failed during the first coronary angiogram. The surgical risk of CABG is increased in the setting of right pneumonectomy and a recent pulmonary embolism.

A PTCA was performed to the mid-LAD and some other septal branches. The repeat coronary angiography pre-PTCA and post-PTCA is shown in Figure C8-10D. The distal LAD is a thin vessel and the success of the PTCA was questionable.

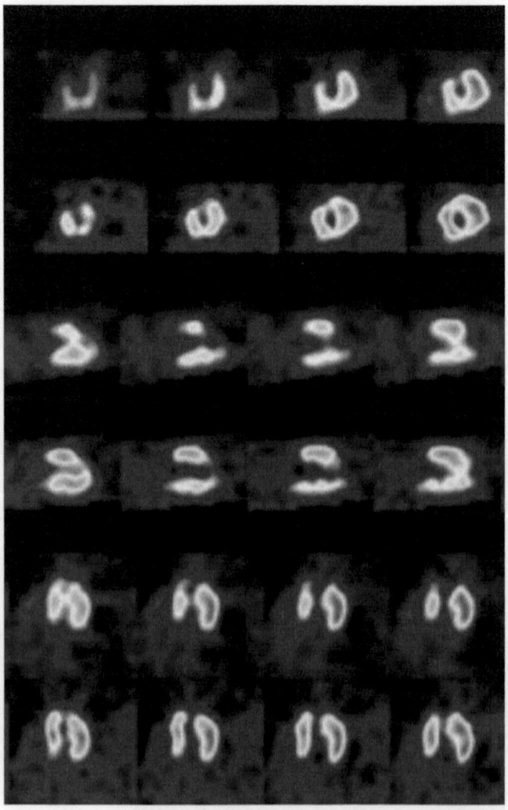
C

FIGURE C8-10. (C)

Discussion

This case presents a difficult dilemma. This patient presented with a mid-LAD occlusion and questionable MI with some viability. The SPECT images clearly demonstrated ischemic but viable myocardium in the LAD territory associated with some degree of scarring. Detection of ischemic but viable myocardium was improved with administration of nitrate before acquisition of the resting images. This was discussed in Case 8.9. Because of dysrhythmia, gated images could not be acquired and there is no information about LV function. The patient was referred for a repeat coronary angiography that revealed some degree of spontaneous recanalization of the LAD.

In this patient, it would be important to have information about the LV function. The LVEF is a strong prognostic indicator of survival as demonstrated in the coronary artery surgery (CASS) study.[146] In the CASS study, a subgroup of 780 patients with stable ischemic heart disease was randomized to receive surgical or nonsurgical treatment. This study demonstrated a correlation between LVEF and survival, regardless of therapy.

Strong evidence in the literature indicates that patients with viable ischemic myocardium do benefit from revascularization compared with medical treatment when anatomically feasible. For example, Cuocolo et al.[130] evaluated the effects of successful revascularization on survival and LV function in 76 patients with previous MI and evidence of dysfunctional but still viable myocardium at rest-redistribution ^{201}Tl imaging. During the 17 months follow-up, the survival rate was 97% in the group of patients who underwent revascularization and 66% in the group of patients treated medically ($p < 0.01$). DiCarli et al.[121] evaluated the prog-

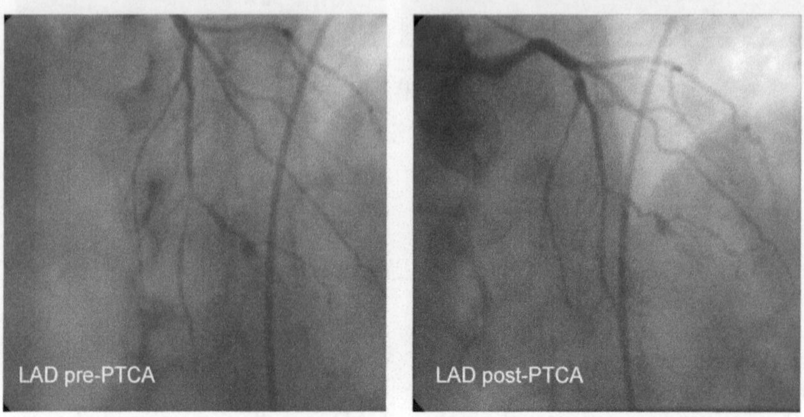

D

FIGURE C8-10. (D)

nostic value of PET for predicting survival and improvement in symptoms of heart failure in 93 patients with CAD and LV dysfunction (mean LVEF of 25%). The annual survival probability of patients with a mismatched perfusion/metabolism pattern receiving medical therapy was lower than those without mismatch (50% versus 92%, $p = 0.007$).

Interpretation

Ischemic viable myocardium in the territory of the occluded mid-LAD demonstrated with adenosine/nitrate-enhanced rest ^{99m}Tc-MIBI SPECT.

Case 8.11

History

A 60-year-old man with a history of CAD, remote MI, and CABG presented with angina and CHF. His coronary angiogram revealed severe native multivessel disease, an occluded SVG to the RCA, an open left internal mammary graft to the LAD, and an LVEF of 39%. The resting echocardiogram revealed severe anteroseptal hypokinesis and akinesis of the apex, lateral, and inferior wall of the heart. The results of the dobutamine echocardiogram are shown in Figure C8-11A.

Findings

Dobutamine echocardiography demonstrated viability in the LAD territory that was expected as the internal mammary graft to the LAD was patent on coronary angiography. On the other hand, wall motion in the inferior and lateral wall did not improve with low-dose dobutamine infusion indicating nonviability by dobutamine echocardiographic criteria.

Discussion

This patient may have potentially several levels of myocardial injury: stunned, hibernating, and infarcted myocardium. Dobutamine echocardiography is less sensitive but somewhat more specific than radionuclide studies, as demonstrated in the metaanalysis on the prediction of functional recovery post-revascularization published by Bax et al.[104] In total, 105 studies between 1980 and 2001, with 3034 patients, were included. When all studies were pooled, a sensitivity of 84% and a specificity of 69% were obtained. An important discrepancy was noted between the sensitivity/specificity of dobutamine stress echocardiography and nuclear imaging. When the metaanalysis was restricted to 11 studies with 325 patients who underwent both low-dose dobutamine echocardiography and some form of rest nuclear imaging (thus both protocols only focusing on viability without ischemia), nuclear imaging appeared significantly more sensitive in the prediction of functional recovery, whereas dobutamine echocardiography was more specific.

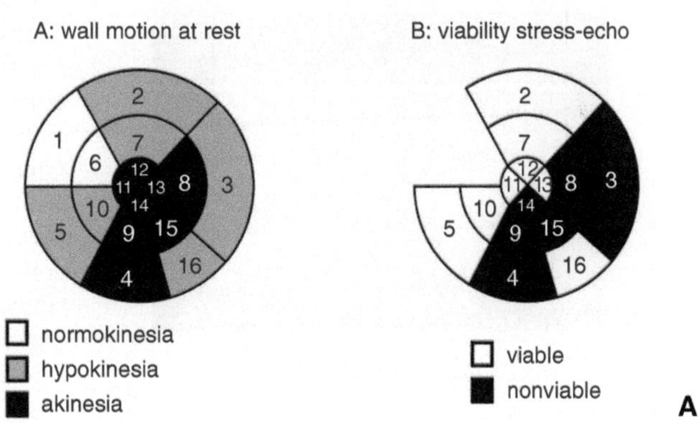

FIGURE C8-11. (A)

This patient was referred for a follow-up scintigraphic study for further evaluation of viability in the inferior and lateral myocardium using a more sensitive technique. Resting perfusion was evaluated with ^{99m}Tc-tetrofosmin and viability with myocardial glucose metabolism using FDG. FDG imaging was performed after administration of acipimox (500 mg, oral dose) and a low-fat, carbohydrate-rich meal to enhance myocardial FDG uptake. Sixty minutes after the meal, FDG was injected, and after an additional 45 minutes to allow cardiac FDG uptake, dual-isotope simultaneous acquisition SPECT was performed. A triple-head gamma camera system equipped with high-energy 511-keV collimators was used to acquire the images. The energies were centered on the 140-keV photon peak of ^{99m}Tc-tetrofosmin with a 15% window and on the 511-keV photon peak of ^{18}F-FDG with a 15% window. From the raw scintigraphic data, 6-mm thick (1 pixel) transaxial slices, as well as standard short- and long-axis projections perpendicular to the heart axis were reconstructed. For an exact alignment of the perfusion and FDG images, these data were reconstructed simultaneously. ^{99m}Tc-tetrofosmin FDG SPECT images are displayed in Figure C8-11B.

The perfusion images showed a defect in the inferior, posterior, and lateral segments, and FDG uptake was preserved in these segments. Hence, both perfusion and FDG uptake were normal in the anterior, septal, and apical segments, whereas a perfusion-FDG mismatch was present in the inferior, posterior, and lateral segments, indicating ischemic viable tissue in these segments.

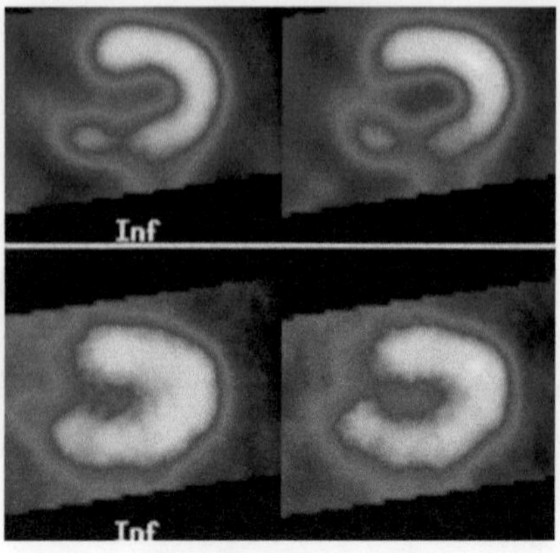

B

FIGURE C8-11. (B)

Assessment of hibernating myocardium in patients with ischemic cardiomyopathy is important for clinical decision making.[147] It allows for the selection of patients who will benefit most from revascularization procedures. Currently, several noninvasive techniques are available for the assessment of hibernating myocardium.[9] Although, MRI, dobutamine echocardiography and several radiopharmaceuticals can be used to assess viability, the most sensitive technique and current standard of care, when available, is the evaluation of myocardial glucose metabolism with FDG PET or SPECT. The metabolic conditions are extremely important in determining cardiac FDG uptake because the myocardium can use various substrates for its metabolism. ^{201}Tl scintigraphy (using rest-redistribution or reinjection protocols) can be used to evaluate cell membrane integrity. ^{99m}Tc-MIBI uptake reflects the integrity of the mitochondrial membrane. Low-dose dobutamine echocardiography is used to assess contractile reserve.

Although each of these techniques reflects a different feature of the hibernating myocardium, all of them have been demonstrated to predict improvement of function after revascularization. In general, the nuclear techniques tend to be more sensitive for the assessment of hibernating myocardium. This was demonstrated recently by Cornel et al.[148] comparing directly FDG SPECT with dobutamine stress echocardiography in 40 patients with ischemic cardiomyopathy. The results indicated that virtually all segments with contractile reserve demonstrated intact FDG uptake. On the contrary, 27% of the segments without contractile reserve also exhibited preserved FDG uptake. Similar findings were reported by Chan et al.[149] comparing FDG PET imaging with dobutamine stress echocardiography. Hence, some patients may not demonstrate contractile reserve, but may still have other signs of viability (residual glucose utilization, preserved cell/mitochondrial membrane integrity), as is also the case in the patient discussed. The exact clinical value of this discrepancy is unknown. ^{201}Tl seems to require smaller volume of viable tissue than dobutamine echocardiography or MRI to detect viability.[150,151] Preliminary data have shown that myocardium with preserved FDG uptake but without contractile reserve has more severe ultrastructural damage as compared with myocardium with FDG uptake and contractile reserve.[152] A study comparing dobutamine echocardiography, PET, and ^{201}Tl SPECT with correlation of the percent of viable myocytes in the explanted hearts demonstrated that 50% of myocytes must be viable to see evidence of contractile reserve by dobutamine echocardiography, whereas scintigraphic methods identify segments with less viable myocytes.[153] While myocardium with preserved FDG uptake and contractile reserve may improve in function early after revascularization, myocardium with preserved FDG uptake but without contractile reserve may take longer to improve in function after revascularization, perhaps longer than 3 months. Larger follow-up series of these patients are needed to fully elucidate this interesting observation.

MRI does also provide accurate evaluation of myocardial viability using delayed Gd enhancement or late enhancement. Delayed enhancement MRI can precisely delineate old and new MI (and even microinfarcts post-PTCA).[154]

Interpretation

Ischemic but viable myocardium in the inferolateral wall of the myocardium demonstrated with ^{99m}Tc-tetrofosmin/FDG SPECT despite absent contractile reserve with dobutamine echocardiography.

Case 8.12

History

A 69-year-old man with diabetes and prior inferoseptal wall MI was admitted to the coronary care unit for recurrent episodes of CHF; on admission he was in NYHA class IV; he had no accompanying angina. Additional comorbidity included impaired renal function and peripheral vascular disease. The resting ECG showed Q waves in leads II, III, and AVF. A coronary angiogram revealed extensive, diffuse three-vessel disease, with an occluded RCA and an LVEF of 23%. Resting 2-D echocardiography, performed on admission, showed akinesia of the inferolateral, inferior, septal, and apical segments. A resting ^{201}Tl study (imaging was started <10min after administration of ^{201}Tl) revealed severe hypoperfusion in all the akinetic segments on resting echocardiography (inferolateral, inferior, septal, and apical regions). He was referred for a viability study with FDG SPECT. FDG was injected after 60 minutes of hyperinsulinemic euglycemic clamping. Representative, mid-ventricular short-axis slices are displayed in Figure C8-12A. The polar maps are displayed in Figure C8-12B; in these maps, green represents severely reduced tracer uptake, whereas red is indicative of preserved tracer uptake.

Findings

Severe defects matching hypoperfusion are seen in the inferolateral and inferior regions indicating scar tissue. However, the other regions (septal, apical) exhibited relatively preserved FDG uptake, which is increased relative to perfusion, indicating viable myocardium.

Although the findings on ^{201}Tl SPECT/FDG PET imaging suggested a large area of viable myocardium in dysfunctional regions, the patient was treated medically. The reasons for this decision were twofold: (1) the patient had a high comorbidity, placing the patient at high risk during revascularization, and (2) in the presence of diabetes, the anatomy of the coronary arteries did not allow adequate revascularization. The patient died suddenly, a few months after discharge from the hospital.

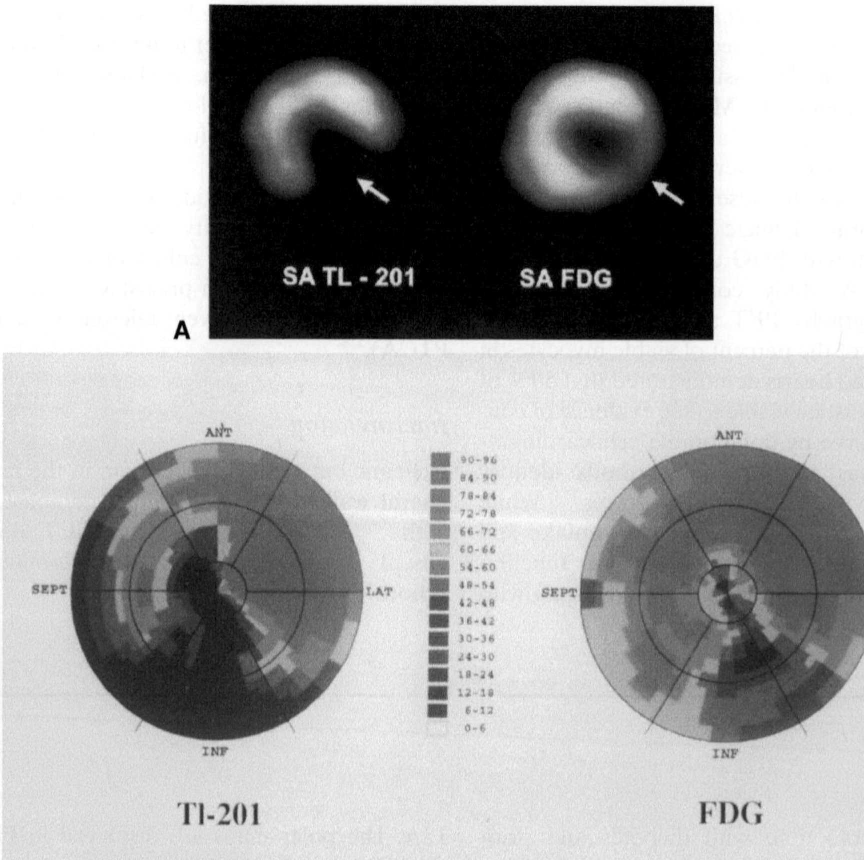

FIGURE C8-12. (A and B, from Bax, Visser, and Poldermans [155], by permission of *J Nucl Cardiol.*)

Discussion

Based on the SPECT findings, the patient was at high risk for future cardiac events. Pooling of the available studies focusing on the prognostic value of FDG imaging has shown that patients with viable myocardium at risk, who were treated medically, had an extremely high event-rate. This was in sharp contrast to the very low event-rate in the patients with viable myocardium who underwent revascularization. These prognostic studies were limited by their retrospective character and the nonrandomized aspect.[11] In other words, the reason why patients with viable myocardium did not undergo revascularization is unknown and may have influenced the results. For this reason, a prospective, randomized trial (STICH) was recently initiated, to further evaluate the prognostic value of viability testing. Patients with heart failure due to chronic CAD and depressed LV function need evaluation for the presence or absence of viable myocardium. Based on the available data in the literature, revascularization should be attempted when viable myocardium is present. However, comorbidity and anatomy of target vessels (in particular in patients with diabetes) should be considered also in the decision to revascularize or not. In addition, the results of the prospective, randomized trial (STICH) are awaited to draw definitive conclusions related to viability and subsequent treatment.

Interpretation

Ischemic but viable myocardium in the apex and septum demonstrated with ^{201}Tl SPECT/FDG SPECT imaging. Patients with ischemic viable myocardium have a poor prognosis if they cannot be revascularized.

Case 8.13

History

A 64-year-old man with a prior lateral MI was evaluated for recurrent episodes of heart failure. At the time of evaluation he was in NYHA class III, expressing dyspnea on minimal exertion. He did not experience concomitant angina. The resting ECG showed Q waves in the leads I, AVL, and V4-6. A coronary angiogram showed three-vessel disease, with significant stenoses (70% to 90%) in the LAD and RCA. The LCX was occluded proximally, with collateral filling.

Resting 2-D echocardiography showed akinesia of the anterolateral and inferolateral segments and hypokinesia of the septal, inferior, and apical segments. In addition, the LV was severely dilated with an LV end-diastolic diameter of 74 mm. The LVEF was 18%. He was referred for evaluation of viability. Rest-4-hour redistribution ^{201}Tl SPECT and FDG SPECT images (during hyperinsulinemic euglycemic clamping) are displayed in Figure C8-13.

Findings

The immediate resting perfusion ^{201}Tl images (Figure C8-13, upper row) demonstrated virtually absent uptake in the lateral segments that are akinetic on 2-D echocardiography. Perfusion is decreased to a lesser extent in the inferior segment. The 4-hour delayed resting ^{201}Tl images (middle row), assessing intact cell membranes (and thus viability) demonstrate virtually no fill-in in the hypoperfused regions. Because tracer uptake in part of the inferior wall is equal to 50%, it should be considered viable; the lateral wall, however, has tracer uptake <50% and should be considered nonviable.

FDG SPECT (Figure C8-13, bottom row) confirmed viability in the inferior, septal, and apical segments (also observed on ^{201}Tl rest-redistribution). In addition, the lateral segments also showed partial fill-in on FDG imaging, thus suggesting residual viable tissue in these segments.

Discussion

Characteristics of viability on ^{201}Tl rest-redistribution imaging include (1) significant redistribution (observed on the delayed images) of hypoperfused regions; significant redistribution is defined as equal to 10% increase in tracer uptake, and (2) equal to 50% tracer uptake on the delayed images, independent of the presence or absence of redistribution. Accordingly, hypoperfused segments with tracer uptake <50% are considered scar tissue.

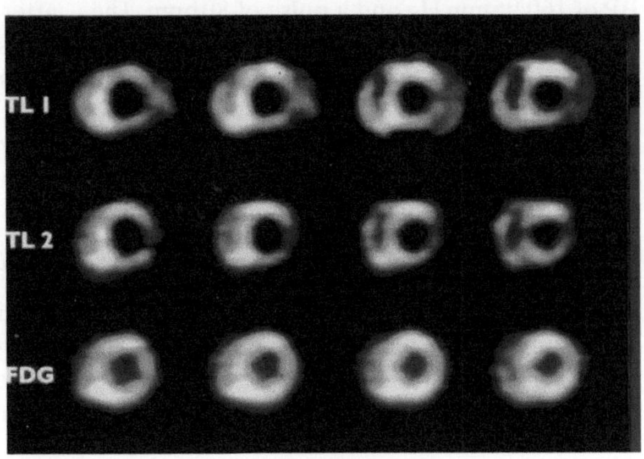

FIGURE C8-13.

When quantitative analysis was applied to the data of the current patient, only the lateral segments were considered nonviable, since tracer uptake on the delayed images in these segments was <50%. The other hypoperfused segments (inferior) still had tracer uptake equal to 50% on the delayed images. Thus, according to ^{201}Tl rest-redistribution imaging, scar tissue was present in the lateral wall, whereas the other segments contained viable myocardium.

Based on the findings on both rest-redistribution ^{201}Tl and FDG SPECT images, indicating the presence of viable myocardium in the majority of the dysfunctional segments, the patients underwent complete surgical revascularization. The procedure was uncomplicated, and functional follow-up was performed with resting echocardiography at 3 months and 12 months following revascularization. Although symptoms had improved, the LVEF did not improve (20% on late follow-up) and the regional wall motion abnormalities remained unchanged.

It has been suggested that in the presence of severe dilatation and remodeling of the LV, functional recovery cannot be achieved by revascularization, despite the presence of viable myocardium in the dysfunctional regions.[139,140] The exact cutoff value of LV diameter (beyond which no recovery can be expected) is currently unclear and needs further study. It is plausible that an LV end-diastolic diameter >70 mm has a low likelihood of recovery. Still, revascularization of viable myocardium may be of clinical importance, since revascularization of viable regions may prevent ischemic events, and also revascularization may prevent further remodeling.

Besides assessment of viability, other issues may be important in the prediction of recovery of function. The current case illustrates that extensive remodeling may prevent recovery of function despite the presence of viable myocardium.

Interpretation

1. Large areas of ischemic viable myocardium demonstrated with rest-redistribution ^{201}Tl and FDG SPECT imaging.
2. Extensive remodeling and dilatation of the LV may prevent recovery of function post-revascularization but improve symptoms and prognosis.

Case 8.14

History

A 62-year-old man was admitted with an episode of acute chest pain lasting for 4 hours. He had no history of cardiac or other disease. Risk factors for CAD included smoking and hypertension. Physical examination revealed a BP of 160/95 mm Hg and a pulse of 80 bpm. The ECG showed an ST-T segment elevation in leads II, III, and AVF, indicative of acute inferior MI. The patient received intravenous thrombolysis and recovered well. Follow-up ECG showed Q waves and negative T waves in leads II, III, and AVF. He did not complain of angina or symptoms of heart failure. TMT before discharge showed no ischemia. Resting 2-D echocardiography showed mildly depressed LVEF (42%) with akinesia of the inferior segments. He was referred for viability assessment with an MRI. A resting baseline MRI was performed first, followed by MR images obtained during low-dose dobutamine infusion (10 mcg/kg/min for 5 minutes) (Figure C8-14A). Next, contrast-enhanced images (Figure C8-14B) were acquired approximately 20 minutes after a bolus injection of Gd-DTPA (Magnevist; Schering/Berlex, Berlin, Germany, 0.1 mmol/kg). The MRIs were acquired with a 1.5 Tesla system (1.5-T, Gyroscan NT Intera, Philips Medical Systems, Best, The Netherlands).

Findings

Resting cine MRIs (short-axis slices, Figure C8-14A) showed a thinned inferior wall with akinesia; the other regions showed normal contraction. No improvement of contractile

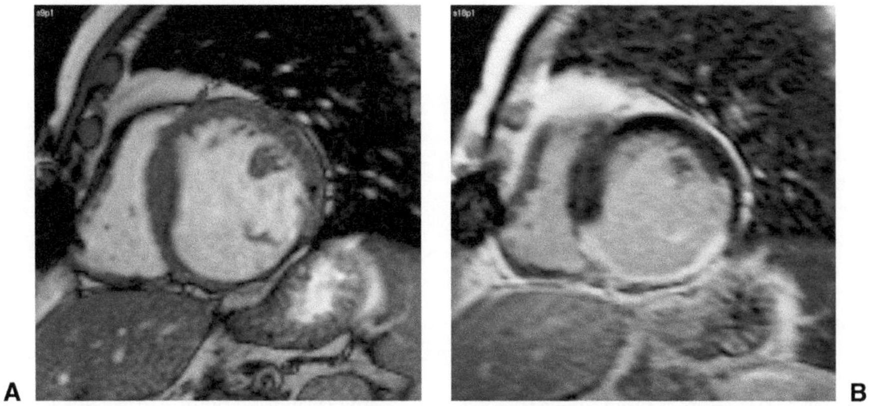

FIGURE C8-14. (A and B)

function was observed during low-dose dobutamine infusion, indicating absence of viable tissue in the inferior wall. The inferior wall showed hyper-enhancement on the delayed images, extending over the entire inferior wall, indicating transmural scar tissue (Figure C8-14B).

Discussion

The patient recovered well, without cardiac events during follow-up. Since the inferior wall contained predominantly scar tissue on MRI, revascularization was not considered. This case demonstrated the use of contrast-enhanced MRI for the assessment of scar tissue; in contrast to other viability techniques, this approach allows delineation of scar tissue. The great advantage of the technique is the superb resolution, allowing precise assessment of the extent of transmurality of scar tissue. A disadvantage is that it provides no information on the remaining *viable* tissue, whether this is normal or hibernating or stunned. However, in combination with dobutamine, it may become possible to provide precise information on the tissue characterization of dysfunctional segments. Cardiac MRI is further discussed in Chapter 14.

Interpretation

Inferior wall MI demonstrated with baseline/low-dose dobutamine/delayed Gd-enhanced MRI.

References

1. Gheorghiade M, Bonow RO. Chronic heart failure in the United States. A manifestation of coronary artery disease. *Circulation.* 1998;97:282–289.
2. Challapalli S, Bonow RO, Gheorghiade M. Medical management of heart failure secondary to coronary artery disease. *Coron Artery Disease.* 1998;9:659–674.
3. Bax JJ, Poldermans D, Elhendy A, et al. Improvement of left ventricular ejection fraction, heart failure symptoms and prognosis after revascularization in patients with chronic coronary artery disease and viable myocardium detected by dobutamine stress echocardiography. *J Am Coll Cardiol.* 1999;34:163–169.
4. Baker DW, Jones R, Hodges J, et al. Management of heart failure. III. The role of revascularization in treatment of patients with moderate or severe left ventricular systolic dysfunction. *JAMA.* 1994;272:1528–1534.
5. Wijns W, Vatner SF, Camici PG. Hibernating myocardium. *N Engl J Med.* 1998;339:173–181.
6. Beller GA. Noninvasive assessment of myocardial viability. *N Engl J Med.* 2000;343:1488–1490.
7. Dilsizian V, Bonow RO. Current diagnostic techniques of assessing viability in patients with hibernating and stunned myocardium. *Circulation.* 1993;87:1–20.
8. Marwick TH. The viable myocardium. Epidemiology, detection, and clinical implications. *Lancet.* 1998;351:815–819.
9. Bax JJ, Wijns W, Cornel JH, et al. Accuracy of currently available techniques for prediction of functional recovery after revascularization in

patients with left ventricular dysfunction due to chronic coronary artery disease: Comparison of pooled data. *J Am Coll Cardiol.* 1997;30:1451–1460.
10. Haas F, Haehnel CJ, Picker W, et al. Preoperative positron emission tomographic viability assessment and perioperative and postoperative risk in patients with advanced ischemic heart disease. *J Am Coll Cardiol.* 1997; 30: 1693–1700.
11. Allman KC, Shaw LJ, Hachamovitch R, Udelson JE. Myocardial viability testing and impact of revascularization on prognosis in patients with coronary artery disease and left ventricular dysfunction: a meta-analysis. *J Am Coll Cardiol.* 2002;39:1151–1158.
12. Bax JJ, Wijns W. FDG imaging to assess myocardial viability: PET, SPECT or gamma camera coincidence imaging? *J Nucl Med.* 1999; 40:1893–1895.
13. Rahimtoola SH. The hibernating myocardium. *Am Heart J.* 1989;117:211–221.
14. Braunwald E, Kloner RA. The stunned myocardium: prolonged post-ischemic ventricular dysfunction. *Circulation.* 1982;66:1146–1148.
15. Schinkel AF, Bax JJ, Boersma E, Elhendy A, Roelandt JRTC, Poldermans D. How many patients with ischemic cardiomyopathy exhibit viable myocardium? *Am J Cardiol.* 2001;88: 561–564.
16. Auerbach MA, Schoder H, Gambhir SS et al. Prevalence of myocardial viability as detected by positron emission tomography in patients with ischemic cardiomyopathy. *Circulation.* 1999;99:2921–2926.
17. Fox KF, Cowie MR, Wood DA, et al. Coronary artery disease as the cause of incident heart failure in the population. *Eur Heart J.* 2001;22: 221–236.
18. Al-Mohammad A, Mahy IR, Norton MY, et al. Prevalence of hibernating myocardium in patients with severely impaired ischaemic left ventricles. *Heart.* 1998;80:559–564.
19. Beanlands RS, DeKemp RA, Smith S, Johansen HL, Ruddy TD. F-18-fluorodeoxyglucose PET imaging alters clinical decision making in patients with impaired ventricular function. *Am J Cardiol.* 1997;79:1092–1095.
20. Bax JJ, Van Eck-Smit BL, van der Wall EE. Assessment of tissue viability: Clinical demand and problems. *Eur Heart J.* 1998;19:847–858.
21. Dilsizian V, Borrow RO. Current diagnostic techniques for assessing myocardial viability in patients with hibernating and stunned myocardium. *Circulation.* 1993;87:1–20.
22. Bonow RO, Dilsizian V. Thallium-201 for assessing myocardial viability. *Semin Nucl Med.* 1991;21:230–241.
23. Cloninger KG, DePuey EG, Garcia E, et al. Incomplete redistribution in delayed thallium-201 single photon emission computed tomography SPECT imaging images: Overestimation of myocardial scarring. *J Am Coll Cardiol.* 1988; 12:955–963.
24. Kiat H, Berman DS, Maddahi J, et al. Late reversibility of tomographic myocardial thallium-201 defects: An accurate marker of myocardial viability. *J Am Coll Cardiol.* 1988; 12:1456–1463.
25. Yang LD, Berman DS, Kiat H, et al. The frequency of late redistribution in SPECT thallium-201 stress-redistribution studies. *J Am Coll Cardiol.* 1990;15:334–340.
26. Dilsizian V, Rocco TP, Freedman NM, Leon MB, Bonow RO. Enhanced detection of ischemic but viable myocardium by the reinjection of thallium after stress-redistribution imaging. *N Engl J Med.* 1990;323:141–146.
27. Bonow RO, Dilsizian V, Cuocolo A, et al. Identification of viable myocardium in patients with coronary artery disease and left ventricular dysfunction: Comparison of thallium scintigraphy with reinjection and PET imaging with ^{18}F-fluorodeoxyglucose. *Circulation.* 1991;83:26–37.
28. Kitsiou AN, Srinivasan G, Quyyumi AA, Summers RM, Bacharach SL, Dilsizian V. Stress-induced reversible and mild-to-moderate irreversible thallium defects: Are they equally accurate for predicting recovery of regional left ventricular function after revascularization? *Circulation.* 1998;98:501–508.
29. Marin-Neto JA, Dilsizian V, Arrighi JA, et al. Thallium scintigraphy compared with 18F-fluorodeoxyglucose positron emission tomography for assessing myocardial viability in patients with moderate versus severe left ventricular dysfunction. *Am J Cardiol.* 1998;82:1001–1007.
30. Dilsizian V, Smeltzer WR, Freedman NM, et al. Thallium reinjection after stress-redistribution imaging: Does 24H delayed imaging following reinjection enhance detection of viable myocardium? *Circulation.* 1991; 83:1247–1255.
31. Bax JJ, Cornel JH, Visser FC, et al. Comparison of fluorine-18-FDG with rest-redistribution thallium-201 SPECT to delineate viable myocardium and predict functional recovery

after revascularization. *J Nucl Med.* 1998;39: 1481–1486.
32. Bax JJ, Visser FC, Van Lingen A, et al. Comparison between 360° and 180° data sampling in thallium-201 rest-redistribution single-photon emission tomography to predict functional recovery after revascularization. *Eur J Nucl Med.* 1997;24:516–522.
33. Wagdy HM, Christian TF, Miller TD, Gibbons RJ. The value of 24-hour images after rest thallium injection. *Nucl Med Commun.* 2002;23:629–637.
34. Matsunari I, Fujino S, Taki J, et al. Significance of late redistribution thallium-201 imaging after rest injection for detection of viable myocardium. *J Nucl Med.* 1997;38:1073–1078.
35. Bonow RO, Dilsizian V. Thallium-201 and technetium-99m-MIBI for assessing viable myocardium. *J Nucl Med.* 1992;33:815–818.
36. Matsunari I, Fujino, Taki J, et al. Quantitative rest technetium-99m tetrofosmin imaging in predicting functional recovery after revascularization: Comparison with rest–redistribution thallium-201. *J Am Coll Cardiol.* 1997;29: 1226–1233.
37. Matsunari I, Böning G, Ziegler SI, et al. Attenuation-corrected ^{99m}Tc-tetrofosmin single-photon emission computed tomography in the detection of viable myocardium: Comparison with positron emission tomography using ^{18}F-fluorodeoxyglucose. *J Am Coll Cardiol.* 1998; 32:927–935.
38. Cuocolo A, Pace L, Ricciardelli B, et al. Identification of viable myocardium in patients with chronic coronary artery disease: comparison of thallium-201 scintigraphy with reinjection and technetium-99m-methoxyisobutyl isonitrile. *J Nucl Med.* 1992;33:505–511.
39. Soufer R, Dey HM, Ng CK, Zaret BL. Comparison of MIBI single-photon emission computed tomography with positron emission tomography for estimating left ventricular myocardial viability. *Am J Cardiol.* 1995;75: 1214–1219.
40. Sawada S, Allman KC, Muzik O, et al. Positron emission tomography detects evidence of viability in rest technetium-99m MIBI defects. *J Am Coll Cardiol.* 1994;23:92–98.
41. Altehoefer C, Vom Dahl J, Biedermann M, et al. Significance of defect severity in technetium-99m-MIBI SPECT at rest to assess myocardial viability: comparison with fluorine-18-FDG PET. *J Nucl Med.* 1994;35:569–574.
42. Schneider CA, Voth E, Gawlich S, et al. Significance of rest technetium-99m sestamibi imaging for the prediction of improvement of left ventricular dysfunction after Q wave myocardial infarction: Importance of infarct location adjusted thresholds. *J Am Coll Cardiol.* 1998;32:648–654.
43. Smanio PE, Watson DD, Segalla DL, Vinson EL, Smith WH, Beller GA. Value of gating of technetium-99m sestamibi single-photon emission computed tomographic imaging. *J Am Coll Cardiol.* 1997;30:1687–1692.
44. Bisi G, Sciagra R, Santoro GM, Fazzini PF. Rest technetium-99m sestamibi tomography in combination with short-term administration of nitrates: Feasibility and reliability for prediction of postrevascularization outcome of asynergic territories. *J Am Coll Cardiol.* 1994;24:1282–1289.
45. Senior R, Kaul S, Raval U, Lahiri A. Impact of revascularization and myocardial viability determined by nitrate-enhanced ^{99m}Tc sestamibi and ^{201}Tl imaging on mortality and functional outcome in ischemic cardiomyopathy. *J Nucl Cardiol.* 2002;9:454–462.
46. Sciagra R, Bisi G, Santoro GM, et al. Comparison of baseline-nitrate technetium-99m sestamibi with rest-redistribution thallium-201 tomography in detecting viable hibernating myocardium and predicting postrevascularization recovery. *J Am Coll Cardiol.* 1997;30: 384–391.
47. Sciagra R, Leoncini M, Marcucci G, et al. Technetium-99m sestamibi imaging to predict left ventricular ejection fraction outcome after revascularization in patients with chronic coronary artery disease and left ventricular dysfunction: comparison between baseline and nitrate-enhanced imaging. *Eur J Nucl Med.* 2001;28:680–687.
48. Batista JF, Pereztol O, Valdes JA, et al. Improved detection of myocardial perfusion reversibility by rest-nitroglycerin ^{99m}Tc-MIBI: Comparison with ^{201}Tl reinjection. *J Nucl Cardiol.* 1999;6:480–486.
49. Oudiz RJ, Smith DE, Pollack AJ, et al. Nitrate-enhanced thallium-201 single photon emission tomography imaging in hibernating myocardium. *Am Heart J.* 1999;138:206–209.
50. Narula J, Dawson MS, Singh BK, et al. Noninvasive characterization of stunned, hibernating, remodeled and nonviable myocardium in ischemic cardiomyopathy. *J Am Coll Cardiol.* 2002;36:1913–1919.
51. Everaert H, Vanhove C, Franken PR. Effects of low-dose dobutamine on left ventricular func-

tion in normal subjects as assessed by gated single-photon emission tomography myocardial perfusion studies. *Eur J Nucl Med.* 1999; 26:1298–1303.

52. Leoncini M, Sciagra R, Bellandi F, et al. Low-dose dobutamine nitrate-enhanced technetium 99m sestamibi gated SPECT versus low-dose dobutamine echocardiography for detecting reversible dysfunction in ischemic cardiomyopathy. *J Nucl Cardiol.* 2002;9:402–406.
53. Bax JJ, Patton JA, Poldermans D, Elhendy A, Sandler MP. 18-Fluorodeoxyglucose imaging with PET and SPECT: Cardiac applications. *Semin Nucl Med.* 2000;30:281–298.
54. Ding HJ, Shiau YC, Wang JJ, Ho ST, Kao A. The influences of blood glucose and duration of fasting on myocardial glucose uptake of [18F]fluoro-2-deoxy-D-glucose. *Nucl Med Commun.* 2002;23:961–965.
55. Martin WH, Jones RC, Delbeke D, et al. A simplified intravenous glucose loading protocol for fluorine-18 fluorodeoxyglucose cardiac single-photon emission tomography. *Eur J Nucl Med.* 1997;24:1291–1297.
56. Knuuti MJ, et al. Euglycemic Hyperinsulinemic Clamp and Oral Glucose-Load in Stimulating Myocardial Glucose-Utilization During Positron Emission Tomography. *J Nucl Med.* 1992;33(7):1255–1262.
57. Knuuti MJ, Yki-J, Rvinen H, Voipio-Pulkki LM, et al. Enhancement of myocardial [fluorine-18] fluorodeoxyglucose uptake by a nicotinic acid derivative. *J Nucl Med.* 1994;35:989–998.
58. Musatti L, Maggi E, Moro E, et al. Bioavailability and pharmacokinetics of acipimox, a new antilipolytic and hypolipidaemic agent. *J Int Med Res.* 1981;9:381–386.
59. Stone CK, et al. Effect of Nicotinic-Acid on Exogenous Myocardial Glucose-Utilization. *J Nucl Med.* 1995;36(6):996–1002.
60. Bax JJ, Veening MA, Visser FC, et al. Optimal metabolic conditions during fluorine-18 fluorodeoxyglucose imaging; a comparative study using different protocols. *Eur J Nucl Med.* 1997;23:35–41.
61. Kam BL, Valkena R, Poldermans D, et al. Feasibility and image quality of dual-isotope SPECT using ^{18}F-FDG and ^{99m}Tc-tetrofosmin after acipimox administration. *J Nucl Med.* 2003;44:140–145.
62. Hasegawa S, Kusuoka H, Uehara T, et al. Glucose tolerance and myocardial ^{18}F fluorodeoxyglucose uptake in normal regions in coronary heart disease patients. *Ann Nucl Med.* 1998;12:363–368.
63. Vom Dahl J, Hermann WH, Hicks RJ, et al. Myocardial glucose uptake in patients with insulin-dependent diabetes mellitus assessed by positron emission tomography. *Circulation.* 1993;88:395–404.
64. Ohtake T, et al. Myocardial Glucose-Metabolism in Noninsulin-Dependent Diabetes-Mellitus Patients Evaluated by FDG-PET. *J Nucl Med.* 1995;36(3):456–463.
65. Vitale GD, et al. Myocardial glucose utilization and optimization of ^{18}F-FDG PET imaging in patients with non-insulin-dependent diabetes mellitus, coronary artery disease, and left ventricular dysfunction. *J Nucl Med.* 2001; 42(12):1730–1736.
66. Marshall RC, Tillisch JH, Phelps ME, et al. Identification and differentiation of resting myocardial ischemia and infarction in man with positron computed tomography, ^{18}F-labeled fluorodeoxyglucose and ^{13}N ammonia. *Circulation.* 1983;67:766–778.
67. Brunken R, Tillish J, Schwaiger M, et al. Regional perfusion, glucose metabolism, and wall motion in patients with chronic electrocardiographic Q wave infarctions: Evidence for persistence of viable tissue in some infarct regions by positron emission tomography. *Circulation.* 1986;73(5):951–963.
68. Brunken R, Schwaiger M, Grover-McKay M, et al. Positron emission tomography detects tissue metabolic activity in myocardial segments with persistent thallium perfusion defects. *J Am Coll Cardiol.* 1987;10:557–567.
69. Van Lingen A, Huijgens PC, Visser FC, et al. Performance characteristics of a 511-keV collimator for imaging positron emitters with a standard gamma-camera. *Eur J Nucl Med.* 1992;19:315–321.
70. Sandler MP, Patton JA. Fluorine 18-labeled fluorodeoxyglucose myocardial single-photon emission computed tomography: An alternative for determining myocardial viability. *J Nucl Cardiol.* 1996;3:342–349.
71. Sandler MP, Videlefsky S, Delbeke D, et al. Evaluation of myocardial ischemia using a rest metabolism/stress perfusion protocol with fluorine-18 deoxyglucose/technetium-99m MIBI and dual-isotope simultaneous-acquisition single-photon emission computed tomography. *J Am Coll Cardiol.* 1995;26:870–888.
72. Delbeke D, Videlefsky SW, Patton JA, Campbell MG, Martin WH, Ohana I, Sandler MP.

Rest myocardial perfusion/metabolism imaging using simultaneous dual-isotope acquisition SPECT with Technetium-99m-MIBI and fluorine-18-FDG. *J Nucl Med.* 1995;36:2110–2119.

73. Sandler MP, Bax JJ, Patton JA, et al. Fluorine-18-fluorodeoxyglucose cardiac imaging using a modified scintillation camera. *J Nucl Med.* 1998;39:2035–2043.
74. Stoll HP, Helwig N, Alexander C, et al. Myocardial metabolic imaging by means of fluorine-18 deoxyglucose/technetium-99m sestamibi dual-isotope single-photon emission tomography. *Eur J Nucl Med.* 1994;21:1085–1093.
75. Burt RW, Perkins OW, Oppenheim BE, et al. Direct comparison of fluorine-18-FDG SPECT, fluorine-18-FDG PET and rest thallium-201 SPECT for the detection of myocardial viability. *J Nucl Med.* 1995;36:176–179.
76. Martin WH, Delbeke D, Patton JA, et al. FDG-SPECT: correlation with FDG-PET. *J Nucl Med.* 1995;36:988–995.
77. Bax JJ, Visser FC, Blanksma PK, et al. Comparison of myocardial uptake of F18-fluorodeoxyglucose imaged with positron emission tomography and single photon emission computed tomography. *J Nucl Med.* 1996;37:1631–1636.
78. Chen EQ, MacIntyre J, Go RT, et al. Myocardial viability studies using fluorine-18-FDG SPECT: A comparison with fluorine-18-FDG PET. *J Nucl Med.* 1997;38:582–586.
79. Srinivasan G, Kitsiou AN, Bacharach SL, Bartlett ML, Miller-Davis C, Dilsizian V. [^{18}F]fluorodeoxyglucose single photon emission computed tomography. Can it replace PET and thallium SPECT for the assessment of myocardial viability? *Circulation.* 1998;97:843–850.
80. Hasegawa S, Uehara T, Yamaguchi H, et al. Validity of ^{18}F fluorodeoxyglucose imaging with a dual-head coincidence gamma camera for detection of myocardial viability. *J Nucl Med.* 1999;40:1884–1892.
81. De Sutter J, de Winter F, Van de Wiele C, et al. Cardiac fluorine-18 fluorodeoxyglucose imaging using a dual-head gamma camera with coincidence detection: A clinical pilot study. *Eur J Nucl Med.* 2000;27:676–685.
82. Nowak B, Zimny M, Schwarz ER, et al. Diagnosis of myocardial viability by dual-head coincidence gamma camera fluorine-18 fluorodeoxyglucose positron emission tomography with and without nonuniform attenuation correction. *Eur J Nucl Med.* 2000;27: 1501–1508.
83. Pagano D, Bonser RS, Townend JN, Ordoubadi F, Lorenzoni R, Camici PG. Predictive value of dobutamine echocardiography and positron emission tomography in identifying hibernating myocardium in patients with postischaemic heart failure. *Heart.* 1998;79:281–288.
84. Tillisch J, Brunken R, Marshall R, et al. Reversibility of cardiac wall-motion abnormalities predicted by positron tomography. *N Engl J Med.* 1986;314:884–888.
85. Marwick TH, MacIntyre WJ, Lafont A, et al. Metabolic responses of hibernating and infarcted myocardium to revascularization. *Circulation.* 1992;85:1347–1353.
86. Gropler RJ, Geltman EM, Sampathkumaran K, et al. Comparison of carbon-11-acetate with fluorine-18-fluorodeoxyglucose for delineating viable myocardium by positron emission tomography. *J Am Coll Cardiol.* 1993;22:1587–1597.
87. Knuuti MJ, Saraste M, Nuutila P, et al. Myocardial viability: Fluorine-18-deoxyglucose PET in prediction of wall motion recovery after revascularization. *Am Heart J.* 1994;127:785–796.
88. Depr C, Vanoverschelde JL, Melin JA, et al. Structural and metabolic correlates of the reversibility of chronic left ventricular ischemic dysfunction in humans. *Am J Physiol.* 1995; 268:H1265–H1275.
89. Tamaki N, Kawamoto M, Tadamura E, et al. Prediction of reversible ischemia after revascularization. Perfusion and metabolic studies with positron emission tomography. *Circulation.* 1995;91:1697–1705.
90. Vom Dahl J, Altehoefer C, Sheehan FH, et al. Recovery of regional left ventricular dysfunction after coronary revascularization. Impact of myocardial viability assessed by nuclear imaging and vessel patency at follow-up angiography. *J Am Coll Cardiol.* 1996;28:948–958.
91. Gerber BL, Vanoverschelde JL, Bol A, et al. Myocardial blood flow, glucose uptake and recruitment of inotropic reserve in chronic left ventricular ischemic dysfunction. Implications for the pathophysiology of chronic hibernation. *Circulation.* 1996;94:651–659.
92. Maes AF, Borgers M, Flameng W, et al. Assessment of myocardial viability in chronic coronary artery disease using technetium-99m sestamibi SPECT. Correlation with histologic and positron emission tomographic studies and functional follow-up. *J Am Coll Cardiol.* 1997; 29:62–68.

93. Vanoverschelde JL, Wijns W, Depre C, et al. Mechanisms of chronic regional postischemic dysfunction in humans. New insights from the study of noninfarcted collateral-dependent myocardium. *Circulation.* 1993;87:1513–1523.
94. Baer FM, Voth E, Deutsch HJ, Schneider CA, et al. Predictive value of low dose dobutamine transesophageal echocardiography and fluorine-18 fluorodeoxyglucose PET for recovery of regional left ventricular function after successful revascularization. *J Am Coll Cardiol.* 1996;28:60–69.
95. Bax JJ, Visser FC, Elhendy A, et al. Prediction of improvement of regional left ventricular function after revascularization using different perfusion-metabolism criteria. *J Nucl Med.* 1999;40:1866–1873.
96. Knuuti MJ, Nuutila P, Ruotsalainen U, et al. The value of quantitative analysis of glucose utilization in detection of myocardial viability by PET. *J Nucl Med.* 1993;34:2068–2075.
97. Fath-Ordoubadi F, Pagano D, Marinho NVS, Keogh BE, Bonser RS, Camici PG. Coronary revascularization in the treatment of moderate and severe postischemic left ventricular dysfunction. *Am J Cardiol.* 1998;82:26–31.
98. Knapp FF Jr, Kropp J. Iodine—123 labeled fatty acids for myocardial single-photon emission tomography: current status and future perspectives. *Eur J Nucl Med.* 1995;22:361–381.
99. Kawai Y, Tsukamoto E, Nozaki Y, et al. Significance of reduced uptake of iodinated fatty acid analogue for the evaluation of patients with chest pain. *J Am Coll Cardiol.* 2001;38: 1888–1894.
100. Matsuki T, Takano M, Iwata M, et al. Prognostic significance of normal BMIPP imaging in patients with angina pectoris without prior myocardial infarction: comparison with stress myocardial perfusion imaging. *J Nucl Med.* 2002;43(Suppl):143P.
101. Kawamoto M, Tamaki N, Yonekura Y, et al. Combined study with ^{123}I fatty acid and thallium-201 to assess ischemic myocardium. *Ann Nucl Med.* 1994;8:47–54.
102. Tamaki N, Tadamua E, Kawamoto M, et al. Decreased uptake of iodinated branched fatty acid analog indicated metabolic alterations in ischemic myocardium. *J Nucl Med.* 1995;36: 1974–1980.
103. Fukuzawa S, Ozawa S, Shimada K, et al. Prognostic values of perfusion-metabolic mismatch in ^{201}Tl and BMIPP scintigraphic imaging in patients with chronic coronary artery disease and left ventricular dysfunction undergoing revascularization. *Ann Nucl Med.* 2002;16:109–115.
104. Bax JJ, Poldermans D, Elhendy A, Boersma E, Rahimtoola SH. Sensitivity, specificity, and predictive accuracies of various noninvasive techniques for detecting hibernating myocardium. *Curr Probl Cardiol.* 2001;26:142–186.
105. Poldermans D, Rambaldi R, Bax JJ, et al. Safety and utility of atropine addition during dobutamine stress echocardiography for the assessment of viable myocardium in patients with severe left ventricular dysfunction. *Eur Heart J.* 1998;19:1712–1718.
106. Van der Wall EE, Bax JJ. Current clinical relevance of cardiovascular magnetic resonance and its relationship to nuclear cardiology. *J Nucl Cardiol.* 1999;6:462–469.
107. Baer FM, Theissen P, Schneider CA, Voth E, Sechtem U, Schicha H, Erdmann E. Dobutamine magnetic resonance imaging predicts contractile recovery of chronically dysfunctional myocardium after successful revascularization. *J Am Coll Cardiol.* 1998;31:1040–1048.
108. Baer FM, Crnac J, Schmidt M, et al. Magnetic resonance pharmacological stress for detecting coronary disease. Comparison with echocardiography. *Herz.* 2000;25:400–408.
109. Kim RJ, Wu E, Rafael A, et al. The use of contrast-enhanced magnetic resonance imaging to identify reversible myocardial dysfunction. *N Engl J Med.* 2000;343:1445–1453.
110. Klein C, Nekolla SG, Bengel FM, et al. Assessment of myocardial viability with contrast-enhanced magnetic resonance imaging: Comparison with Positron emission tomography. *Circulation.* 2002;105:162.
111. Bax JJ, Maddahi J, Poldermans D, et al. Sequential ^{201}Tl imaging and dobutamine echocardiography to enhance accuracy of predicting improved left ventricular ejection fraction after revascularization. *J Nucl Med.* 2002;43:795–802.
112. Bax JJ, Visser FC, Poldermans D, et al. Relationship between preoperative viability and postoperative improvement in LVEF and heart failure symptoms. *J Nucl Med.* 2001;42:79–86.
113. Dreyfus GD, Duboc D, Blasco A, et al. Myocardial viability assessment in ischemic cardiomyopathy: benefits of coronary revascularization. *Ann Thorac Surg.* 1994;57:1402–1408.
114. Marwick TH, Zuchowski C, Lauer MS, Secknus MA, Williams MJ, Lytle BW. Functional status and quality of life in patients with heart failure undergoing coronary bypass surgery after

assessment of myocardial viability. *J Am Coll Cardiol.* 1999;33:750–758.
115. Beanlands RS, Hendry PJ, Masters RG, et al. Delay in revascularization is associated with increased mortality rate in patients with severe left ventricular dysfunction and viable myocardium on fluorine 18-fluorordeoxyglucose positron emission tomography. *Circulation.* 1998;98:II-51–II-56.
116. Schwarz ER, Schoendube FA, Kostin S, et al. Prolonged myocardial hibernation exacerbates cardiomyocyte degeneration and impairs recovery of function after revascularization. *J Am Coll Cardiol.* 1998;31:1018–1026.
117. Gunning MG, Chua TP, Harrington D, et al. Hibernating myocardium: Clinical and functional response to revascularisation. *Eur J Cardio-Thorac Surg.* 1997;11:1105–1112.
118. DiCarli MF, Asgarzadie F, Schelbert HR, et al. Quantitative relation between myocardial viability and improvement in heart failure symptoms after revascularization in patients with ischemic cardiomyopathy. *Circulation.* 1995;92: 3436–3444.
119. Marwick TH, Nemec JJ, Lafont A, Salcedo EE, MacIntyre WJ. Prediction by postexercise fluoro-18 deoxyglucose positron emission tomography of improvement in exercise capacity after revascularization. *Am J Cardiol.* 1992; 69:854–859.
120. Eitzman D, Al-Aouar ZR, Kanter HL, et al. Clinical outcome of patients with advanced coronary artery disease after viability studies with positron emission tomography. *J Am Coll Cardiol.* 1992;20:559–565.
121. Di Carli M, Davidson M, Little R, et al. Value of metabolic imaging with positron emission tomography for evaluating prognosis in patients with coronary artery disease and left ventricular dysfunction. *Am J Cardiol.* 1994;73: 527–533.
122. vom Dahl J, Altehoefer C, Sheehan FH, et al. Effect of myocardial viability assessed by technetium-99m-sestamibi SPECT and fluorine-18-FDG PET on clinical outcome in coronary artery disease. *J Nucl Med.* 1997;38:742–748.
123. Yoshida K, Gould KL. Quantitative relation of myocardial infarct size and myocardial viability by positron emission tomography to left ventricular ejection fraction and 3-year mortality with and without revascularization. *J Am Coll Cardiol.* 1993;22:984–987.
124. Lee KS, Marwick TH, Cook SA, et al. Prognosis of patients with left ventricular dysfunction, with and without viable myocardium after myocardial infarction. Relative efficacy of medical therapy and revascularization. *Circulation.* 1994;90:2687–2694.
125. Pagano D, Lewis ME, Townend JN, Davies P, Camici PG, Bonser RS. Coronary revascularization for postischemic heart failure: How myocardial viability affects survival. *Heart.* 1999;82:684–688.
126. Tamaki N, Kawamoto M, Takahashi N, et al. Prognostic value of an increase in fluorine-18 deoxyglucose uptake in patients with myocardial infarction: comparison with stress thallium imaging. *J Am Coll Cardiol.* 1993;22:1621–1627.
127. Gioia G, Powers J, Heo J, Iskandrian AS. Prognostic value of rest-redistribution tomographic thallium-201 imaging in ischemic cardiomyopathy. *Am J Cardiol.* 1995;75:759–762.
128. Pagley PR, Beller GA, Watson DD, Gimple LW, Ragosta M. Improved outcome after coronary bypass surgery in patients with ischemic cardiomyopathy and residual myocardial viability. *Circulation.* 1997;96:793–800.
129. Zafrir N, Leppo JA, Reinhardt CP, Dahlberg ST. Thallium reinjection versus standard stress/delay redistribution imaging for prediction of cardiac events. *J Am Coll Cardiol.* 1998;31: 1280–1285.
130. Cuocolo A, Petretta M, Nicolai E, et al. Successful coronary revascularization improves prognosis in patients with previous myocardial infarction and evidence of viable myocardium at thallium-201 imaging. *Eur J Nucl Med.* 1998; 25:60–68.
131. Chaudhry FA, Tauke JT, Alessandrini RS, et al. Prognostic implications of myocardial contractile reserve in patients with coronary artery disease and left ventricular dysfunction. *J Am Coll Cardiol.* 1999;34:730–738.
132. Senior R, Kaul S, Lahiri A. Myocardial viability on echocardiography predicts long-term survival after revascularization in patients with ischemic congestive heart failure. *J Am Coll Cardiol.* 1999;33:1848–1854.
133. Afridi I, Grayburn PA, Panza J, Oh JK, Zoghbi WA, Marwick TH. Myocardial viability during dobutamine echocardiography predicts survival in patients with coronary artery disease and severe left ventricular systolic dysfunction. *J Am Coll Cardiol.* 1998;32:921–926.
134. Meluzin J, Cerny J, Frelich M, et al. Prognostic value of the amount of dysfunctional but viable myocardium in revascularized patients with

coronary artery disease and left ventricular dysfunction. *J Am Coll Cardiol.* 1998;32:912–920.

135. Williams MJ, Odabashian J, Laurer MS, Thomas JD, Marwick TH. Prognostic value of dobutamine echocardiography in patients with left ventricular dysfunction. *J Am Coll Cardiol.* 1996;27:132–139.
136. Elasser A, Schlepper M, Klovekorn WP, et al. Hibernating myocardium, an incomplete adaptation to ischemia. *Circulation.* 1997;96:2920–2931.
137. Schwartz ER, Schaper J, vom Dahl J, et al. Myocyte degeneration and cell death in hibernating human myocardium. *J Am Coll Cardiol* 1996;27:1577–1585.
138. DiCarli MF. Assessment of myocardial viability after myocardial infarction. *J Nucl Cardiol.* 2002;9:229–235.
139. Louie HW, Laks H, Milgalter E, et al. Ischemic cardiomyopathy. Criteria for coronary revascularization and cardiac transplantation. *Circulation.* 1991;84:III290–III295.
140. Yamagushi A, Ino T, Adachi H, et al. Left ventricular volume predicts postoperative course in patients with ischemic cardiomyopathy. *Ann Thorac Surg.* 1998;65:434–438.
141. Bacharach SL, Bax JJ, Case J, et al. PET myocardial glucose metabolism and perfusion imaging: Part 1-Guidelines for data acquisition and patient preparation. *J Nucl Cardiol.* 2003; 10(5):543–556.
142. Schelbert HR, Beanlands R, Bengel F, et al. PET myocardial perfusion and glucose metabolism imaging: Part 2-Guidelines for interpretation and reporting. *J Nucl Cardiol.* 2003;10(5): 557–571.
143. Pagano D, Townend JN, Little WA, et al. Coronary artery bypass surgery as treatment for ischemic heart failure: The predictive value of viability assessment with quantitative positron emission tomography for symptomatic and functional outcome. *J Thorac Cardiovasc Surg.* 1998;115:791–799.
144. Bax JJ, Visser FC, Poldermans D, et al. Long-term prognostic value of FDG SPECT in patients with ischaemic left ventricular dysfunction. *Eur Heart J.* 1999;20:257 [Abstract].
145. Wijffels E, Wijns W, Verheye S, et al. Prognostic value of FDG imaging using SPECT in patients with severe left ventricular dysfunction. *J Am Coll Cardiol.* 1999;33:416A, [Abstract].
146. Coronary artery surgery study (CASS): A randomized trial of coronary bypass surgery. Survival data. *Circulation.* 1983;68:939–950.
147. Harwick TH. The viable myocardium: epidemiology, detection, and clinical implications. *Lancet.* 1998;351:815–819.
148. Cornel JH, Bax JJ, Elhendy A, Visser FC, Boersma E, Poldermans D, Sloof GW, Fioretti PM. Agreement and disagreement between "metabolic viability" and "contractile reserve" in akinetic myocardium. *J Nucl Cardiol.* 1999;6: 383–388.
149. Chan RK, Lee KJ, Calafiore P, Berlangieri SU, McKay WJ, Tonkin AM. Comparison of dobutamine echocardiography and positron emission tomography in patients with chronic ischemic left ventricular dysfunction. *J Am Coll Cardiol.* 1996;27:1601–1607.
150. Zamorano J, Delgado J, Almeria C, et al. Reason for discrepancies in identifying myocardial viability by thallium-201 redistribution, magnetic resonance imaging and dobutamine echocardiography. *Am J Cardiol.* 2002;90:455–459.
151. Zamorano JL, Delgado J, Almeria C, et al. Assessment of cardiac viability by thallium-201 redistribution and dobutamine echocardiography. *Am Heart J.* 2002;143:157–162.
152. Pagano D, Bonser DS, Townend JN, Parums D, Camici PG. Histopathological correlates of dobutamine echocardiography in hibernating myocardium. *Circulation.* 1996;94:I-543 [abstract].
153. Baumgartner H, Porenta G, Lau YK, et al. Assessment of myocardial viability by dobutamine echocardiography, positron emission tomography and thallium-201 SPECT: Correlation with histopathology in explanted hearts. *J Am Coll Cardiol.* 1998;32:1701–1708.
154. Ricciardi MJ, Wu E, Davidson CJ, et al. Visualization of discrete microinfarction after percutaneous coronary intervention associated with mild creatine kinase-MB elevation. *Circulation.* 2001;103:2780–2783.
155. Bax JJ, Visser FC, Poldermans D, et al. Prognostic value of perfusion-FDG mismatch in ischemic cardiomyopathy. *J Nucl Cardiol.* 2002; 9:675–677.

9
Myocardial Perfusion Imaging for Cardiac Risk Stratification

Sean W. Hayes, Daniel S. Berman, Rory Hachamovitch, and Guido Germano

Coronary artery disease (CAD) is the number one cause of death for both men and women in the United States, causing 1 out of every 5 deaths.[1] Stress single photon emission computed tomography (SPECT) myocardial perfusion scintigraphy (MPS) has been shown to effectively stratify risk of patients for cardiac death and nonfatal myocardial infarction (MI). At our institution, we advocate a semiquantitative scoring system to standardize the visual interpretation of stress MPS scans, providing semiquantitative global indices for overall assessment of extent and severity of perfusion abnormality.[2,3] This approach is more systematic and reproducible than simple qualitative evaluation.

Twenty-Segment Model

A 20-segment scoring method, first developed at Cedars-Sinai Medical Center, is based on three short-axis slices [distal (apical), mid, and basal] representing the entire left ventricle (LV), with the 2 apical segments visualized in a midvertical long-axis image. Each of the 20 segments has a distinct name and is scored using a 5 point system (0 = normal, 4 = absence of detectable tracer uptake).[2,3] Severe perfusion defects with scores of 3 or 4 can be reported as consistent with a critical (≥90 percent) coronary stenosis.[4]

Seventeen-Segment Model

A 17-segment scoring system is now recommended by the American Heart Association, American College of Cardiology, and the American Society for Nuclear Cardiology (AHA, ACC, and ASNC).[5,6] The only differences from the 20-segment model are that the smaller size of the distal short-axis slice is accounted for by 4 instead of 6 segments and the apex is 1 segment instead of 2 segments. For laboratories interested in converting from 20- to 17-segment systems, an approach has been developed and preliminarily validated.[7]

Summed Scores

Segmental scoring systems lend themselves to the derivation of summed scores from the 17 to 20 segments (i.e., global indices of perfusion).[3] The overall extent and severity of perfusion defects are reflected by the summed stress score (SSS), the summed rest score (SRS), and the summed differences score (SDS), the latter defined as SSS-SRS and representing an index of the degree of reversibility. For the 20-segment model, risk groups have been defined using SSS categories with SSS of 0 to 3 being normal; 4 to 8 mildly abnormal; 9 to 13 moderately abnormal; and >13 severely abnormal.[7–9]

Percent Myocardium

More recently, we have shifted to a segmental scoring system that reports a semiquantitative estimation of the % myocardium involved, hence expressing overall perfusion defects as % stress, % reversible, and % fixed. This is accomplished by dividing the summed scores by the worst segmental score possible (80 for 20 segments; 68 for 17 segments).[10] The benefits of this approach include the following: It provides a measure with intuitive implications (% myocardium hypoperfused), not possible with the unit-less summed scores; it can easily be applied (yielding numerically equivalent values) to scoring systems that use different numbers of segments (e.g., 20, 17, 13); and it is applicable to quantitative methods that directly measure these abnormalities as % myocardium. Risk groups by % stress abnormal that correlate with the established SSS risk groups are <5% (normal or minimally abnormal), 5% to 9% (mildly abnormal), 10% to 14% (moderately abnormal), and ≥15% (severely abnormal).[11,12]

Polar Maps

A variety of commercially available software packages are available to assist in image interpretation.[13] These computer approaches generally operate by automatic determination of the amount of radioactivity at rest and stress within each pixel or small zone of the myocardium, scaling this amount by the maximal amount of radioactivity in the myocardium (normalization), and then comparing this scaled amount to the lower limit of normal. The change between rest and stress is usually also assessed, and compared with normal, providing information about perfusion defect reversibility. The results are most commonly displayed using polar maps.

Because these computer-based quantitative programs do not take into account artifacts that may be easily detected visually (such as marked breast attenuation), it is generally recommended that they be used as a *second expert* opinion, with the principal and final interpretation based on the visual assessment.

Case Presentations

Case 9.1

History

A 71-year-old man with a history of hypertension and hypercholesterolemia presented with typical angina. He was referred for exercise MPS. He exercised for 8:52 minutes to a heart rate (HR) of 133 (89% of maximum predicted HR [MPHR]). The clinical response was ischemic with chest discomfort occurring at 8 minutes into exercise. The stress ECG was also ischemic with 3.1 mm downsloping ST-segment depression in lead V6. The supine dual-isotope rest ^{201}Tl/stress ^{99m}Tc-MIBI MPS images as well as the quantitative perfusion SPECT (QPS) analysis are displayed in Figures C9-1A and C9-1B, respectively.

Findings

The MPS images demonstrate a large reversible defect in the anterior, septal, and apical walls in the left anterior descending (LAD) distribution; there is also a large reversible defect in the inferior and inferoseptal walls in the right coronary artery (RCA) distribution. Based on the summed perfusion index scores, the % stress, % reversible, and % fixed myocardial defects were 36%, 36%, and 0%, respectively. Transient ischemic dilation (TID) is seen in the left ventricle, which is a marker for severe and extensive CAD. On the gated SPECT images (not shown) there was evidence of stunning, with the post-stress left

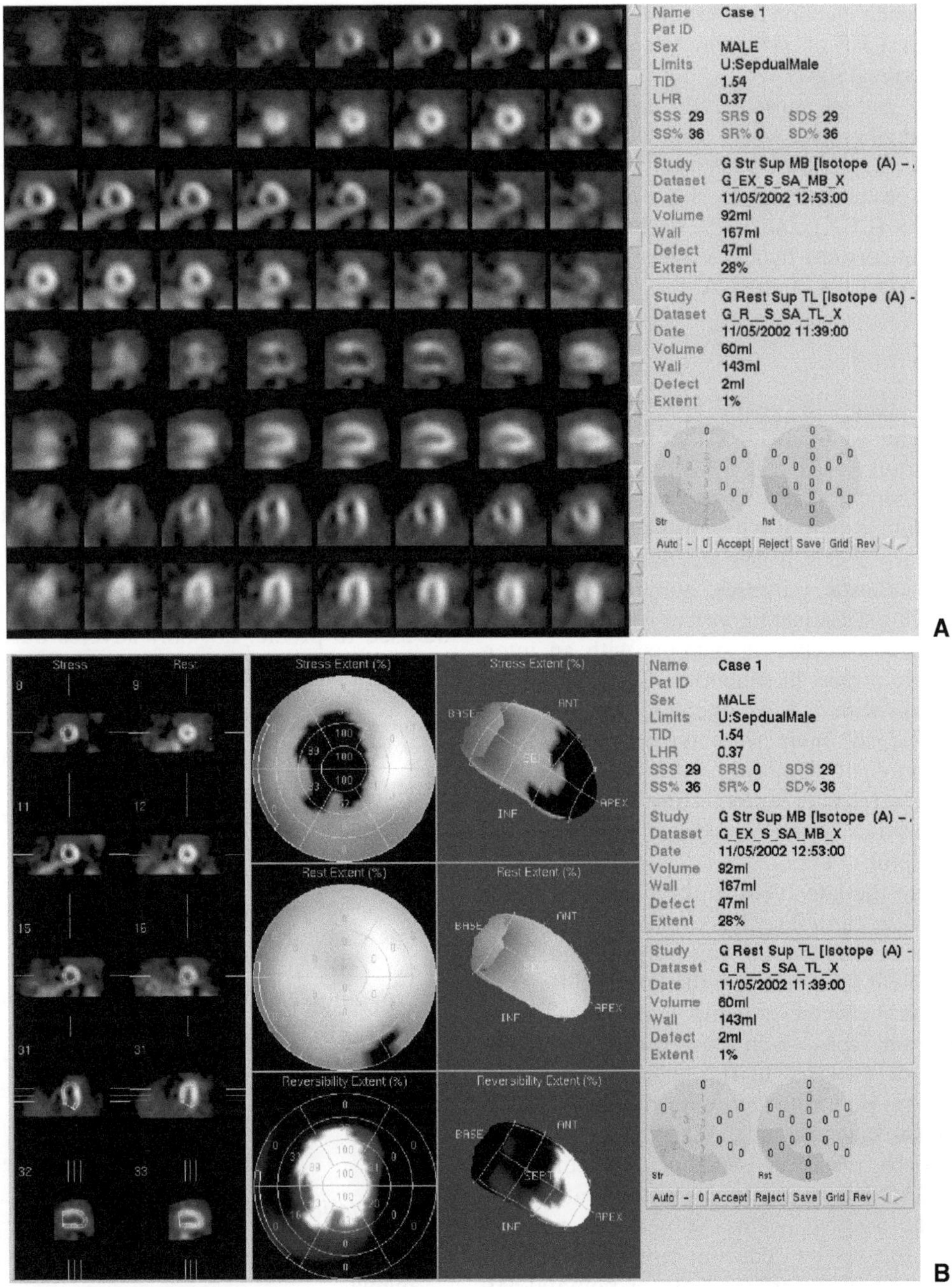

FIGURE C9-1. (A and B)

ventricular ejection fraction (EF) of 46% worse than rest EF of 53%, which is also consistent with critical CAD.

The patient subsequently underwent coronary angiography, which revealed severe triple-vessel disease, with a subtotal proximal LAD, 100% occluded diagonal, 90% occluded left circumflex (LCX), and 100% occluded RCA. He then underwent bypass surgery with grafts to the LAD, LCX, and RCA.

Discussion

More than 20 years ago, Diamond and Forrester[14] demonstrated that the likelihood of significant CAD can be estimated based on age, gender, and symptom presentation determined before stress testing. In the 1970s and early 1980s, it was widely advocated that for diagnostic purposes, noninvasive testing, including stress testing with or without imaging, would be effective in patients with an intermediate pretest likelihood of CAD, but not in patients with a high likelihood of CAD. In this elderly man with typical angina, the likelihood of significant CAD was very high before referral to stress testing, so for diagnostic purposes testing would not be expected to be helpful.

From the late 1980s to the present, the role of nuclear cardiology has expanded to the area of risk assessment. For this purpose, the greatest benefit from testing—the largest difference in risk between patients with normal and abnormal scans—is in those with a high likelihood of CAD.[3,15] In this elderly gentleman, MPS was performed more for risk stratification than for diagnosis of CAD. With a risk-based approach, the focus is not on predicting who has CAD but on identifying patients at risk for specific adverse events. Subsequent management focuses on reducing risk of these outcomes, whether cardiac death or nonfatal MI. Invasive diagnostic and therapeutic procedures are limited to those patients who are most likely to benefit from them.

Hachamovitch et al.[9] have previously demonstrated that stress MPS effectively risk stratifies patients for cardiac events. In a study looking at over 5,000 patients, the rates for both myocardical infarction (MI) and cardiac death were found to increase significantly with worsening scan abnormalities (Table 9-1).

Table 9-1. Rates of Cardiac Death and Myocardial Infarction as a Function of Perfusion Results in 5000 Patients

Summed Stress Score (SSS)	Annual Event Rate (%)	
	Myocardial Infarction	Cardiac Death
<4 (normal)	0.5	0.3
4–8 (mildly abnormal)	2.7	0.8
9–13 (moderately abnormal)	2.9	2.3
>13 (severely abnormal)	4.2	2.9

Data from Hachamovitch R, Berman DS, Shaw LJ, et al. (9). *Circulation*.

More recently, Hachamovitch et al.[10] demonstrated that the extent of ischemia can further be used to predict not only adverse outcome, but also which patients will benefit from revascularization compared with medical management.

The SSS of 29 (36% stress defect) in this patient signifies a very high risk for cardiac events. Since the defect was entirely reversible (36% reversible defect, 0% fixed), coronary angiography was indicated as performed above. The presence of TID and stunning in this case, along with the severe extensive defects, all would lead to the prediction of severe multivessel disease as was found on angiography. Based on the extensive reversibility, one would also predict that the patient's survival would be improved by successful revascularization.

Interpretation

1. Presentation: elderly man with typical angina.
2. Exercise MPS: ischemic clinical and ECG responses, large reversible defect in LAD distribution, large reversible defect in RCA distribution, TID, stunning.
3. Coronary angiography: severe 3-vessel disease.

Case 9.2

History

A 74-year-old man with a history of diabetes and smoking presented with shortness of breath. He was referred for adenosine MPS. The resting ECG demonstrated right bundle branch block. The ECG response to adenosine stress was nondiagnostic secondary to right bundle branch block. The supine and prone dual-isotope rest ^{201}Tl/stress ^{99m}Tc-MIBI MPS images in the supine and prone positions are displayed in Figures C9-2A and C9-2B, respectively and the QPS analysis in Figure C9-2C.

Findings

The MPS images demonstrate normal stress myocardial perfusion. Based on the summed perfusion index scores, the % stress, % reversible, and % fixed myocardial defects were 0%, 0%, and 0%, respectively. There was TID, however, which is a marker for severe and extensive CAD. In addition, on the gated SPECT images (not shown) there was evidence of stunning, with the post-stress EF of 36% worse than rest EF of 60%, which is also consistent with critical CAD. The patient subsequently underwent coronary angiography, which revealed severe triple vessel disease, with a 75% proximal LAD, 50% mid LCX, 90% first obtuse marginal (OM1), and 75% mid-RCA stenoses. He then underwent angioplasty with stent insertion of the LAD and OM1.

Discussion

Assessing the amount of stress-induced ischemia and the post-stress EF can enhance the prediction of cardiac death and nonfatal MI. In a study by Sharir et al.,[16] 2,686 patients underwent dual isotope rest ^{201}Tl/stress ^{99m}Tc-MIBI MPS. By Cox regression analysis, the most powerful predictor of cardiac death was the post-stress EF, whereas the most powerful

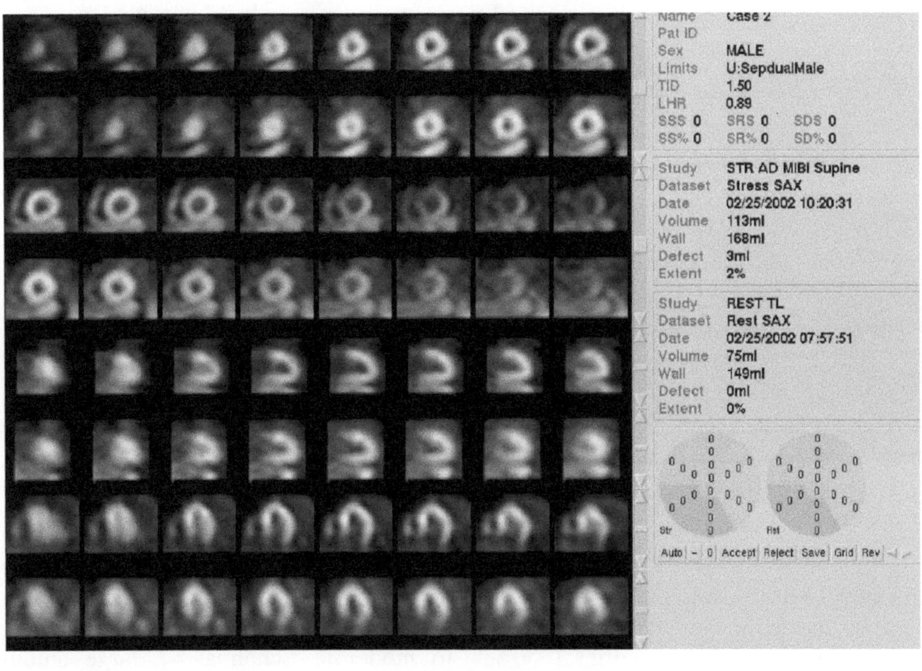

A

FIGURE C9-2. (A)

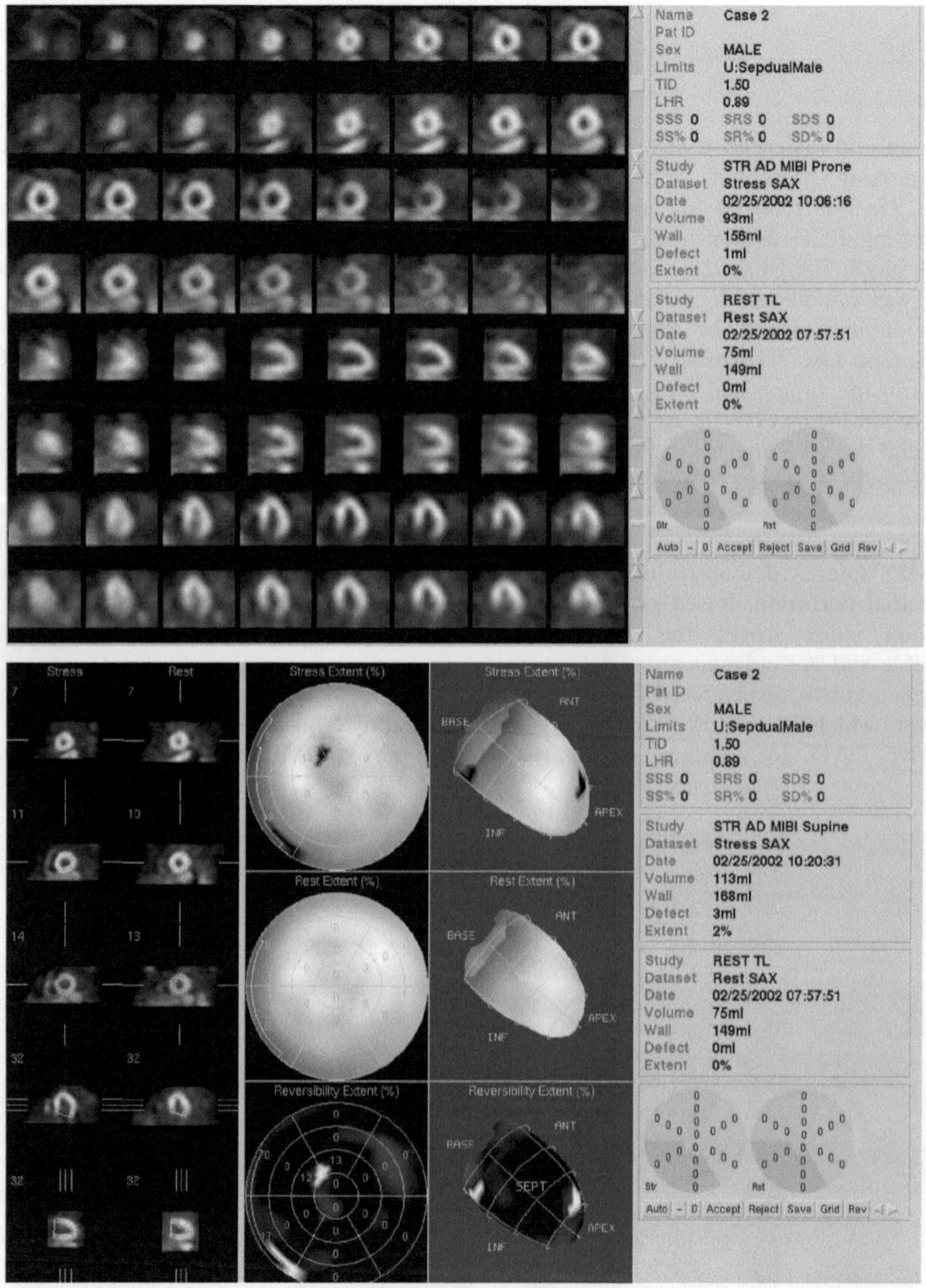

FIGURE C9-2. (B and C)

predictor of MI was the amount of ischemia as measured by the SDS. Patients were divided into subsets based on EF categories (>50%, normal; 30% to 50%, mild to moderate LV dysfunction; <30%, severe LV dysfunction) and SDS categories (0 to 1, no ischemia; 2 to 7, mild to moderate ischemia; >7, large amount of ischemia), which allowed patients to be divided into low- (<1%/year), intermediate- (1% to 3%/ year), and high-risk (>3%/year) subgroups for cardiac death. Patients with EF >50% were at low risk for cardiac death, unless they had a large amount of ischemia (SDS > 7), which put them in the intermediate risk group (2% to 3%/year). Patients with EF 30% to 50% and SDS ≥2 were intermediate risk. Patients with EF <30% were high risk regardless of the amount of ischemia.

Although the patient in this case would have been identified as low risk based on EF 30% to 50% and no ischemia (SDS 0 to 1), the presence of shortness of breath and diabetes are high risk markers of increased risk of cardiac death in patients undergoing adenosine stress MPS.[17] In spite of normal myocardial perfusion and normal resting left ventricular function, the presence of TID and stunning raised the possibility of balanced reduction in flow during adenosine stress. This was confirmed on angiography, which revealed triple-vessel disease. The study points out the need for taking into account the nonnuclear and nonperfusion SPECT results when applying MPS for purposes of risk-stratification and guiding clinical management decisions.[18]

Interpretation

1. Presentation: elderly diabetic man with shortness of breath.
2. Adenosine MPS: nondiagnostic ECG response, normal myocardial perfusion, TID, stunning.
3. Coronary angiography: severe 3-vessel disease.

Case 9.3

History

A 67-year-old woman with a history of hypertension, insulin-requiring diabetes, and hypercholesterolemia presented with shortness of breath and nonanginal chest pain. She was referred for adenosine MPS. The resting ECG demonstrated poor R wave progression and possible lateral MI. The baseline and end of adenosine infusion HR and blood pressure (BP) were 84 vs. 93 bpm and 150/70 vs. 138/66 mmHg, respectively. The clinical and ECG responses to adenosine stress were nonischemic. The supine dual-isotope rest ^{201}Tl/stress ^{99m}Tc-MIBI MPS images as well as the QPS analysis are displayed in Figures C9-3A and C9-3B, respectively.

Findings

The MPS images demonstrate, in the LAD distribution, a small to medium sized reversible defect in the anteroapical and distal anterior walls; and in the LCX distribution, a small to medium sized reversible defect in the distal lateral wall. Based on the summed perfusion index scores, the % stress, % reversible, and % fixed myocardial defects were 10%, 9%, and 1%, respectively. In addition, on the gated SPECT images (not shown) there was evidence of stunning, with the post-stress EF of 57% worse than rest EF of 64% and new post-stress wall motion abnormalities in the distal lateral wall, which is consistent with critical CAD. The patient subsequently underwent coronary angiography, which revealed a subtotal left main stenosis. She then underwent bypass surgery with grafts to the LAD and OM1.

Discussion

Patients undergoing adenosine stress are known to be higher risk than patients who are able to undergo exercise stress.[9] Berman et al.[11] designed a study to assess the incremental prognostic value of adenosine stress MPS in women versus men, and to explore the prognostic value impact of diabetes mellitus. Consecutive patients (n = 6,173) who underwent rest ^{201}Tl/adenosine ^{99m}Tc-MIBI MPS were followed for 27.0 ± 8.8 months. The cardiac death rates were lower in women than men (2.0%/year vs. 2.7%/year, respectively, $p < 0.05$). Even after risk adjustment, cardiac death risk

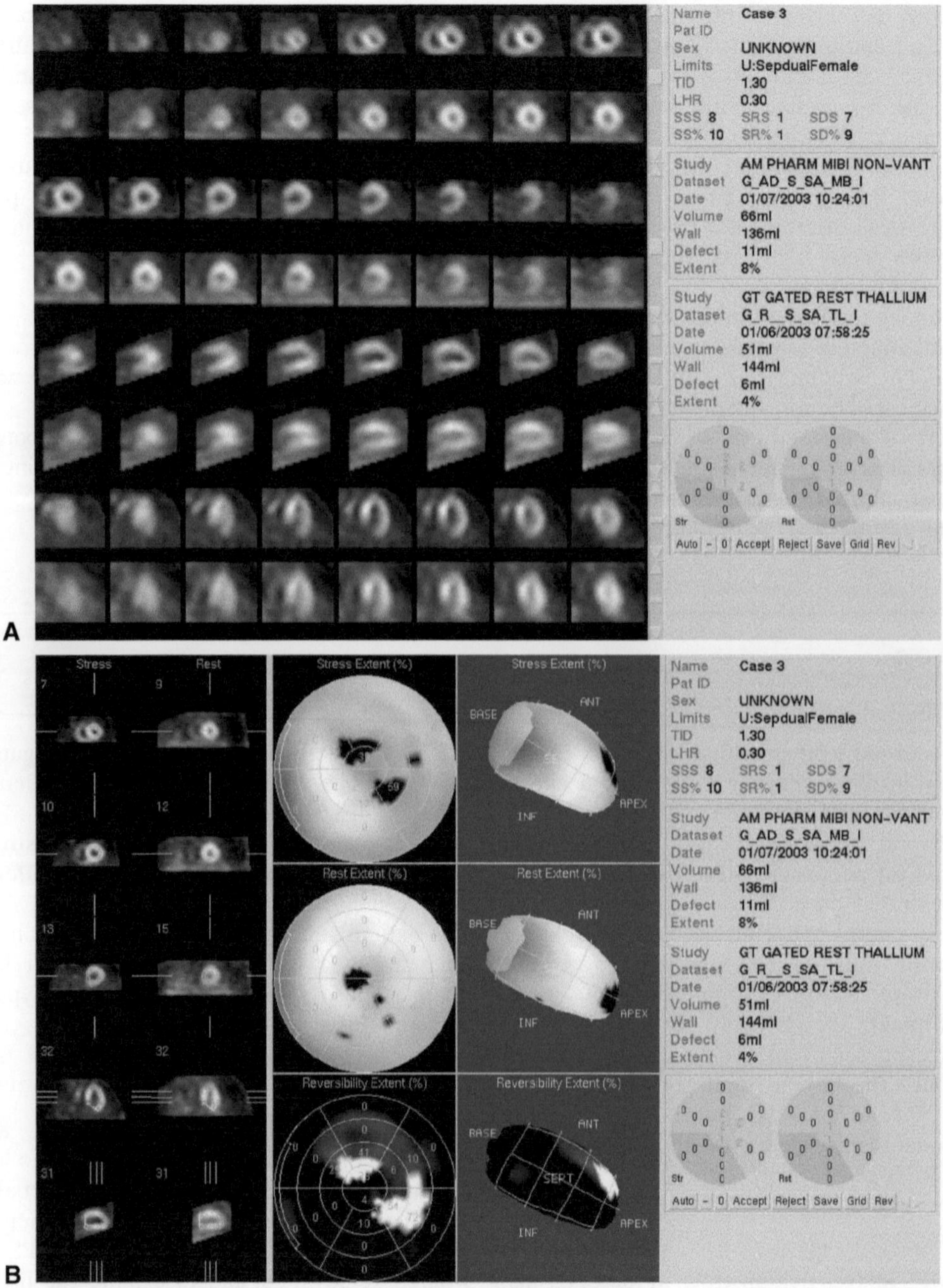

FIGURE C9-3. (A and B)

increased significantly in both men and women as a function of MPS results. One important finding was that diabetic women had a significantly greater risk of cardiac death over nondiabetic women as well as diabetic men. A second finding was that for any MPS result, diabetic patients requiring insulin were higher risk for cardiac death than diabetic patients not requiring insulin. The patient in this case had an SSS of 8 (mildly abnormal), but in a diabetic woman undergoing adenosine stress, this MPS result predicted a high cardiac mortality of 3.3%/year.

Until recently, the prognostic importance of the hemodynamic response to adenosine infusion in patients undergoing adenosine stress MPS was not known. Abidov et al.[19] identified 3,444 patients older than age 55 years who underwent adenosine (without low-level treadmill exercise) stress MPS. Two hundred twenty-four cardiac deaths occurred during follow-up of 2.0 ± 0.8 years. Peak HR was defined as the HR at the end of adenosine infusion. Both high rest HR and to a lesser extent low peak HR were markers of cardiac death. In multivariable analysis, peak/rest HR ratio was an independent predictor of cardiac death, with the highest cardiac mortality in patients with the lowest ratios. Patients whose peak HR increased less than 12% over the resting HR (peak/rest HR ratio <1.12) were at the highest risk. In addition, peak/rest HR ratio further risk stratified patients within MPS categories.

The patient in this case had a low peak/rest HR ratio of 93/84 = 1.11 and thus provides another high-risk marker for cardiac death. Hachamovitch et al.[17] have developed an adenosine prognostic score that incorporates all the known high-risk markers in patients undergoing adenosine stress MPS (age, diabetes, shortness of breath, rest HR, peak HR, rest ECG, % myocardium ischemic, and % myocardium fixed). Although this score would be cumbersome for the busy clinician to calculate on a regular basis, the score can be automated as part of a reporting program, making the routine reporting of predicted risks feasible.

Interpretation

1. Presentation: Diabetic woman with shortness of breath and nonanginal chest pain.
2. Adenosine MPS: nonischemic ECG response, small to medium size reversible defects in both the LAD and LCX distributions, stunning.
3. Coronary angiography: subtotal left main stenosis.

Case 9.4

History

A 71-year-old woman with hypertension was referred for adenosine MPS for evaluation of typical angina. The resting ECG showed early repolarization abnormality. The stress ECG revealed no ST-segment depression. Both the clinical and ECG response to adenosine stress were nonischemic. The supine dual-isotope rest ^{201}Tl/stress ^{99m}Tc-MIBI MPS images as well as the QPS analysis are displayed in Figures C9-4A and C9-4B, respectively.

Findings

The MPS images demonstrate normal myocardial perfusion. Based on the summed perfusion index scores, the % stress, % reversible, and % fixed myocardial defects were 0%, 0%, and 0%, respectively. On the post-adenosine stress gated SPECT images (not shown) there was normal left ventricular wall motion with an EF of 64%.

Discussion

The normal summed stress score (SSS ≤ 3) suggests a low risk for cardiac death or MI.[9] In this elderly woman with typical angina, the likelihood of significant obstructive CAD is intermediate, but the likelihood of a cardiac event (cardiac death or MI) is <1%/year. Unless her symptoms are intractable, given her good prognosis, she would be an excellent candidate for aggressive medical therapy.

Previously, patients with a high likelihood of having significant CAD were often considered already risk stratified and thus sent directly to angiography. Hachamovitch et al.[15] evaluated

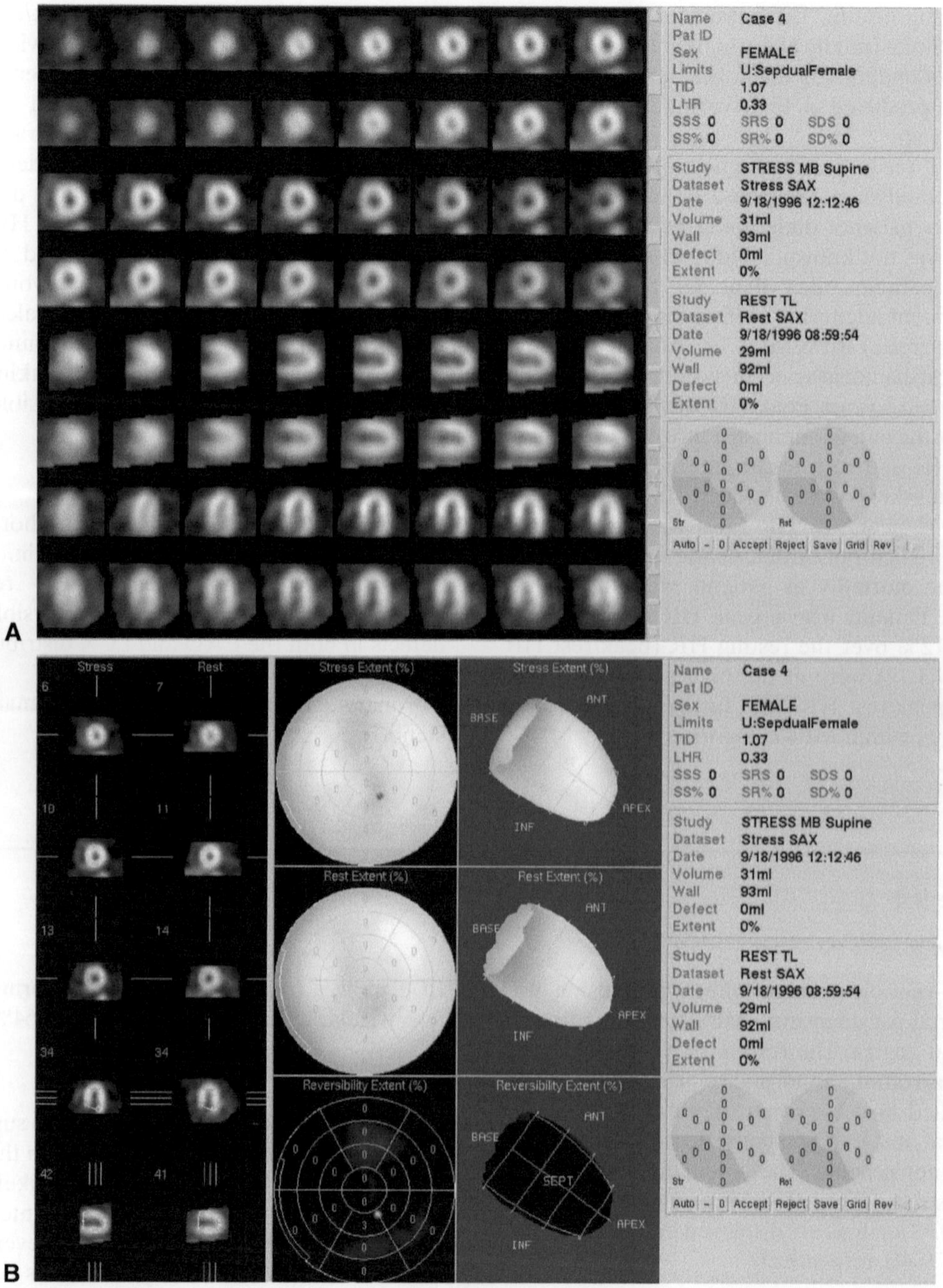

FIGURE C9-4. (A and B)

the prognostic and cost implications of stress MPS in 1,270 patients undergoing exercise or adenosine MPS with high pre-test likelihood of CAD (>0.85) but no prior CAD. Ninety-five percent of the patients had typical angina. Patients with normal MPS had a low risk of cardiac death (0.6%/year). With increasing extent and severity of MPS defects, the risk of cardiac death or MI increased significantly. Stress MPS was cost-effective compared with initial referral to exercise treadmill testing without imaging, and it saved money compared with direct referral to angiography. The study results suggest that patients with typical angina and no history of prior CAD benefit from referral to stress MPS over exercise treadmill testing alone.

In another report, Poornima et al.[20] found that a clinical score (CS) can help identify patients who would benefit from stress MPS over exercise treadmill alone. The CS was computed by assigning 1 point each to the following: diabetes, insulin use, male sex, history of MI, typical angina, and each decade over age 40. A CS ≥5 identified a group with a hard event (HE) rate of cardiac death or MI of 9% over 5 years; this group was further risk stratified through based on severity of SSS (14-segment model), with patients having normal, moderately abnormal, and severely abnormal scans having 5-year HE rates of 6%, 3%, and 22%, respectively. Based on this clinical score, elderly patients with typical angina, diabetes, or history of MI frequently have a CS ≥5 and thus make up a group in which stress MPS will be useful. Although the patient in the current case has a CS of 4 (based on age and typical angina), which is below the threshold of 5, since she required adenosine stress, stress MPS was necessary. In brief, then, the study of Hachamovitch et al.[15] illustrates that even patients with a high likelihood of CAD benefit from stress MPS for purposes of cost-effective risk stratification, and the study of Poornima et al.[20] shows that when patients have a high clinical risk (which is closely related to a high likelihood of CAD), even if they are able to exercise, a "low-risk" treadmill exercise test is insufficient to reach a true low risk state, and direct referral for a stress imaging procedure may be appropriate. Since neither of these papers was published as a full manuscript at the time of the writing of the most recent guidelines for stable angina[21] or those for the use of radionuclide procedures,[22] the use of MPS in this category of patients did not achieve the Class I indication; however, this may well change with the next series of guidelines based on these large studies.

One important goal of stress MPS is not just identifying who is at high risk of cardiac events, but determining who would benefit from early revascularization instead of medical therapy (MT). Hachamovitch et al.[10] followed 10,627 consecutive patients who underwent exercise or adenosine MPS and had no prior MI or revascularization; mean follow-up, 1.9 ± 0.6 years. Cardiac death occurred in 146 patients (1.4%). Treatment received within 60 days post-MPS defined subgroups undergoing revascularization (671 patients, 2.8% mortality) or medical therapy (MT; 9,956 patients, 1.3% mortality; $p = 0.0004$). Based on the Cox proportional hazards model predicting cardiac death ($\chi^2 = 539$, $p < 0.0001$), patients undergoing MT demonstrated a survival advantage over patients undergoing revascularization in the setting of no or mild ischemia, whereas patients undergoing revascularization had an increasing survival benefit over patients undergoing MT when moderate to severe ischemia was present. Further, increasing survival benefit for revascularization over MT was noted in higher risk patients (elderly, those with adenosine stress, and women, especially diabetics).

The incremental prognostic value of gated SPECT in elderly patients has also been assessed. Hayes et al.[23] followed 2,003 consecutive patients ≥70 years old who underwent exercise or adenosine gated MPS; mean follow-up was 662 ± 238 days (all ≥1 year). The mean age was 77.1 ± 5.2 years, 44.1% were woman, and 54.3% underwent adenosine stress. SDS categories were no ischemia (0 to 1), mild to moderate ischemia (2 to 7), and severe ischemia (>7). EF categories were ≥45% and <45%. EF ($\chi^2 = 13.8$, $p = 0.0002$) added incremental value to SDS ($\chi^2 = 9.0$, $p = 0.011$), SRS ($\chi^2 = 7.4$, $p = 0.006$), and type of stress ($\chi^2 = 9.1$, $p = 0.002$) for the prediction of cardiac death. Patients with normal scans (SSS 0 to 3) were at low risk for cardiac death (0.4%/yr), but patients with mild to moderately abnormal studies (SSS 4 to 13) were at intermediate risk (2%/yr) and those with severely abnormal scan (SSS > 13) were at high risk (4.7%). Patients with EF >45% and no more than moderate ischemia (SDS 0 to 7) were low risk for cardiac death (<1%/yr), whereas patients with a large amount of ischemia were intermediate risk (2.0%/yr). Patients with EF <45% were high risk (>5%/yr) regardless of the amount of ischemia. The combined assessment of SDS and EF identified more patients (64.6%) as low risk for CAD (<1% annual risk) than assessment of SSS (49.9%) alone. Thus, the combined assessment of function and perfusion identifies significantly more low-risk elderly patients than perfusion alone.

Interpretation

1. Presentation: elderly woman with typical angina.
2. Adenosine MPS: normal myocardial perfusion and function.

Case 9.5

History

A 58-year-old man presented with atypical angina. He had a history of MI treated with primary angioplasty of the LAD 10 months earlier. He was referred for exercise MPS. He exercised for 7:23 minutes to an HR of 178 bpm (110% of MPHR). The ECG response was ischemic with the stress ECG demonstrating 1.7 mm upsloping ST-segment depression in lead AVF. The supine dual-isotope rest ^{201}Tl/stress ^{99m}Tc-MIBI MPS images as well as the QPS analysis are displayed in Figures C9-5A and C9-5B, respectively.

Findings

The MPS images demonstrate a medium sized nonreversible defect in the anteroseptal wall in the LAD distribution. Based on the summed perfusion index scores, the % stress, % reversible, and % fixed myocardial defects were 10%, 0%, and 10%, respectively. On the post-stress gated SPECT images (not shown), there was hypokinesis of the septal wall with an EF of 49%. The patient subsequently underwent coronary angiography, which revealed no significant coronary stenoses.

Discussion

This patient with known CAD requires aggressive secondary prevention to prevent recurrent cardiac events over the long term. Based on the results of stress MPS, he would have been identified as low risk based on EF 30% to 50% and no ischemia (SDS 0 to 1).[16]

Zellweger et al.[24] identified 1,413 consecutive patients with remote prior MI who underwent rest ^{201}Tl/stress ^{99m}Tc-MIBI MPS. Infarct size was determined by the number of nonreversible segments (20-segment model). Patients with small MI (<4 nonreversible segments) and no or mild ischemia (SDS ≤ 6) had low risk of cardiac death (0.6%/yr). Patients with small MI and moderate to severe ischemia (SDS > 6) had a cardiac death rate of 1.6%/yr, and patients with large MI (≥4 nonreversible segments) had moderate to high annual cardiac death rates (3.7% to 6.6%) regardless of the extent of ischemia. The patient in the current case had three nonreversible segments and no ischemia and thus would be considered low risk for cardiac death. Based on these considerations, the costs and risks of coronary angiography in this patient could have been avoided.

Interpretation

1. Presentation: atypical chest pain, prior MI and angioplasty of LAD.
2. Exercise MPS: medium sized nonreversible defect in the anteroseptal wall in the LAD distribution; post-stress EF 49%.
3. Coronary angiography: no significant stenosis.

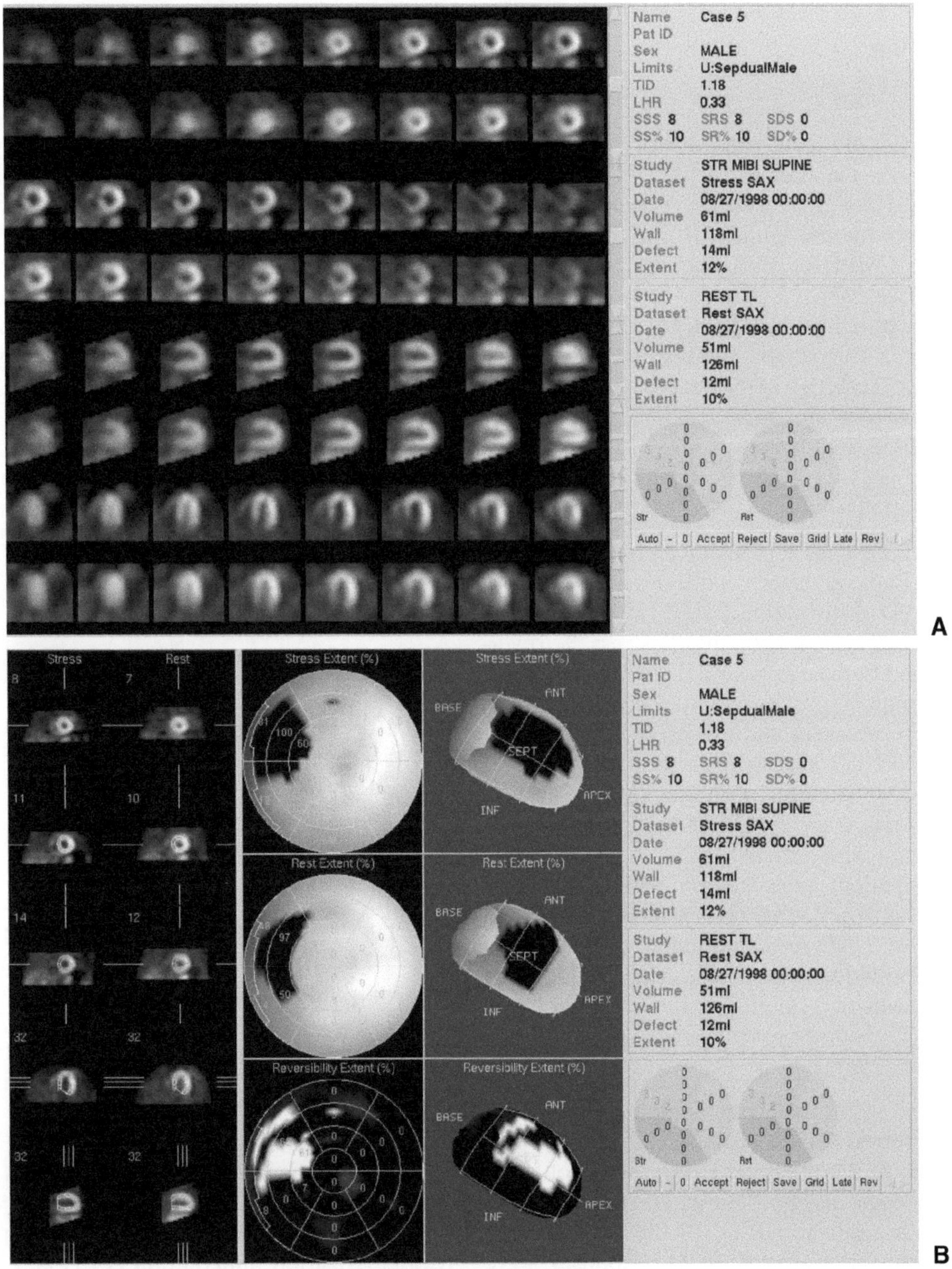

FIGURE C9-5. (A and B)

Case 9.6

History: Part 1

A 60-year-old man with a history of hypertension and diabetes presented with atypical angina. He was referred for exercise MPS. He exercised for 4:47 minutes to an HR of 139 bpm (87% of MPHR). Both the clinical and ECG responses were ischemic; the stress ECG demonstrated 2.4-mm ST-segment elevation in lead V2. The supine dual-isotope rest ^{201}Tl/stress ^{99m}Tc-MIBI MPS images as well as the QPS analysis are displayed in Figures C9-6A and C9-6B, respectively.

Findings: Part 1

The MPS images demonstrate a large reversible defect in the anterior, septal, and apical walls in the LAD distribution. Based on the summed perfusion index scores, the % stress, % reversible, and % fixed myocardial defects were 39%, 35%, and 4%, respectively. There is TID, a marker for severe and extensive CAD. On the gated SPECT images (not shown) there was evidence of stunning, with the post-stress EF of 41% worse than rest EF of 46%, which is also consistent with critical CAD.

The patient subsequently underwent coronary angiography, which revealed an occluded proximal LAD, 60% occluded diagonal, and 50% occluded RCA. He then underwent angioplasty and stenting of the proximal LAD.

History: Part 2

Because of the high-risk anatomy, the patient was referred for exercise MPS 2 months post stenting of the proximal LAD, even though he had become asymptomatic. He exercised for 6:51 minutes to an HR of 137 (86% of MPHR). Both the clinical and ECG responses were nonischemic. The supine dual-isotope rest ^{201}Tl/stress ^{99m}Tc-MIBI MPS images as well as the QPS analysis are displayed in Figures C9-6C and C9-6D, respectively.

Findings: Part 2

The MPS images are now normal. Based on the summed perfusion index scores, the % stress, % reversible, and % fixed myocardial defects were 0%, 0%, and 0%, respectively. TID is no longer present. On the gated SPECT images (not shown) there was no longer evidence of stunning and the post-stress EF of 53% has improved from 41% on the previous study.

History: Part 3

Four months post-angioplasty, the patient developed mild chest pain that was nonexertional and was classified as nonanginal. He was referred for exercise MPS. He exercised for 6:59 minutes to an HR of 125 (78% of MPHR). The ECG response was ischemic with 1.0-mm downsloping ST-segment depression in lead V5. The supine dual-isotope rest ^{201}Tl/stress ^{99m}Tc-MIBI MPS images as well as the QPS analysis are displayed in Figures C9-6E and C9-6F, respectively.

Findings: Part 3

The MPS images demonstrate a large reversible defect in the anterior, septal, and apical walls in the LAD distribution. Based on the summed perfusion index scores, the % stress, % reversible, and % fixed myocardial defects were 28%, 28%, and 0%, respectively. There is TID, a marker for severe and extensive CAD. On the gated SPECT images (not shown) there was evidence of stunning, with the post-stress EF of 48% worse than rest EF of 55%, which is also consistent with critical CAD. The findings were similar to those observed before percutaneous revascularization intervention (PCI) and were considered to indicate likely restenosis.

The patient underwent repeat coronary angiography, which revealed subtotal in-stent restenosis in the LAD and 50% occluded RCA.

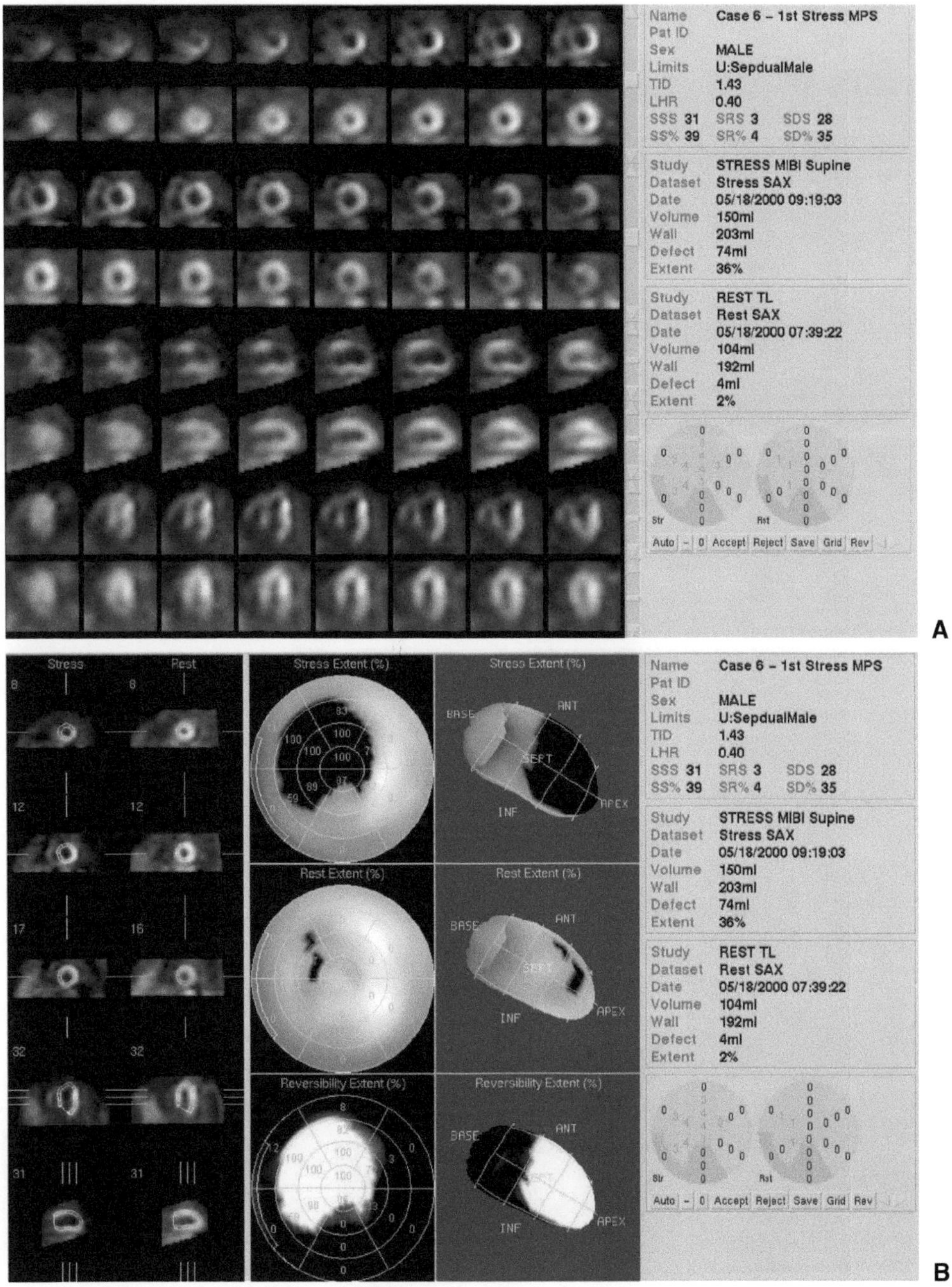

FIGURE C9-6. (A and B)

He then underwent repeat PCI of the LAD, which was successful with no subsequent events.

Discussion

On initial evaluation, this patient had a mildly decreased EF and a large amount of ischemia

C

D

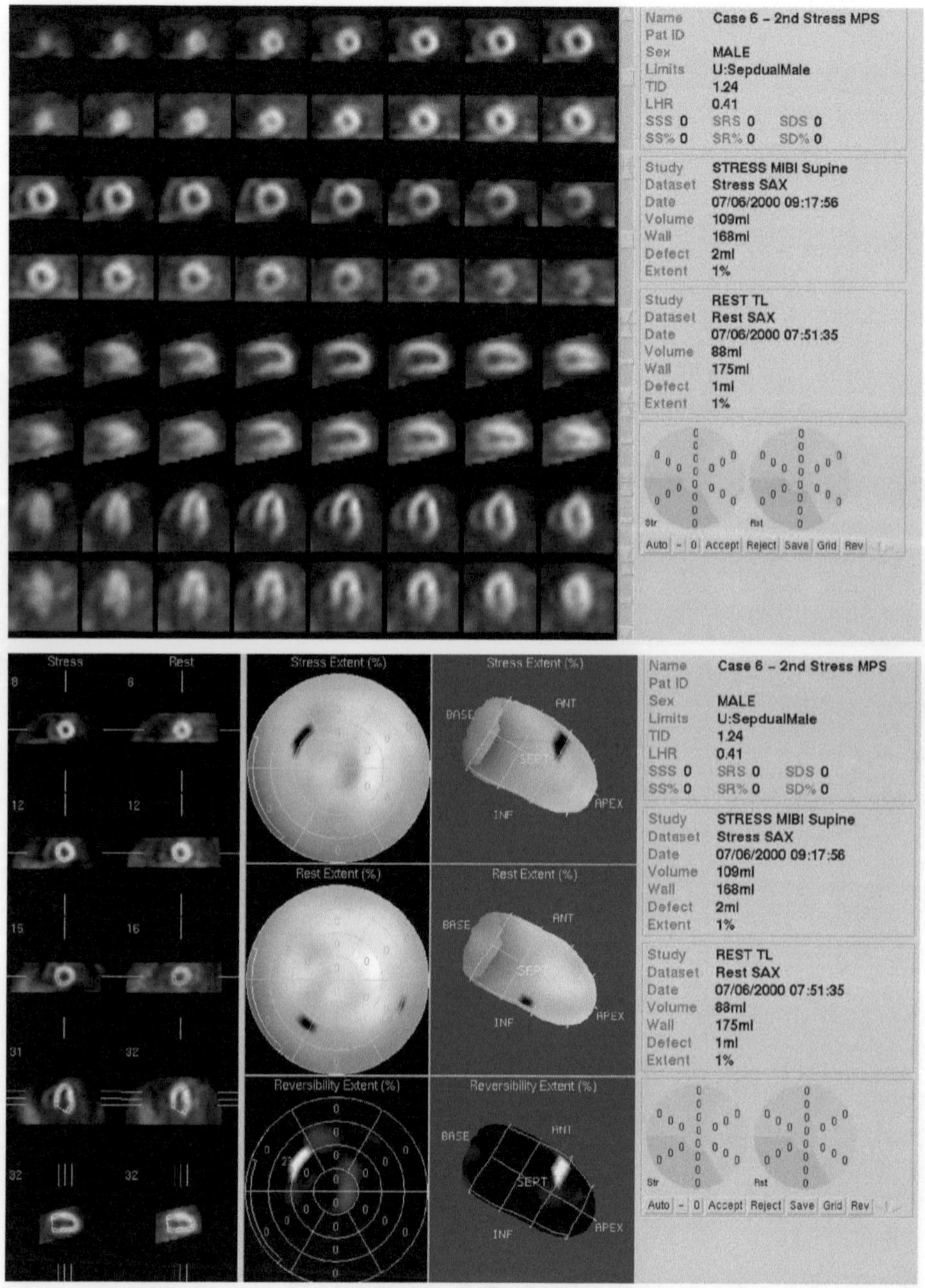

FIGURE C9-6. (C and D)

and thus would be considered to be at intermediate to high risk of cardiac death.[16] Other high-risk markers are the presence of diabetes, TID, and stunning, each of which increases the likelihood of severe CAD. This is consistent with the subsequent finding of an occluded proximal LAD.

After the first PCI, the patient was asymptomatic. Although recurrent symptoms are an indication for stress MPS in the first 12 months

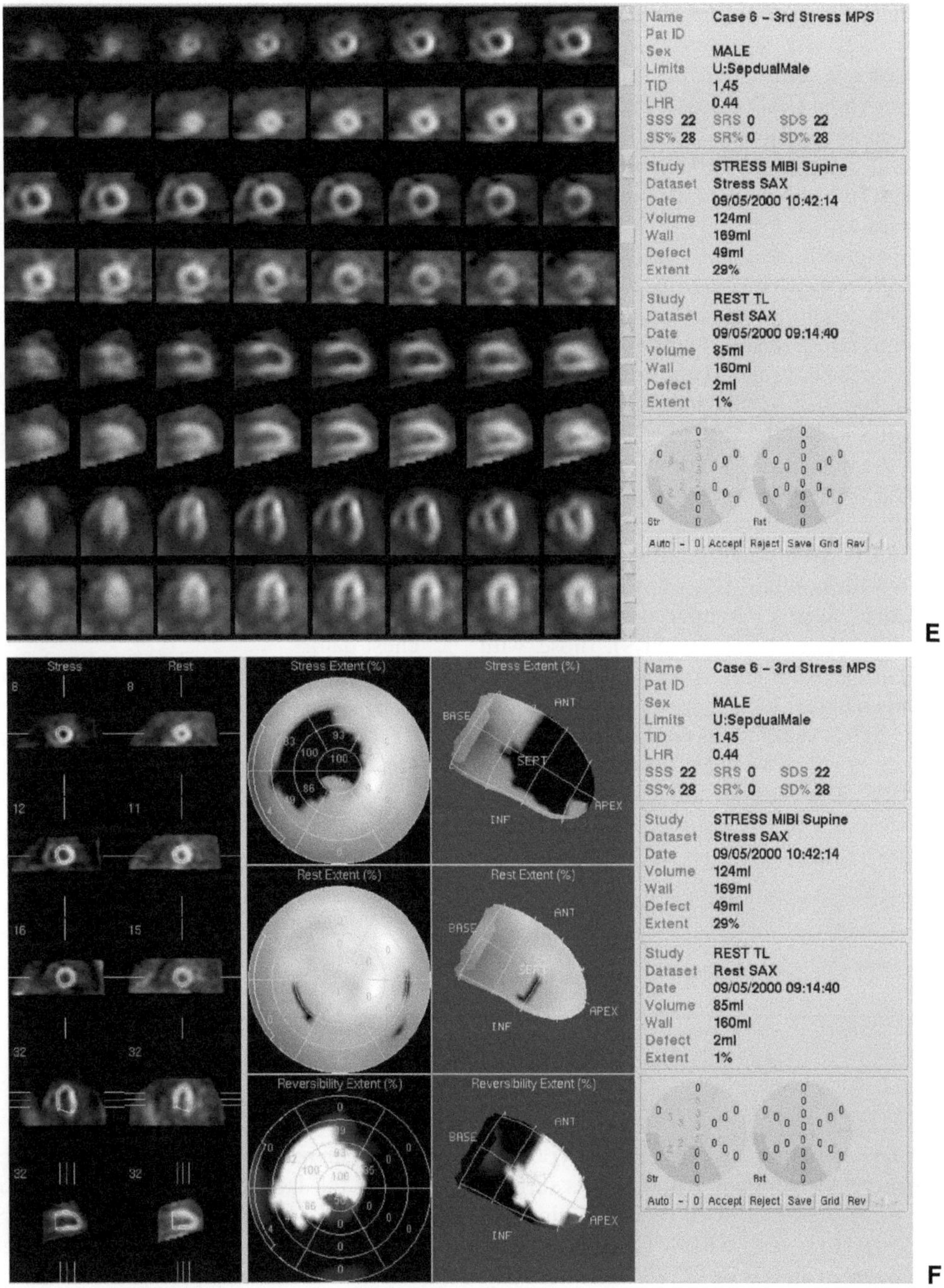

FIGURE C9-6. (E and F)

after PCI, most asymptomatic patients do not require early risk stratification. Patients with decreased left ventricular function, multivessel CAD, proximal LAD disease, previous sudden death, diabetes mellitus, hazardous occupations, and suboptimal PCI results are considered high risk and may be candidates for early risk stratification.[25]

The patient in this study underwent repeat stress MPS very early, 2 months after successful PCI with stenting of the proximal LAD. Although stress testing within the first 12 months can be considered appropriate for high-risk patients such as this one (proximal LAD), stress MPS within the first 2 months is still well within the restenosis window. Hayes et al.[26] identified 2,692 consecutive patients with previous PCI who underwent rest ^{201}Tl/stress ^{99m}Tc-MIBI MPS. Six hundred forty-seven patients with normal MPS were then followed for cardiac events. Compared with patients tested late after PCI (>60 days), those with normal stress MPS early post PCI (<60 days) had a much higher incidence of repeat catheterization (26.6% vs. 6.7%) as well as repeat revascularization (21% vs. 2.5%) within 180 days after MPS. The findings suggest that normal MPS early post PCI does not predict a low incidence of restenosis.

The patient in this case did return at 4 months after PCI when he developed mild recurrent chest pain. He again had the high-risk MPS findings of a large reversible defect in the LAD distribution, stunning, and TID, which were consistent with the finding of subtotal in-stent restenosis in the LAD, which required repeat angioplasty. The series of three serial studies in this case are an excellent example of stress MPS in patients with recurrent symptoms or high-risk features that can help stratify risk in patients and that normal MPS early after PCI does not mean that the likelihood of subsequent restenosis is low.

Interpretation

1. Presentation: diabetic man with atypical chest pain.
2. Exercise MPS: large reversible defect in the LAD distribution; TID, stunning.
3. Coronary angiography: occluded proximal LAD and subsequent restenosis.

Case 9.7

History

A 69-year-old man with a history of hypertension, hypercholesterolemia, and bypass surgery 1 year prior presented with typical angina. He was referred for exercise MPS. He exercised for 6:54 minutes to an HR of 125 (83% of MPHR). The clinical response was ischemic but the stress ECG was nondiagnostic secondary to baseline nonspecific ST-T wave abnormalities. The supine dual-isotope rest ^{201}Tl/stress ^{99m}Tc-MIBI MPS images as well as the QPS analysis are displayed in Figures C9-7A and C9-7B, respectively.

Findings

The MPS images demonstrate a large reversible defect in the lateral wall in the LCX distribution. There is a small reversible defect in the mid anterior wall in the diagonal distribution. There is a small nonreversible defect in the basal inferior wall with a small amount of peri-infarction ischemia in the mid inferior wall in the RCA distribution. Based on the summed perfusion index scores, the % stress, % reversible, and % fixed myocardial defects were 24%, 20%, and 4%, respectively. On the post-stress gated SPECT images (not shown) there was

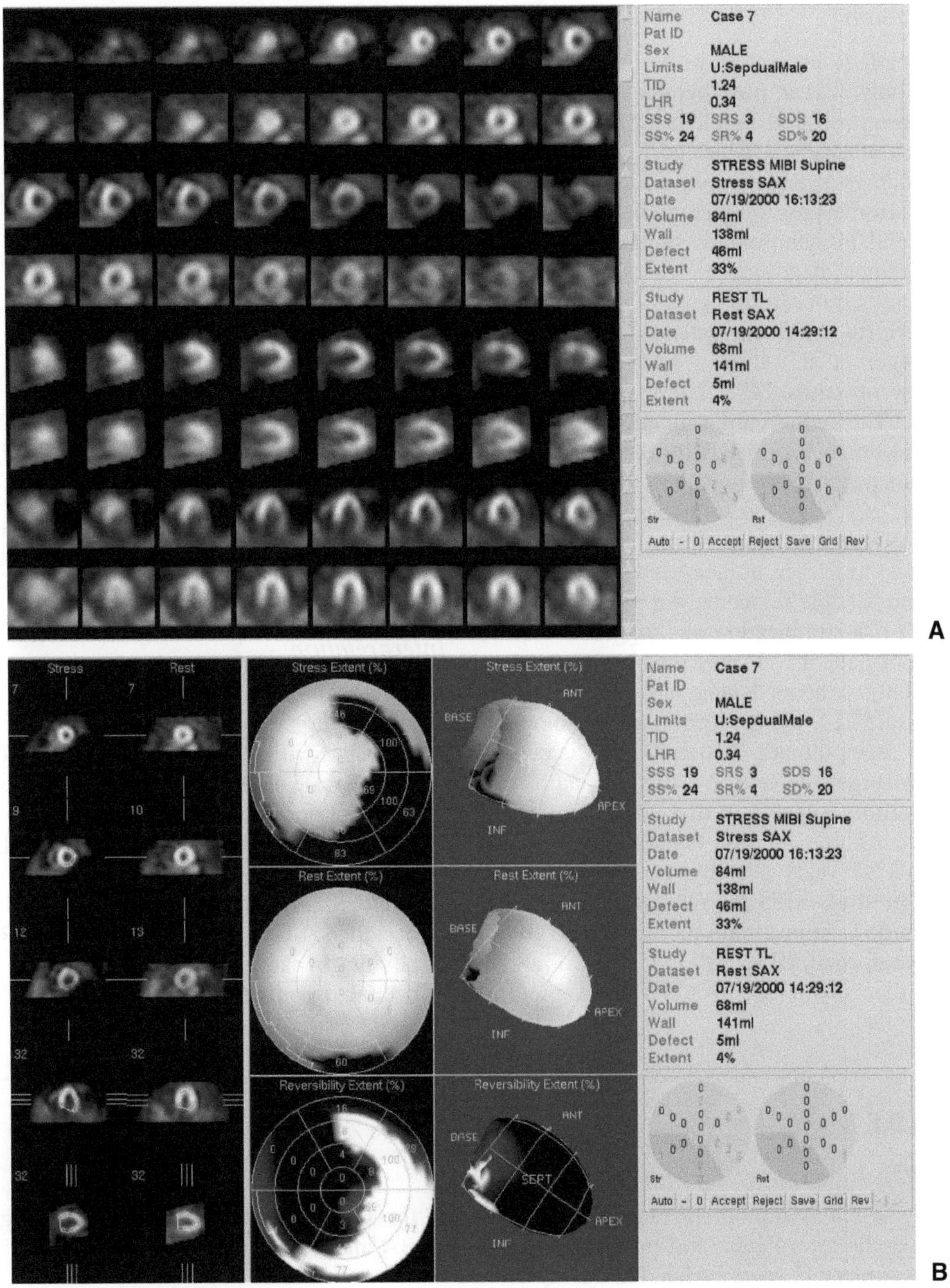

FIGURE C9-7. (A and B)

inferior and inferolateral hypokinesis with a poststress EF of 43%. The patient subsequently underwent coronary angiography, which revealed a 50% occluded mid LAD, 100% occluded proximal LCX and 70% occluded RCA, a patent bypass graft to the LAD, and occluded grafts to the LCX and RCA.

Discussion

This patient presented with recurrent symptoms only 1 year post bypass surgery. Stress MPS demonstrated a small prior MI and a large amount of ischemia, which correlated well with the findings at angiography, thus showing that early after bypass surgery, nuclear testing can be useful in symptomatic patients in guiding management decisions.

There is no uniform agreement about when to perform MPS in patients after CABG. Zellweger et al.[27] studied 1,544 patients who underwent stress MPS 7.1 ± 5.0 years post CABG. The annual cardiac death rate increased as a function of SSS in patients both ≤5 years and >5 years post bypass surgery. In the 628 patients studied ≤5 years post bypass surgery, the independent predictors of cardiac death were age and infarct size, as measured by the number of nonreversible segments. An optimized strategy for risk stratification was suggested for this group of patients ≤5 years post bypass surgery, with only patients having an annual cardiac death rate ≥1% being referred for angiography. Since asymptomatic patients ≤5 years post bypass surgery have a low cardiac death rate, the authors suggested that they would not require routine nuclear testing. Symptomatic patients ≤5 years post bypass surgery would undergo stress MPS for risk stratification and as a guide to appropriate therapy. Those found to have normal MPS (SSS < 4) had a low risk of cardiac death and would receive medical therapy. Those with <4 nonreversible segments or EF ≥ 45% had a low risk of cardiac death if the SDS was ≤6 (0.6%/yr) and thus would generally also receive medical management, but if SDS was >6, the risk of cardiac death was 2%/year, and angiography would be considered. Patients with ≥4 nonreversible segments or EF < 45% were high risk for cardiac death (5.4%/yr). If the SDS is ≥2, then the patient would be referred for angiography for potential revascularization. If no ischemia (SDS < 2) was present, in general medical management without repeat catheterization might be considered unless viability assessment (e.g., late redistribution ^{201}Tl, dobutamine-enhanced contractile function, or FDG/perfusion mismatch) demonstrated viability. Note that this discussion is directed toward those patients who are studied by MPS early after CABG (<5 years).

Interpretation

1. Presentation: typical angina, 1 year post bypass surgery.
2. Exercise MPS: large reversible defect in lateral wall, small reversible defect in anterior wall, and small reversible and small nonreversible defects in the inferior wall, EF 43%.
3. Angiography: 50% occluded LAD, 100% occluded LCx, and 70% occluded RCA, patent bypass graft to the LAD, and occluded grafts to the LCX and RCA.

Case 9.8

History

A 73-year-old asymptomatic man had a history of hypercholesterolemia and previous MI and bypass surgery 11 years earlier. He was referred for exercise MPS. He exercised for 8:43 minutes to an HR of 139 (95% of MPHR). The clinical response was abnormal secondary to exertional hypotension. The stress ECG was ischemic with 1.4-mm horizontal ST-segment depression in lead V5. The supine dual-isotope rest ^{201}Tl/stress ^{99m}Tc-MIBI MPS images as well as the QPS analysis are displayed in Figures C9-8A and C9-8B, respectively.

Findings

The MPS images demonstrate a small to medium sized reversible defect in the basal anterior and anteroseptal walls in the LAD distribution; there is also a small to medium sized reversible defect in the basal inferior and

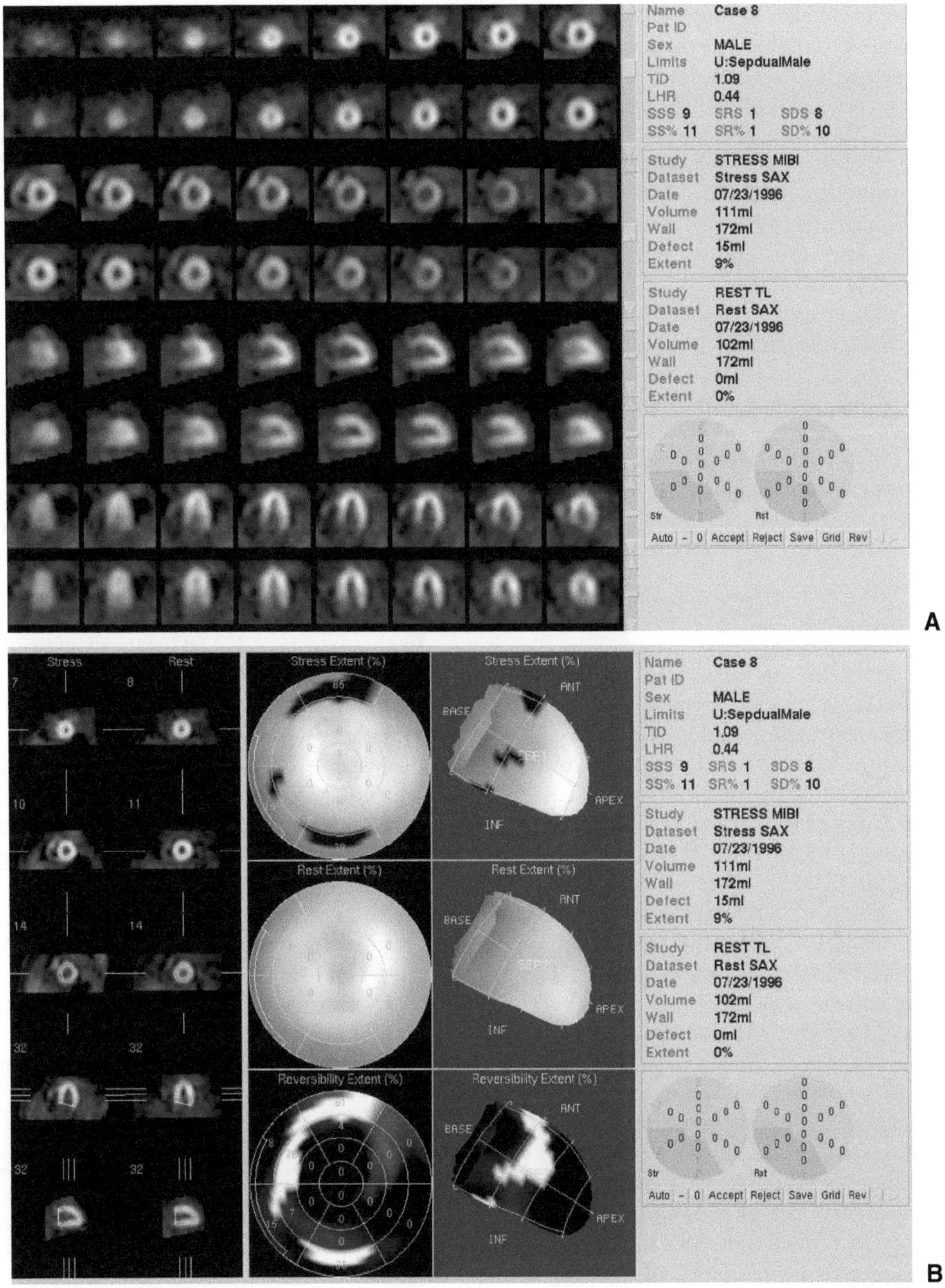

FIGURE C9-8. (A and B)

inferoseptal walls in the RCA distribution. Based on the summed perfusion index scores, the % stress, % reversible, and % fixed myocardial defects were 11%, 10%, and 1%, respectively. On the poststress gated SPECT images (not shown) there was hypokinesis of the basal septal wall and akinesis of the basal inferior wall; the poststress EF was severely decreased at 32% and the end-systolic volume was increased at 107 ml.

The patient did not undergo early coronary angiography. Seven months after the stress MPS study, he had a large acute anterior MI. Coronary angiography at that time revealed 100% occluded left main, 100% occluded RCA, and occluded bypass grafts to the LAD and LCX. He then underwent repeat bypass surgery but suffered an intraoperative cardiac death.

Discussion

This patient in this case was asymptomatic, but was 11 years post bypass surgery. Stress MPS demonstrated a moderately large amount of ischemia (SDS 8) and a poststress EF of 32%. In the study by Sharir et al.[16] discussed in Case 9.2, patients with mildly to moderately decreased EF (30% to 50%) and a large amount of ischemia (SDS > 7) are at increased risk of cardiac death (2.5%/year) and may benefit from coronary angiography. In a previous study by Sharir et al.[28] increased end-systolic volume was shown to further stratify patients in the normal and low post-stress EF groups.

In the study by Zellweger et al.[27] studying patients post bypass surgery undergoing stress MPS discussed in the previous case, there were 916 patients studied more than 5 years post bypass surgery. The annual cardiac death rate increased as a function of SSS. In this subgroup, the independent predictors of cardiac death were age, the extent and severity of ischemia as measured by the SDS, and infarct size (number of nonreversible segments). As discussed in the early post CABG group (previous case), an optimized strategy for risk stratification was proposed, with only patients having an annual cardiac death rate ≥1% being referred for angiography. In this strategy, all patients >5 years post bypass surgery, even if asymptomatic, would benefit for risk stratification with stress MPS. Patients with less than 4 nonreversible segments (<20% of myocardium infarcted) or EF ≥45% had a low risk of cardiac death if there was no ischemia or mild ischemia (SDS ≤ 6) (0.6%/yr) and thus would be treated conservatively, but if there was moderate to large amount of ischemia (SDS > 6), the risk of cardiac death was intermediate, and those patients may benefit from angiography. Patients with 4 or more nonreversible segments or EF <45% were at high risk for cardiac death (5.4%/yr). If the SDS is ≥2, then the patient would be referred for angiography for potential revascularization. If no ischemia (SDS < 2) was present, the patient would receive medical management unless viability assessment demonstrated hibernating myocardium.

In this late post-CABG patient with a 32% EF and a large amount of ischemia (SDS 8), the risk of cardiac death was high. He did not undergo early angiography and 7 months later had a large MI. This case highlights that nuclear testing late (>5 years) after bypass surgery, even in asymptomatic patients, can be useful in guiding management decisions. Another nuclear sign of high risk in this patient was the increase in end-systolic volume.

From the nonnuclear standpoint, the finding of exertional hypotension was itself a high-risk marker. This case again shows the importance of integrating the clinical, perfusion, and nonperfusion nuclear variables in assessing patient risk.

Interpretation

1. Presentation: asymptomatic, 11 years post bypass surgery.
2. Exercise MPS: small to medium sized reversible defect in the basal anterior and anteroseptal; small to medium sized reversible defect in the basal inferior and inferoseptal walls; EF 32%.
3. Angiography: 100% occluded left main, 100% occluded RCA, and occluded bypass grafts to the LAD and LCX.

Case 9.9

History

A 66-year-old man with a history of hypercholesterolemia and family history of CAD presented with nonanginal chest pain. He underwent coronary calcium CT scanning, which revealed extensive coronary atherosclerosis; his total coronary calcium score was 1722.9 with scores of 682.2 in the LAD, 159.6 in the LCX, and 881.1 in the RCA. He was then referred for exercise MPS. He exercised for 6:54 minutes to an HR of 161 (105% of MPHR). The clinical and ECG response to exercise stress were nonischemic. The supine dual-isotope rest ^{201}Tl/stress ^{99m}Tc-MIBI MPS images as well as the QPS analysis are shown in Figures C9-9A and C9-9B, respectively.

Findings

The MPS images demonstrate normal myocardial perfusion. Based on the summed perfusion index scores, the % stress, % reversible, and % fixed myocardial defects were 0%, 0%, and 0%, respectively. On the post-stress gated SPECT images (not shown) there was normal wall motion; the post-stress EF was 66%.

Discussion

The extent and severity of coronary atherosclerosis on coronary calcium imaging (via electron beam CT or helical CT) has generally been categorized based on the coronary calcium score (CCS), with CCS of 0, normal; ≤100, mild; 101 to 400; moderate; and >400, extensive. Shaw et al.[29] demonstrated that all cause mortality rose by category of CCS in both men and women. This and several other studies have illustrated that the CCS provides incremental prognostic value over risk factor assessment alone. However, the presence of coronary artery calcium alone does not imply the need for coronary angiography. Most investigators recommend the use of stress myocardial perfusion imaging in patients who exceed a certain threshold of risk based on the CCS. He et al.[30] evaluated whether the severity of coronary artery calcification predicted silent ischemia on stress MPS. No subject with CCS < 10 had an abnormal SPECT compared with 2.6% of those with scores from 11 to 100, 11.3% of those with scores from 101 to 399, and 46% of those with scores >400. Another study from the same group found that 70% of MIs occur in patients with CCS >75th percentile for age and gender.[31] Thus, patients with CCS above 400, or above 100 especially if above 75th percentile, would be candidates for further risk stratification via stress MPS. Then, if the MPS demonstrated high risk, coronary angiography would be indicated.

Conversely, while normal stress MPS is associated with a low risk of cardiac events, it may not imply the absence of subclinical coronary atherosclerosis. In such patients with a low to intermediate likelihood of CAD, a normal MPS could lead to a less aggressive approach to CAD prevention. In contrast, moderate amounts of coronary atherosclerosis by EBCT (CCS > 100) or above the 75th percentile for age and gender may define patients warranting aggressive medical management. Berman et al.[32] recruited 318 patients without known CAD, with low to intermediate (≤85%) likelihood of CAD and normal stress MPS to undergo EBCT. Sixty patients (19%) had moderate atherosclerosis (CCS 100 to 399) and 61 (19%) had extensive atherosclerosis (CCS ≥400). Thus, while normal MPS is associated with a low short-term risk for cardiac events, patients with normal MPS often have extensive atherosclerosis by CCS criteria. These findings suggest that such patients should not be given a *clean bill of health* and frequently merit aggressive preventive therapy to defer the development of clinical CAD. While no large long-term studies have yet reported prognosis of asymptomatic patients with extensive coronary calcification and normal MPS, standard clinical practice is that these patients are generally not sent for coronary angiography unless they become symptomatic or have nonnuclear findings suggestive of ischemia (e.g., marked ST-segment depression, exercise hypotension).

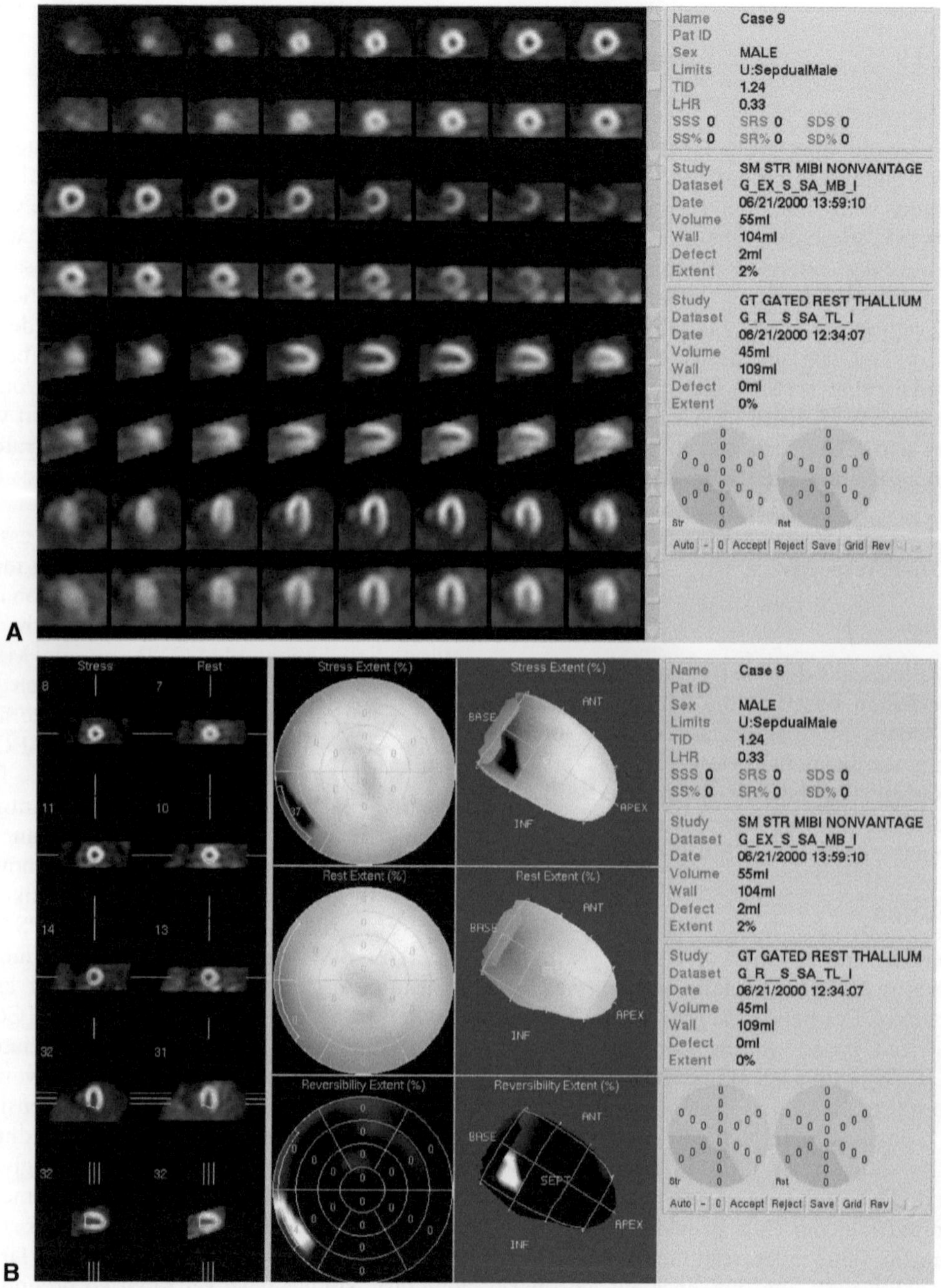

FIGURE C9-9. (A and B)

Interpretation

1. Presentation: extensive coronary atherosclerosis and nonanginal chest pain.
2. Exercise MPS: normal perfusion and function.

References

1. American Heart Association. *Heart Disease and Stroke Statistics—2004 Update.* Dallas: American Heart Association; 2003:1–48.
2. Berman DS, Kiat H, Van Train K, Garcia E, Friedman J, Maddahi J. Technetium 99m sestamibi in the assessment of chronic coronary artery disease. *Semin Nucl Med.* 1991;21:190–212.
3. Berman DS, Hachamovitch R, Kiat H, et al. Incremental value of prognostic testing in patients with known or suspected ischemic heart disease: a basis for optimal utilization of exercise technetium-99m sestamibi myocardial perfusion single-photon emission computed tomography. *J Am Coll Cardiol.* 1995;26:639–647.
4. Matzer L, Kiat H, Van Train K, et al. Quantitative severity of stress thallium-201 myocardial perfusion single-photon emission computed tomography defects in one-vessel coronary artery disease. *Am J Cardiol.* 1993;72:273–279.
5. Cerqueira MD, Weissman NJ, Dilsizian V, et al. Standardized myocardial segmentation and nomenclature for tomographic imaging of the heart. A statement for healthcare professionals from the Cardiac Imaging Committee of the Council on Clinical Cardiology of the American Heart Association. *Int J Cardiovasc Imaging.* 2002;18:539–542.
6. Port S. Imaging guidelines for nuclear cardiology procedures: Part 2. *J Nucl Cardiol.* 1999;6:G49–G84.
7. Berman DS, Kang X, Abidov A, et al. Prognostic value of myocardial perfusion SPECT comparing 17-segment and 20-segment scoring systems. *J Am Coll Cardiol.* 2003;41:445A.
8. Hachamovitch R, Berman DS, Kiat H, et al. Exercise myocardial perfusion SPECT in patients without known coronary artery disease: incremental prognostic value and use in risk stratification. *Circulation.* 1996;93:905–914.
9. Hachamovitch R, Berman DS, Shaw LJ, et al. Incremental prognostic value of myocardial perfusion single photon emission computed tomography for the prediction of cardiac death: differential stratification for risk of cardiac death and myocardial infarction. *Circulation.* 1998;97:535–543.
10. Hachamovitch R, Hayes SW, Friedman JD, Cohen I, Berman DS. Comparison of the short-term survival benefit associated with revascularization compared with medical therapy in patients with no prior coronary artery disease undergoing stress myocardial perfusion single photon emission computed tomography. *Circulation.* 2003;107:2900–2907.
11. Berman DS, Kang X, Hayes SW, et al. Adenosine myocardial perfusion single-photon emission computed tomography in women compared with men. Impact of diabetes mellitus on incremental prognostic value and effect on patient management. *J Am Coll Cardiol.* 2003;41:1125–1133.
12. Berman DS, Germano G. Myocardial perfusion single photon approaches. In Pohost GM, O'Rourke RA, Berman DS, Shah PM (eds). *Imaging in Cardiovascular Disease.* Philadelphia: Lippincott Williams & Wilkins; 2000:159–194.
13. Germano G, Berman DS. Quantitative gated perfusion SPECT. In Germano G, Berman DS (eds). *Clinical Gated Cardiac SPECT.* Armonk, NY: Futura Publishing Company; 1999:115–146.
14. Diamond GA, Forrester JS. Analysis of probability as an aid in the clinical diagnosis of coronary artery disease. *N Engl J Med.* 1979; 300:1350–1358.
15. Hachamovitch R, Hayes SW, Friedman JD, Cohen I, Berman DS. Stress myocardial perfusion SPECT is clinically effective and cost-effective in risk-stratification of patients with a high likelihood of CAD but no known CAD. *J Am Coll Cardiol.* 2004;43(2):200–208.
16. Sharir T, Germano G, Kang X, et al. Prediction of myocardial infarction versus cardiac death by gated myocardial perfusion SPECT: risk stratification by the amount of stress-induced ischemia and the poststress ejection fraction. *J Nucl Med.* 2001;42:831–837.
17. Hachamovitch R, Hayes SW, Friedman JD, Cohen I, Berman DS. A prognostic score for prediction of cardiac mortality risk after adenosine myocardial perfusion scintigraphy. *J Am Coll Cardiol.* (manuscript under review).
18. Beller GA, Watson DD. Risk stratification using stress myocardial perfusion imaging: don't neglect the value of clinical variables. *J Am Coll Cardiol.* 2004;43(2):209–212.
19. Abidov A, Hachamovitch R, Hayes SW, et al. Prognostic impact of hemodynamic response to adenosine in patients older than age 55 years

undergoing vasodilator stress myocardial perfusion study. *Circulation.* 2003;107:2894–2899.

20. Poornima IG, Miller TD, Christian TF, Hodge SO, Bailey KR, Gibbons RJ. Utility of myocardial perfusion imaging in patients with low-risk treadmill scores. *J Am Coll Cardiol.* 2004;43(2): 194–199.
21. Gibbons RJ, Abrams J, Chatterjee K, et al. ACC/AHA 2002 guideline update for the management of patients with chronic stable angina: a report of the American College of Cardiology/American Heart Association Task Force on Practice Guidelines (Committee to Update the 1999 Guidelines for the Management of Patients with Chronic Stable Angina). 2002. Available at www.acc.org/clinical/guidelines/stable/stable.pdf.
22. Klocke FJ, Baird MG, Bateman TM, et al. ACC/AHA/ASNC guidelines for the clinical use of cardiac radionuclide imaging: a report of the American College of Cardiology/American Heart Association Task Force on Practice Guidelines (ACC/AHA/ASNC Committee to Revise the 1995 Guidelines for the Clinical Use of Radionuclide Imaging). 2003. American College of Cardiology web site. Available at www.acc.org/clinical/guidelines/radio/dirIndex.htm.
23. Hayes SW, Schisterman EF, Lewin HC, et al. Incremental prognostic value of gated myocardial perfusion SPECT in elderly patients. *J Am Coll Cardiol.* 2001;37:425A.
24. Zellweger MJ, Dubois EA, Lai S, et al. Risk stratification in patients with remote prior myocardial infarction using rest-stress myocardial perfusion SPECT: prognostic value and impact on referral to early catheterization. *J Nucl Cardiol.* 2002;9:23–32.
25. Gibbons RJ, Balady GJ, Bricker JT, et al. ACC/AHA 2002 guideline update for exercise testing: a report of the American College of Cardiology/American Heart Association Task Force on Practice Guidelines Committee on Exercise Testing. 2002. American College of Cardiology Web site. Available at www.acc.org/clinical/guidelines/exercise/dirIndex.htm.
26. Hayes SW, Lewin HC, Schisterman EF, et al. High incidence of repeat catheterization and revascularization in patients with normal stress myocardial perfusion SPECT early after PCI. *J Am Coll Cardiol.* 2001;37:402A.
27. Zellweger MJ, Lewin HC, Lai S, et al. When to stress patients after coronary artery bypass surgery? Risk stratification in patients early and late post-CABG using stress myocardial perfusion SPECT: implications of appropriate clinical strategies. *J Am Coll Cardiol.* 2001;37: 144–152.
28. Sharir T, Germano G, Kavanagh PB, et al. Incremental prognostic value of post-stress left ventricular ejection fraction and volume by gated myocardial perfusion single photon emission computed tomography. *Circulation.* 1999;100: 1035–1042.
29. Shaw LJ, Raggi P, Schisterman E, Berman DS, Callister TQ. Prognostic value of cardiac risk factors and coronary artery calcium screening for all-cause mortality. *Radiology.* 2003;228:826–833.
30. He ZX, Hedrick TD, Pratt CM, et al. Severity of coronary artery calcification by electron beam computed tomography predicts silent myocardial ischemia. *Circulation.* 2000;101:244–251.
31. Raggi P, Callister TQ, Cooil B, et al. Identification of patients at increased risk of first unheralded acute myocardial infarction by electron-beam computed tomography. *Circulation.* 2000;101:850–855.
32. Berman DS, Hayes SW, Friedman J, et al. Normal myocardial perfusion SPECT does not imply the absence of significant atherosclerosis. *Circulation.* 2003;108:iv–S62.

10 Nuclear Cardiology for Imaging the Effects of Therapy

Leslee J. Shaw, Gary V. Heller, Ronald G. Schwartz, Carlos Cunha Pereira Neto, Vinícius Ludwig, João V. Vitola, Dominique Delbeke, and Daniel S. Berman

Background Concepts in Linking Risk Assessment to Tailored Medical Intervention

Coronary artery revascularization and medical intervention have become powerful therapies in the management of ischemic heart disease. Although coronary angiography forms the basis for much of our existing therapies for patients with known coronary artery disease (CAD), its cost and invasive nature preclude its routine and frequent use in the evaluation of all patients. Furthermore, angiography provides predominantly anatomic assessments and does not standardly assess the physiologic significance of an individual coronary stenosis. Nuclear stress imaging, with its ability to provide information about the physiologic significance of stenoses and risk stratification of CAD patients, is ideally suited to provide supplementary information to assess patients after intervention.[1–3]

Risk stratification is related to the extent and severity of scintigraphic perfusion defects.[1–3] Thus, using empiric risk stratification, linking noninvasive measures to effective therapeutic interventions could provide an optimal venue for enhanced event-free survival for patients with known CAD. A risk-based model for screening was advanced in the American College of Cardiology's (ACC) Bethesda conference on secondary prevention.[4] This model described a method for targeting or tailoring intervention based on the risk in the patient cohort. Diverging from past therapeutic strategies that identify key clinical or diagnostic characteristics whereby intervention is effective, this type of strategy is based on outcome data and the proportional risk benefit received for varying patient subsets.

The optimal risk assessment tool would include markers of the amount of ischemic burden and the extent of left ventricular (LV) dysfunction. From noninvasive imaging, recent evidence suggests that varying outcomes may be estimated when using measures of myocardial ischemia as compared with ventricular function data.[3] Measures of the amount of myocardial ischemia (e.g., ST-segment depression, stress-induced perfusion defects) are proposed estimators of ischemic events, including acute ischemic syndromes, unstable angina, or myocardial infarction (MI). Conversely, the extent of LV dysfunction relates to the frequency of cardiac death. Linking risk assessment to tailored therapeutic intervention is based on the estimation of varying outcomes in statistically powered patient samples.

Ischemia-Based Coronary Angiography

The most recent ACC/American Heart Association (AHA) guidelines for the management of stable angina patients uses this principle of risk-based therapeutic intervention.[5] In particular, indications for coronary angiography are based on a number of measures of ischemia. The highest level of evidence from well-controlled clinical trials and large observational series suggests that coronary angiography is indicated for patients who have stable chest pain and *strongly positive* noninvasive test results. From SPECT imaging this would include (1) a stress-induced large perfusion defect (especially anterior); (2) multiple stress-induced perfusion defects of moderate size; (3) a stress-induced perfusion defect of moderate size with LV dilatation or increased lung uptake following ^{201}Tl imaging; (4) peak exercise or immediate poststress left ventricular ejection fraction (LVEF) <35%; or (5) a markedly abnormal exercise electrocardiogram (ECG) defined as >2mm further ST-segment depression in multiple leads at low levels of exercise and/or a drop in systolic blood pressure (BP) suggestive of poor ventricular performance in the setting of multivessel disease.

These indications highlight the specific patient populations for whom percutaneous coronary interventions (PCI) and coronary artery bypass surgery (CABG) have been shown to have the greatest benefit in terms of risk reduction. In addition to optimal patient selection, patients with moderate to severe SPECT perfusion and ventricular function abnormalities benefit in terms of disproportionately greater risk reduction. Furthermore, initial baseline imaging may then allow for sequential monitoring of patients for evidence of resolution of inducible ischemia, effectiveness of anti-ischemic and risk factor modification, and the completeness of revascularization (depending on the initial treatment of choice). The current chapter focuses on sequential imaging and its utility for the patient with chronic CAD.

Evaluation of Patients After Coronary Angiography

Although coronary angiography documents the extent of CAD, evaluating the hemodynamic significance of a coronary artery lesion is not routine.[6] Patients with coronary artery stenosis of >75% narrowing have clear-cut reductions in coronary blood flow reserve (CBFR), and there is a strong inverse correlation between stenosis severity and coronary vasodilator reserve (but there is a marked scatter for values of CBFR for stenoses of 50% to 70% in caliber).[6] However, there is a strong correlation between nuclear myocardial perfusion imaging (MPI) and CBFR. Miller and colleagues[6] studied a cohort of patients comparing the results of quantitative coronary angiography, ^{99m}Tc-MIBI SPECT imaging, and CBFR measured by Doppler flow probe. A high degree of concordance was noted between CBFR measurements and MIBI uptake (89% agreement, kappa statistic = 0.78). Hence, decisions regarding intervention may be aided by incorporating nuclear imaging into the workup of cardiac catheterized patients.

The ACC/AHA guidelines for percutaneous coronary interventions (PCI) note that documentation of stress-induced ischemia is desirable for most patients undergoing evaluation for revascularization, particularly for patients with stable angina.[7] The ACC/AHA guidelines for PCI include criteria based on an assessment of provocative ischemia.[7] According to this guideline, PCI is indicated for patients with moderate to large areas of ischemia on noninvasive testing that have Canadian Cardiovascular Society Class (CCSC) I or II angina. When both pre- and post-PCI studies have been available, it is possible to evaluate an improvement in myocardial perfusion after successful PCI (see Cases 10.1, 10.2, and 10.3, which illustrates this concept). This improvement has been noted with both reversible and nonreversible defects at rest (see Case 10.3).

New Insights into the Value of Gated SPECT

One of the benefits of gated SPECT for its use in serial monitoring is that this procedure is an objective, validated tool for risk assessment and may be effectively applied in estimating cardiac death or MI.[3] Additionally, changes in myocardial perfusion also provide insight into the vasodilator effects of anti-ischemic as well as cholesterol-lowering therapy and changes in flow with PCI and CABG.[8] For example, cholesterol-lowering drugs improve endothelial function and CBFR in CAD patients over several months.[9] It is postulated that the reduction in clinical events is secondary to functional improvement rather than plaque regression in diseased arteries. In fact, it is these mechanisms that may contribute to reduced ischemic events.

Use of SPECT as a Surrogate Outcome

For SPECT imaging to be effectively applied in serial monitoring of treatment effectiveness several key components are necessary: (1) SPECT must be a sensitive, reproducible tool for detection of myocardial ischemia, (2) SPECT must be highly accurate in the estimation of major adverse cardiac events, and (3) detection of changes in perfusion and function should signify a clinical worsening or improvement that is associated with differences in patient outcome. This reasoning sets up the idea of using SPECT as a surrogate outcome, in which changes in SPECT may be used to reflect important modifications on a patients' clinical condition (Figure 10-1).

Background on Serial SPECT Imaging

The use of SPECT imaging in serial monitoring of controlling anginal symptoms and drug efficacy is increasingly being applied in the management of patients with chronic CAD.[10–12] In large part, the use of SPECT in serial management is based on a substantive body of evidence supporting the fact that ischemia-guided therapy is more effective at reducing the risk of major adverse cardiac events and guiding optimal treatment selection.[5] A number of prior reports note that the efficacy of medical therapy and the completeness of revascularization can be accurately assessed with serial SPECT monitoring[10,11,13–18] (see Cases 10.4 and 10.5).

Critical Factors in Serial Monitoring

What Signifies a Real Change in Perfusion? The Reproducibility of SPECT Imaging

Can you identify *real changes* in perfusion? This question has to do with the reproducibility of SPECT imaging, that is, a real change may be defined as inducible ischemia or normalization beyond test-test variability. For patients with CAD, medical therapy is a cornerstone of management. Follow-up monitoring of patients treated medically requires the use of a test with

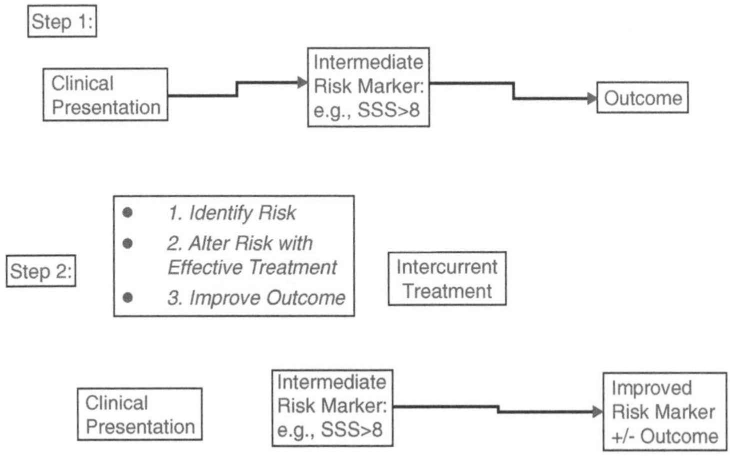

FIGURE 10-1. The evidence-based steps necessary to use SPECT imaging as a surrogate outcome for therapeutic decision-making. Evidence must be established where an imaging marker (e.g., SSS >8) has a well-established association with major adverse cardiac events, that is, SPECT is able to identify risk. The next step in this iterative reasoning is to delineate effective treatments that alter risk. The final step is then for the imaging marker to serve as a surrogate for worsening/improvements in clinical status whereby treatment is initiated based solely on the SPECT imaging results.

highly reproducible results. That is, for a test to be useful in identifying meaningful changes in a patient's disease status, the reproducibility of the test must be defined and limited. Several studies show good reproducibility for nuclear SPECT results. Mahmarian et al.[19] published data showing that quantitative exercise ^{201}Tl SPECT is highly reproducible and can be used to accurately interpret temporal changes in myocardial perfusion in individual patients. A change of 10% or greater in total quantitative perfusion defect size defined the 95% confidence interval for exceeding the variability of that tomographic technique. A previous report from our group showed a high intraobserver agreement in 80 patients with a κ value of 0.82 for stress studies and a κ value of 0.73 for resting studies. Automatic quantitative exercise dual isotope myocardial perfusion SPECT evaluated in 30 patients who had two exercise dual-isotope studies 31 ± 16 days apart, as determined by quantitative perfusion SPECT, is a highly stable measurement and can reliably detect changes of ≥10% from baseline. Using this evidence, it appears that a threshold of change exceeding the reproducibility of the test may then guide clinicians in identifying meaningful cut-off points for clinical worsening, suggesting advancing CAD.

What Is the Optimal Method to Interpret the SPECT Scan to Identify Changes in Perfusion?

Changes in myocardial perfusion, as reported in several prior reports, may be verified through either quantitative or semiquantitative (i.e., 20-segment myocardial model) techniques (Figure 10-2). Using semiquantitative scoring systems, changes that exceed risk-based thresholds can be applied to indicate real changes in myocardial perfusion.[3] Based on prior reports, changes in the summed stress score (SSS) ≥4 indicate significant differences in a patient's risk of cardiac death or MI. Thus, serial monitoring may employ changes based on a semiquantitative approach to SPECT interpretation.

Can Changes in Perfusion Be Linked to Meaningful Differences in Patient Outcome?

A second critical question is whether the changes in perfusion are linked to an improvement or worsening in clinical outcome. As such, a real change may also be defined as changes that equate to significant differences in major adverse cardiac outcomes. Of the patients routinely referred for stress MPI, a

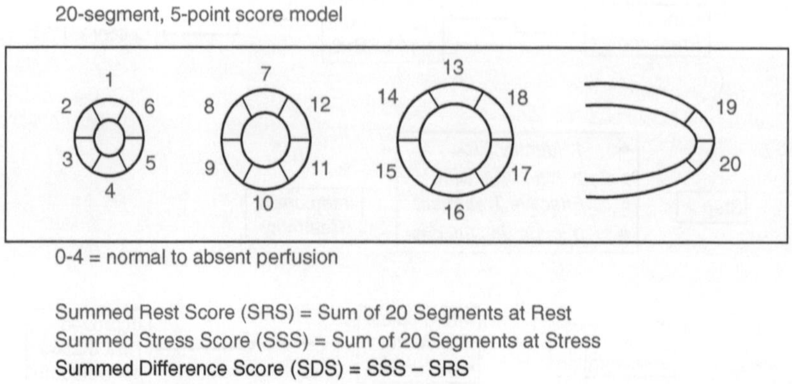

FIGURE 10-2. A 20-segment myocardial model for semiquantitative scoring. Each of the 20 segments is scored for the severity of perfusion reductions using a 5-point score (ranging from 0 = normal to 4 = absent perfusion). Three representative short-axis views are used for scoring as well as the horizontal long-axis view of the apex. The total scores are summed at rest (SRS) and stress (SSS). Inducible ischemia is scored by subtracting the rest from the stress score (SDS). (From Hachamovitch, Berman, Shaw, et al. [3], by permission of *Circulation*.)

TABLE 10-1. Observational 3-Year Death or MI-Free Survival in Coronary Disease Patients from the Economics of Noninvasive Diagnosis Multicenter Registry (n = 2,102)

Number of Vessels with Ischemia	Death or MI-Free Survival (%)
No ischemia	98
1 Vessel ischemia	95
2 Vessel ischemia	92
3 Vessel ischemia	83

Data collected from seven hospitals; analysis includes a Cox multivariable risk-adjusted model of catheterized patients with 1 or 2 vessel disease.

large majority includes patients with a prior history of CAD and worsening clinical symptoms. From large observational series of patients with stable symptoms of CAD, the relative risk of cardiac death is incrementally associated with the extent and severity of a perfusion abnormality.[20] Furthermore, there is also an inverse relationship between peak exercise LVEF and survival.[21] From a recent registry of patients with stable chest pain referred to nuclear MPI, there was an incremental risk of cardiac death or MI as a function of the extent of ischemia on MPI in patients with coronary angiography ≤90 days of stress testing (n = 2,102 from seven hospital multicenter registries).[21] Table 10-1 depicts the results of this analysis. As such, it is likely that the extent and severity of perfusion abnormalities may be used to risk stratify patients who are low to high risk. In a prior publication by Hachamovitch and colleagues,[3] the severity and extent of SPECT myocardial perfusion abnormalities risk stratified 5,183 patients as to their likelihood of cardiac death and MI (Table 10-2). Imaging data allowed identification of patients who were at low risk of cardiac death yet at intermediate risk of nonfatal MI. Patients with mildly abnormal scans after stress testing may benefit from a noninvasive strategy of aggressive medical therapy and may not require revascularization. These results were similar for patients with known and suspected CAD.

How can an Equivalent Level of Stress for Comparison Be Ensured?

When comparing changes in myocardial perfusion and ventricular function, the level of stress must be considered. That is, for true comparisons to be made, the level of stress must be similar for the baseline and comparative scan. One way to accomplish this is to use a pharmacologic stress agent, such as adenosine. But another method is to inject the radioisotope at a similar workload or heart rate (HR) during exercise testing. If maximal testing is performed during both the baseline (off anti-ischemic or other medications) and follow-up (off anti-ischemic or other medications) sessions, then it is likely that the second test may have similar amounts of inducible ischemia but at higher levels of physical work capacity. Thus, for an optimal comparison both the baseline and follow-up test, the stress modality should

TABLE 10-2. Incidence of Major Adverse Cardiac Events by Summed Stress Score Risk Groups

			Expected Event Rate for Improvement	
	Expected Rate of Cardiac Death or MI	Expected Improvement with Treatment	Mild Improvement	Moderate to Marked Improvement
Low risk	0.8%	None-Minimal	0.75%	0.7%
Mildly abnormal	3.5%	~25%–35% of patients experience some improvement	3.2%	2.8%
Moderately abnormal	5.2%	~50%–60% of patients	3.9%	2.7%
Severely abnormal	6.6%	experience moderate improvement	5.0%	3.3%

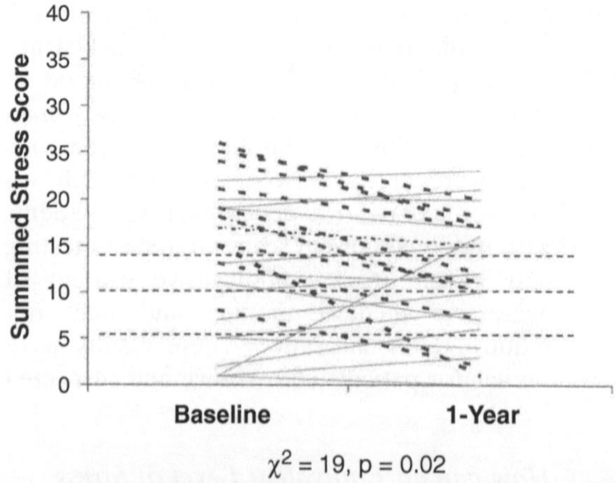

FIGURE 10-3. Baseline and 1-year SSS in 50 patients enrolled in the COURAGE trial. The dotted line indicates patients exhibiting significant improvements at 1 year following treatment initiation. Improvement is defined as a change in the patient's risk group or an SSS change ≥4.

be the same: (1) exercise—exercise, or (2) adenosine—adenosine.

What Is Optimal Utilization of SPECT for Patients with Chronic CAD?

For patients who present with inducible ischemia, a number of medical management decisions are required after testing that include referral to coronary angiography and the use of coronary revascularization procedures (as appropriate). In addition, optimal management also includes secondary prevention strategies to control risk factors as well as the use of an array of anti-ischemic therapies. Thus, the second or follow-up scan may be optimally indicated upon adequate titration of therapeutic regimens and indications that risk factors are adequately controlled achieving target goals. Changes in perfusion defects may be visualized by examining segmental differences in the extent and severity of inducible ischemia as a means to track risk estimations.

How Do You Define an Optimal Improvement in Outcome?

A general tenet of therapeutic intervention is that higher risk patients (e.g., quantitative ischemic defect ≥10%) receive a greater proportional benefit in terms of risk reduction. That is, the higher risk subsets of the population receive a greater proportional reduction in events. For perfusion imaging, this means that a greater percentage of patients with moderate to severe SSS or multivessel abnormalities would elicit more favorable changes in perfusion after therapy when compared with those with single vessel or mild perfusion abnormalities. For example, in a preliminary report from the Clinical Outcomes Utilizing Revascularization and Aggressive Drug Evaluation (COURAGE) trial, approximately half of the patients with moderate-severely abnormal SPECT scans (or those with a SSS >8) had improvements in perfusion following anti-ischemic therapy, risk factor modification, and/or PCI.[22] From this study, a significant improvement in perfusion is defined as a change in the SSS by one or more risk groups (i.e., Δ SSS ≥4), as shown in Figure 10-3. Concomitant to improvements in perfusion, >90% of patients had demonstrable improvements in symptoms, as defined by a CCSC class 0 or 1.

Table 10-2 depicts not only the expected death rates by a patient's SSS but the expected improvement with treatment. Using this outcome-based reasoning, moderate-marked improvement in perfusion noted on the second scan is associated with greater proportional risk reduction than for those patients that exhibit only mild improvements in their SPECT scan. Additionally, there is a proportional relationship between the extent and severity of ischemia at baseline and the resulting therapeutic benefit. Those patients with moderately to severely abnormal SPECT scans at baseline generally exhibit a greater degree and frequency of normalization than would be noted for patients with only mild ischemia.

What Is the Evidence Base for Serial Monitoring Using SPECT Imaging?

A number of controlled clinical trials using serial monitoring with SPECT imaging are ongoing within the context of state-of-the-art medical management strategies, including Bypass Angioplasty Investigation 2-D (in diabetics) (BARI 2-D), COURAGE, and AdenosINe Sestamibi SPECT Post-InfaRction Evaluation (INSPIRE).[22–24] The INSPIRE trial is a randomized prospective multicenter trial to evaluate the role of nuclear cardiac imaging with adenosine ^{99m}Tc-MIBI SPECT for assessing risk and therapeutic outcomes in survivors of acute MI. The COURAGE trial is a clinical trial involving over 3,000 chronic CAD patients randomized to optimal medical therapy (including anti-ischemic and risk factor modification) as compared with PCI. Figures 10-4 through 10-6 present algorithms for serial testing post-MI and chronic CAD patients as used in the INSPIRE and COURAGE clinical trials.

Serial SPECT Imaging

Patient Selection

Since SPECT is capable of detecting flow-limiting lesions from intermediate stenosis to multivessel CAD, there are arrays of patients who may be included in serial monitoring. A benefit of using SPECT is the possibility of localizing the perfusion defect location in correlation with coronary anatomy. SPECT can accurately identify the culprit lesion, and changes in perfusion or function may be used to define which patients are most likely to benefit from coronary revascularization procedures.

Sequential SPECT

Generally, serial imaging is performed at some predetermined time period after the baseline scan. The exact time period has been incompletely defined but depends on the type of therapy. For post-MI patients, repeat imaging has been evaluated at 6 to 12 weeks after discharge (see Case 10.3). A key to evaluating the

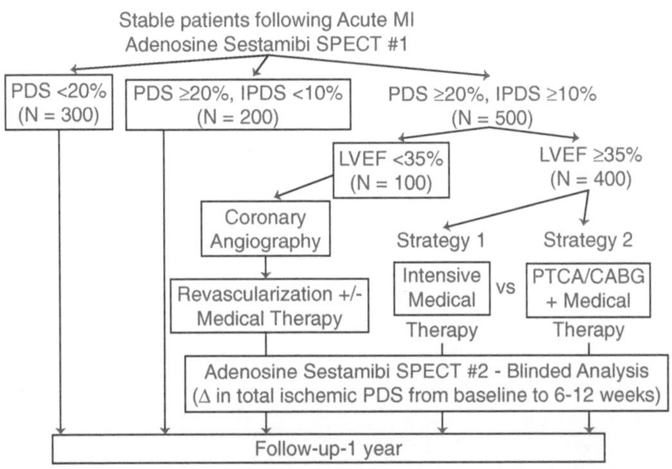

FIGURE 10-4. Algorithm for SPECT imaging employed in the INSPIRE trial. Patients undergo initial adenosine MIBI SPECT at days 2 to 5 post-MI. Based on the initial quantitative perfusion defect size (PDS), patients are allocated to risk groups. A low-risk patient is defined as a PDS <20% of the LV myocardium. However, additional allocation is based on the amount of ischemia (IPDS). Intermediate-risk patients are defined as PDS ≥20% with <10% IPDS. High-risk patients have a PDS ≥20% and IPDS ≥10%. For the high-risk patient group, those with an immediate post-stress left ventricular ejection fraction (LVEF) <35% are referred directly to angiography. For those high-risk patients with an LVEF ≥35%, patients were randomized to intensive medical therapy versus medical therapy plus coronary revascularization (PTCA/CABG, as appropriate). A second scan was performed at 6 to 12 weeks to assess changes in IPDS. All patients were followed for 1 year for the occurrence of major adverse cardiac events.

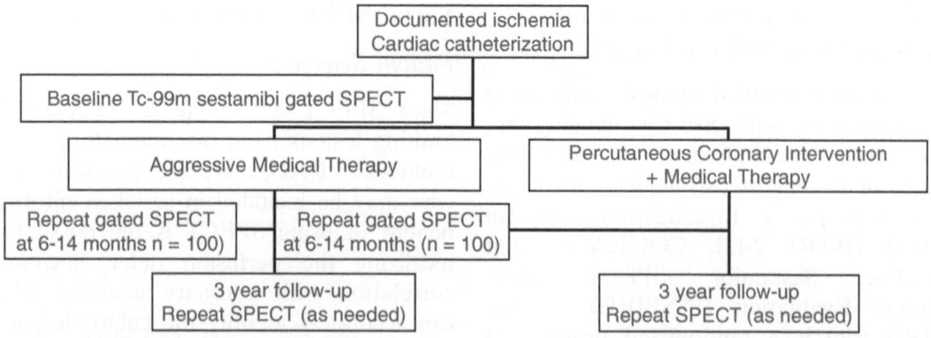

FIGURE 10-5. For the chronic coronary disease patients, serial SPECT imaging is being evaluated in the Clinical Outcomes Using Revascularization and Aggressive Drug Evaluation (COURAGE) trial. For those patients with stable chest pain, enrollment is limited to those with documented ischemia on SPECT imaging. Additionally, patients must have significant disease at coronary angiography and are then randomized to aggressive medical therapy as compared with PCI plus medical therapy. The nuclear substudy of this trial includes serial testing at 6 to 14 months after treatment initiation. All patients are then followed for 3 years for the occurrence of cardiac death or nonfatal MI. Repeat SPECT imaging is performed based on clinical need.

effectiveness of any therapeutic regimen is that all patients *take* their prescribed anti-ischemic medications the morning of the second SPECT study. That is, the first study patients are off any anti-ischemic or statin drugs, whereas they are tested with their medications *on board* at the time of their second study. Thus, this answers the specific question as to whether their current

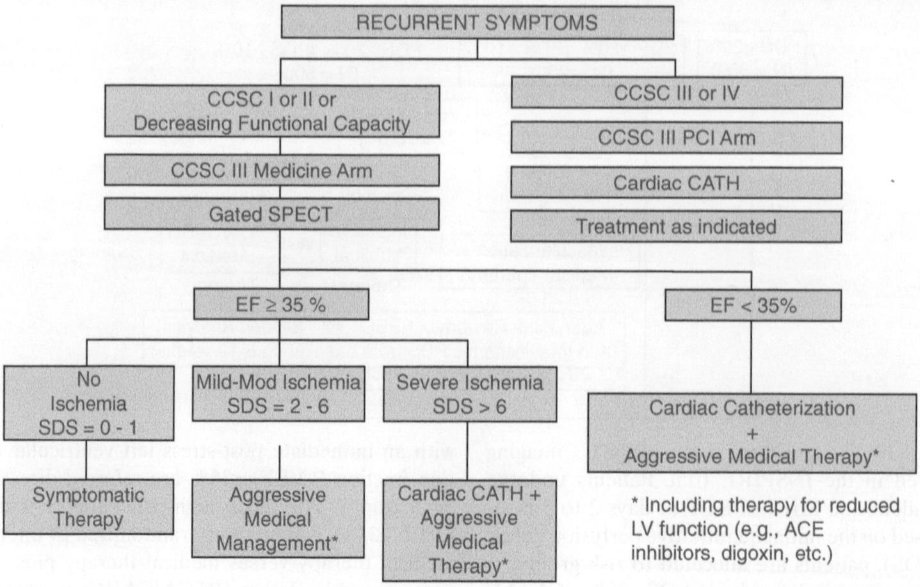

FIGURE 10-6. Algorithm for recurrent angina employed in the Clinical Outcomes Utilizing Revascularization and Aggressive Drug Evaluation (COURAGE) trial. ACE = angiotensin-converting enzyme inhibitor; CATH = catheterization; CCSC = Canadian Cardiovascular Society Class; EF = ejection fraction; LV = left ventricular.

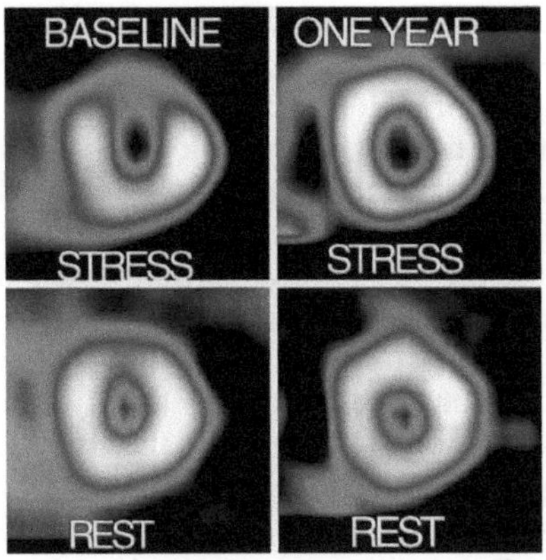

FIGURE 10-7. The baseline clinical history in this 50-year-old man included a 6-week history of typical exertional angina. His ECG was normal on presentation, and a diagnostic coronary angiography revealed an 80% stenosis in the mid-LAD, a 50% ostial stenosis in the RCA, and a 90% stenosis in the distal PDA. His LVEF was 49%. Additionally, his LDL and HDL cholesterol were 166 mg/dL and 38 mg/dL, respectively, at baseline. He was also hypertensive with a blood pressure of 166/120 mm Hg. He had a body mass index of 35.0. At 2 years following aggressive medical management, he was asymptomatic with adequate control of his lipids and blood pressure. He also followed the American Heart Association's step 2 diet and performed 45 minutes of exercise 5 times per week. The baseline scan revealed marked ischemia with an SSS of 18. He exhibited normalization of his perfusion images through 2 years after treatment initiation. (From O'Rourke, Chaudhuri, Shaw, et al. [8], by permission of *Circulation*.)

regimen is effective at controlling both symptoms as well as inducible perfusion abnormalities. An example of serial imaging is reported in Figure 10-7.[8]

Utility of Nuclear Imaging Following Initiation of Medical Therapy

A number of prior reports have noted changes in the extent and severity of stress-induced SPECT ischemia with an array of medical therapies (e.g., nitrates, calcium antagonists, and beta-blocker) as well as coronary revascularization procedures; albeit in small patient samples. The remainder of this chapter provides a synopsis of available evidence on the effects of varying medical management strategies on inducible perfusion abnormalities.

Plaque rupture or erosion has been implicated in acute coronary ischemic syndromes. Impaired vasomotion accompanying atherosclerotic plaque rupture in the setting of a subcritical stenosis has been advocated as a major factor contributing to acute ischemic syndromes. Atherosclerosis is now considered to be a complex process of inflammation within the coronary wall imposed by acute plaque rupture and reduced blood flow to the myocardium. This understanding of the underlying pathophysiology of ischemic heart disease has been used to develop medical therapies aimed at reducing lipids available for deposition in the vessel wall, vasodilatation, in addition to other factors that reduce the risk of cardiac events. Statins, for example, exhibit a beneficial effect by modifying endothelial function, inflammatory responses, plaque stability, and thrombus formation.[25] Radionuclide perfusion defect size and severity have been shown in large multicenter observational series to be strongly correlated with the presence and extent of a high-grade coronary stenosis, but most importantly, for medical therapy, to document the large territories perfused by these vessels.[3,21] Because coronary vasodilation is affected by the chronic inflammatory atherosclerotic process, CAD progression and the response of therapeutic interventions may be monitored with nuclear techniques. A growing body of data on the use of nuclear imaging documents the effectiveness of medical management.[12,14,16,26,27] MPI may prove useful in assessing agents that alter vasomotor tone and coronary endothelial function, such as lipid-lowering drugs.[8] In small patient samples, nitrates, calcium antagonists, and beta-blocker therapy, used alone or in combination, can effectively reduce the extent of stress-induced scintigraphic ischemia.[8,11,12,14,15,26,28–30]

Myocardial Perfusion and Nitrates

Therapy with nitrates significantly reduces myocardial ischemia documented by nuclear imaging. Lewin and Berman.[14] collected data that showed a decrease in defect extent in patients treated once daily with extended-release isosorbide mononitrate (120 mg/day) for 30 to 35 days. Total defect extent was decreased by 13% from baseline to the last study and total defect severity was reduced by 14%. They used a rest ^{201}Tl/exercise ^{99m}Tc-MIBI separate acquisition dual-isotope myocardial perfusion SPECT protocol. Mahmarian et al.[11] tested transdermal nitroglycerin in a randomized, double-blind, placebo-controlled trial using quantitative ^{201}Tl tomography. Patients in the active group had a significant reduction in their total perfusion defect size by an average size of 8.9%, which was most apparent in those with the largest (≥20%) baseline defects, with an average reduction of 11.4%. A significant reduction in total (82% reduction) and ischemic (88% reduction) perfusion defect size was observed for patients receiving active patch therapy. Importantly, a ≥9% reduction in perfusion defect size with sequential SPECT imaging defines the 95% confidence interval exceeding technique variability.[19]

Myocardial Perfusion and Anti-Ischemic Drugs

Combination anti-ischemic calcium antagonists, beta-blockers, and nitrate therapy are more commonly used for patients. A number of studies have also documented the effects of acute administration of therapy during active stress.[31–33] Cid et al.[33] demonstrated that patients taking one or more anti-ischemic medications during dobutamine SPECT had a significant reduction in the likelihood of an abnormal scan. Furthermore, Shehata et al.[32] reported the acute effects of propranolol administration on dobutamine-induced perfusion defects in CAD patients. For this series, dobutamine SPECT was performed on separate days with and without pretreatment of intravenous propranolol. The results indicated that total and ischemic perfusion defect size was reduced by 22% and 32%, respectively, following propranolol administration.

When using pharmacologic vasodilator stress, Dakik and colleagues[12] reported the results of sequential adenosine SPECT to compare the efficacy of medical therapy versus coronary angioplasty for suppressing ischemia in 44 post-MI patients whose initial perfusion scan exhibited a large area of ischemia. Approximately 30 days after the initiation of therapy, the reduction in total (12% to 15%) and ischemic (12%) perfusion defect size was similar for patients randomized to intensive medical therapy versus coronary angioplasty. Sharir et al.[31] studied the effects of combination anti-ischemic medications on perfusion defect size in 21 patients with chronic CAD who underwent dipyridamole ^{201}Tl SPECT. Baseline SPECT was performed off anti-ischemic medications and then repeated following administration of calcium channel antagonists, nitrates, or beta-blockers. The results indicated a 24% to 33% reduction in defect size with anti-ischemic medications.

Prognostic Value of Nuclear Imaging in Medical Management

Despite the reported benefit of medical therapies on reducing stress-induced defect patterns, it is important to determine how reductions in the extent of abnormalities affect event-free survival. In the Angioplasty compared to Medicine Study (ACME) study, 270 patients were randomized to receive anti-ischemic therapy or coronary angioplasty.[15] ^{201}Tl planar scintigraphy was performed at baseline and after 6 months of therapy. Survival was significantly improved for patients who had normalized perfusion with either therapy as compared with those with persistent ischemia (92% versus 82%, $p = 0.02$). A more recent study in acute MI patients reported that event-free survival was 96% for patients who had a significant reduction in perfusion defect size, compared with 65% for those who exhibited no major reduction in perfusion defect size on nuclear imaging.[12]

Lipid-Lowering Drugs

In dyslipidemic patients, effective cholesterol lowering has been shown to improve myocardial perfusion reserve by nuclear imaging.[34,35] These results indicate that impairment of reactive hyperemia may play a role in identifying cardiac outcomes and for targeting medical therapy. The supporting rationale may be related to the fact that alterations in CBFR may result not only from fixed stenosis but also from intrinsic wall elasticity, integrity of the endothelium, and vasodilator responsiveness within the arterial wall. Worsening of defect size and severity may identify patients for whom additional *medical revascularization therapy* with lipid-lowering agents or angiotensin enzyme inhibitor or receptor blocker therapy or mechanical coronary revascularization may be warranted. Eichstadt et al.[36] demonstrated improvement of myocardial perfusion by short-term fluvastatin therapy. They reported 17 male subjects who were treated for 12 weeks and then followed up by ^{201}Tl SPECT scintigraphy. In ischemic segments myocardial perfusion increased by 30%, whereas in normal segments perfusion increased by only 5% and this was statistically significant. In 15 asymptomatic subjects with elevated cholesterol levels, fluvastatin treatment significantly increased CBFR, documented by serial ^{13}N-ammonia PET imaging at rest and during pharmacological stress. Mostaza et al.[10] revealed an 18% reduction in the amount of defect reversibility in randomized, placebo-controlled study with a cross-over design that included 16 weeks of 20 mg of pravastatin and placebo. (See Figure 10-8.) And most recently, Schwartz et al.[37] reported serial stress SPECT MPI studies showing resolution of stress perfusion defects, over a 6-month time course of pravastatin therapy and diet, in 25 patients with known CAD and proven hypercholesterolemia. This study demonstrated that a 42% reduction of mean low-density lipoprotein (LDL) cholesterol was associated with a 53% reduction of mean stress perfusion score. (See Figures 10-9A and 10-9B.)[37] Improvements in stress perfusion were observed in 48% of patients, with complete normalization in 22%. Resolution of the stress perfusion defects by SPECT MPI was noted with either exercise or pharmacologic vasodilator (adenosine) stress and could not be accounted for on the basis of the use of other medications. Similar to a prior PET MPI study of Guethlin et al.[38] that measured quantitative CBFR during the first 6

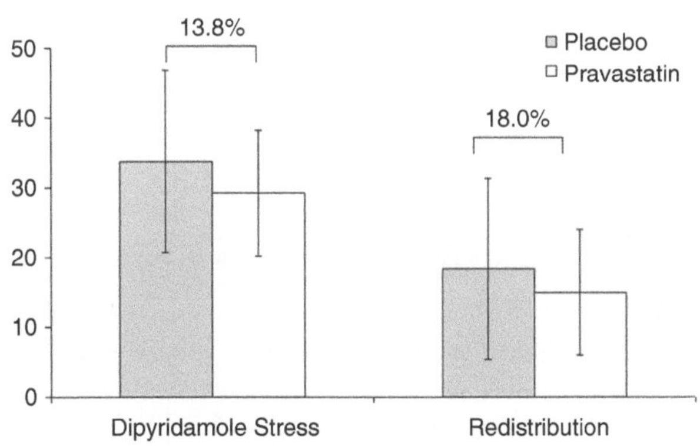

FIGURE 10-8. Results from a randomized, placebo-controlled study with a crossover design employing 16 weeks of 20 mg of pravastatin and placebo revealed improved dipyridamole ^{201}Tl SPECT myocardial perfusion with pravastatin in a total of 18 patients. The y-axis represents quantitative analysis performed according to the Cedars-Sinai method using a commercially available software. The results are expressed as a percentage of perfusion defects in the LV and in each vascular territory. A territory was considered ischemic if the magnitude of the perfusion defect exceeded 20%. A global percentage defect was calculated per patient as the average of the defects in each territory.

A

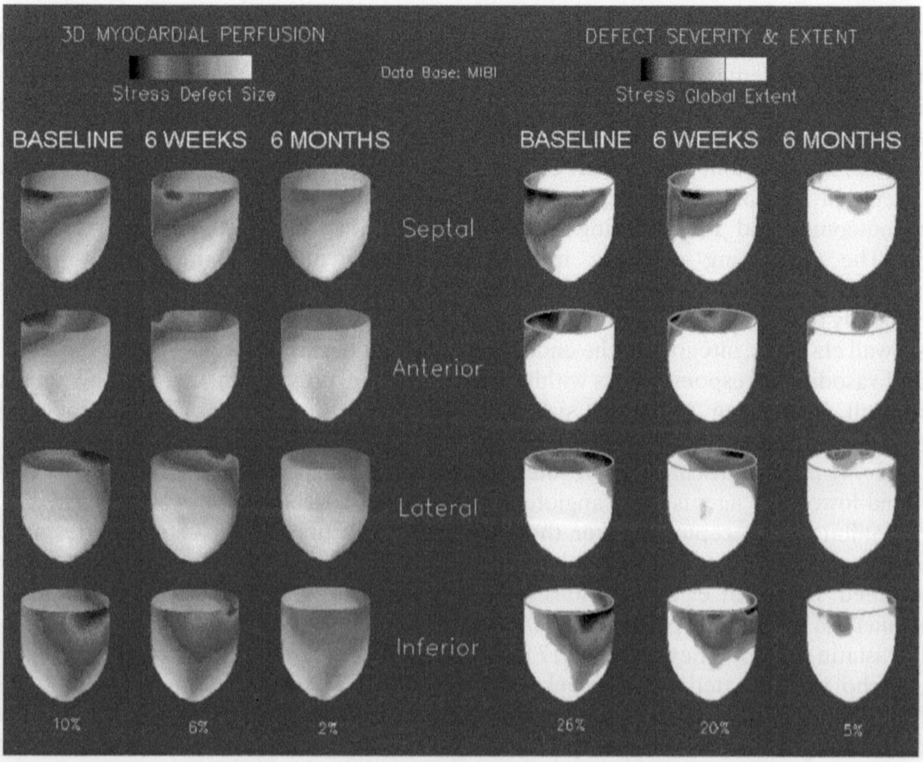

B

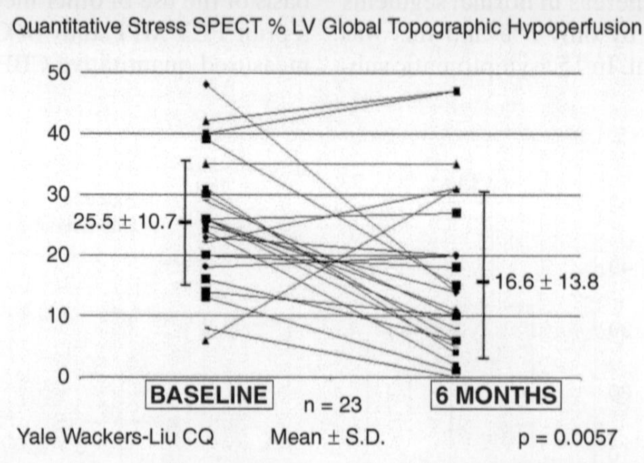

FIGURE 10-9. (A) Automated quantitative analyses of defect (% LV hypoperfusion) size (left images) and global extent (right images) at baseline, 6 weeks and 6 months of pravastatin therapy. Quantitative analyses verified improved average stress perfusion by six months in the study population. (B) Automated analyses of the stress SPECT myocardial perfusion defect size and topographic extent quantified by % LV hypoperfusion. No differences were found between baseline and 6 week studies (not shown). Lines track individual patient values from baseline to the 6-month study, which showed significantly reduced stress induced hypoperfusion. (From Schwartz, Pearson, Kalaria, et al. [37] by permission of *J Am Coll Cardiol.*)

months of fluvastatin therapy, improvement in stress SPECT abnormalities was seen at 6 months, but not at the earlier study time points of 6 weeks or 2 months at which time substantial lipid responses were evident. The time course of scintigraphic response is consistent with the time course of clinical coronary event reduction identified in a number of large, randomized controlled trials of statin therapy and lags behind the serum lipid responses. In both these latter radionuclide tomographic statin monitoring trials, changes in stress perfusion did not positively correlate with the magnitude of changes in serum levels of the total cholesterol or the lipid fractions, including LDL cholesterol. This observation is potentially important, since annual morbid coronary event rates in the active treatment arm of the large statin trials may reach 7.8% despite favorable lipid responses, and opportunities to prevent events of clinical nonresponders who appear to have a favorable lipid response may be lost. The value of radionuclide tomographic monitoring of effectiveness of treatment response has also been reported by Sdringola et al.,[39] who monitored 409 CAD patients with ^{82}Rb PET MPI. Baseline and 2.6-year follow-up PET MPI studies were obtained and patients were subsequently followed for coronary events for 5 more years. Very low fat, low calorie food, weight control, and regular exercise combined with lipid active drugs dosed to target goals substantially reduced hard and soft cardiac events. Predictably, size and severity of radionuclide tomographic myocardial perfusion abnormalities paralleled treatment intensity and predicted outcomes.

In summary, preliminary evidence in a growing number of small to intermediate sized pilot studies demonstrates that radionuclide SPECT and PET MPI may provide assessment of the potential effectiveness of anti-ischemic and risk factor modification therapy that is incremental to standard clinical and laboratory monitoring strategies. Further investigation is warranted to demonstrate the value of this approach, and to determine if it is incremental to existing examination and laboratory monitoring approaches, including biomarkers of atherothrombosis, in order to (1) quantify residual, on-treatment risk of morbid clinical events, and (2) permit adjustment of the therapeutic strategy in nonresponders to effect a more favorable clinical outcome before morbid clinical events. Ultimately, clinical and cost effectiveness of this approach in selected patient populations must be demonstrated before guidelines can incorporate a strategy with an apparent high initial cost for baseline and follow-up testing.

Utility of Nuclear Imaging Evaluating Patients Post-Revascularization

When compared with other modalities, MPI has an advantage due to its ability to localize disease, as well as to provide more direct evidence of CBFR under stressful conditions. Several studies have evaluated the role of nuclear imaging in the evaluation of patients after PCI.[16,40] In general, for patients with a marked improvement in luminal flow or change in percent stenosis, routine cardiac imaging post-PCI is not recommended. However, in the setting of recurrent symptoms (excluding CCSC III–IV), cardiac imaging has been reported to be useful in discerning the necessity for repeat coronary angiography.[7] Furthermore, for patients who have incomplete revascularization, routine post-PCI imaging may also be used to determine the extent of remodeling or if post-procedural restenosis has occurred. Recurrence of symptoms or limitations in function would be an indication for nuclear testing, excluding patients with unstable angina (i.e., CCSC III or IV). The occurrence of atypical symptoms is also an indication for nuclear imaging (see Cases 10.4 and 10.5).

A number of reports have indicated that nuclear imaging is accurate for the detection of restenosis. Using ^{201}Tl SPECT, Hecht et al.[41,42] demonstrated that nuclear testing is accurate in defining the presence of restenosis, whether or not complete revascularization was achieved with PCI. They compared the sensitivity and specificity for detecting restenosis by exercise ECG and ^{201}Tl SPECT in 116 patients. The sensitivity was 93% vs. 52% and the specificity

77% vs. 64% for SPECT and exercise ECG, respectively.[42] Pfisterer et al.[43] described ischemia on ^{201}Tl scintigraphy in 28% of 490 patients who underwent PCI at 6 months before nuclear testing. Ischemia was associated with significant stenosis in 97% of the patients. Conversely, the results of exercise ECG were negative in 74% of patients with scintigraphic ischemia and angiographic stenosis[43] (see Case 10.1). Angiographic restenosis was similarly high for patients with symptomatic and silent ischemia. A similar report was published by Milan et al.[44] on the detection of restenosis by ^{99m}Tc-MIBI as well as ^{201}Tl after successful angioplasty in 37 patients. They reported a sensitivity of 87.5% and a specificity of 78% for the detection of restenosis. Overall sensitivity rates ranging from 76% to 94% (mean = 89%) and specificity rates ranging from 46% to 84% (mean = 75%) have been published.[41–44]

The use of nuclear testing very early after angioplasty is controversial. Early data suggested that improved myocardial perfusion could be documented very early after PCI (see Cases 10.1 and 10.6). Stress ^{201}Tl scintigraphy may predict late restenosis even if it is performed within 24 hours after angioplasty (sensitivity 77%, specificity 67%).[45] Other reports showed that the nuclear test result may more likely be false positive early following PCI.[46,47] It has been reported that partially reversible or persistent defects might be noted shortly after PCI, with no angiographic evidence of abnormality in the vessels. Resolution of reversible defects is often observed on subsequent tests.[46,48] Several explanations for the higher false-positive rate of stress myocardial perfusion SPECT early following PCI have been proposed, including stunned vasa vasorum in the coronary artery undergoing angioplasty affecting vasodilator reserve, distal embolization of atheromatous material, and local vascular trauma, to name only a few.

Nuclear imaging had a high positive and negative predictive value for restenosis when imaging was delayed approximately 2 to 4 weeks following the index procedure.[45] From this review, there was a steady decline in the rate of false-positive scan results as time from the index procedure elapsed, although median sample sizes were small (n = 63 patients). Despite the observation of increased false-positive rate, recent experience has suggested that the frequency of the early post PCI false-positive myocardial perfusion study result is much lower than previously observed. Miller and Verani.[45] proposed that post-PCI false-positive rates may be less common today due to improved resolution with ^{99m}Tc-agents, as well as improved restoration of blood flow with newer interventional techniques, such as stenting (see Case 10.1). Nevertheless, it is recommended that the use of nuclear imaging be symptom driven, and that early testing for all patients following PCI be discouraged, unless the clinical scenario warrants otherwise. The role of MPI following PCI and CABG is further discussed in the case presentations.

Prognostic Value of Nuclear Imaging Post-PCI

In addition to assessing the recurrence of a significant lesion, another important question for patients with CAD deals with risk assessment. Limited reports have been made on risk assessment of the post-PCI patient. In a preliminary report assessing the cardiac event rate and referral to coronary angiography in patients undergoing stress ^{99m}Tc-MIBI SPECT 1 month to 1 year following PCI, we showed the results in 539 patients studied with rest ^{201}Tl/stress ^{99m}Tc-MIBI dual isotope SPECT. The hard event rate (cardiac death or MI) and total event rate (hard events plus late bypass surgery occurring more than 60 days following testing) increase significantly as a function of SPECT abnormality. The SSS, derived from the stress perfusion scores of 20 SPECT segments, in a Cox proportional hazards model, as well as the type of stress (adenosine versus treadmill exercise test) performed, were the only significant predictors of hard events. Furthermore, the referral rates to early coronary angiography following SPECT were directly proportional to the degree of scan abnormality. For patients without angina, the total event rate was comparable to those with angina. The relationships between scan findings and event rates were similar for patients with and without angina.

From these preliminary results, we conclude that stress MPI plays an important role in the clinical management of the post-PCI patient. There appears to be an appropriate use of nuclear scan results in guiding decisions after coronary angiography, with low coronary angiography rates following MPI in patients with little evidence of ischemia. In addition to assessing the ability of MPI to detect restenosis, the previously mentioned work of Pfisterer et al.[43] also evaluated the prognostic implications of silent ischemia. These investigators have shown that the prognosis for patients with silent ischemia was remarkably similar to that of symptomatic patients. These observations suggest that silent ischemia due to restenosis after angioplasty has a significant prognostic importance that may be reduced by repeat angioplasty and, therefore, should be aggressively excluded. For example, diabetic patients are known to have more silent ischemia than nondiabetic patients, and this topic is addressed further in Chapter 12.

In addition to providing perfusion information, gated SPECT can be used to assess regional and global ventricular function after PCI (see Cases 10.2 and 10.3). This technique provides accurate measurements of LVEF and LV volumes as well as a semiquantitative assessment of regional wall motion. To date, there have been no reports of the use of gated SPECT in the post-PCI patient. In Figure 10-6, we present the algorithm for testing employed in the COURAGE trial.[21] These results indicate that patients with impaired LVEF poststress require aggressive management (regardless of the extent of ischemia) due to their high rate of cardiac events. By comparison, in patients with preserved LV function, the extent of ischemia may be used to guide posttest risk-reducing therapy. Given the powerful prognostic content of perfusion stress EF, the techniques of gated SPECT may also prove superior to perfusion SPECT alone in risk stratification of the post-PCI patient. Thus, on the basis of the available evidence, MPI after PCI is useful in identifying restenosis and in stratifying patient risk, and appears to have an appropriate impact on the clinical management of post-PCI patients.

Development of a Nuclear-Driven Patient Management Strategy

Using an evidence-based approach to medicine, published reports were then synthesized for use in the COURAGE trial (see Figure 10-6). Patients with known CAD post-initiation of therapy or post-PCI with recurrent mild to moderate symptoms (i.e., CCSC I or II) should undergo gated SPECT imaging. From the nuclear scan results, the recommended management strategy for patients with poor LV function (i.e., EF ≤35%) or those with >1 area of provocative ischemia is coronary angiography. As the degree of risk reduction with therapy is greatest for high-risk patients, it is likely that patients with marked ischemia and systolic dysfunction will receive the greatest benefit from an aggressive, intervention-based care post-nuclear imaging (see Case 10.4). Medical management and secondary prevention strategies should be undertaken for the remaining patient cohorts. For low-risk patients with known CAD, a large body of evidence suggests that they have an excellent survival rate and do not need further evaluation.

Conclusion

Use of SPECT imaging in clinical trials builds on our current evidence. This body of evidence supports the utility of serial monitoring of treatment effectiveness with gated SPECT. Changes in both myocardial perfusion and ventricular function can aid in assessing global risk and the adequacy of current treatment, and act as a corollary to changes in symptoms or functional capabilities. This method of using gated SPECT truly integrates SPECT into patient management. The data help to provide supportive evidence to shape medical society and clinical guidelines of care as well as clinical indications for reimbursement, and, most importantly, to provide physician confidence in guidelines for patient management decisions.

Case Presentations

Case 10.1

History

A 61-year-old man with no cardiac risk factors presented with three episodes of atypical chest pain within the last 10 days. He was referred for a rest/stress same day ^{99m}Tc-MIBI study. He exercised 11 minutes on a standard Bruce protocol. His HR rose from 88 to 159 bpm, and BP from 110/70 to 160/90 mmHg, although there was a slight decrease of BP at peak exercise. There were no ischemic changes on the ECG during exercise, and he did not develop chest pain. The stress/rest ^{99m}Tc-MIBI images (vertical long axis = VLA) are displayed in Figure C10-1A.

Findings

The stress ^{99m}Tc-MIBI SPECT images demonstrated moderately decreased uptake along the anterior wall, septum, and the inferior wall, with evidence of reversibility at rest (Figure C10-1A). The gated images revealed normal wall motion and an LVEF of 64%.

Coronary angiography confirmed the presence of a severe obstructive lesion at the mid-left anterior descending (LAD) coronary artery (Figure C10-1B) and milder stenoses in the right coronary artery (RCA) (Figure C10-1C).

Two stents were placed, one in the LAD and one in the RCA. A repeat rest/stress MPI performed 8 days later, for atypical chest pain, showed significant improvement with normal myocardial perfusion (Figure C10-1D).

Discussion

This case illustrates two interesting points. First is the atypical presentation of CAD and negative exercise ECG while multivessel ischemia was detected by MPI. MPI identified multivessel ischemia, which prompted a therapeutic intervention to reduce the high risk for subsequent cardiac events. However, a slightly decreased BP at peak exercise was indicative of severe CAD.[49] Certainly, MPI added incremental prognostic information to that of clinical presentation and normal exercise ECG, as well documented in the literature.[2,50]

Second is the possibility of using MPI to evaluate the results of interventional therapy. In this case, we discuss evaluation of MPI early after PCI (8 days), whereas in Case 10.3 at a

A 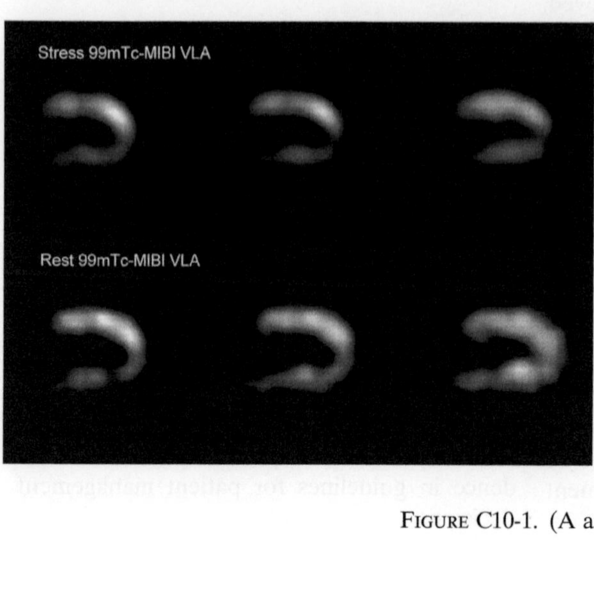

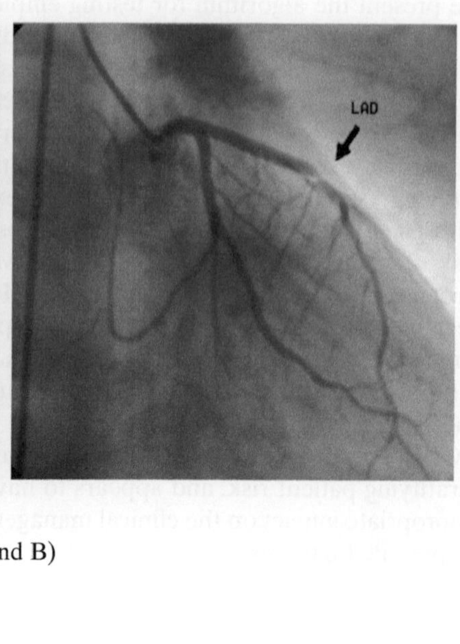 B

FIGURE C10-1. (A and B)

later period (75 days). One question that may be raised is: what is the ideal time to evaluate results of coronary stenting with MPI?

A review of the literature from 1980 through 2001 was conducted to identify studies examining post-PTCA functional testing for diagnosing restenosis.[51] The pretest probability of restenosis in symptomatic patients increases in a nonlinear fashion from 20% or less at 1 month, to nearly 90% at 1 year post angioplasty. The approximated accuracy of the exercise stress testing, MPI, and stress-echocardiography for detecting restenosis was 62%, 82%, and 84%, respectively. The authors concluded that in symptomatic patients during the first month after PTCA, none of the noninvasive modalities are able to accurately detect restenosis. Late after PTCA (7 to 9 months), the pretest probability of restenosis is high and therefore the non-invasive tests can be spared. The authors recommend performing MPI or stress echocardiography in symptomatic patients during the 1- to 6-month period when the pretest probability is intermediate.

A debate exists regarding the routine use of MPI following stenting for asymptomatic patients. Compared with balloon angioplasty alone, coronary stenting has been shown to decrease significantly the rate of restenosis,[52] supporting the idea that routine evaluation of asymptomatic patients may not be necessary. However, routine evaluation with MPI is recommended in diabetic patients as they can have ischemia without symptoms of chest pain, and the rate of restenosis is higher in this population. MPI has been considered a reliable method for the detection of restenosis[53] and has a higher accuracy for detection of restenosis than occurrence of angina or exercise-induced ECG changes.[54] Galassi et al.[54] studied 97 patients 3 to 5 months post-stent placement and found a sensitivity of 82% with a specificity of 84% using stress/rest MPI. Milavetz et al.[55] studied 209 patients who underwent MPI within 1 year of stent placement and found a sensitivity of 95% and a specificity of 75% for lesions causing greater than 70% obstruction. In addition, ischemia due to endothelial dysfunction can be demonstrated by MPI, whereas coronary angiography can be normal (see discussion of Case 10.6).

Rodés-Cabau et al.[56] found a higher rate of restenosis when ischemic findings were present on MPI performed early after stenting. Georgoulias et al.[53] studied 41 patients and found a negative predictive value for MPI of 83.3% 6 months following stenting.

Others have evaluated whether or not early MPI following stenting can yield any information regarding future events. A negative MPI performed more than 3 months after coronary angioplasty is also associated with an excel-

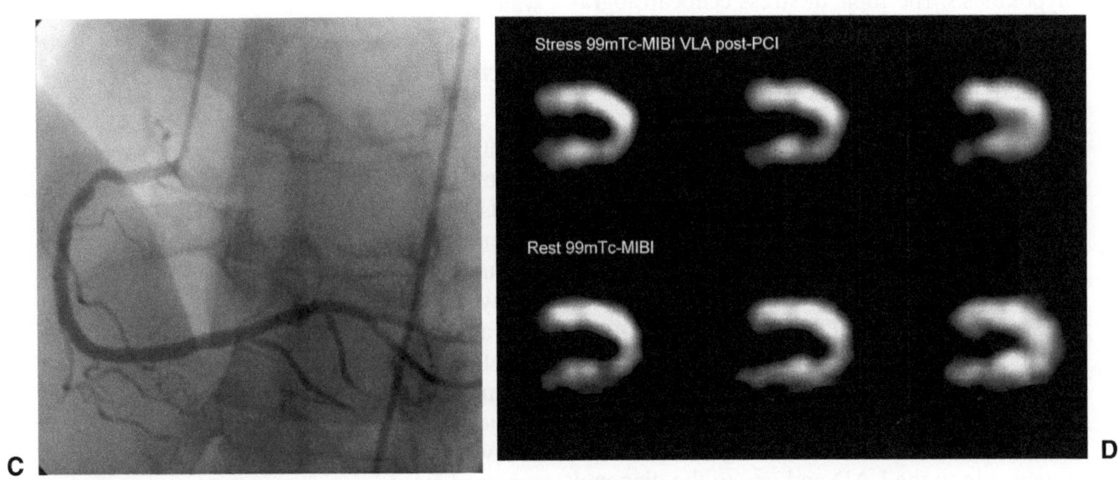

Figure C10-1. (C and D)

lent prognosis,[57] and the extent and severity of myocardial ischemia at exercise SPECT performed between 12 and 18 months after PCI predicts cardiac events during long-term follow-up in symptomatic and symptom-free patients.[58] Baseline MPI performed before coronary stenting is important for comparison with the follow-up studies.

The guidelines from the ACC and AHA for assessment of diagnostic and therapeutic cardiovascular procedures were published in 1995[59] but with some of the new evidence in the literature, the current recommendations for MPI in patients post PCI can be summarized the following way:

1. For symptomatic patients, MPI should be performed in the interval of 1 to 6 months post PCI and even earlier if complications from the procedure itself is suspected, i.e., acute or subacute occlusion.

2. For asymptomatic patients, the routine performance of MPI post-PCI is more controversial but may be helpful for risk stratification in patients with a higher probability of silent ischemia, i.e., diabetics.

Interpretations

1. Significant LAD and RCA ischemia identified by MPI in a patient with atypical symptoms and a negative exercise ECG but depressed BP response at peak exercise.

2. Noncardiac chest pain 8 days post stent placement accurately demonstrated by postprocedural MPI.

Case 10.2

History

A 73-year-old asymptomatic man with hypertension, tobacco use, and a family history of CAD was referred for evaluation of a positive exercise ECG performed as a routine screening. An adenosine stress echocardiography using microbubbles as a myocardial contrast agent revealed inferior and anteroseptal hypokinesis. The topic of stress echocardiography is further discussed in Chapter 16. A rest/stress ^{99m}Tc-MIBI SPECT study was performed for further risk stratification and is displayed in Figure C10-2A.

Findings

MPI revealed a mild reversible perfusion defect in the anterior, anterolateral, and lateral walls. The LVEF was slightly depressed at 44% with mild global hypokinesia. Coronary angiography confirmed the presence of a stenosis in the LAD (Figure C10-2B) and a critical lesion on a large diagonal branch. He was treated with two drug-eluting stents with rapamycin to the LAD and one to the diagonal branch, with good immediate results as shown on Figure C10-2C.

A rest/stress ^{99m}Tc-MIBI SPECT study performed 2 months later as part of an investigational protocol to assess stent patency demonstrated significant improvement with a normal perfusion pattern (Figure C10-2D). Gated SPECT images showed an increase in the LVEF from 44% to 53% with normal LV wall motion.

Discussion

This case illustrates the use of MPI to evaluate results of therapy with percutaneous revascularization using the new generation drug-eluting stents with rapamycin. A 20% to 40% rate of restenosis is observed in patients after balloon percutaneous transluminal coronary angioplasty (PTCA).[52,60–62] The use of stents reduced the rate of restenosis to approximately 20%. In a preliminary study, the new generation of drug-eluting stents with rapamycin reduce even further the rate of restenosis to 0% at a 1-year follow-up observed compared with 26.6% in the standard-stent group.[63]

Whether or not MPI should be performed routinely for the evaluation of patients after

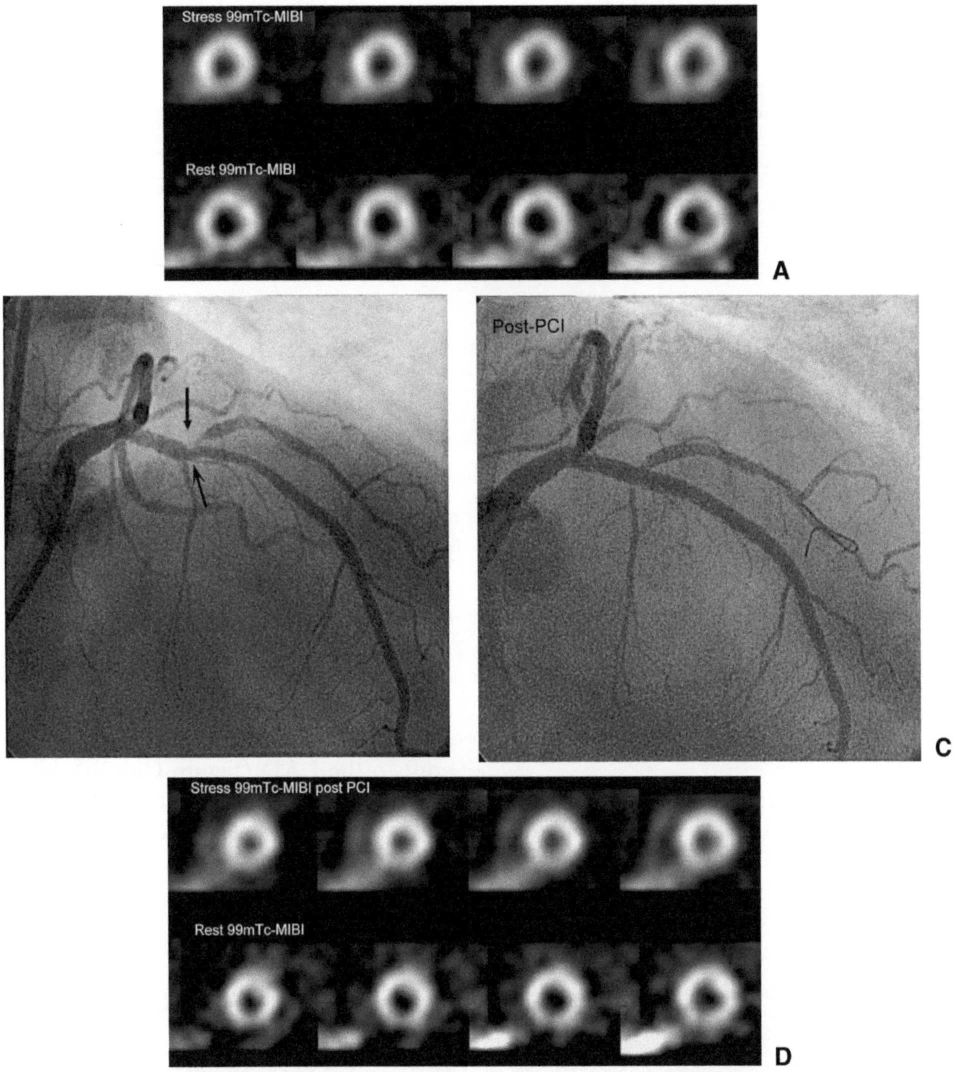

FIGURE C10-2. (A–D) (B and C, courtesy of Drs. Costantino Costantini and Marcelo Freitas, Clinica Cardiologyca Costantini, Curitiba, Brazil.)

revascularization procedures is a controversial issue. According to the guidelines for clinical use of cardiac radionuclide imaging,[59] routine evaluation is not indicated for asymptomatic patients. A literature search was conducted to identify studies with MPI 6 months after PTCA was performed for the diagnosis of restenosis and revealed a sensitivity of 87% to 95% and a specificity of 78% to 95%.[64] Cottin et al.[65] studied 152 patients 3 to 7 months after coronary stenting and concluded that the absence of ischemia after MPI indicates low risk for cardiovascular events. Milavetz et al.[55] studied 209 patients within 1 year of stenting showing a sensitivity, specificity, positive predictive value, negative predictive value, and accuracy of MPI for detection of significant angiographic restenosis (>70%) of 95%, 73%, 88%, 89%, and 88%, respectively.

It is known that CBFR remains impaired early after successful PTCA or stenting because of significant loss of microvascular integrity.[66,67] A study evaluating 83 patients with dipyridamole ^{201}Tl (88 lesions—38 PTCA, and 50 stents) 12 to 48 hours after PCI revealed reversible defects in the territories supplied by 36% of the stented lesions and 32% of the lesions treated by balloon angioplasty.[68]

Interpretations

1. LAD and diagonal lesions identified by MPI.
2. Normalization of perfusion pattern seen 2 months after PCI and treatment with a drug-eluting stent.

Case 10.3

History

Case 10.3 emphasizes the response to therapy of the patient previously presented in Case 6.6. This patient is a 74-year-old man with known CAD presenting to the ED with atypical epigastric pain and diaphoresis. He had a past medical history of CABG 14 years earlier but no prior MI. His ECG was unchanged compared with 4 years earlier. A rest/stress ^{99m}Tc-MIBI SPECT study was performed and is displayed in Figure C10-3A.

Findings and Discussion

The resting ^{99m}Tc-MIBI SPECT images showed a very large area of severely decreased myocardial perfusion involving the anterior wall, septum, and apex (entire LAD territory), and also the inferior wall and inferoseptal regions (entire RCA territory). Gated SPECT images demonstrated global hypokinesis and an enlarged LV with an EDV of 140 ml, an ESV of 85 ml, and LVEF of 39%. Considering the findings on the rest images, this patient was classified as very high risk, and the stress component of MPI was cancelled.

The patient underwent coronary angiography that revealed an occluded LAD and RCA, an occluded saphenous graft to the RCA, and a severe elongated stenosis on the saphenous graft to the LAD (Figure C10-3B), filled with thrombus. A stent was placed in the LAD graft with good results and good flow to the native LAD, as shown in Figure C10-3C. In Figure C10-3D, complete filling of the RCA is seen

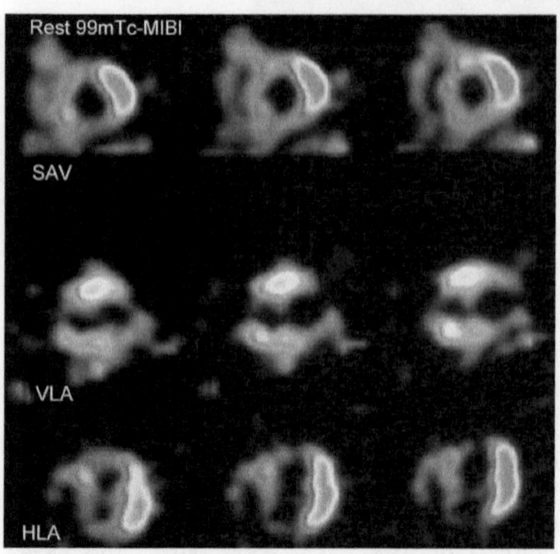

A

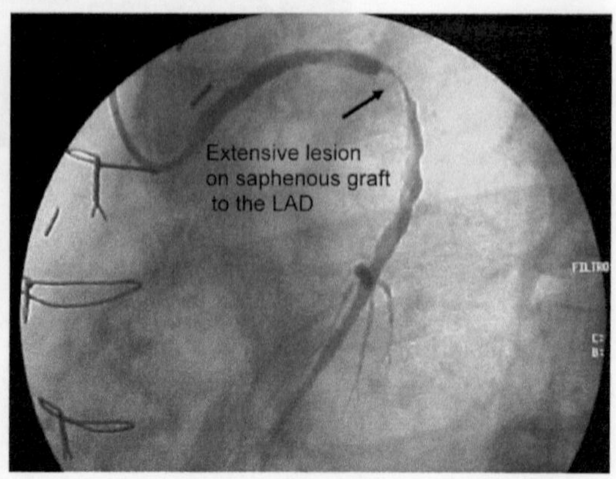

B

FIGURE C10-3. (A and B) (B–D, courtesy of Drs. Augusto Franco de Oliveira and Luiz Lessa, Hospital do Conação, Curitiba, Brazil.)

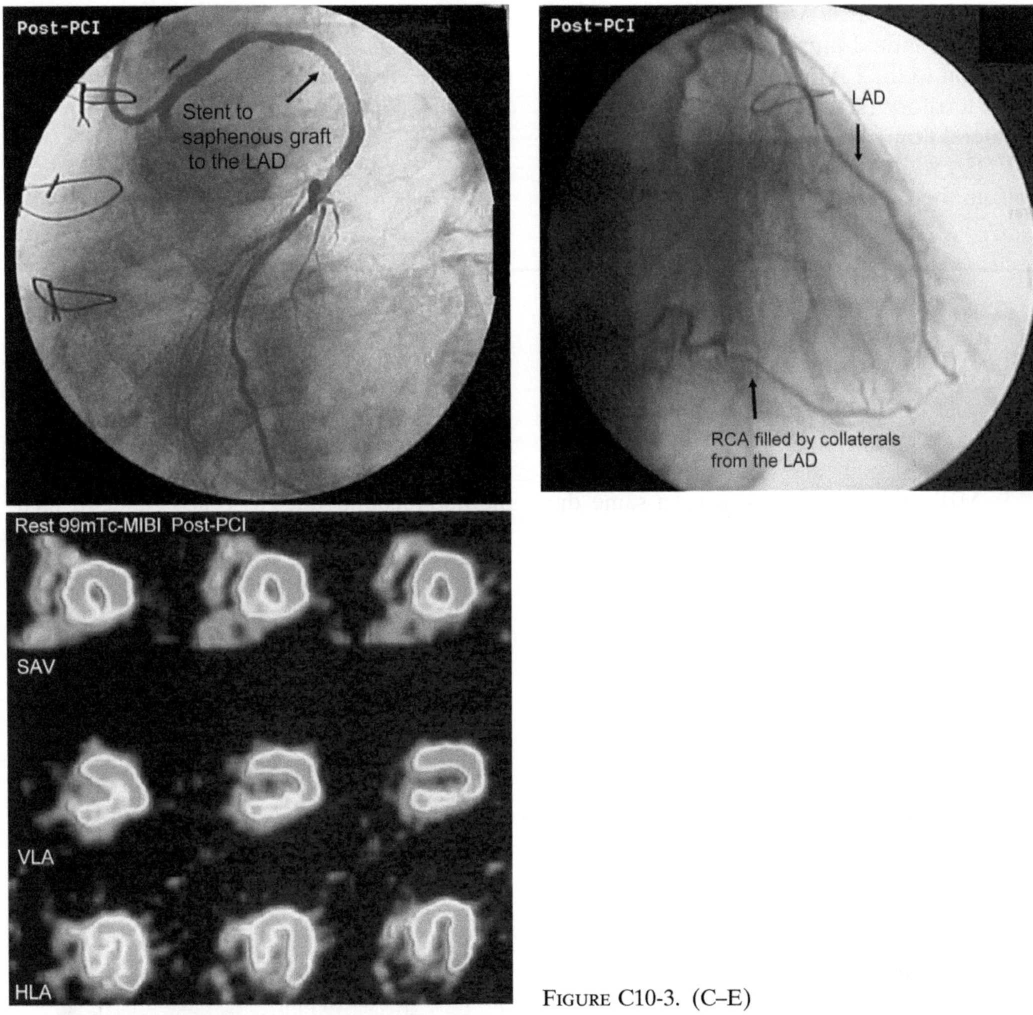

FIGURE C10-3. (C–E)

when contrast is injected in the LAD graft, due to significant collateral flow coming from the reperfused LAD.

At day 75 following graft stenting, a rest ^{99m}Tc-MIBI SPECT study (Figure C10-3E) was performed for evaluation of stent patency and the degree of possible recovery of LV function. Compared with the pre-PC1 MPI study there was a remarkable improvement of rest perfusion to the entire LAD territory and also significant but incomplete improvement of perfusion to the RCA territory. This finding indicates that the stent placed in the LAD graft allowed improvement of perfusion to an extensive area involving the entire LAD territory, and provided collateral flow to the RCA territory. Gated SPECT showed remarkable improvement of LV function, including a significant decrease of LV size, now with an EDV of 84 ml, an ESV of 30 ml, and a major increase in LVEF from 39% to 64%.

This case illustrates the use of ^{99m}Tc-MIBI to assess the dramatic response to emergency interventional therapy with coronary stenting in the setting of AMI. The role of MPI in the evaluation of patients post PCI is discussed in more detail in Case 10.1.

Interpretations

1. Rest MPI identifying acute MI, successfully treated with saphenous graft PTCA and stent placement.

2. Follow-up rest MPI 75 days after PCI revealing marked improvement in myocardial perfusion to the LAD territory and also to the RCA territory (secondary to improvement of collateral flow from the LAD), both as a result of PTCA with stent placement in the saphenous graft to the LAD.

3. Major improvement of LV function 75 days following PTCA with stent placement, with a decrease of LV cavity size and increase of LVEF from 39% to 64%.

Case 10.4

History

A 41-year-old man, a former smoker, with no additional coronary risk factors presented with atypical chest pain and anxiety. Exercise/rest ^{99m}Tc-MIBI SPECT images using a same day protocol are displayed in Figure C10-4A.

Findings

A large, moderately severe, reversible perfusion defect was seen along the anterior wall, septum, and apex, consistent with ischemia in the LAD distribution, and confirmed by coronary angiography. He was initially managed by PTCA with stent placement in the LAD but due to complex anatomy and complications, he required a CABG. His symptoms resolved after surgery but he returned 9 months later with episodes of anxiety, pallor, and sweating.

A recent CT angiography revealed a patent left internal mammary artery (LIMA) graft to the LAD and a severely diseased native artery with 70% to 80% stenosis proximal to the LIMA where a stent was initially placed (Figure C10-4B). He was referred for a repeat rest/exercise stress ^{99m}Tc-MIBI SPECT study to evaluate the results of therapy (Figure C10-4C).

Both the exercise stress and rest ^{99m}Tc-MIBI images demonstrated homogeneous perfusion of the LV. The gated images demonstrated normal LVEF and normal wall motion and systolic wall thickening. The symptoms were therefore attributed to a noncardiac etiology, and medical management was recommended.

Discussion

MPI can be used to follow-up the results of CABG. The long-term effectiveness of CABG to maintain myocardial perfusion has been limited by graft stenosis and progression of CAD in native vessels.[69] MPI is a noninvasive method recommended as a class I imaging technique by the guidelines for clinical cardiac

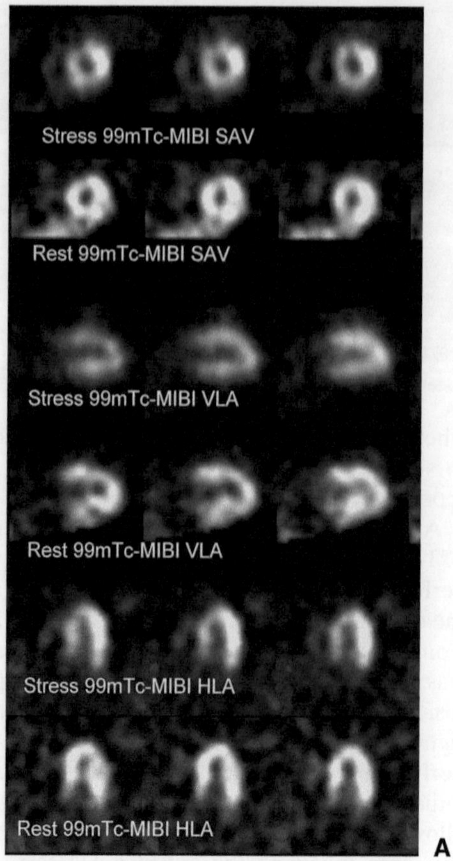

FIGURE C10-4. (A)

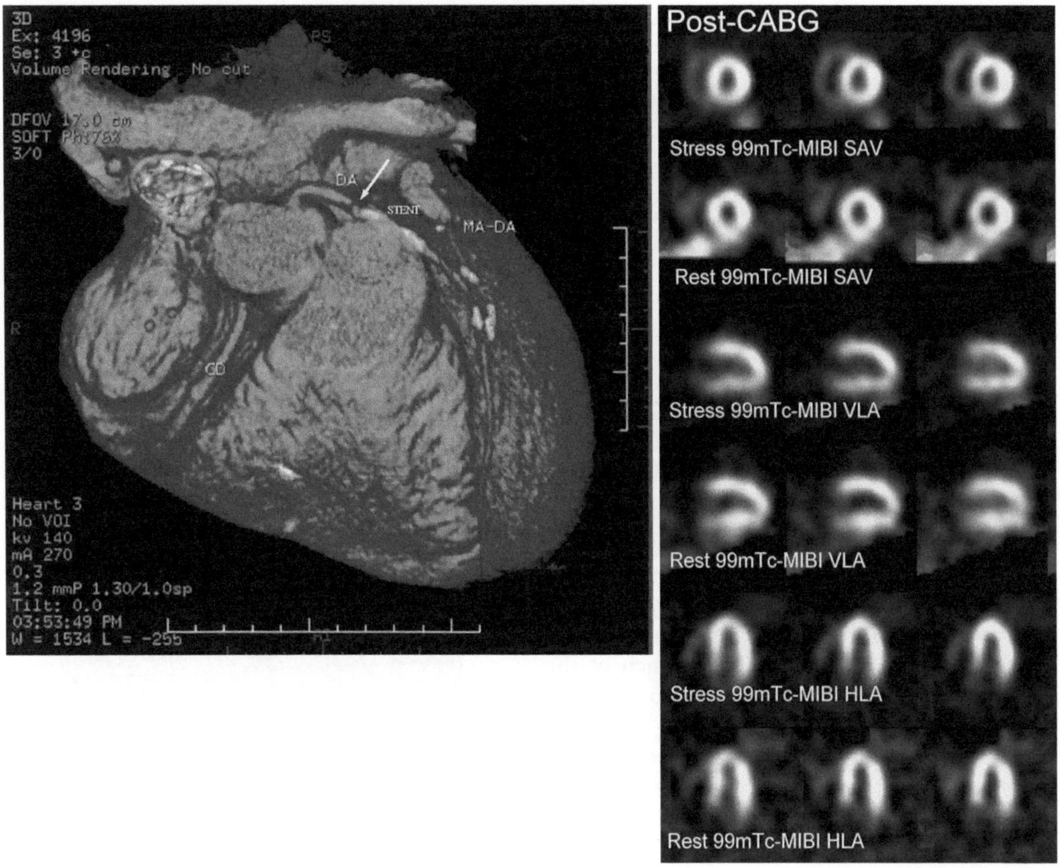

FIGURE C10-4. (B and C)

radionuclide imaging to evaluate symptomatic patients who previously underwent CABG.[59] This patient was symptomatic, 9 months after CABG despite the atypical initial presentation. Zellweger et al.[17] suggested that symptomatic patients who are less than 5 years out from CABG would benefit from MPI, determining the severity and extent of ischemia and providing guidance to therapy. This same study demonstrated that all patients, independent of the presence of symptoms, would benefit from MPI when they were more than 5 years after CABG.

Other studies have evaluated whether or not MPI following CABG can provide prognostic information.[69–71] Lauer et al.[69] reviewed 873 symptom-free patients who underwent exercise ^{201}Tl SPECT following CABG to evaluate the prognostic value of MPI for prediction of cardiac death and nonfatal MI. They concluded that perfusion defects and impaired exercise capacity (less than 6 METs) were strong and independent predictors of adverse events and that routine screening exercise MPI post CABG should be considered in asymptomatic patients, especially in patients with poor exercise tolerance.

The guidelines from the ACC and AHA for assessment and therapeutic cardiovascular procedures were published in 1995[59] but with some of the new evidence in the literature, the current recommendations for MPI in patients post-CABG can be summarized in the following way:

1. For symptomatic patients, MPI should be performed and provides diagnostic and prognostic information.

2. For asymptomatic patients, periodic MPI is recommended if the patient is more than 5 years post CABG, and before 5 years if exercise capacity is limited or if there is a possibility of silent ischemia.

Interpretations

1. LAD ischemia in a young man with atypical symptoms identified by MPI and requiring treatment with CABG.
2. Evaluation for recurrence of atypical symptoms 9 months after CABG.

Case 10.5

History

A 75-year-old woman with a history of PTCA and stent placement in the LAD and diagonal branch 6 months earlier presented with unstable angina. Coronary angiography revealed a severe stenosis of the marginal branch of the LCX, a severe lesion in the LAD, and in a diagonal branch. A dipyridamole ^{99m}Tc-MIBI SPECT study was performed for therapy planning. Significant ST-segment changes were seen on the ECG during dipyridamole infusion. The SPECT images revealed anterolateral and inferolateral ischemia and the patient underwent CABG. Due to recurrent chest pain 9 months later, a ^{99m}Tc-MIBI SPECT study was performed to evaluate response to therapy (Figure C10-5). At this time the ECG showed no changes during dipyridamole infusion.

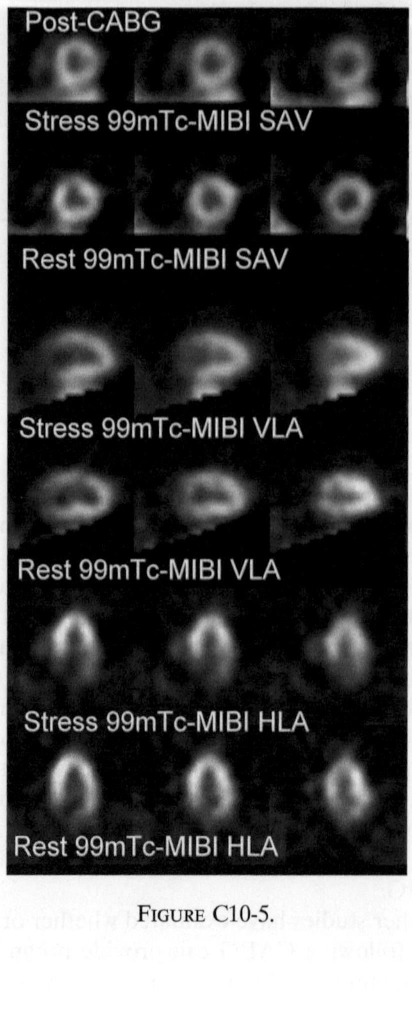

FIGURE C10-5.

Findings

The ^{99m}Tc-MIBI SPECT images showed reversible hypoperfusion in the anterior, septal, anterolateral, and lateral walls. Poststress gated SPECT images revealed normal LV motion, wall thickening, and volumes with an LVEF of 59%.

Discussion

This case illustrates the use of MPI to evaluate results of therapy 6 months after PCI and again 9 months after CABG. As in the previous case (Case 10.4), this patient presented with symptoms 9 months after revascularization. This is a class I indication based on the Guidelines for the clinical use of cardiac radionuclide imaging,[59] considering the presence of symptoms. Despite revascularization on two separate occasions, the patient remained symptomatic with clear evidence of ischemia on MPI. One important advantage of MPI over other methods is its ability to identify regional perfusion defects and determine the culprit lesion most of the time (see discussion of Case 10.4). Localization of ischemia on MPI can guide additional treatment using percutaneous techniques such as PTCA and stent placement. Improved myocardial perfusion after successful CABG results in several benefits, including increased survival in patients with left main disease or 3-vessel disease with LV dysfunction. Successful CABG is also associated with more favorable ventricular remodeling in patients with ischemic cardiomyopathy, reducing the incidence of malignant and potentially life-threatening arrhythmias.[72]

Interpretations

1. Value of MPI to evaluate results of therapy 6 months after PTCA and 9 months after CABG in a patient with recurrent chest pain.
2. Multivessel ischemia detected by MPI post-PCI and CABG.

Case 10.6

History

A 61-year-old man with multiple risk factors for CAD experienced typical angina 8 days following an acute MI that had been managed by PTCA with stent placement in the mid-LAD. He was referred for a same-day rest ^{201}Tl/adenosine ^{99m}Tc-MIBI protocol. His rest ECG revealed inverted T waves in V2 through V5. During the adenosine infusion the patient experienced typical angina accompanied by new inferior T-wave inversion. The adenosine/rest gated SPECT images are displayed in Figure C10-6.

Findings

The poststress SPECT images showed marked hypoperfusion of the anterior wall, septum, apex, and the distal inferior wall, with partial reversibility on the resting images, consistent with ischemia. The gated images showed hypokinesis of the distal anterior wall and apex, with an LVEF of 45% (images not shown). In view of these findings the patient underwent repeat coronary angiography showing a patent stent in the mid-LAD, with no evidence of restenosis.

Discussion

SPECT images revealed reversible perfusion defects in the absence of in-stent restenosis by angiography. Coronary endothelial dysfunction may be responsible for this phenomenon.[56] Endothelial dysfunction leads to impairment of coronary dilatation and CBFR.[73] This can play a role in myocardial malperfusion even though an anatomical lesion cannot be demonstrated. The pathophysiology of endothelial dysfunction is still unclear. The effect of vasoactive agents released at the site of dilatation due to mechanical trauma, coronary spasm, endothelial dysfunction,[56] or the dynamic recoil of the artery wall at the site of the earlier stenosis[74] can play a role. Endothelial dysfunction may certainly cause impairment of the coronary dilatation and may lead to ischemic events.[73] The inability of the artery to function normally to provide adequate blood flow, to the increased metabolic needs of the myocardium,[75,76] may result in clinically apparent ischemia and anginal symptoms.[77]

PTCA with stent placement procedures produces a greater degree of endothelial dysfunction when compared with balloon angioplasty alone,[78] and this can persist for several months.[68] The degree and the duration of the endothelial dysfunction appear to be proportional to the severity of the injury.[78] To deter-

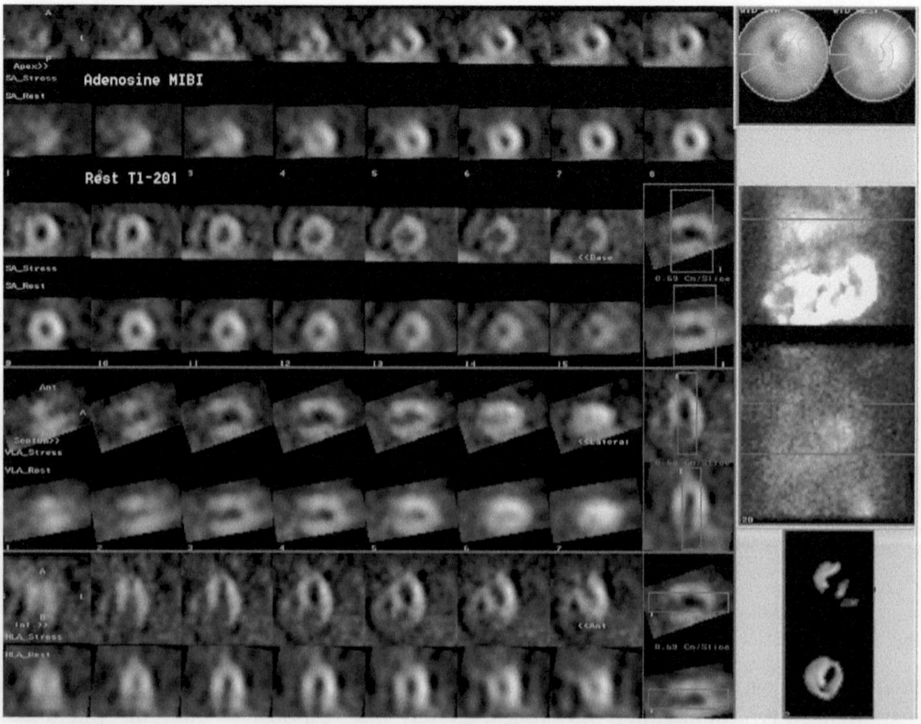

FIGURE C10-6.

mine the mechanisms of flow abnormalities after stent implantation, Kern et al.[79] measured CBFR in arteries containing the stent and in angiographically normal reference vessels and found that at least half of the flow abnormalities were caused by global microvascular disease. Another study investigated 57 patients with stable angina who underwent successful stent implantation.[80] During follow-up, 15 of 57 patients complained of chest pain and six of those exhibited evidence of ischemia on exercise MPI with in-stent restenosis on coronary angiography. In eight of the remaining nine patients, chest pain occurred without evidence of ischemia on MPI or in-stent restenosis at angiography. Intracoronary ergonovine reproduced their chest pain, and there was more intense coronary vasoreactivity to ergonovine and nitroglycerin. The authors concluded that chest pain occurs in the absence of in-stent restenosis in 20% of patients after stent implantation and appears to be associated with more intense coronary vasoreactivity.

We should keep in mind that even though an anatomical lesion is not found on coronary angiography, microvascular disease may still exist, including endothelial dysfunction that can cause diminished regional coronary flow and perfusion defects on MPI. This information is important and crucial for patient follow-up. The issue of endothelial dysfunction is further discussed in Chapter 17.

Interpretations

1. Use of MPI to follow-up therapy post-PTCA with stent placement.
2. Ischemia shown by MPI with patent vessels on coronary angiography thought to be due to endothelial dysfunction after stent placement in the LAD.

References

1. Berman DS, Hachamovitch R, Kiat H, Cohen I, Cabico JA, Wang FP, et al. Incremental value of

prognostic testing in patients with known or suspected ischemic heart disease: a basis for optimal utilization of exercise technetium-99m sestamibi myocardial perfusion single-photon emission computed tomography. *J Am Coll Cardiol.* 1995; 26(3):639–647.
2. Hachamovitch R, Berman DS, Kiat H, Cohen I, Cabico JA, Friedman J, et al. Exercise myocardial perfusion SPECT in patients without known coronary artery disease: incremental prognostic value and use in risk stratification. *Circulation.* 1996;93(5):905–914.
3. Hachamovitch R, Berman DS, Shaw LJ, Kiat H, Cohen I, Cabico JA, et al. Incremental prognostic value of myocardial perfusion single photon emission computed tomography for the prediction of cardiac death: differential stratification for risk of cardiac death and myocardial infarction [published erratum appears in *Circulation.* 1998 Jul 14;98(2):190]. *Circulation.* 1998;97(6): 535–543.
4. Califf RM, Armstrong PW, Carver JR, D'Agostino RB, Strauss WE. Stratification of patients into high, medium, and low risk subgroups for purposes of risk factor management. *J Am Coll Cardiol.* 1996;27:964–1047.
5. Gibbons RJ, Abrams J, Chatterjee K, et al. ACC/AHA 2002 guideline update for the management of patients with chronic stable angina—summary article. *J Am Coll Cardiol.* 2003; 41:159–168.
6. Miller DD, Younis LT, Bach RG, et al. Correlation of pharmacological ^{99m}Tc-sestamibi myocardial perfusion imaging with poststenotic coronary flow reserve in patients with angiographically intermediate coronary artery stenoses. *Circulation.* 1994;89(5):2150–2160.
7. Ryan TJ, Kennedy JW, Keriakes DJ, King SB III, McCallister BD, Smith SC Jr, Ullyot DJ. Guidelines for percutaneous transluminal coronary angioplasty. A report of the American Heart Association/American College of Cardiology Task Force on assessment of diagnostic and therapeutic cardiovascular procedures. *Circulation.* 1993;88:2987–3007.
8. O'Rourke RA, Chaudhuri T, Shaw L, Berman DS. Resolution of stress-induced myocardial ischemia during aggressive medical therapy as demonstrated by single photon emission computed tomography imaging. *Circulation.* 2001; 103:2315.
9. Kinlay S, Libby P, Ganz P. Endothelial function and coronary artery disease. *Curr Opin Lipidol.* 2001;12(4):383–389.
10. Mostaza JM, Gomez MV, Gallardo F, et al. Cholesterol reduction improves myocardial perfusion abnormalities in patients with coronary artery disease and average cholesterol levels. *J Am Coll Cardiol.* 2000;35:76–82.
11. Mahmarian JJ, Fenimore NL, Marks GF, et al. Transdermal nitroglycerin patch therapy reduces the extent of exercise-induced myocardial ischemia: results of a double-blind, placebo-controlled trial using quantitative thallium-201 tomography. *J Am Coll Cardiol.* 1994;24(1): 25–32.
12. Dakik HA, Kleiman NS, Farmer NS, et al. Intensive medical therapy versus coronary angioplasty for suppression of myocardial ischemia in survivors of acute myocardial infarction: a prospective randomized pilot study. *Circulation.* 1998;98(19):1985–1996.
13. Lauer MS, Lytle B, Pashkow F, et al. Prediction of death and myocardial infarction by screening with exercise-thallium testing after coronary-artery-bypass grafting. *Lancet.* 1998;351:615–622.
14. Lewin HC, Berman DS. Achieving sustained improvement in myocardial perfusion: role of isosorbide mononitrate. *Am J Cardiol.* 1997; 79(12B):31–35.
15. Parisi AF, Hartigan PM, Folland ED. Evaluation of exercise thallium scintigraphy versus exercise electrocardiography in predicting survival outcomes and morbid cardiac events in patients with single- and double-vessel disease. Findings from the Angioplasty Compared to Medicine (ACME) Study. *J Am Coll Cardiol.* 1997;30(5): 1256–1263.
16. Zellweger MJ, Berman D, Shaw L, et al. Evaluation of patients after intervention. In Polhost G, et al. (eds). *Imaging in Cardiovascular Medicine.* Philadelphia: Lippincott Williams & Wilkins; 2000.
17. Zellweger MJ, Lewin HC, Lai S, et al. When to stress patients after coronary artery bypass surgery? Risk stratification in patients early and late post-CABG using stress myocardial perfusion SPECT: implications of appropriate clinical strategies. *J Am Coll Cardiol.* 2001;37:144–152.
18. Zellweger MJ, Lewin H, Lai S, et al. Risk stratification in patients early and late post-CABG using stress myocardial perfusion SPECT: Implications of appropriate clinical strategies. *J Am Coll Cardiol.* (in press).
19. Mahmarian JJ, Moye LA, Verani MS, Bloom MF, Pratt CM. High reproducibility of myocardial

perfusion defects in patients undergoing serial exercise thallium-201 tomography. *Am J Cardiol.* 1995;75(16):1116–1119.
20. Shaw LJ, Miller DD, Berman DS, Hachamovitch R. Clinical and economic outcomes assessment in nuclear cardiology. *Q J Nuc Med.* 2000;44(2): 138–152.
21. Shaw LJ, Berman DS, Hachamovitch R, Heller GV, Travin M, Kesler K, Miller DD. Noninvasive strategies for the estimation of cardiac risk: An observational assessment of outcome in stable chest pain patients. *Am J Cardiol.* 2000;86(1): 1–7.
22. Hayes SW, Shaw LJ, O'Rourke RA, et al. COURAGE investigators. Relationship between clinical site and core lab assessments of perfusion and function on stress gated myocardial perfusion SPECT. *J Am Coll Cardiol.* 2001;37: 438A.
23. Boden WE, Weintraub WS, O'Rourke RA, et al. Review of the trials comparing medical therapy versus angioplasty and the rationale/design of the clinical outcomes utilizing percutaneous coronary revascularization and aggressive drug evaluation (COURAGE) trial. *Am Heart J.* 2003 (in press).
24. Iskander S, Pratt CM, Filipchuk NG, et al. Medical and revascularization therapies for suppression of post-infarction myocardial ischemia. Preliminary results from the Adenosine Sestamibi Post-Infarction Evaluation (INSPIRE) trial. *Circulation.* 2001;104:II-455.
25. LaRosa JC. Understanding risk in hypercholesterolemia. *Clin Cardiol.* 2003;26(1 Suppl 1):I3–6.
26. Yokoyama I, Ohtake T, Momomura S, et al. Reduced coronary flow reserve in hypercholesterolemic patients without overt coronary stenosis. *Circulation.* 1996;94(12):3232–3238.
27. Zeiher AM, Krause T, Schachinger V, et al. Impaired endothelium-dependent vasodilation of coronary resistance vessels is associated with exercise-induced myocardial ischemia. *Circulation.* 1995;91:2345–2352.
28. Aoki M, Sakai K, Koyanagi S, Takeshita A, Nakamura M. Effect of nitroglycerin on coronary collateral function during exercise evaluated by quantitative analysis of thallium-201 single photon emission computed tomography. *Am Heart J.* 1991;121(5):1361–1366.
29. Stegaru B, Loose R, Keller H, Buss J, Wetzel E. Effects of long-term treatment with 120 mg of sustained-release isosorbide dinitrate and 60 mg of sustained-release nifedipine on myocardial perfusion. *Am J Cardiol.* 1988;61(9):74E–77E.
30. Zacca NM, Verani MS, Chahine RA, Miller RR. Effect of nifedipine on exercise-induced left ventricular dysfunction and myocardial hypoperfusion in stable angina. *Am J Cardiol.* 1982;50(4): 689–695.
31. Sharir T, Rabinowitz B, Chouraqui P. Anti-ischemic drugs reduce size of reversible defects in dipyridamole/submaximal exercise ^{201}Tl SPECT imaging. *J Nucl Cardiol.* 1997;4:S71.
32. Shehata AR, Mascitelli VA, Herman SD, et al. Impact of acute propranolol administration on dobutamine-induced myocardial ischemia as evaluated by myocardial perfusion imaging and echocardiography. *Am J Cardiol.* 1997;80: 268–272.
33. Cid E, Mahmarian JJ. Factors affecting the diagnostic accuracy of quantitative single photon tomography combined with dobutamine stress. *J Nucl Med.* 1996;37:58P.
34. Gould KL, Ornish D, Scherwitz L, et al. Changes in myocardial perfusion abnormalities by positron emission tomography after long-term, intense risk factor modification. *JAMA.* 1995; 274(11):894–901.
35. Gould KL. Reversal of coronary atherosclerosis. Clinical promise as the basis for noninvasive management of coronary artery disease. *Circulation.* 1994;90(3):1558–1571.
36. Eichstadt HW, Eskotter H, Hoffman I, Amthauer HW, Weidinger G. Improvement of myocardial perfusion by short-term fluvastatin therapy in coronary artery disease. *Am J Cardiol.* 1995;76(2):122A–125A.
37. Schwartz RG, Pearson TA, Kalaria V, et al. Prospective serial evaluation of myocardial perfusion and lipids during the first six months of pravastatin therapy: coronary artery disease regression single photon emission computed tomography monitoring trial. *J Am Coll Cardiol.* 2003;42:600–610.
38. Guethlin M, Kasel AM, Coppenrath K, Ziegler S, Delius W, Schwaiger M. Delayed response of myocardial flow reserve to lipid-lowering therapy with fluvastatin. *Circulation.* 1999;99: 475–481.
39. Sdringola S, Nakagawa K, Nakagawa Y, et al. Combined intense lifestyle and pharmacologic lipid treatment further reduce coronary events and myocardial perfusion abnormalities compared with usual-care cholesterol-lowering drugs in coronary artery disease. *J Am Coll Cardiol.* 2003;41:263–272.
40. Alazraki NP, Krawczynska EG, Kosinski AS, et al. Prognostic value of ^{201}Tl SPECT for

patients with multivessel coronary disease post-revascularization: results from the Emory angioplasty-surgery trial. *Am J Cardiol.* 1999;84(12):1369–1374.
41. Hecht HS, Shaw RE, Bruce TR, Ryan C, Stertzer SH, Myler RK. Usefulness of tomographic thallium-201 imaging for detection of restenosis after percutaneous transluminal coronary angioplasty. *Am J Cardiol.* 1990;66(19):1314–1318.
42. Hecht HS, Shaw RE, Chin HL, Ryan C, Stertzer SH, Myler RK. Silent ischemia after coronary angioplasty: evaluation of restenosis and extent of ischemia in asymptomatic patients by tomographic thallium-201 exercise imaging and comparison with symptomatic patients. *J Am Coll Cardiol.* 1991;17(3):670–677.
43. Pfisterer M, Rickenbacher P, Kiowski W, Muller-Brand J, Burkart F. Silent ischemia after percutaneous transluminal coronary angioplasty: incidence and prognostic significance. *J Am Coll Cardiol.* 1993;22(5):1446–1454.
44. Milan E, Zoccarato O, Terzi A, et al. Technetium-99m-sestamibi SPECT to detect restenosis after successful percutaneous coronary angioplasty. *J Nuc Med.* 1996;37(8):1300–1305.
45. Miller DD, Verani MS. Current status of myocardial perfusion imaging after percutaneous transluminal coronary angioplasty. *J Am Coll Cardiol.* 1994;24(1):260–266.
46. Breisblatt WM, Barnes JV, Weiland F, Spaccavento LJ. Incomplete revascularization in multivessel percutaneous transluminal coronary angioplasty: the role for stress thallium-201 imaging. *J Am Coll Cardiol.* 1988;11(6):1183–1390.
47. Manyari DE, Knudtson M, Kloiber R, Roth D. Sequential thallium-201 myocardial perfusion studies after successful percutaneous transluminal coronary artery angioplasty: delayed resolution of exercise-induced scintigraphic abnormalities. *Circulation.* 1988;77(1):86–95.
48. Hirzel HO, Nuesch K, Gruentzig AR, Luetolf UM. Short- and long-term changes in myocardial perfusion after percutaneous transluminal coronary angioplasty assessed by thallium-201 exercise scintigraphy. *Circulation.* 1981;63:1001–1007.
49. Hammermeister KE, DeRouen TA, Dodge HT, et al. Prognostic and predictive value of exertional hypotension in suspected coronary artery disease. *Am J Cardiol.* 1983;51:1261–1266.
50. Hachamovitch R, Berman DS, Kiat H, Cohen I, Friedman JD, Shaw LJ. Value of stress myocardial perfusion single photon emission computed tomography in patients with normal resting electrocardiograms. An evaluation of incremental prognostic value and cost-effectiveness. *Circulation.* 2002;105:823–829.
51. Dori G, Denekamp Y, Fishman S, Bitterman H. Exercise stress testing, myocardial perfusion imaging and stress echocardiography for detecting restenosis after successful percutaneous transluminal coronary angioplasty: a review of performance. *J Intern Med.* 2003;253:253–262.
52. Fischman DL, Leon M, Baim DS, et al. A randomized comparison of coronary stent placement and balloon angioplasty in the treatment of coronary artery disease. *N Engl J Med.* 1994;331:496–501.
53. Georgoulias P, Demakopoulos N, Kontos A, et al. ^{99m}Tc tetrofosmin myocardial perfusion imaging before and six months after percutaneous transluminal coronary angioplasty. *Clin Nucl Med.* 1998;23:678–682.
54. Galassi AR, Rosario F, Azzarelli S, et al. Usefulness of exercise tomographic myocardial perfusion imaging for detection of restenosis after coronary stent implantation. *Am J Cardiol.* 2000;85:1362–1364.
55. Milavetz JJ, Miller TD, Hodge DO, Holmes DR, Gibbons RJ. Accuracy of single-photon emission computed tomography myocardial perfusion imaging in patients with stents in native coronary arteries. *Am J Cardiol.* 1998;82:857–861.
56. Rodés-Cabau J, Candell-Riera J, Domingo E, et al. Frequency and clinical significance of myocardial ischemia detected early after coronary stent implantation. *J Nucl Med.* 2001;42:1768–1772.
57. Teles RC, Reis-Santos K, Gil V, et al. A negative myocardial perfusion scintigram after coronary angioplasty confers benign long-term prognosis. *Rev Port Cardiol.* 2002;21:1393–1402.
58. Acampa W, Peretta M, Florimonte L, et al. Prognostic value of exercise cardiac tomography performed late after percutaneous coronary intervention in symptomatic and symptom-free patients. *Am J Cardiol.* 2003;91:259–263.
59. Ritchie JL, Bateman TM, Bonow RO, et al. Guidelines for clinical use of cardiac radionuclide imaging: A report of the American College of Cardiology/American Heart Association task force on assessment of diagnostic and therapeutic cardiovascular procedures (Committee on Radionuclide Imaging)—developed in collaboration with the American Society of Nuclear Cardiology. *J Nucl Cardiol.* 1995;Mar–Apr;2(2 Pt1):172–192.

60. Serruys PW, de Jaegere P, Kiemeneij F, et al. A comparison of balloon-expandable-stent implantation with balloon angioplasty in patients with coronary artery disease. Benestent Study Group. *N Engl J Med.* 1994;Aug 25;331(8):489–495.
61. Schomig A, Kastrati A, Mudra H, et al. Four-year experience with Palmaz-Schatz stenting in coronary angioplasty complicated by dissection with threatened or present vessel closure. *Circulation.* 1994;Dec;90(6):2716–2724.
62. Fenton SH, Fischman DL, Savage MP, et al. Long-term angiographic and clinical outcome after implantation of balloon-expandable stents in aortocoronary saphenous vein grafts. *Am J Cardiol.* 1994;Dec 15;74(12):1187–1191.
63. Morice MC, Serruys PW, Sousa JE, et al., and the RAVEL Study Group. A randomized comparison of a sirolimus-eluting stent with a standard stent for coronary revascularization. *N Engl J Med.* 2002;Jun 6;346(23):1773–1780.
64. Garzon PP, Eisenberg MJ. Functional testing for the detection of restenosis after percutaneous transluminal coronary angioplasty: a meta-analysis. *Can J Cardiol.* 2001;Jan;17(1):41–48.
65. Cottin Y, Rezaizadeh K, Touzery C, et al. Long-term prognostic value of ^{201}Tl single-photon emission computed tomographic myocardial perfusion imaging after coronary stenting. *Am Heart J.* 2001;Jun;141(6):999–1006.
66. Stempfle HU, Schmid R, Tausig A, et al. Early detection of myocardial microcirculatory disturbances after primary PTCA in patients with acute myocardial infarction: coronary blood flow velocity versus sestamibi perfusion imaging. *Z Kardiol.* 2002;91 Suppl 3:126–131.
67. Fram DB, Azar RR, Ahlberg AW, et al. Duration of abnormal SPECT myocardial perfusion imaging following resolution of acute ischemia: an angioplasty model. *J Am Coll Cardiol.* 2003; Feb 5;41(3):452–459.
68. Jaffe R, Haim SB, Karkabi B, et al. Myocardial perfusion abnormalities early (12–24h) after coronary stenting or balloon angioplasty: implications regarding pathophysiology and late clinical outcome. *Cardiology.* 2002;98(1–2):60–66.
69. Lauer MS, Lytle B, Pashkow F, Snader CE, Marwick TH. Prediction of death and myocardial infarction by screening with exercise-thallium testing after coronary-artery-bypass grafting. *Lancet.* 1998;351:615–622.
70. Miller TD, Christian TF, Hodge DO, et al. Prognostic value of exercise thallium-201 imaging performed within 2 years of coronary artery bypass graft surgery. *J Am Coll Cardiol.* 1998; 31(4):848–854.
71. Desideri A, Candelpergher G, Zanco P, et al. Exercise technetium 99m sestamibi single-photon emission computed tomography late after coronary bypass surgery: long-term follow-up. *Clin Cardiol.* 1997;20(9):779–784.
72. Elhendy A, Cornel JH, Domburg RT, et al. Effect of coronary artery bypass surgery on myocardial perfusion and ejection fraction response to inotropic stimulation in patients without improvement in resting ejection fraction. *Am J Cardiol.* 2000;86:490–494.
73. Kjaer A, Meyer C, Nielsen FS, Parving HH, Hesse B. Dipyridamole, cold pressor test and demonstration of endothelial dysfunction: a PET study of myocardial perfusion in diabetes. *J Nucl Med.* 2003;44:19–23.
74. Kosa I, Blasini R, Schneider-Eicke J, et al. Early recovery of coronary flow reserve after stent implantation as assessed by positron emission tomography. *J Am Coll Cardiol.* 1999;34(4): 1036–1041.
75. Fleming RM, Harrington GM. Quantitative coronary arteriography and its assessment of atherosclerosis. Part 1. Examining the independent variables. *Angiology.* 1994;45:829–833.
76. Fleming RM, Harrington GM. Quantitative coronary arteriography and its assessment of atherosclerosis. Part 2. Calculating stenosis flow reserve directly from percent diameter stenosis. *Angiology.* 1994;45:835–840.
77. Fleming RM, Boyd L, Forster M. Angina is caused by regional blood flow differences-proof of a physiologic (not anatomic) narrowing. Joint ACC-ESC Session, 49th Annual Scientific Sessions, Anaheim, CA 12 March 2000.
78. Caramori PR, Lima VC, Seidelin PH, Newton GE, Parker JD, Adelman AG. Long term endothelial dysfunction after coronary artery stenting. *J Am Coll Cardiol.* 1999;34: 1675–1679.
79. Kern MJ, Puri S, Bach RG, et al. Abnormal coronary flow abnormality reserve after coronary stenting in patients: role of relative coronary reserve to assess potential mechanisms. *Circulation.* 1999;100:2491–2498.
80. Versaci F, Gaspardone A, Tomai F, et al. Chest pain after coronary artery stent implantation. *Am J Cardiol.* 2002;89:500–504.

11
Risk Assessment Before Noncardiac Surgery

Jeffrey A. Leppo and Seth Dahlberg

The evaluation of preoperative cardiac risk in patients undergoing noncardiac surgery has been a challenging and important topic over the past 25 years. Given the growing prevalence of both coronary artery disease (CAD) and noncardiac surgical procedures in the United States,[1] the preoperative evaluation for cardiac risk becomes more important. The medical parameters and clinical factors first reported by Goldman et al.[2] have evolved into a more systematic approach and recently into American College of Cardiology/American Heart Association guidelines.[3] Although controlled prospective or randomized clinical trials are lacking in this clinical area, there are many retrospective reports and a few metaanalyses that demonstrate the utility of nuclear cardiology testing in this evaluation process.

The goals of this chapter are to review the current preoperative guidelines as they deal with nuclear cardiology studies and to review the prognostic utility of such evaluation for both short-term (preoperative) and long-term follow-up. This chapter focuses on CAD as the main feature of preoperative cardiac assessment. In patients with CAD, the evaluations of ischemia and left ventricular (LV) function have been shown to have significant prognostic utility for cardiac events such as myocardial infarction (MI) or cardiac death.[4]

Perioperative Cardiac Assessment for Noncardiac Surgery

As recently reviewed by Mukherjee and Eagle,[5] it is possible to divide the perioperative cardiac assessment for noncardiac surgery into 8 steps to achieve an optimal medical outcome.

First Step: Clinical Evaluation of Preoperative Cardiac Risk

There have been reports[2,6,7] that have shown that cardiac risk for noncardiac surgery can be determined by a careful history and physical examination, which often are summarized as clinical indices. Typical clinical parameters that have been shown to have useful prognostic importance in predicting perioperative events include a history of angina, congestive heart failure (CHF), MI, and diabetes. If the symptomatic level of angina or cardiac failure is moderate to severe and the MI is recent (less than 3 months), then most guidelines would suggest that the cardiac problem requires attention and resolution before the patient undergoes elective surgery. In contrast, the absence of these clinical parameters in an otherwise low-risk

Table 11-1. Risk of Various Types of Surgery

High surgical risk
Emergent major operations, particularly in the elderly
Aortic and other major vascular surgery
Peripheral vascular surgery
Anticipated prolonged surgical procedures associated with large fluid shifts and/or blood loss
Intermediate surgical risk
Carotid endarterectomy
Head and neck surgery
Intraperitoneal and intrathoracic
Orthopedic surgery
Prostate surgery
Low surgical risk
Endoscopic procedures
Superficial procedures
Cataract surgery
Breast surgery
Prostate surgery

Data from Eagle KA, Berger PB, Calkins H, et al. ACC/AHA guideline update for perioperative cardiovascular evaluation for noncardiac surgery–executive summary: a report of the American College of Cardiology/American Heart Association Task Force on Practice Guidelines (Committee to Update the 1996 Guidelines on Perioperative Cardiovascular Evaluation for Noncardiac Surgery). *J Am Coll Cardiol.* 2002;39:542–553.

surgical patient is often associated with a low cardiac event rate after elective surgery. As in most types of risk assessment, it is also important to consider the specific patient population that you are evaluating.

Second Step: Evaluate Functional Capacity

The cardiology evaluation should include objective or historical information to appropriate and evaluate functional capacity. The Duke activity status index[8] can be used to approximate the metabolic equivalents (METs) for many daily activities. If the patient can exceed 4 METs with daily activity (climbs 1 to 2 flights of stairs, performs their own housework, or exercises regularly), then the patient will typically have sufficient cardiovascular reserve to tolerate the stress of surgery. In contrast, those patients who have limited functional capacity may have poor cardiovascular reserve, which could increase their surgical risk. Those patients with poor functional capacity have worse perioperative and long-term outcomes after noncardiac surgery.

Third Step: Evaluate the Specific Surgery Risk

The type of surgery also has an important impact on perioperative risk. In Table 11-1,[3] the major types of surgical procedures are divided into high-, intermediate-, and low-risk groups.

Fourth Step: When to Obtain Additional Noninvasive Testing

A recommendation for further testing can be made on the basis of the first three steps. Table 11-2 shows how the guidelines can be simplified based on functional capacity, intermediate clinical risk factors, and type of surgery. The greatest benefit to a noninvasive approach appears to be in patients with intermediate risk, and this type of testing has both short- and long-term prognostic utility.

Fifth Step: When to Recommend Invasive Procedures

It is typical to recommend coronary angiography for preoperative patients who have unstable or class IV angina, as well as ischemia after a recent MI. It is generally recommended to perform preoperative coronary angiography in a similar fashion as the nonoperative situation

Table 11-2. Shortcut to Noninvasive Testing in Preoperative Patients If Any Two Factors Are Present

1. Intermediate clinical predictors are present (Canadian class 1 or 2 angina, prior MI based on history or pathological Q waves, compensated or prior CHF, or diabetes)
2. Poor functional capacity (<4 METS)
3. High surgical risk procedure (emergency major operations; aortic repair or peripheral vascular; prolonged surgical procedures with large fluid shifts and/or blood loss)

(evidence of high ischemic or heart failure risk based on poorly controlled symptoms or very positive noninvasive test results). Froehlich et al.[9] have proposed a stepwise, judicious use of both noninvasive and invasive procedures to provide a low rate of cardiac events. In addition, there are now recommendations in the guidelines to wait at least 2 weeks and, if possible, 4 weeks after coronary artery stent placement before performing any elective noncardiac surgery.[10] This is done to permit more complete endothelialization of the coronary intervention site and a full course of antiplatelet therapy to be administered.

Sixth Step: Medical Therapy Optimization

Based on the patient's cardiac condition, the patient should be on an optimal medical therapy both perioperatively and for the long term. Most CAD patients with anginal symptoms should benefit from aspirin, beta-blockers, nitrates, and probably statin therapy. The addition of angiotensin-converting enzyme inhibitor or receptor blocker should be used when left ventricular ejection fraction (LVEF) is reduced (<40%) or the patient has clinical heart failure. In higher-risk CAD patients, efforts should be made to correct anemia and electrolyte imbalances, as well as to promptly correct postoperative pain to reduce catecholamine release. Inotropic agents that elevate myocardial oxygen demand should generally be avoided. A detailed discussion of beta-blocker therapy follows in the specific clinical risk section.

Seventh Step: Practice Appropriate Perioperative Care and Monitoring

In perioperative patients with known or suspected CAD, electrocardiograms (ECGs) should be collected preoperatively and immediately after surgery. Perioperative ECG monitoring (especially of leads that showed ST-segment depression during preoperative stress testing) should be performed for the initial 2 days after surgery. Serum biomarkers (creatinine kinase and troponin) should be measured in the first 24 hours after surgery in high-risk CAD patients. Antiplatelet agents should be restarted as soon as possible, and any patient who develops ST-segment elevation MI should be evaluated for urgent coronary angiography and percutaneous coronary intervention (PCI).

Eighth Step: Develop Long-Term Cardiac Therapy and Follow-Up

The process of cardiac consultation and risk assessment for the preoperative patient should be viewed as an opportunity to practice good medical care. Cardiac risk factors should be appropriately treated (hypertension, diabetes, hyperlipidemia, smoking, cardiac murmurs, ischemia, heart failure, and so forth). This evaluation and recommendations should be communicated to the patient and the primary care physician, so that it becomes part of the long-term health plan. This is especially important for any patient who sustains a severe ischemic episode, heart failure, or nonfatal MI in the perioperative period. All of these events carry high risk for future cardiac events over the next 2 to 4 years.

Specific Clinical Risk Assessment

Although the clinical question that is often posed to the medical or cardiac consultant is whether or not to *clear* the patient for noncardiac surgery, the ACC/AHA guidelines[3] suggest an overall conservative approach to the use of expensive tests and interventions. Specific algorithms describe a clinical pathway for the medical consultant to use, but these should be viewed in the setting of a team approach involving the primary care physician, surgeon, anesthesiologist, and patient.

Little can be done for patients who must undergo emergency surgery, other than attempting to manage acute medical problems in the perioperative period. However, after surgical recovery it may be helpful in long-term follow-up to complete an appropriate evaluation in those patients with significant or major cardiac problems. For instance, a patient with unstable angina or a nontransmural MI during emergency abdominal surgery should undergo routine diagnostic studies to assess cardiac function and residual ischemia before discharge.

The real challenge is in symptomatic or mildly symptomatic patients who are being evaluated for elective surgical procedures. It is best to begin by obtaining a detailed medical history, physical examination, and ECG. Particular attention should be paid to obtaining information about angina, MI, CHF, symptomatic arrhythmia, diabetes, peripheral vascular disease, and prior history of coronary angiography or revascularization procedures. Even in the presence of a known history of CAD, it is recommended to proceed with elective surgery if the patient has had successful coronary revascularization within the previous 5 years[11] and is without recurrent signs or symptoms. It is also reasonable to proceed to surgery if the patient has had a recent coronary angiography or stress test that reveals favorable results or a stable (low-risk) clinical situation. However, the presence of major cardiac symptoms, as noted previously, should alert the consulting physician to reconsider a decision to allow the patient to undergo any elective procedure.

Vascular Surgery

Although it is important to detect CAD and assess its severity in most routine preoperative evaluations,[2] it is clearly a prominent feature of elective vascular surgery. This is the result of the high prevalence (approximately 60%) of CAD in many large series of vascular surgery patients[12] and has been well documented in a series of 1,000 patients who routinely underwent coronary angiography before vascular surgery.[13] The incidence of nonfatal MI or cardiac death in this population has been summarized in Table 11-3. It is clear that cardiac death was a relatively high risk in the earlier published literature but, in the early 1990s, the death rate had fallen to less than 2%. During the same time period, the rate of nonfatal MIs has generally decreased, but the incidence is still twofold to threefold higher than cardiac death. Although it appears that overall patient care (involving preselection and more intense perioperative management) has resulted in a lower death rate, the ability to predict and prevent infarctions is much more difficult. It would seem reasonable at this point to conclude that aggressive interventions to further lower the death rate will be difficult and will

TABLE 11-3. Perioperative Cardiac Events in Noncardiac Surgery ($n \geq 100$ Patients)

		Incidence of	
Vascular Surgery	No. Patients	NFMI (%)	CV Death (%)
Young 1977[47] 1958–68	75	12.5	8.0
1968–76	143	12.5	8.0
Hertzer 1981[48] Aortic	343	NA	6.1
Peripheral	273	NA	3.3
Cutler 1987[49]	116	7.8	0
Raby 1989[50]	176	2.3	0.6
Eagle 1989[7]	200	4.5	3.0
Younis 1990[51]	111	3.6	3.6
Hendel 1992[52]	327	6.7	2.1
Taylor 1991[53]	491	3.5	0.8
Kresowik 1993[54]	170	2.4	0.6
McFalls 1993[55]	116	17.0	1.7
Baron 1994[17]	457	4.8	2.2
Bry 1994[56]	237	5.9	1.3
Seeger 1994[57]	172 (no test)	1.1	0.6
	146 (test)	3.4	0.7
Fleisher 1995[58]	109	3.7	0.9

NFMI: nonfatal myocardial infarction; CV: cardiovascular, No = number.

probably fail to be cost-effective because of the low incidence. However, the observation that nonfatal MI in the postoperative period is a powerful predictor of late cardiac events[14] suggests the need to combine preoperative screening plans with longer-term coronary management.

Shaw et al.[15] reviewed the utility of preoperative noninvasive testing in a large metaanalysis. These authors reviewed studies from 1985 to 1994 in which either dipyridamole thallium (n = 1994) or dobutamine echocardiography (n = 455) was used as a pharmacologic stressor. Reversible perfusion defects were noted in 26% of patients, and nonfatal MI or cardiovascular death occurred in 9% of these postoperative cases. In contrast, 430 (22%) patients had normal perfusion scans and an event rate of 1.4%. Similar prognostic utility was noted in the dobutamine echocardiography studies. New wall motion abnormalities during dobutamine-induced stress were noted in 39% of the patients, and 11% of these cases had a major cardiac event. In the 270 (61%) patients without new regional wall motion abnormalities, the event rate was 0.4%. The authors of this metaanalysis concluded that (1) reversible perfusion defects have significant positive predictive accuracy; (2) dobutamine-induced wall motion abnormalities predict adverse outcomes; (3) the use of semiquantitative image analysis for perfusion imaging should improve its prognostic utility; and (4) fixed defects predict long-term cardiac events with an accuracy equal to reversible defects for perioperative events.

In summary, this background review confirms that cardiac events are a significant risk during elective surgery. In certain high-risk surgery populations (vascular), CAD is quite common. It is also clear that the most common perioperative cardiac event is a nonfatal MI, which implies that the extent of ischemic burden would be a useful predictor of these types of outcomes. Therefore, the addition of noninvasive testing in this population should be able to definitively quantify the degree of ischemia to enhance the clinical information. If LV function can also be evaluated, it will prove helpful in the long-term evaluation of cardiac risk as well.

Specific Issues Related to Preoperative Testing

The preoperative guidelines[3] are fairly straightforward about recommendations for patients having emergency surgery and for those with major cardiac predictors. However, the majority of patients fall into the large group of patients who have either intermediate or minor clinical predictors of increased perioperative cardiovascular risk. Table 11-2 presents a shortcut approach to a large number of patients in whom the decision to recommend testing before surgery can be difficult. Basically, if 2 of the 3 listed factors are true, then the guidelines suggest the use of noninvasive cardiac testing as part of the preoperative evaluation. In any patients with an intermediate clinical predictor, the presence of either a low functional capacity or high surgical risk should lead the consulting physician to perform noninvasive testing.

In the absence of intermediate clinical predictors, noninvasive testing should be performed when both the surgical risk is high and the functional capacity is low. The guidelines define minor clinical predictors as advanced age, abnormal ECG, rhythm other than sinus, history of stroke, or uncontrolled systemic hypertension. These factors do not by themselves suggest the need for further testing but, when combined with low functional capacity and high-risk surgery, preoperative testing is recommended.

A summary of pharmacologic (dipyridamole or adenosine) myocardial perfusion imaging (MPI) in more than 3,000 patients is shown in Table 11-4. In the upper section, all studies involved vascular surgery, and the incidence of thallium redistribution was 42%. The overall positive predictive accuracy is 12%, but its value has clearly decreased over the past decades (from the mid-1980s). In this vascular surgery population, the prevalence of CAD is 60% to 70%, and 38% (930 of 2417) of these patients have a normal stress perfusion scan. It is important to note that the average negative predictive accuracy is 99%, which implies that a normal stress perfusion study has powerful

TABLE 11-4. Pharmacologic Perfusion Imaging for Preoperative Assessment of Cardiac Risk

Author Vascular Surgery Only	Thallium redist (%)	Periop events MI/Dead (%)	Ischemia Pos. Pred(%)	Normal Scan Neg. Pred (%)
Boucher 1985[59]	33	6	19	100
Cutler 1987[49]	47	10	20	100
Fletcher 1988[60]	22	4	37	100
Sachs 1988[61]	31	4	14	100
Eagle 1989[7]	41	8	16	98
Younis 1990[51]	36	7	15	100
Mangano 1991[16]	37	5	5	95
Lette 1992[36]	45	8	17	99
Hendel 1992[52]	51	9	14	99
Kresowik 1993[54]	39	3	4	98
Baron 1994[17]	35	5	4	96
Bry 1994[56]	46	7	11	100
Koutelou 1995[62]	44	3	6	100
Marshall 1995[63]	47	10	16	97
Total (weighted avg)	42	7	12	99
2417 Total patients				
Other Surgery Author	**Thallium redist (%)**	**Periop events MI/Dead (%)**	**Ischemia Pos. Pred(%)**	**Normal Scan Neg. Pred (%)**
Coley 1992[64]	36	4	11	99
Shaw 1992[65]	47	10	21	100
Brown 1993[66]	33	5	13	99
Younis 1994[67]	31	9	18	98
Stratmann 1996[68]	29	4	6	99
Van Damme 1997[69]	34	2	NA	NA
Total (weighted avg)	33	6	13	99
923 Total patients				

prognostic utility during the perioperative period.

The importance of negative predictive accuracy is emphasized by the observation that 2 of these publications concluded that perfusion imaging was not accurate in detecting risk. In studies by Mangano et al.[16] and Baron et al.,[17] event sensitivity and negative predictive accuracy were relatively low, which suggests that the application of MPI is not universally appropriate. In laboratories where the sensitivity for CAD is low and the cardiac event rate in patients with normal scans exceeds 2%, the prognostic utility for perfusion imaging will not be this good. There may also be a bias in patient selection for noninvasive testing, as well as whether the studies were prospective or retrospective. In addition, there are probably differences in imaging techniques and expertise.

In the lower section of Table 11-4, the population has been expanded to include patients who did not have vascular surgery. Most patients in this section were studied because there was an increased risk of CAD, and the overall event rate (7%) was the same as in the vascular surgery group. It is interesting to note that the incidence of thallium redistribution was somewhat lower, but the positive predictive value was similar to that noted in the nonvascular surgery group.

Clinical Application of the Preoperative Guidelines

Although there are no randomized studies that have initially tested the guidelines, there are some studies that demonstrate the clinical consequences of using these guidelines in a practical way. Lee et al.[18] evaluated a total of 4,315 patients undergoing elective noncardiac surgery. They reported a simple clinical index of 6 factors that could predict perioperative cardiac events. Specifically, the presence of high-risk surgery, a history of CAD, CHF, or cerebrovascular disease, as well as treatment with insulin or a creatinemia of greater than 2.0 mg/dl were useful for risk assessment. In a validation population trial, the authors noted that when none or only one of these 6 factors were present (74% of all patients), the postoperative cardiac event rate was less than 1%. In contrast, the event rate in patients with any 2 factors was 7% (18% of all patients) and in those patients with 3 or more factors (8% of all patients), the event rate was 11%.

In another study, Vanzetto et al.[19] conducted a prospective clinical trial of patients undergoing abdominal aortic surgery and identified a subgroup of high-risk CAD. This classification of high risk was based on the presence of 2 or more clinical predictors. Of 457 patients, 32% (147) were classified as high risk, and subsequently 134 (of the 147) patients underwent surgery after dipyridamole (SPECT) thallium scans. The remaining 317 patients underwent elective aortic surgery without any further testing based on the presence of no more than a single high-risk parameter. On the basis of these clinical criteria alone, 9% of the high-risk patients had cardiac events. In contrast, there was a 4% event rate in patients with one risk factor and a rate of approximately 2% in patients without any CAD risk predictors. In this study the classification of high risk is equivalent to intermediate clinical predictors in the ACC/AHA preoperative guidelines.[3] The combination of aortic vascular surgery with these clinical risk factors should result in preoperative testing, and the observed event rate of 23% in patients with thallium redistribution confirms the prognostic utility of scintigraphy in this subgroup. It is also important to add that Vanzetto et al.[19] performed a multivariate analysis that showed that the number of ischemic segments was the single best predictor of perioperative events.

It is equally important to note that a normal perfusion scan in this clinical high-risk group is associated with a low event rate, which is equivalent to that observed in patients without any clinical risk predictors. Therefore, the presence of a normal stress perfusion scan in high-risk vascular surgery patients appears to identify an otherwise undetected low-risk subgroup that is equivalent to a group with no clinical risk factors. In comparison with the observations of Lee et al.,[18] this report emphasizes the higher inherent cardiac risk when the evaluations involve only vascular surgery patients.

In another preoperative cardiac risk study, Bartels et al.[20] evaluated a strategy that emulated the ACC/AHA recommendations. Clinical risk classifications were assigned to 201 patients who were to undergo major vascular surgery. Approximately 10% of the patients were defined as high risk based on the presence of an MI within the prior 6 months, decompensated CHF, Canadian class 3-4 angina, significant arrhythmias, or severe valvular disease. This is consistent with major clinical CAD risk predictors in the guidelines.[3]

In 40% of the patients, an intermediate cardiac risk was assigned based on the presence of a remote MI, compensated CHF, Canadian class 1-2 angina, diabetes (insulin-dependent), or elevated serum creatine level. In the remaining half of the patients, none of these factors were present, and they were defined as low risk. All the low-risk patients and the intermediate-risk patients (52%) with a functional capacity of >5 METs based on a questionnaire (Duke Activity Status Index)[8] proceeded directly to major aortic surgery without further testing. The remaining intermediate-risk patients (48%) who had a functional capacity of <5 METs on the questionnaire underwent noninvasive testing (40%) or intensified medical care (60%) before surgery. In the high-risk group, approximately one-half underwent noninvasive testing, and the other half received intensified medical treatment. Subsequently 5 (6%) intermediate- and 2 (9%) high-risk patients underwent preoperative coronary angiography, resulting in one coronary artery bypass graft (CABG) procedure and 2 cancellations of further elective surgery.

Cardiac events occurred in 5% of the high-risk group and in 9% of the intermediate-risk group patients. The low-risk group had an event rate of 2%. In addition, intensified medical treatment or additional testing and intervention in the high-risk patients can also be appropriately guided by test results. Furthermore, this report confirms the value of testing to evaluate intermediate-risk patients. Overall, this study does support the clinical algorithm suggested by the published guidelines, but there were some protocol alterations that resulted in poor outcomes. Further studies are needed to determine whether preoperative patients at higher risk can be appropriately treated and have a lower event rate during the perioperative period.

These 2 imaging articles support the use of selective testing of vascular surgery patients according to a clinical algorithm that is similar to the ACC/AHA guidelines. These data also suggest that increased risk is associated with larger segmental abnormalities. However, some more recent articles[21–23] have suggested that the use of beta-blockers alone is sufficient to adequately manage most preoperative patients. In these reports, the results of the Dutch Echocardiographic Cardiac Risk Evaluation Applying Stress Echocardiography (DECREASE) trial show that intermediate-risk (based on the extent of dobutamine-induced segmental wall motion abnormalities) vascular surgery patients have a significantly lower event rate if treated with bisoprolol before surgery. These articles have several limitations that include a retrospective methodology and high prevalence of prior MIs, as well as a relatively high postoperative cardiac death rate.

In addition, other reports by Wallace et al.[24] and Mangano et al.[25] using prospective, random, and blinded methodology, show that beta-blockers given intravenously just before surgery do not decrease perioperative cardiac events. Presently, it would still seem quite reasonable to use or continue beta-blockers in the perioperative period in all patients with known or suspected CAD.

Special Subgroups and Gender Considerations

The question of routine screening for all patients undergoing renal or liver transplants is more an issue of long-term follow-up and cardiac prognosis. There is little immediate risk to performing the transplant surgery, but it is clear that cardiac morbidity and mortality can have a significant impact during the postoperative follow-up period. This seems to be especially true for patients with diabetes[26] and can result in routine noninvasive or coronary angiography testing in many patients before transplantation. Heston et al.[27] have shown that an "expert system" using clinical risk predictors and thallium stress testing can achieve an overall accuracy of 89% in predicting 4-year cardiac mortality among 189 renal transplant candidates. This observation is supported by prior publications[28,29] and suggests that no further cardiac evaluation is needed if there are no clinical risk predictors such as a history of CHF, angina, insulin-dependent diabetes, age >50 years, or an abnormal ECG (excluding LV hypertrophy).

In patients being evaluated for cardiac problems before liver transplantation, there has been little published experience. There is a long-term cardiac risk, but a recent study from Kryzhanovski and Beller[30] suggests that this risk is too low to warrant routine stress MPI or radionuclide angiogram in all patients. There were no cardiac events in 63 liver transplant procedures, and only one patient had a high-risk scan. Therefore, cardiac evaluations should be used in this patient subgroup only when there is clear evidence for CAD or when significant (intermediate) clinical risk predictors are present.

The effect of gender differences was reviewed by Hendel et al.,[31] and it is clear from this study of vascular surgery patients that overall cardiac events in both the perioperative and the long-term follow-up period were similar for men and women. However, significant differences in various clinical factors for the prediction of cardiac events were noted. Multivariate analysis of clinical and scintigraphic factors for perioperative MI or cardiac death showed that Q waves, a history of CHF, thallium redistribution, and ST-segment depression during parenteral dipyridamole administration were the best predictors in men. In contrast, only thallium redistribution was a significant predictor in women, and the presence of angina (not significant in men) was also of value.

These observations on gender differences suggest that overall clinical risk assessment might be improved by application of different specific predictors for each subpopulation. For instance, ST depression is a powerful predictor of perioperative events in male patients, but lacks such an impact in a female population. In contrast, perfusion imaging has a significant prognostic ability for both male and female patients and may well explain why this factor is the best overall predictor in the entire population. This report by Hendel et al.[31] also evaluated long-term (4- to 5-year) follow-up in this population and again noted gender differences in clinical but not scintigraphic predictors of cardiac events. Overall, this study suggests that scintigraphic findings are effective in both male and female populations, but clinical factors need to be specific for gender differences. In addition, scintigraphic findings that correlate with ischemia (transient defects) are more powerful predictors of perioperative events, whereas late events are best predicted by the extent of injured myocardium or scar (fixed defects).

TABLE 11-5. Proposed Prognostic Gradient of Abnormal Results from Stress (Pharmacologic or Exercise) Perfusion Imaging in All Patients Even Those With Suspected or Proven CAD

Very low risk
Normal stress perfusion study
Low risk
Stress induced or fixed perfusion defects of small size
Intermediate risk
Stress induced or fixed perfusion defects of moderate size
Stress induced perfusion defects of small to moderate size with LVEF < 35%
High risk
Stress induced perfusion defects (ischemia) of greater than moderate size
Fixed perfusion defects (scar) of greater than moderate size with LVEF < 35%
Moderate size stress-induced perfusion defects in any patients with diabetes or LVEF < 35%

Data from Beller, Brown, Hendel, et al. (45). *J Nuc Cardiol.*

Preoperative Evaluations and Referral to Coronary Angiography

The presence of a positive test result should not be used simply as a justification to proceed with coronary angiography and revascularization. An example of a proposed prognostic gradient for perfusion imaging is shown in Table 11-5. There are no controlled studies or randomized data to properly evaluate the utility of coronary angiography. In addition, the precise role of CABG or angioplasty in patients undergoing coronary angiography is as yet undetermined and consequently unclear. However, some recommendations have been made in the ACC/AHA guidelines.[3]

In patients with known or suspected CAD, there are class I (strongly supported) indications for coronary angiography when there is (1) evidence for high risk or adverse outcomes based on noninvasive test results; (2) angina that is unresponsive to medical therapy; (3) unstable angina in situations in which there are intermediate- or high-risk noncardiac surgery; and (4) nondiagnostic noninvasive test results in those patients with high clinical risk who are undergoing high-risk surgery. The guidelines also make it clear that antithrombolytic therapy should be given for 3 to 4 and preferably 6 weeks after any PCI procedure before elective surgery is performed. This is based in part on a study[10] that reported catastrophic outcomes after coronary stenting in patients who went to surgery too quickly after their PCIs.

There are class II (moderately supported) indications for coronary angiography when there are (1) multiple intermediate clinical risk parameters and planned vascular surgery even though noninvasive testing should be the first consideration; (2) moderate to large ischemic areas on noninvasive testing but without high risk findings or reduced LVEF; (3) nondiagnostic noninvasive test results in intermediate clinical risk patients who are undergoing high-risk noncardiac surgery; (4) urgent noncardiac surgery in patients recovering from an acute MI; (5) patients having a perioperative MI; and (6) patients who are medically stable with class II or IV angina who are having low-risk or minor surgery.

These guidelines also suggest that there is no indication (class III) for coronary angiography in patients (1) with low-risk noncardiac surgery, who have a known history of CAD and demonstrate no high-risk noninvasive test results; (2) with no symptoms after coronary revascularization with excellent exercise capacity (≥7 METs); (3) with mild stable angina who have good left ventricular function and demonstrate no high-risk noninvasive test results; (4) with concomitant medical illness that precludes coronary revascularization or those who refuse to consider such therapy; and (5) who are candidates for liver, lung, or renal transplant who are less than 40 years old as part of an evaluation for transplant, unless noninvasive testing reveals high risk for adverse outcomes.

Late Follow-Up After Noncardiac Surgery

Background

Once a preoperative consultation for cardiac risk is completed, it is important to consider how any of the clinical or testing data collected for surgical evaluation can be of further use. In fact, it may be even more important to evaluate the long-term risk assessment in contrast to the short-term preoperative consultation. This is especially pertinent to the vascular surgery population, since many longitudinal studies have been published and the future risk of cardiac mortality and morbidity is well recognized.

Table 11-6 summarizes late cardiac events that occurred in a population dominated by vascular surgery procedures. It appears that cardiac mortality during long-term follow-up has been decreasing over the past decade, which was also noted previously for postoperative events (see Table 11-3). The impact of better patient selection and perioperative care for those who undergo vascular surgery has been a likely factor in reducing mortality in these large patient studies. However, despite the trend for reduced event rates over time, it

TABLE 11-6. Cardiac Event Rate in Long-Term Postoperative Follow-Up

Author	Avg FU Years	# Pts	NFMI	CV Death
Hertzer 1980[45]	6–7	286	NA	22.0%
Hertzer 1981[48]	7–8	256	NA	22.0%
Roger 1989[70]	8	75 no CAD	12.0%	12.0%
		47 CAD	28.0%	38.0%
Hertzer 1987[71]	4.6	228	NA	6.1%
Younis 1990[51]	1.5	127	—12%—	
Lette 1992[72]	1.3	355	5.4%	6.8%
Mangano 1992[73]	2	444	2.5%	5.4%
Seeger 1994[57]	2.8	171 (no test)	NA	1.2%
		144 (test)	NA	3.6%
Hendel 1995[31]	4.2	556	5.0%	7.7%
Fleisher 1995[58]	1.4	108	6.5%	3.7%
Poldermans 1997[23]	1.6	316	3.5%	3.5%

Avg FU: average follow-up; # Pts: number patients in each study; NFMI: nonfatal myocardial infarctions; CV death: cardiac death; CAD: coronary artery disease.

is still observed that subgroups with known CAD have a worse prognosis.

In a review of the vascular surgery literature from 1975 to 1987, Hertzer[32] noted that late mortality in patients with aortic aneurysms was 44% in those with probable CAD but was only 22% in those without CAD. This review also noted a large increase in mortality among patients having infrainguinal or carotid surgery based on the presence of symptomatic CAD. L'Italien et al.[33] completed a dual-center comparison of perioperative and long-term follow-up (5 years) based in part on the type of vascular surgery (aortic, infrainguinal, or carotid) performed. These authors noted that patients undergoing infrainguinal or carotid surgery had significantly lower cumulative survival and more perioperative events compared with aortic surgery patients. However, in patients without any CAD risk factors, survival was above 95% in all 3 surgical groups, and perioperative events occurred in less than 1%. When the surgical groups were adjusted for comorbid factors, the differences in cardiac event rates were significantly reduced. These authors concluded that cardiac and diabetic status were critical predictors for long- and short-term cardiac events. Specifically, a history of angina or CHF, diabetes, fixed dipyridamole thallium defects, and perioperative MI were identified as the best predictors of long-term events. Therefore, the type of vascular surgery performed may not be as important as the extent of cardiac risk factors as determined by clinical history and stress scintigraphic results.

Clinical Challenges in Long-Term Follow-Up

Evidence suggests that both the data that are collected, as well as the process of evaluation and subsequent work-up or intervention (medical or surgical) have resulted in better outcomes and predictions. A recent review of a national Medicare population sample identified a cohort of patients (n = 6,895) who underwent elective vascular surgery during a 17-month period in 1991 and 1992. The authors noted a relatively high mortality (14%) at 1 year of follow-up. However, in those patients undergoing preoperative stress testing with or without CABG surgery, the mortality was lower (<6%).[34] In another follow-up study of peripheral vascular surgery patients (n = 343) for a mean of 40 months, cardiac events were significantly more frequent in those who had an LVED of <35% or ischemia on dipyridamole-thallium imaging.[35] Other studies[36,37] also confirm the value of semiquantitative analysis of MPI when using these types of preoperative tests to predict future cardiac events. All these studies have the ability to combine an assessment of myocardial ischemia and left ventricular function into a more useful clinical index.

Using Preoperative Testing for Long-Term Prognosis

In the evaluation of cardiac risk for elective surgery, it is clear that clinical CAD risk factors, noninvasive cardiac imaging, and coronary angiography can all provide useful information in the appropriate patient subgroup. As noted previously, both assessment of LV function and the extent of myocardial ischemia are critical factors in the determination of risk. This is especially pertinent when intermediate or major clinical predictors are present. However, it is also clear that cardiac events are a greater problem in the long-term (3 to 5 years) medical management of these patients and merit attention.

Therefore, we should evaluate which (if any) of the clinical and noninvasive testing parameters could possibly be used to better predict long-term follow-up. If predictive information about perioperative, as well as long-term risk can be combined, it could be more cost-effective and timely to provide all this information to the referring physician before the elective surgery decision is finalized. As previously noted, a large metaanalysis[15] on preoperative testing (echocardiography and scintigraphy) has shown that indices of ischemia (transient perfusion defects and new wall motion abnormalities) are strongly associated with perioperative cardiac risk. Both echocardiographic and scintigraphic techniques can determine whether ischemia and infarction (reduced LV function) are present. Although MPI has previously used indirect measurements of LV function, it is now fairly routine to obtain LVEF calculations from gated cardiac studies using technetium-based perfusion agents.[38]

Table 11-7 displays the prediction of long-term survival after aortic vascular surgery in different patient studies using various clinical parameters that have demonstrated significant preoperative prognostic utility. The clinical risk index[39] can be divided into low-, intermediate-, and high-risk groups, and there is a significant survival difference between low- and high-risk patients. As expected, the mortality is elevated in the high-risk group but the low-risk patients have 22% mortality over 5 years. This is the same group of patients who are often sent directly to elective surgery without cardiac testing and typically have low (2%) perioperative event rates. However, the guidelines (and shortcut) recommend obtaining a functional capacity measurement in low-risk patients if there is high-risk surgery. It is possible that further risk stratification of this group might have helped to detect those low-clinical-risk patients who could have benefited from further cardiac testing. It is evident that intermediate-risk patients also have a fairly high (>50%) mortality over the 5-year follow-up period and may warrant further investigation. It is interesting to note that Hendel and Leppo[40] showed that scintigraphic findings could provide more prognostic information in the follow-up of vascular surgery patients when compared with clinical indices alone.

This is not to suggest that all patients should be tested by cardiac stress imaging; but if the overall guidelines are followed, the resulting information can be used for more surgical patients (especially vascular surgery patients), and it is important for the medical consultant to carefully consider the long-term consequences and risk as well as the immediate ones. Our group has also looked at the short- and long-term impact of coronary angiography referral based on positive test results.[41] Our data suggest that more invasive cardiac intervention does not consistently result in improved short- or long-term follow-up in vascular surgery patients. Therefore, it seems appropriate to continue to recommend that invasive interventions after preoperative clinical or testing evaluation should be based on the ACC/AHA practice guidelines.[42] Specifically, patients with increased clinical or stress-testing

TABLE 11-7. Prediction of Long-Term Survival After Aortic Reconstruction

	Cumulative Survival			
Screening Test	1 yr (%)	2 yr (%)	3 yr (%)	5 yr (%)
White et al. 1988[39]				
Goldman risk index (clinical)				
I (low)	98	90	84	78
II/III (intermediate)	84	78	66	46
IV (high)	55	40	30	18
Kazmers et al. 1988[43]				
Radionuclide ventriculogram				
≥35% LVEF	90	82	82	—
<35% LVEF	56	56	37	—
Hertzer 1987[32]				
CAD by angiography				
≤ single vessel	97	95	92	85
≥ double vessel	83	74	53	22
Cutler et al. 1992[44]				
Dipyridamole thallium-201 scan				
Normal scan	99	97	97	97
Fixed defect	88	79	69	55

LVEF: left ventricular ejection fraction; CAD: coronary artery disease.

risk do not need to be routinely sent for interventions just because elective surgery is contemplated.

LVEF is another powerful predictor of survival in patients with CAD. In Table 11-7, Kazmers et al.[43] noted that at a cut-point of 35%, the 3-year survival was significantly better in those with an LVEF of greater than 35%. This is not surprising, but over the same time period, mortality in those patients with preserved LVEF was approximately 6% per year. Therefore, the observation of having an LVEF of greater than 35% does not necessarily imply an excellent event-free survival.

The long-term prognostic power of multivessel CAD has been demonstrated by Hertzer.[32] In Table 11-7, a summary of data collected after vascular surgery is shown. These investigators noted that patients with 2- or 3-vessel CAD had a 5-year event-free survival of only 22%. In contrast, those patients with only single-vessel CAD or normal coronary angiographies had a survival of 85%. This results in a fairly low-risk group with a 3% per year cardiac event rate, but coronary angiography is no longer a routine perioperative screening methodology.

A long-term follow-up study by Cutler et al.[44] is presented at the bottom of Table 11-7. The authors reported a very low event rate in vascular patients who had a normal stress perfusion scan (<1%/year). Patients in the higher-risk group were noted to have fixed perfusion defects. In a subsequent study, Emlein et al.[37] reported that the extent of LV cavity dilation was the most important factor in predicting cardiac death among patients with abnormal scans. These studies clearly show that patients with a normal scan have a very low risk of long-term follow-up events, and we have already shown (see Table 11-4) that this observation (normal scan) has a high negative predictive value in the preoperative evaluation period. Therefore, pharmacologic stress MPI can be used to assess appropriate patient populations for both perioperative and long-term events by use of slightly different predictors. The extent of transient defects impacts the short-term events, which typically involve nonfatal MI, whereas large cavity size and fixed defects predict long-term events, which usually involve cardiac death. Perhaps the current use of gated perfusion imaging will provide a valuable objective parameter (LVEF) for evaluating long-term cardiac risk. It is likely that a technique that can quantitate the extent of ischemia as well as determine the LVEF should prove to be a most reliable method to evaluate short- and long-term prognosis in patients being considered for elective noncardiac surgery.

Case Presentations

Case 11.1

History

A 76-year-old woman with diabetes presented for preoperative evaluation for a vascular left foot ulcer. She had no angina, dyspnea, CHF, or history of CAD, but had limited activity due to peripheral vascular disease. Given the combination of low functional capacity, diabetes, and major vascular surgery, a dipyridamole/rest ^{201}Tl SPECT gated study was performed and is displayed in Figure C11-1.

Findings

The ^{201}Tl SPECT images showed a large area of stress-induced ischemia in the lateral and anterior wall, apex, and inferolateral region with transient LV cavity dilatation. The gated study revealed an LVEF of 50% with mild anterior and posterolateral wall hypokinesis. Coronary angiography revealed 3-vessel disease and a left main stenosis. She underwent a 3-vessel CABG and then had an aortobifemoral bypass with no cardiac events.

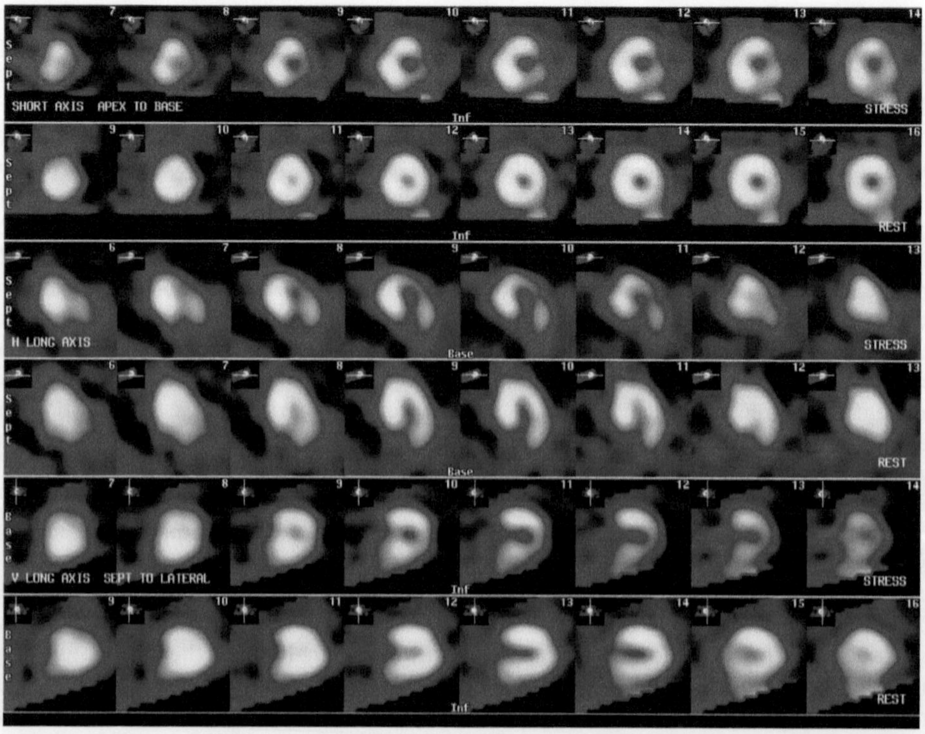

FIGURE C11-1.

Discussion

This case illustrates the need to follow-up on these types of patients with poor exercise tolerance, even if they are asymptomatic for CAD. This patient is asymptomatic but has diabetes, which is a clinical parameter that has been shown to have useful prognostic importance in predicting perioperative events. (See First Step: Clinical Evaluation of Preoperative Cardiac Risk at the beginning of this chapter.) In addition, this patient has limited physical activity and therefore poor cardiovascular reserve, which could increase her surgical risk. (See Second Step: Evaluate Functional Capacity, at the beginning of this chapter.) The contemplation of peripheral vascular surgery is a high-risk surgical procedure (See Third Step: Evaluate the Specific Surgery Risk at the beginning of this chapter, and also Table 11-1.) Presurgical noninvasive testing with stress/rest MPI is indicated in this patient population with intermediate risk. (See Fourth Step: When to Obtain Additional Noninvasive Testing, and also Table 11-2).

The stress/rest MPI demonstrated a large area of stress-induced ischemia. A metaanalysis reviewing 1994 dipyridamole thallium studies demonstrated that reversible perfusion defects have a significant positive predictive accuracy to predict cardiac events during elective surgery.[15] According to a proposed prognostic gradient of abnormal results from stress perfusion imaging based on summary recommendations from the International Nuclear Cardiology Retreat[45] (see Table 11-5), this patient is at high risk for cardiac perioperative events. Although there are no controlled studies or randomized data to properly evaluate the utility of coronary angiography, some recommendations have been made by the ACC/AHA guidelines.[3] Class I (strongly supported) indications for coronary angiography include evidence for high risk based on noninvasive test results. Other indications for coronary angiography are summarized in the Seventh

Step: Practice Appropriate Perioperative Care and Monitoring, at the beginning of this chapter. Coronary angiography revealed 3-vessel CAD in this patient, and she underwent CABG surgery prior to aortobifemoral bypass.

Interpretation

Severe multivessel wall ischemia demonstrated with stress/rest SPECT MPI performed for preoperative evaluation of high-risk surgery in an asymptomatic patient with poor exercise tolerance.

Case 11.2

History

A 61-year-old man with a history of a past MI and CABG 11 years ago presented for cardiac evaluation before peripheral vascular surgery. He had no symptoms of angina or CHF, but had a history of peripheral vascular disease and is status post aortobiiliac bypass and right knee amputation. He could climb 2 flights of stairs with a leg prosthesis and was active walking with no cardiac symptoms. A stress/rest SPECT study was performed for preoperative evaluation (Figure C11-2A) and 6 months later because of atypical symptoms and new preoperative evaluation for carotid surgery (Figure C11-2B).

Findings

The stress/rest SPECT images obtained for preoperative evaluation (Figure C11-2A) showed a moderate area of ischemia and a small infarct in the inferoapical region. The gated study revealed an LVEF of 47% with inferoapical hypokinesis. Medical therapy was reemphasized to him and adjusted to include aspirin, atorvastatin, nicotinic acid, atenolol, and also isosorbide for atypical neck burning.

The follow-up stress/rest SPECT images obtained 6 months later for atypical symptoms and preoperative evaluation for carotid surgery showed less ischemia on this medical therapy, and the LVEF was 48%, with no focal wall motion abnormalities.

Discussion

This case illustrated that medical therapy without invasive coronary angiography can be an appropriate choice in patients with good exercise capacity despite a stress/rest MPI indicating moderate risk. The same rationale algorithm (as in Case 11.1) for preoperative evaluation of patients referred for noncardiac surgery can be followed. This patient is asymptomatic and has none of the clinical parameters (history of angina, CHF, MI, or diabetes) that have been shown to have useful prognostic importance in predicting perioperative events. (See First Step: Clinical Evaluation of Preoperative Cardiac Risk, at the beginning of this chapter.) This patient has a good exercise capacity and therefore good cardiovascular reserve to sustain the surgical risk. (See Second Step: Evaluate Functional Capacity, at the beginning of this chapter.) The contemplation of peripheral vascular surgery is a high-risk surgical procedure. (See Third Step: Evaluate the Specific Surgery Risk, at the beginning of this chapter, and also Table 11-1.) Presurgical noninvasive testing with stress/rest MPI is indicated in this patient population with intermediate risk. (See Fourth Step: When to Obtain Additional Noninvasive Testing, at the beginning of this chapter, and Table 11-2.)

The stress/rest MPI demonstrated a moderate area of stress-induced ischemia. According to a proposed prognostic gradient of abnormal results from stress perfusion imaging based on summary recommendations from International Nuclear Cardiology Retreat[45] (see Table 11-5), this patient is at intermediate risk for cardiac perioperative events.

The indication for coronary angiography is questionable in the group of patients (see Seventh Step: Practice Appropriate Perioperative Care and Monitoring, at the beginning of

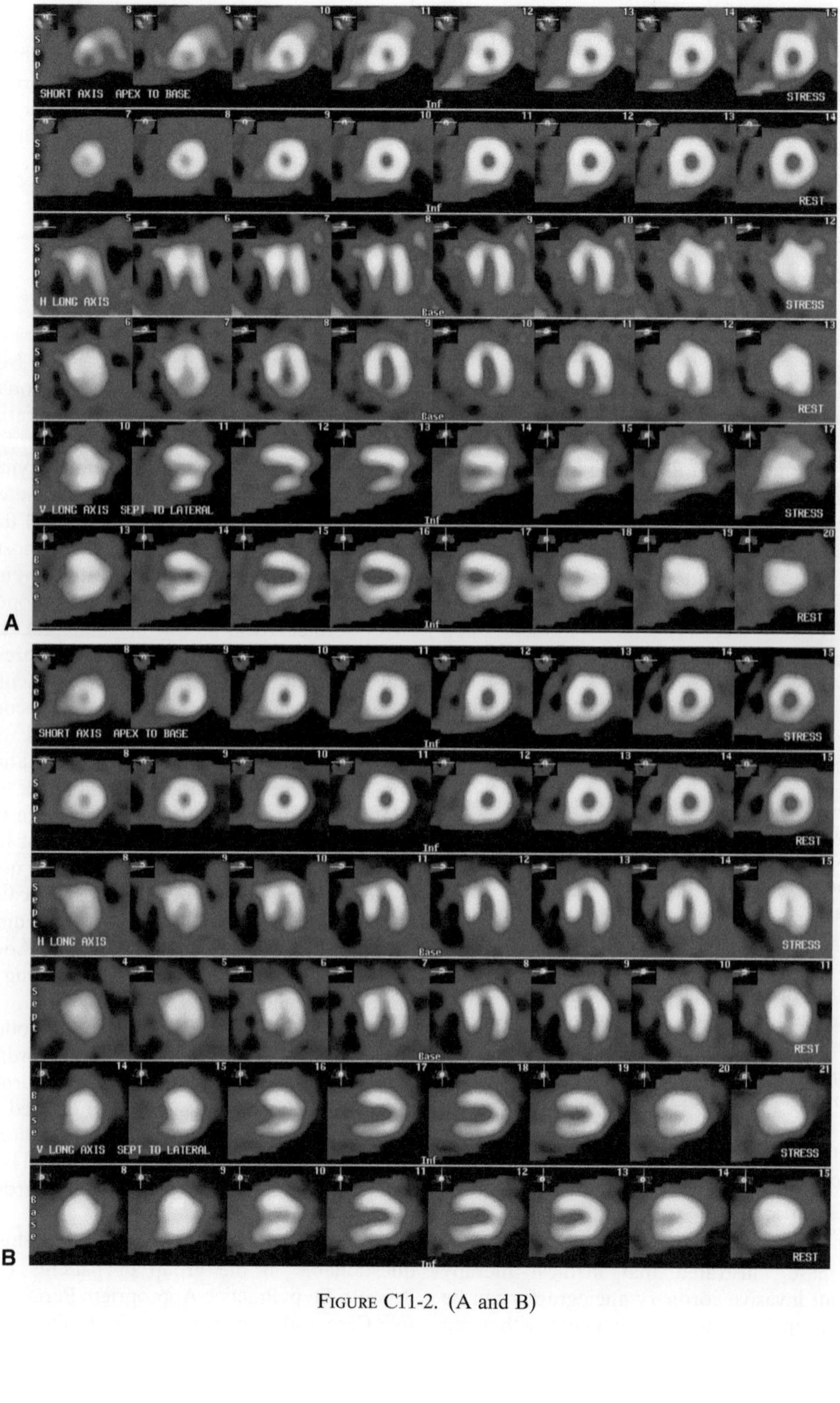

FIGURE C11-2. (A and B)

this chapter) and this was not performed in the patient presented. However, some recent evidence suggests that intensive medical therapy is sufficient to adequately manage most preoperative patients[21–23] and medical therapy was proved to be a good choice in this patient.

Interpretation

Moderate inferoapical ischemia improving with medical therapy in a patient with good exercise tolerance demonstrated with stress/rest SPECT MPI performed for preoperative evaluation and follow-up.

Case 11.3

History

A 71-year-old man needed surgery to repair an inguinal hernia with general anesthesia. A treadmill test showed ST-segment depression and coronary angiography demonstrated a 50% to 60% LAD lesion and a left marginal branch eccentric 70% stenosis. The RCA was a dominant vessel and had a long 70% stenosis just before its bifurcation. A myocardial perfusion stress/rest SPECT study was performed. The patient exercised on a Bruce protocol for 8 minutes, achieving 110% of predicted maximum heart rate. His blood pressure peaked at 192/82 mmHg, and no major ST-segment shifts were seen. He denied chest pain with exertion. The exercise/rest ^{99m}Tc-MIBI SPECT images are displayed in Figure C11-3.

Findings

The stress/rest SPECT images were normal and the LVEF was 60%. This case illustrates the dilemma one often faces with results of coronary angiography.

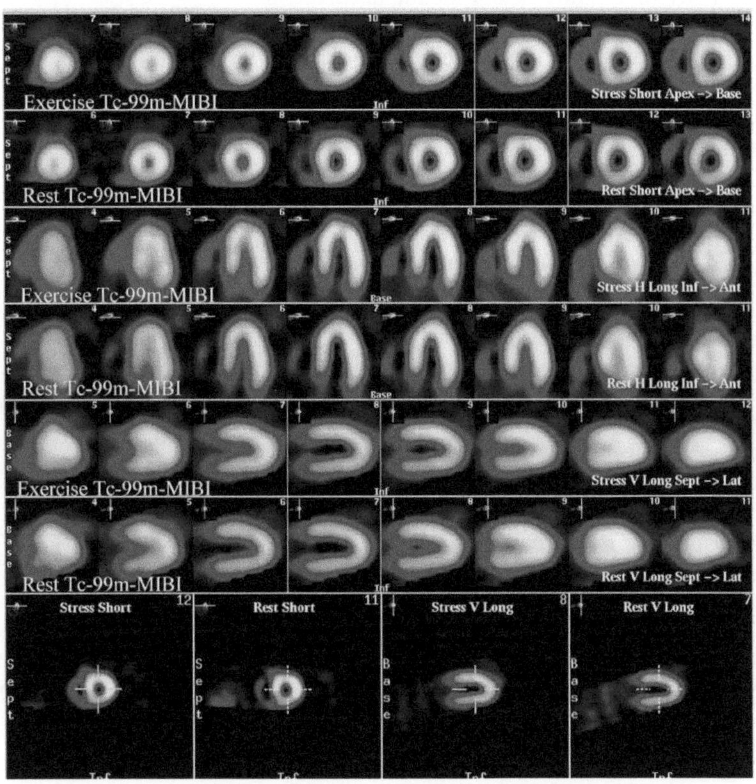

FIGURE C11-3. (Courtesy of Dr. S. V. Shikare, Sharjah, United Arab Emirates.)

Discussion

The most challenging and important question in the preoperative evaluation of cardiac risk is the determination of the patient's current medical status. Specifically, in patients with CAD, the evaluation of both LV function and ischemic burden have been shown to have significant prognostic significance for future cardiac events.[4] Therefore, any attempt to evaluate preoperative risk should include an assessment of these 2 parameters. Unfortunately, a clinical history and physical examination may not have high sensitivity for detection of significant CAD. Accordingly, noninvasive testing should be able to provide a more objective measure of cardiac function and ischemia.

The utility of preoperative noninvasive testing was reviewed in a large metaanalysis by Shaw et al.[15] These authors reviewed studies from 1985 to 1994 in which either dipyridamole ^{201}Tl (n = 1994) or dobutamine echocardiography (n = 455) was used. Reversible perfusion defects were noted in 26% of patients, and nonfatal MI or cardiovascular death occurred in 9% of these preoperative cases. In contrast, 430 (22%) patients had normal perfusion scans and an event rate of 1.4%. Similar prognostic utility was noted in the dobutamine echocardiography studies. New wall motion abnormalities during dobutamine-induced stress were noted in 39% of the patients and 11% of these cases had a major cardiac event. In the 270 (61%) patients without new regional wall motion abnormalities, the event rate was 0.4%.

Clinical Risk Assessment

Although the clinical question that is often posed to the medical or cardiac consultant is whether or not to clear the patient for noncardiac surgery, the ACC/AHA guidelines[3] suggest an overall conservative approach to the use of expensive tests and interventions. In this particular case, the patient did not have a clear guideline indication for presurgical testing. He did not have an intermediate risk factor (angina, MI, CHF, or diabetes), and he appeared to have a good functional capacity. Finally, the risk of surgery is low for an inguinal hernia. Therefore, once the initial stress test is performed, it may be that the test result, rather than the patient, is being treated. The coronary angiography performance appears to be a rather hasty decision, but at least the patient underwent perfusion imaging to evaluate the functional severity of the anatomic disease. The perfusion scan did not really show much in the way of ischemia. The LVEF by gated SPECT was normal, and there was no cavity dilation or other factors to suggest severe general ischemia or poor LV function.

Therefore, what would the purpose of CABG or PCI be in this patient? There was no evidence of ischemia by MPI criteria and no symptoms of angina. The ECG was somewhat equivocal during the exercise stress test performed for MPI, and the functional capacity was quite good (8 minutes, stage 3 of Bruce). If this patient had presented to the cardiology office with "atypical chest pain," the correct management would probably be medical therapy for CAD (aspirin, beta-blocker, and statin therapy if indicated, as suggested in the recent ACC/AHA guideline for stable CAD in asymptomatic patients).

Overall, this patient should be told that appropriate preoperative testing and medical therapy should result in better long-term outcome than no testing at all. As shown in a recent report by Licker et al.,[46] only 10% of abdominal aortic surgery patients needed to undergo coronary revascularization as part of a preoperative study that followed the ACC/AHA preoperative guideline reports. This group emphasized preoperative, intraoperative, and postoperative medical therapy with alpha-agonists, beta-blockers, and appropriate anesthetic regimens. There are no data to support the use of CABG or PCI to prevent perioperative cardiac events, and if PCI is indicated, a 4- to 6-week recovery time is suggested before elective surgery.

Interpretation

Normal stress/rest MPI in a patient with documented CAD stratified as low preoperative risk.

References

1. American Heart Association. *2003 Heart and Stroke Statistical Update.* Dallas: American Heart Association; 2003:1–46.
2. Goldman L, Caldera DL, Nussbaum SR, et al. Multifactorial index of cardiac risk in noncardiac surgical procedures. *N Engl J Med.* 1977;297: 845–850.
3. Eagle KA, Berger PB, Calkins H, et al. ACC/AHA guideline update for perioperative cardiovascular evaluation for noncardiac surgery—executive summary: a report of the American College of Cardiology/American Heart Association Task Force on Practice Guidelines (Committee to Update the 1996 Guidelines on Perioperative Cardiovascular Evaluation for Noncardiac Surgery). *J Am Coll Cardiol.* 2002; 39:542–553.
4. Califf RM, Armstrong PW, Carver JR, D'Agostino RB, Strauss WE. Task force 5: Stratification of patients into high, medium and low risk subgroups for purposes of risk factor management. *J Am Coll Cardiol.* 1996;27:1007–1019.
5. Mukherjee D, Eagle KA. Perioperative cardiac assessment for noncardiac surgery: eight steps to the best possible outcome. *Circulation.* 2003;107: 2771.
6. Detsky AS, Abrams HB, Forbath N, Scott JG, Hilliard JR. Cardiac assessment for patients undergoing noncardiac surgery: A multifactorial clinical risk index. *Arch Intern Med.* 1986;146: 2131–2134.
7. Eagle KA, Coley CM, Newell JB, et al. Combining clinical and thallium data optimizes preoperative assessment of cardiac risk before major vascular surgery. *Ann Intern Med.* 1989; 110:859–866.
8. Hlatky MA, Boineau RE, Higginbotham MB, et al. A brief self-administered questionnaire to determine functional capacity (the Duke Activity Status Index). *Am J Cardiol.* 1989;64:651–654.
9. Froehlich JB, Karavite D, Russman PL, et al. American College of Cardiology/American Heart Association preoperative assessment guidelines reduce resource utilization before aortic surgery. *J Vasc Surg.* 2002;36:758–763.
10. Kaluza GL, Joseph J, Lee JR, Raizner ME, Raizner AE. Catastrophic outcomes of noncardiac surgery soon after coronary stenting. *J Am Coll Cardiol.* 2000;35:1288–1294.
11. Eagle KA, Rihal CS, Mickel MC, Holmes DR, Foster ED, Gersh BJ. Cardiac risk of noncardiac surgery: influence of coronary disease and type of surgery in 3368 operations. *Circulation.* 1997; 96:1882–1887.
12. Gersh BJ, Rihal CS, Rooke TW, Ballard DJ. Evaluation and management of patients with both peripheral vascular and coronary artery disease. *J Am Coll Cardiol.* 1991;18:203–214.
13. Hertzer NR, Beven EG, Young JR, et al. Coronary artery disease in peripheral vascular patients: a classification of 1000 coronary angiograms and results of surgical management. *Ann Surg.* 1984;199:223–233.
14. Hollenberg M, Mangano DT, Browner WS, London MJ, Tubau JF, Tateo IM. Predictors of postoperative myocardial ischemia in patients undergoing noncardiac surgery. *JAMA.* 1992; 268:205–209.
15. Shaw LJ, Eagle KA, Gersh BJ, Miller DD. Meta-analysis of intravenous dipyridamole-thallium-201 imaging (1985 to 1994) and dobutamine echocardiography (1991 to 1994) for risk stratification before vascular surgery. *J Am Coll Cardiol.* 1996;27:787–798.
16. Mangano DT, London MJ, Tubau JF, et al. Study of perioperative ischemia research group: dipyridamole thallium-201 scintigraphy as a preoperative screening test: a reexamination of its predictive potential. *Circulation.* 1991;84: 493–502.
17. Baron JF, Mundler O, Bertrand M, et al. Dipyridamole-thallium scintigraphy and gated radionuclide angiography to assess cardiac risk before abdominal aortic surgery. *N Engl J Med.* 1994;330:663–669.
18. Lee TH, Marcantonio ER, Mangione CM, et al. Derivation and prospective validation of a simple index for prediction of cardiac risk of major noncardiac surgery. *Circulation.* 1999;100: 1043–1049.
19. Vanzetto G, Machecourt J, Blendea D, et al. Additive value of thallium single-photon emission computer tomography myocardial imaging for prediction of perioperative events in clinically selected high cardiac risk patients having abdominal aortic surgery. *Am J Cardiol.* 1996; 77:143–148.
20. Bartels C, Bechtel JF, Hossmann V, Horsch S. Cardiac risk stratification for high-risk vascular surgery. *Circulation.* 1997;95:2473–2475.
21. Poldermans D, Boersma E, Bax JJ, et al. The effect of bisoprolol on perioperative mortality and myocardial infarction in high-risk patients undergoing vascular surgery. Dutch Echocardiographic Cardiac Risk Evaluation Applying

Stress Echocardiography Study Group. *N Engl J Med.* 1999;341:1789–1794.
22. Boersma E, Poldermans D, Bax JJ, et al. Predictors of cardiac events after major vascular surgery: Role of clinical characteristics, dobutamine, echocardiography, and beta-blocker therapy. *JAMA.* 2001;285:1865–1873.
23. Poldermans D, Arnese M, Fioretti PM, et al. Sustained prognostic value of dobutamine stress echocardiography for late cardiac events after major noncardiac vascular surgery. *Circulation.* 1997;95:53–58.
24. Wallace A, Layug B, Tateo I, et al. Prophylactic atenolol reduces postoperative myocardial ischemia. McSPI Research Group. *Anesthesiology.* 1998;88:7–17.
25. Mangano DT, Layug EL, Wallace A, Tateo I. Effect of atenolol on mortality and cardiovascular morbidity after noncardiac surgery. *N Engl J Med.* 1996;335:1713–1720.
26. Weinrauch LA, D'Elia JA, Healy RW, et al. Asymptomatic coronary artery disease: Angiography in diabetic patients before renal transplantation: Relations of findings to postoperative survival. *Ann Intern Med.* 1978;88: 346–348.
27. Heston TF, Norman DJ, Barry JM, Bennett WM, Wilson RA. Cardiac risk stratification in renal transplantation using a form of artificial intelligence. *Am J Cardiol.* 1997;79:415–417.
28. Iqbal A, Gibbons RJ, McGoon MD, Steiroff S, Frohnert PT, Velosa JA. Noninvasive assessment of cardiac risk in insulin-dependent diabetic patients being evaluated for pancreatic transplantation using thallium-201 myocardial perfusion scintigraphy. *Transplant Proc.* 1991;23: 1690–1691.
29. Fattah AA, Kamal AM, Pancholy S, et al. Prognostic implications of normal exercise tomographic thallium images in patients with angiographic evidence of significant coronary artery disease. *Am J Cardiol.* 1994;74:769–771.
30. Kryzhanovski VA, Beller GA. Usefulness of preoperative noninvasive radionuclide testing for detecting coronary artery disease in candidates for liver transplantation. *Am J Cardiol.* 1997;79: 986–988.
31. Hendel RC, Chen MH, L'Italien GJ, et al. Sex differences in perioperative and long-term cardiac event-free survival in vascular surgery patients: an analysis of clinical and scintigraphic variables. *Circulation.* 1995;91:1044–1051.
32. Hertzer NR. Basic data concerning associated coronary artery disease in peripheral vascular patients. *Ann Vasc Surg.* 1987;1:616–620.
33. L'Italien GJ, Cambria RP, Cutler BS, et al. Comparative early and late cardiac morbidity among patients requiring different vascular surgery procedures. *J Vasc Surg.* 1995;21:935–944.
34. Fleisher LA, Eagle KA, Shaffer T, Anderson GF. Perioperative- and long-term mortality rates after major vascular surgery: the relationship to preoperative testing in the Medicare population. *Anesth Analg.* 1999;89:849–855.
35. Schueppert MT, Kresowik TF, Corry DC, et al. Selection of patients for cardiac evaluation before peripheral vascular operations. *J Vasc Surg.* 1996;23:802–808.
36. Lette J, Waters D, Cerino M, Picard M, Champagne P, Lapointe J. Preoperative coronary artery disease risk stratification based on dipyridamole imaging and a simple three-step, three-segment model for patients undergoing noncardiac vascular surgery or major general surgery. *Am J Cardiol.* 1992;69:1553–1558.
37. Emlein G, Villegas B, Dahlberg S, Leppo J. Left ventricular cavity size determined by preoperative dipyridamole thallium scintigraphy as a predictor of late cardiac events in vascular surgery patients. *Am Heart J.* 1996;131:907–914.
38. Garcia EV, Bacharach SL, Mahmarian JJ, et al. Imaging guidelines for nuclear cardiology procedures. Part 1. *J Nucl Cardiol.* 1996;3:G1–G46.
39. White GH, Advani SM, Williams RA, Wilson SE. Cardiac risk index as a predictor of long-term survival after repair of abdominal aortic aneurysm. *Am J Surg.* 1988;156:103–107.
40. Hendel RC, Leppo JA. The value of perioperative clinical indexes and dipyridamole thallium scintigraphy for the prediction of myocardial infarction and cardiac death in patients undergoing vascular surgery. *J Nucl Cardiol.* 1995;2: 18–225.
41. Massie MT, Rohrer MJ, Leppo JA, Cutler BS. Is coronary angiography necessary for vascular surgery patients who have positive results of dipyridamole thallium scans? *J Vasc Surg.* 1997; 25:975–983.
42. Pepine CJ, Allen HD, Bashore TM, et al. ACC/AHA guidelines for cardiac catheterization and cardiac catheterization laboratories. *J Am Coll Cardiol.* 1991;18:1149–1182.
43. Kazmers A, Cerqueira MD, Zierler RE. Perioperative and late outcome in patients with left ventricular ejection fraction of 35% or less who

require major vascular surgery. *J Vasc Surg*. 1988; 8:307–315.
44. Cutler BS, Hendel RC, Leppo JA. Dipyridamole-thallium scintigraphy predicts perioperative and long-term survival after major vascular surgery. *J Vasc Surg*. 1992;15:972–981.
45. Beller GA, Brown KA, Hendel RC, Shaw LJ, Williams KA. Unresolved issues in risk stratification: Chronic coronary artery disease including preoperative testing. *J Nucl Cardiol*. 1997; 4:92–95.
46. Licker M, Khatchatourian G, Schweizer A, Bednarkiewicz M, Tassaux D, Chevalley C. The impact of a cardioprotective protocol on the incidence of cardiac complications after aortic abdominal surgery. *Anesth Analg*. 2002; 95(6):1525–1533.
47. Young AE, Sandberg GW, Couch NP. The reduction of mortality of abdominal aortic aneurysm resection. *Am J Surg*. 1977;134:585–590.
48. Hertzer NR. Fatal myocardial infarction following lower extremity revascularization: two hundred seventy-three patients followed six to eleven postoperative years. *Ann Surg*. 1981;193: 492–498.
49. Cutler BS, Leppo JA. Dipyridamole thallium 201 scintigraphy to detect coronary artery disease before abdominal aortic surgery. *J Vasc Surg*. 1987;5:91–100.
50. Raby KE, Goldman L, Creager MA, et al. Correlation between preoperative ischemia and major cardiac events after peripheral vascular surgery. *N Engl J Med*. 1989;321:1296–1300.
51. Younis LT, Aguirre F, Byers S, et al. Perioperative and long-term prognostic value of intravenous dipyridamole thallium scintigraphy in patients with peripheral vascular disease. *Am Heart J*. 1990;119:1287–1292.
52. Hendel RC, Whitfield SS, Villegas BJ, Cutler BS, Leppo JA. Prediction of late cardiac events by dipyridamole thallium imaging in patients undergoing elective vascular surgery. *Am J Cardiol*. 1992;70:1243–1249.
53. Taylor LM Jr, Yeager RA, Moneta GL, McConnell DB, Porter JM. The incidence of perioperative myocardial infarction in general vascular surgery. *J Vasc Surg*. 1991;15:52–61.
54. Kresowik TF, Bower TR, Garner SA, et al. Dipyridamole thallium imaging in patients being considered for vascular procedures. *Arch Surg*. 1993;128:299–302.
55. McFalls EO, Doliszny KM, Grund F, Chute E, Chesler E. Angina and persistent exercise thallium defects: Independent risk factors in elective vascular surgery. *J Am Coll Cardiol*. 1993;21:1347–1352.
56. Bry JD, Belkin M, O'Donnell TF Jr, et al. An assessment of the positive predictive value and cost-effectiveness of dipyridamole myocardial scintigraphy in patients undergoing vascular surgery. *J Vasc Surg*. 1994;19:112–124.
57. Seeger JM, Rosenthal GR, Self SB, Flynn TC, Limacher MC, Harward TR. Does routine stress-thallium cardiac scanning reduce postoperative cardiac complications? *Ann Surg*. 1994;219:654–663.
58. Fleisher LA, Rosenbaum SH, Nelson AH, Jain D, Wackers FJ, Zaret BL. Preoperative dipyridamole thallium imaging and ambulatory electrocardiographic monitoring as a predictor of perioperative cardiac events and long term outcome. *Anesthesiology*. 1995;83:906–917.
59. Boucher CA, Brewster DC, Darling C, Okada R, Strauss HW, Pohost GM. Determination of cardiac risk by dipyridamole-thallium imaging before peripheral vascular surgery. *N Engl J Med*. 1985;312:389–394.
60. Fletcher JP, Antico VF, Gruenewald S, Kershaw LZ. Dipyridamole-thallium scan for screening of coronary artery disease prior to vascular surgery. *J Cardiovasc Surg*. 1988;29:666–669.
61. Sachs RN, Tellier P, Larmignat P, et al. Assessment by dipyridamole-thallium-201 myocardial scintigraphy of coronary risk before peripheral vascular surgery. *Surgery*. 1988;103:584–587.
62. Koutelou MG, Asimacopoulos PJ, Mahmarian JJ, Kimball KT, Verani MS. Preoperative risk stratification by adenosine thallium 201 single-photon emission computed tomography in patients undergoing vascular surgery. *J Nucl Med*. 1995;2:389–394.
63. Marshall ES, Raichlen JS, Forman S, Heyrich GP, Keen WD, Weitz HH. Adenosine radionuclide perfusion imaging in the preoperative evaluation of patients undergoing peripheral vascular surgery. *Am J Cardiol*. 1995;76:817–821.
64. Coley CM, Field TS, Abraham SA, Boucher CA, Eagle KA. Usefulness of dipyridamole-thallium scanning for preoperative evaluation of cardiac risk for nonvascular surgery. *Am J Cardiol*. 1992; 69:1280–1285.
65. Shaw L, Miller DD, Kong BA, et al. Determination of perioperative cardiac risk by adenosine thallium-201 myocardial imaging. *Am Heart J*. 1992;124:861–869.
66. Brown KA, Rowen M. Extent of jeopardized viable myocardium determined by myocardial perfusion imaging best predicts perioperative

cardiac events in patients undergoing noncardiac surgery. *J Am Coll Cardiol.* 1993;21:325–330.

67. Younis L, Stratmann H, Takase B, Byers S, Chaitman BR, Miller DD. Preoperative clinical assessment and dipyridamole thallium-201 scintigraphy for prediction and prevention of cardiac events in patients having major noncardiovascular surgery and known or suspected coronary artery disease. *Am J Cardiol.* 1994; 74:311–317.
68. Stratmann HG, Younis LT, Wittry MD, Amato M, Mark AL, Miller DD. Dipyridamole technetium 99m sestamibi myocardial tomography for preoperative cardiac risk stratification before major or minor nonvascular surgery. *Am Heart J.* 1996;132:536–541.
69. Van Damme H, Pierard L, Gillain D, Benoit T, Rigo P, Limet R. Cardiac risk assessment before vascular surgery: a prospective study comparing clinical evaluation, dobutamine stress echocardiography, and dobutamine ^{99m}Tc sestamibi tomoscintigraphy. *Cardiovasc Surg.* 1997;5:54–64.
70. Roger VL, Ballard DJ, Hallett JW Jr, Osmundson PJ, Puetz PA, Gersh BJ. Influence of coronary artery disease on morbidity and mortality after abdominal aortic aneurysmectomy: a population-based study, 1971–1987. *J Am Coll Cardiol.* 1989;14:1245–1252.
71. Hertzer NR, Young JR, Beven EG, et al. Late results of coronary bypass in patients with infrarenal aortic aneurysms: the Cleveland Clinic study. *Ann Surg.* 1987;205:360–367.
72. Lette J, Waters D, Champagne P, Picard M, Cerino M, Lapointe J. Prognostic implications of a negative dipyridamole-thallium scan: results in 360 patients. *Am J Med.* 1992;92:615–620.
73. Mangano DT, Browner WS, Hollenberg M, Li J, Tateo IM. Long-term cardiac prognosis following noncardiac surgery. *JAMA.* 1992;268:233–239.

12
Applications of Myocardial Perfusion Imaging in Special Populations

Jennifer H. Mieres, Jean M. Cacciabaudo, and Mikhail Levin

The continuous and dramatic growth in the field of nuclear cardiology over the past two decades has accounted for its central role in the clinical evaluation of patients with known or suspected coronary artery disease (CAD). The development of gated single photon emission tomography (SPECT) has facilitated the expansion of nuclear cardiology studies from the evaluation of myocardial perfusion alone to the evaluation of both perfusion and ventricular function data in a single study.

This chapter focuses on the role of myocardial perfusion and function imaging in the evaluation of CAD in special populations: (1) women with suspected CAD; (2) left bundle branch block (LBBB) on ECG; (3) diabetes mellitus; (4) congestive heart failure (CHF); and (5) asymptomatic patients at risk for CAD.

Case Presentations

Case 12.1

History

A 55-year-old woman with hypertension and hypercholesterolemia was referred for exercise myocardial perfusion imaging (MPI) before elective foot surgery. Her past medical history was significant for systemic lupus erythematosus (SLE). Her SLE was well controlled on intermittent small doses of prednisone. She was noted to have a mildly abnormal preoperative electrocardiogram (ECG). She had no history of cardiac disease; however, for the previous 3 months, she had noted intermittent symptoms of chest burning and dyspnea with exertion. The baseline ECG was significant for tall R wave in precordial lead V2 and mild T-wave inversion in leads V3 and V4. She had been asymptomatic for the past week before the exercise MPI. She completed 5 minutes of a standard Bruce protocol, and the test was terminated due to fatigue. She had symptoms of dyspnea, normal blood pressure (BP) response to exercise, and reached 87% of maximum predicted heart rate (HR). The exercise ^{99m}Tc-MIBI/rest ^{201}Tl SPECT images are displayed in Figure C12-1A.

Findings

Ventricular dilatation was evident on the stress images but not on the rest images. The transient ischemic dilatation (TID) index on quantitative analysis was 1.30 (normal <1.20). On the stress images, there were moderate perfusion defects in the apical, anterior, anteroseptal, and distal inferior walls. The rest images demonstrated improvement of uptake in the areas described previously, consistent with ischemia. The sum stress score (SSS) by quantitative analysis using

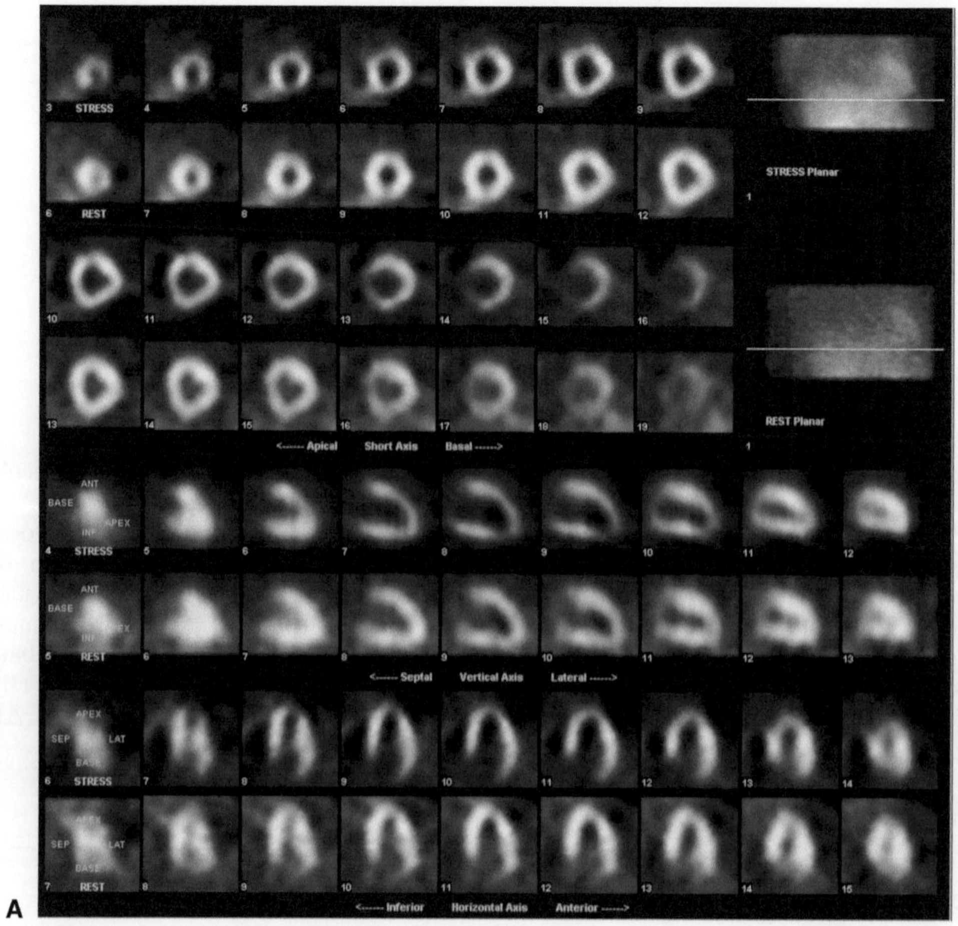

FIGURE C12-1. (A)

a 20-segment LV model was calculated at 10, consistent with a moderate amount of exercise induced ischemia of those regions. SSS of 9 to 13 indicates a moderately abnormal study.[1] The postexercise gated SPECT study demonstrated mild hypokinesis of the distal anterior, apical, and distal anteroseptal walls.

Discussion

The patient's symptoms of intermittent episodes of chest burning and dyspnea were atypical and not believed to be related to CAD. The pretest likelihood of CAD in a 55-year old woman with atypical angina is intermediate.[2] Exercise MPI is indicated for diagnosis and prognosis in patients with an intermediate pretest likelihood of CAD, and was instrumental in the accurate diagnosis of severe stenosis of the proximal left anterior descending (LAD) coronary artery in this patient.

A) Heart Disease in Women

Coronary artery disease (CAD) is the leading cause of death of women in the United States and the western world. Gender differences exist in the presentation and manifestations of heart disease, with a higher mortality for women with myocardial infarction (MI) compared with men.[3] The key to reduction in mortality from CAD is early detection. TMT is less accurate in women than in men due to a higher number of false-positive exercise ECG results.[4] A meta-analysis determined that MPI is more accurate than exercise ECG in women.[5] The lower specificities may be due to a digoxin-like effect of circulating estrogens resulting in varying changes in the ST-segment, leading to a higher false-positive rate of exercise ECG stress testing in women.[6]

It is important to realize that women with CAD may present with less classic symptoms of CAD. Women do not infrequently present with symptoms of nausea, dizziness, indigestion, and back pain as a manifestation of CAD, as was true in this case.

B) Role of MPI in the Evaluation of Women with Suspected CAD

A growing body of evidence supports the incremental value of MPI to the use of clinical variables or exercise stress testing in the evaluation of women with suspected CAD.[7] The high diagnostic accuracy of stress SPECT MPI has been confirmed in more than 3,000 women[8–11] and stress SPECT MPI with gated SPECT has been validated in women.[12–14] The combination of perfusion and functional data provides event-specific risk stratification that can aid in treatment selection. Perfusion data indicate risk of MI and death, while data on cardiac function offer information on risk of cardiac death. In women with suspected CAD, MPI with gated SPECT adds incremental value to the use of clinical variables or exercise stress testing (Figure C12-1B).

Interpretations

1. Exercise-induced ischemia of the anteroseptal, apical, and distal inferior walls, consistent with an LAD lesion confirmed by angiography.
2. Evidence for mild stunning of the areas supplied by the left anterior descending coronary artery (LAD) on the postexercise gated SPECT images.
3. Transient ischemic dilatation of the LV, a marker of severe CAD believed to be due to subendocardial ischemia in the setting of severe coronary artery stenosis and associated with a poor prognosis.

Outcome

Based on a markedly abnormal exercise myocardial perfusion study, the patient was referred for coronary angiography, which demonstrated 90% stenosis of the proximal LAD and prompted percutaneous transluminal coronary angioplasty (PTCA) and stent placement in the proximal LAD.

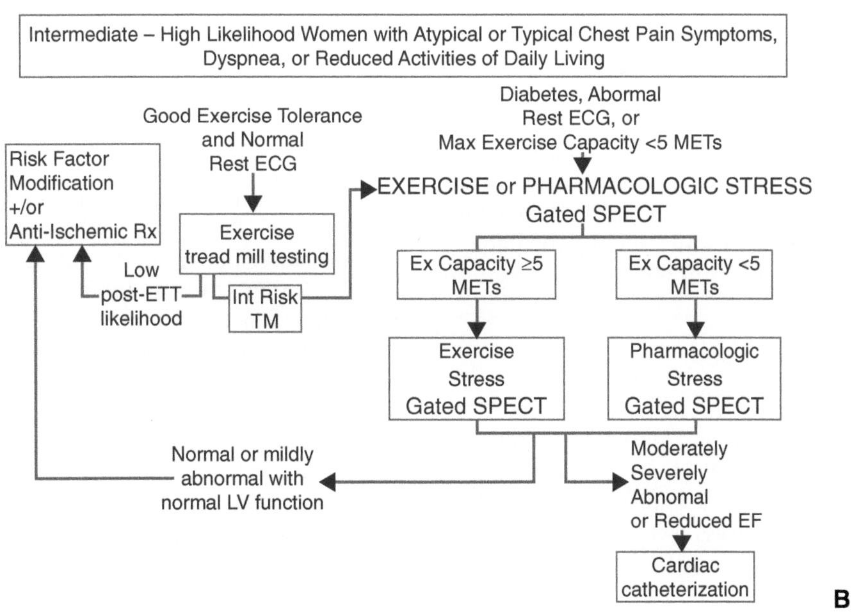

FIGURE C12-1. (B, from Mieres, Shaw, Hendel, et al. [14], by permission of *J Nucl Cardiol.*)

Case 12.2

History

A 60-year-old woman was referred for MPI because of intermittent episodes of palpitations and the finding of a new left bundle branch block (LBBB) on ECG. She had no additional risk factors for CAD besides age, and denied any history or symptoms of heart disease. A dual isotope rest ^{201}Tl/adenosine ^{99m}Tc-MIBI/SPECT was performed. There were no symptoms of chest pain; however, the patient complained of palpitations during the injection of ^{201}Tl. The ECG after the injection ^{201}Tl is shown in Figure C12-2A. There were no complaints of chest pain or palpitations during adenosine infusion. The ECG was significant for LBBB. The adenosine ^{99m}Tc-MIBI/rest ^{201}Tl SPECT images are displayed in Figure C12-2B.

Findings

The resting ECG acquired at the time of ^{201}Tl injection demonstrated atrial fibrillation and LBBB, at an average HR of approximately 135 beats per minute (bpm). The patient continued to complain of palpitations during the acquisition of the resting images. The resting SPECT images demonstrated decreased ^{201}Tl uptake in the septal wall. The pharmacologic stress images demonstrated homogeneous uptake of radiotracer in all areas of the LV, consistent with no evidence for MI or pharmacologic stress-induced ischemia. The postpharmacologic gated SPECT images demonstrated normal LV function with a left ventricular ejection fraction (LVEF) of 60%.

Discussion

In this patient ^{201}Tl was injected and rest images were acquired during a period of rapid atrial fibrillation and LBBB. Heart rate at the time of injection with ^{201}Tl was approximately 135 bpm. Pharmacologic stress was performed with adenosine and ^{99m}Tc-MIBI was injected at a peak HR of 85. Therefore, the rest images reflected septal asynchrony at a high HR, while the pharmacologic stress images were acquired at a much lower HR with resultant homogenous radiotracer uptake in the septal wall and all regions of the LV.

Coronary artery disease, hypertensive heart disease, and nonischemic cardiomyopathy are among the common causes of LBBB.[15] Because the left bundle receives its blood supply from both the LAD and right coronary arteries, the presence of an LBBB due to CAD implies significant CAD in both coronary arteries. Therefore, early identification of CAD in the setting of an LBBB is crucial for decreasing mortality and morbidity due to CAD.

Myocardial perfusion imaging (MPI) has played an important role in the identification of patients with LBBB and CAD. However, a review of the literature demonstrates that 40% to 50% of patients with LBBB may develop septal defects during exercise MPI in the absence of significant CAD of the LAD.[16–18] In patients who undergo exercise MPI in the setting of a baseline LBBB on ECG, reversible septal perfusion defects may occur, mimicking exercise-induced septal ischemia. Based on animal experiments, Hirzel and colleagues[19] summarized that at high heart rates in the setting of an LBBB, there is asynchronous relaxation of the septum, which is out of phase with the diastolic filling of the remainder of the LV (phase during which coronary flow is maximal) with resultant relative decrease in septal blood flow. This mechanism suggests that the delay between left and right ventricular activation results in reduced diastolic filling time for the septum. Therefore, at high heart rates, in the setting of an LBBB, the degree of septal asynchrony relative to the ECG R-R interval is greater than at rest, making septal perfusion defects appear reversible.[20] It has been reported that vasodilator stress with adenosine or dipyridamole can minimize the septal defects associated with exercise MPI in the presence of an LBBB.[20–23] This topic is also discussed in Cases 5.3 and 13.9.

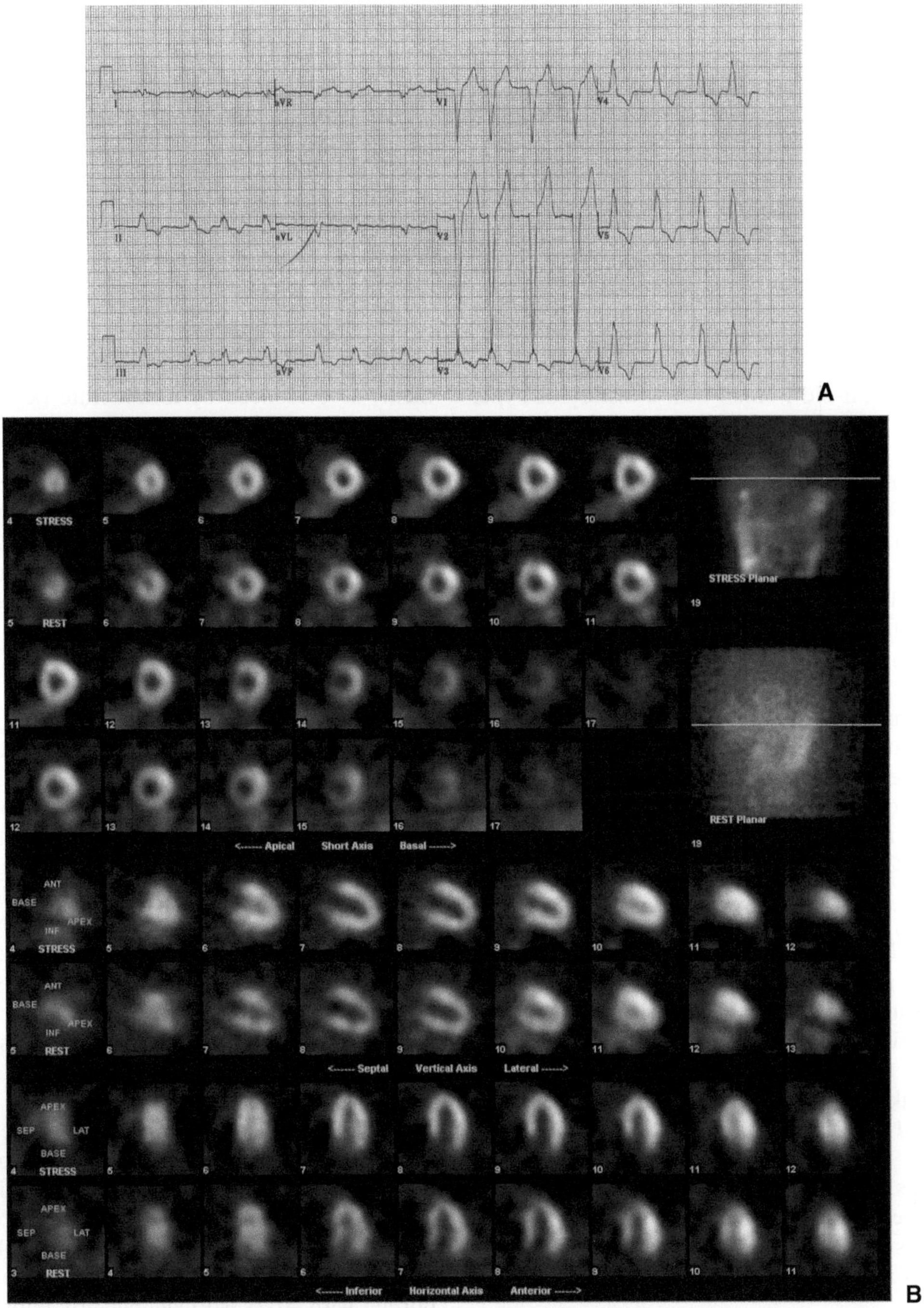

FIGURE C12-2. (A and B)

Diagnosis

1. Artifactual defect on the resting images due to LBBB and infection of the radiopharmaceutical during rapid atrial fibrillation at 135 bpm.
2. Normal perfusion on the adenosine images acquired at a lower HR of 85 bpm.

Outcome

Despite a normal pharmacologic stress MPI study, persistent complaints of chest pain lead to coronary angiography. No significant stenosis was demonstrated.

Case 12.3

History

A 65-year-old woman with a history of hypertension and type II diabetes mellitus presented with a 3-month history of episodic exertional dyspnea. A dual isotope rest ^{201}Tl/exercise ^{99m}Tc-MIBI SPECT was performed. She exercised 6 minutes on a standard Bruce protocol and achieved an HR of 130 bpm (84% of MPHR) without the occurrence of chest pain. The test was terminated due to fatigue and significant dyspnea at peak exercise. She reached only 84% of MPHR, suggesting a depressed chronotropic response considering her intense fatigue. At this HR, the exercise ECG demonstrated 1.5-mm downsloping ST-segment depression in leads V4–V6, consistent with ischemia. The exercise ^{99m}Tc-MIBI/rest ^{201}Tl SPECT images are displayed in Figure C12-3A.

Findings

The images in Figure C12-3A demonstrated perfusion defects on the stress images in the inferior and inferolateral walls, whereas the rest images demonstrated homogeneous uptake throughout the LV. The SSS was calculated at 12. Thus, there were reversible perfusion defects in the inferior and inferolateral walls, consistent with a moderate degree of exercise-induced ischemia of those regions. The poststress gated SPECT images were normal with an LVEF of 60%.

Discussion

In this 65-year-old woman with multiple risk factors, the symptoms of exertional dyspnea are most likely secondary to CAD (anginal equivalent) as evidenced by a moderate degree of exercise-induced ischemia of the inferior and inferolateral walls. Despite the paucity of symptoms in this patient, diabetes is a major and potent risk factor for CAD. Patients with both diabetes and CAD have a higher incidence of premature CAD.[24] For example, diabetic patients with normal MPI have a threefold increase in cardiac events compared with nondiabetic patients.[25]

Stress MPI has recently been shown to have diagnostic and prognostic accuracy in the evaluation of symptomatic diabetic patients.[26–28] Data from Kang and colleagues[28] suggest similar sensitivity and specificity in diabetic patients in comparison with those without diabetes. This study demonstrated a sensitivity of 90% and normalcy rate of 95% for the detection of CAD in patients with diabetes. More recently, Giri and colleagues[27] demonstrated a powerful prognostic value of MPI in a large cohort of diabetic patients. In this group of diabetic patients who had stress MPI, the presence and extent of perfusion defects independently predicted cardiac events. The presence and extent of perfusion abnormalities were the strongest predictors of cardiac events among diabetic women with a significantly higher cardiac events rate among diabetic women compared with nondiabetic women. In a large cohort of women, estimate of ischemic burden with stress MPI significantly improved risk stratification in diabetic women compared with clinical assessment alone, and stratification by the number of ischemic vessels demonstrated a significant linear increase in cardiac events.

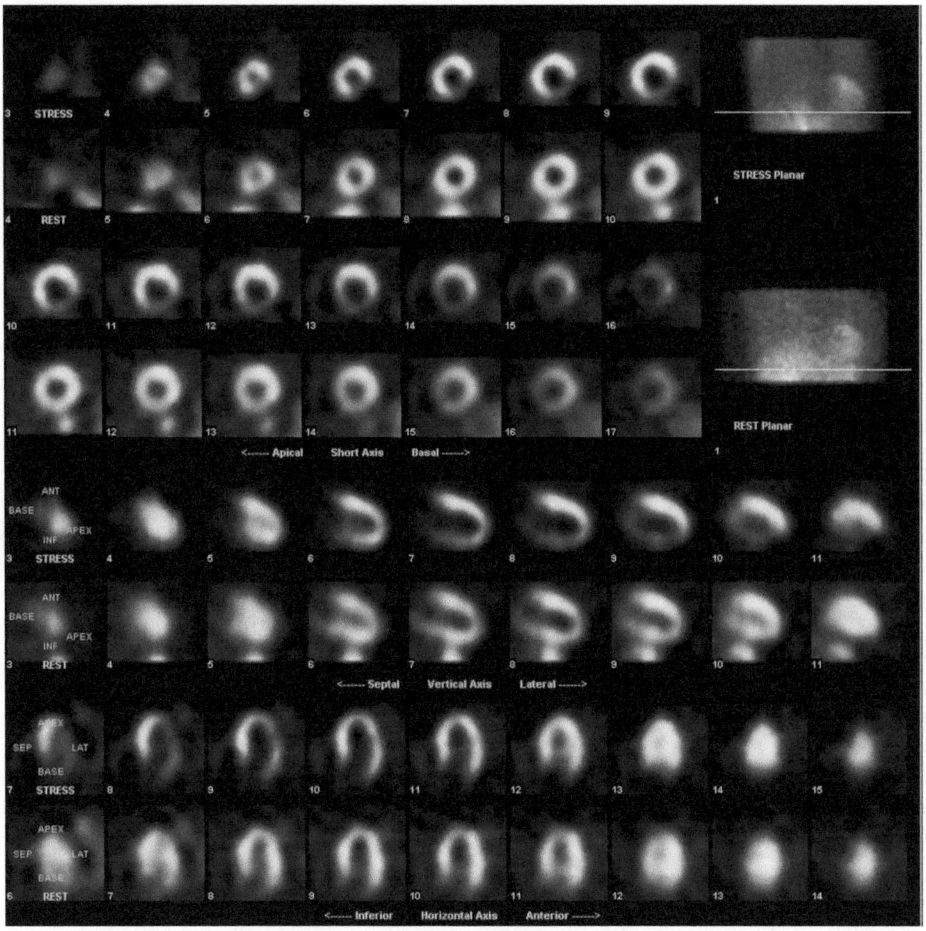

A

FIGURE C12-3. (A)

Thus, in the symptomatic diabetic patient, stress MPI plays an important role in the diagnosis and risk stratification of those patients with an increased risk of CAD (Figure C12-3B). As data are collected in the asymptomatic diabetic population, it is anticipated that stress MPI will have an increasingly relevant role.[29]

Diagnosis

Stress myocardial perfusion images consistent with a moderate amount of exercise-induced ischemia of the inferior and inferolateral walls.

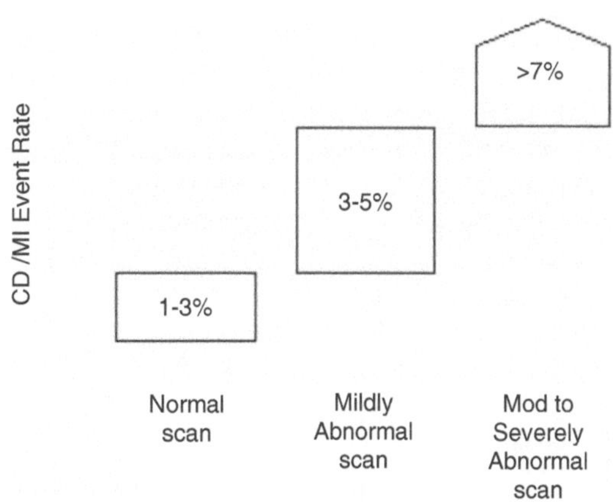

B

FIGURE C12-3. (B, from Kang, Berman, Lewin, et al. [28], by permission of *Am Heart J.*)

Outcome

Coronary angiography demonstrated a left dominant coronary system with a 90% stenosis of the proximal LCX, which was treated with successful placement of a stent. There was 40% stenosis of the mid LAD and 30% stenosis of the RCA.

Case 12.4

History

A 45-year-old man was admitted to the hospital with new onset of congestive heart failure (CHF) and a history of progressive symptoms of exertional dyspnea for 1 month before admission. He denied any history of heart disease or symptoms of chest pain. His admission ECG was significant for sinus rhythm with Q waves in leads V2–V4, suggesting an anterior wall MI in the past (despite having no history of prior MI). The ECG also demonstrated an intraventricular conduction delay and left anterior hemiblock. Admission chest radiography demonstrated cardiomegaly. He was referred for an exercise MPI study on day 4 of admission after treatment for heart failure. He completed 6 minutes of a standard Bruce protocol, reaching 85% of his maximum predicted HR. There was no evidence of ischemic changes on the ECG, and the test was terminated due to fatigue and dyspnea. The exercise ^{99m}Tc-MIBI/rest ^{99m}Tc-MIBI SPECT images are displayed in Figure C12-4.

Findings

The exercise ^{99m}Tc-MIBI SPECT images demonstrated a dilated LV cavity and some mild decreased uptake of radiotracer in the anteroseptal, inferior, inferoseptal, and inferoapical walls that are reversible on the resting images. The SSS was quantitatively calculated at 5, consistent with mild ischemia.[1] Both the rest and the postexercise gated SPECT images demonstrated severe global hypokinesis of the LV and an LVEF of 11%.

Discussion

Heart failure is the final common pathway of a large majority of cardiovascular disorders.[30] In a patient who presents with new onset of CHF, determination of the underlying etiology of LV dysfunction is a crucial first step in deciding on patient management. The identification of CAD as the underlying etiology of CHF and LV dysfunction has important diagnostic and therapeutic implications, especially for the prevention of future ischemic events.[31] If CAD is suspected as the underlying cause, two distinct diagnostic paradigms can be implemented to detect the presence or absence of CAD: either noninvasive imaging with stress gated SPECT MPI or coronary angiography. The current ACC/AHA guidelines for CHF recommend coronary angiography for the group of patients with CHF and a history of angina.[32] In this group of patients, studies have demonstrated a better long-term survival with surgical coronary artery revascularization compared with medical therapy.[33,34]

The choice of a diagnostic strategy for the patient described in this case is less clear as there is a paucity of published data on the best diagnostic approach to the patient with no history of MI and no angina. MPI with gated SPECT has been shown to be useful in differentiating CAD from a nonischemic etiology of CHF. In a cohort of 37 patients with CHF and reduced LVEF, Danias and colleagues[35] found that patients with ischemic heart disease as the etiology of CHF had evidence of more severe and extensive perfusion defects (evidenced by a higher SSS) and regional wall motion abnormalities compared with those patients with nonischemic cardiomyopathy. This study also demonstrated that patients with nonischemic cardiomyopathy may have small, mild perfusion abnormalities with diffuse wall motion abnormalities on gated SPECT MPI.

Data thus far demonstrate a high negative predictive value of MPI in the detection of the

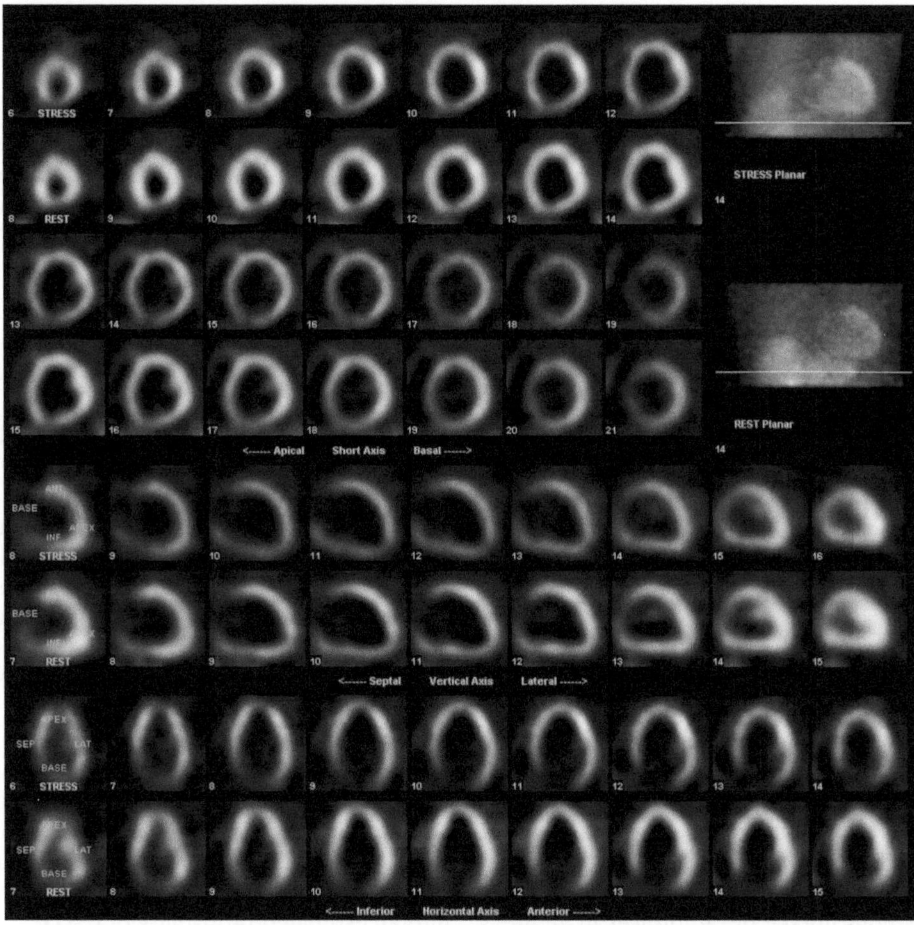

FIGURE C12-4.

presence or absence of CAD in patients with CHF. Ischemic heart disease as the cause of CHF and LV dysfunction is unlikely in the setting of a normal or mildly abnormal perfusion scan.[31]

Interpretation

Abnormal MPI with a dilated LV and an LVEF of 11% on both the rest and on postexercise ^{99m}Tc-MIBI gated SPECT study was seen. Although the pattern of perfusion abnormality is mild, in the presence of severe global LV dysfunction on the rest and post-stress gated SPECT studies ischemic cardiomyopathy should be considered, but nonischemic cardiomyopathy would still be a possible diagnosis for this patient.

Outcome

Coronary angiography demonstrated normal coronary arteries. Myocardial biopsy was suspicious for Chagas' disease. The working diagnosis was nonischemic cardiomyopathy possibly secondary to Chagas' disease in this patient from Guyana. This patient also had a left anterior hemiblock on ECG, which is a conduction abnormality frequently found in patients with cardiac Chagas' disease, usually in combination with right bundle branch block. Chagas disease can also lead to perfusion abnormalities mimicking CAD.

Case 12.5

History

A 45-year-old asymptomatic man was referred for exercise MPI because of an abnormal exercise stress test that he underwent before the start of an exercise program. He is 5 ft, 10 inches and weighs 220 lbs. His medical history is significant for a 5-year history of hypertension, 15-year history of smoking, and a family history of CAD. He completed 9 minutes of a standard Bruce protocol to an HR of 150 bpm and a peak BP of 230/110 mmHg. The test was terminated due a hypertensive response to exercise. He had no symptoms of chest pain or dyspnea with exercise. His post exercise ECG and exercise ^{99m}Tc-MIBI/rest ^{201}Tl dual isotope SPECT images are displayed in Figures C12-5A and C12-5B, respectively.

Findings

The postexercise ECG demonstrated 1.0 mm flat ST-segment depression in leads V4–V6, which actually started at 8 minutes of exercise and persisted until 10 minutes into recovery (Figure C12-5A), suggesting ischemia; however, the dual isotope exercise myocardial perfusion imaging study demonstrated unequivocally homogenous uptake of radiotracer in all areas of the LV. This is consistent with normal myocardial perfusion with no evidence for MI or exercise-induced myocardial ischemia at this level of exercise.

Discussion

Coronary artery disease continues to be the leading cause of death of men and women in the western world. While a large percentage of cardiac events (MI and death) occur in patients who have risk factors and are symptomatic from ischemic heart disease, a moderate percentage of cardiac events occur in patients who are asymptomatic.[3] Occult CAD always precedes the onset of clinically manifest disease and can present as sudden cardiac death or acute MI (Figure C12-5C).

Therefore, the noninvasive detection of silent CAD is an important clinical goal in individuals who are potentially at high risk for cardiac death or MI based on the presence of cardiac risk factors. The detection of high risk may be accomplished by integrating a number of traditional risk factors, e.g., age, family history of premature CAD, hypertension, and smoking into an estimated probability of CAD.[36]

A

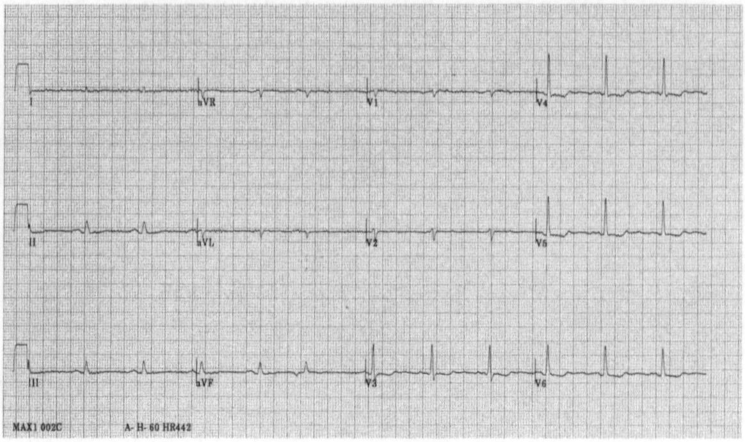

FIGURE C12-5. (A)

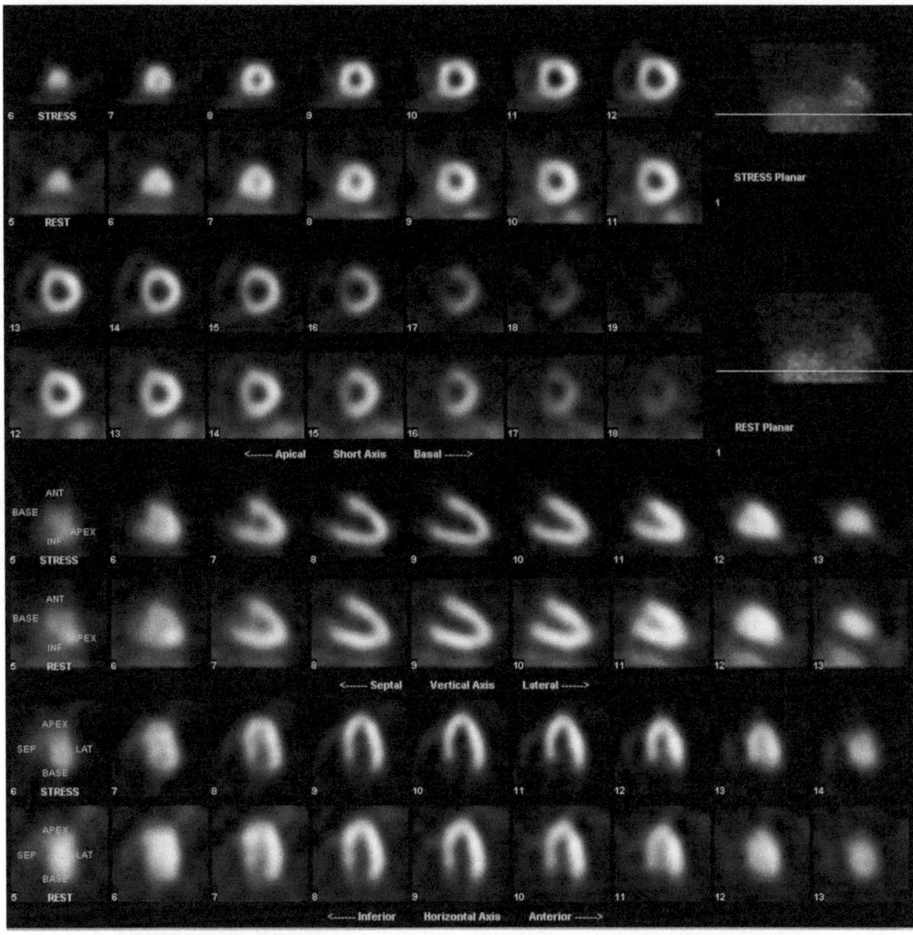

B

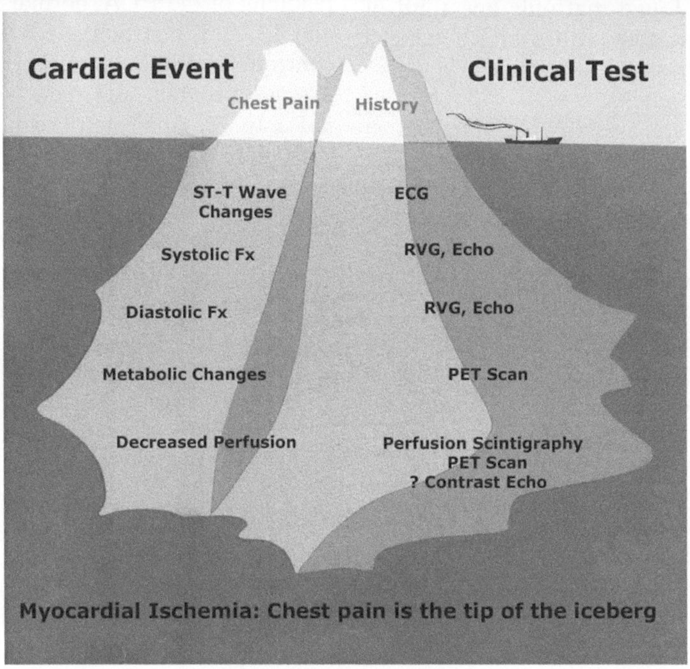

C

FIGURE C12-5. (B and C)

Which Asymptomatic Individual Should Be Screened for CAD?

Bayesian analysis indicates that detection of occult CAD by noninvasive testing should be most accurate in asymptomatic groups with a high prevalence of CAD.[37] Studies of treadmill exercise ECG testing and MPI studies demonstrate that the positive predictive accuracy is much worse in symptom-free, low-prevalence cohorts than in clinically symptomatic patients.[38,39]

Therefore, screening for occult CAD is recommended for selected cohorts who are at high risk for ischemic heart disease. This includes patients with high risk factor levels for CAD, such as family history of premature CAD, diabetes, and familial hypercholesterolemia. Screening may also be indicated for populations at moderately high risk who are about to begin strenuous exercise programs.

A large body of evidence is available on treadmill exercise testing for detecting CAD in an asymptomatic population.[40] An abnormal exercise test is associated with subsequent CAD events and therefore predicts increased cardiac risk. In studies that have evaluated the relation between abnormal exercise ECG and the results of coronary angiography, Froelicher and colleagues[41] found that only one third of 111 asymptomatic men with exercise-induced ST-segment depression had coronary artery lesions of ≥50% stenosis.

Limited data are available on the role of nuclear cardiology studies in asymptomatic patients. In a cohort of 264 aymptomatic siblings of patients with premature CAD (The Johns Hopkins Sibling Study), ^{201}Tl SPECT was more sensitive than exercise ECG for identifying future cardiac events.[42]

It is important to realize that exercise MPI reflects the obstruction of coronary blood flow that exists at the time of maximal exercise, which is a function of both the severity of coronary artery lesion, the vasomotor tone of the epicardial arteries, collateral circulation, and the coronary microcirculation (endothelial function) at peak exercise.[43] A mild coronary artery lesion may become flow limiting during exercise, if it is located in a segment of the artery that undergoes constriction, or if it involves the vessel wall significantly affecting the coronary reserve.

It is well recognized that acute MI resulting from atherosclerotic plaque rupture and arterial thrombosis occurs very often at the site of mild coronary artery stenosis than at severe flow-limiting stenoses.[44] Therefore, identification of mild disease may predict which high-risk individuals will be at risk for future cardiac events.

In the previous case, this asymptomatic patient with a high clinical risk for CAD and an abnormal exercise ECG, exercise myocardial perfusion was indicated and useful in his risk assessment.[45] The normal exercise myocardial perfusion study places him at a low risk for a cardiac event in the next year.[46]

Interpretations

1. Ischemic ECG response to exercise.
2. Hypertensive response to exercise.
3. Normal myocardial perfusion imaging study predictive of good prognosis.

Outcome

Coronary angiography demonstrated mild plaquing of the RCA, normal LAD, left main, and LCX. The patient's BP was aggressively controlled with beta-blockers. He began his exercise program and reduced his body mass index to 25. Cholesterol, which was elevated with LDL of 180, was controlled on pravastatin.

References

1. Berman DS, German G. Clinical applications of nuclear cardiology. In Berman DS, Germano G (Eds). *Clinical Gated Cardiac SPECT.* Armonk, NY: Futura Publications; 1999:1–63.
2. Gibbons RJ, Balady GJ, Beasley JW, et al. ACC/AHA guidelines for exercise testing: Executive summary. *J Am Coll Cardiol.* 1997;96:345–354.
3. American Heart Association. *Heart and Stroke Statistical Update 2003.* Dallas: American Heart Association; 2003:1–46.
4. Miller TD, Roger VL, Milavetz JJ, et al. Assessment of the exercise electrocardiogram in

women versus men using tomographic myocardial perfusion imaging as the reference standard. *Am J Cardiol.* 2001;87:868–873.

5. Kwok Y, Kim C, Grady D, et al. Analysis of exercise testing to detect coronary artery disease in women. *Am J Cardiol.* 1999;83:660–666.
6. Morise AP, Dalal JN, Duval RD. Value of a simple measure of estrogen status for improving the diagnosis of coronary artery disease in women. *Am J Med.* 1993;94:491–496.
7. Heller GV, Fossati AT. Detection of coronary artery disease in women. In Zaret B, Beller G (Eds). *Nuclear Cardiology: State of the Art and Future Directions* 2nd ed. St. Louis: Mosby; 1999:298–311.
8. Travin MI, Duca MD, Kline GM, et al. Relation of gender to physician use of test results and to the prognostic value of stress technetium 99m sestamibi myocardial single-photon emission computed tomography scintigraphy. *Am Heart J.* 1997;134:73–82.
9. Hachamovitch R, Berman DS, Kiat H, et al. Effective risk stratification using exercise myocardial perfusion SPECT in women: gender-related differences in prognostic nuclear testing. *J Am Coll Cardiol.* 1996;28:34–44.
10. Taillefer R, DePuey EG, Udelson JE, et al. Comparative diagnostic accuracy of ^{201}Tl and ^{99m}Tc sestamibi SPECT imaging (perfusion and ECG-gated SPECT) in detecting coronary artery disease in women. *J Am Coll Cardiol.* 1997;29:69–77.
11. Marwick T, Shaw LJ, Lauer MS, et al. The noninvasive prediction of cardiac mortality in men and women with known or suspected coronary artery disease. Economics of Noninvasive Diagnosis (END) Study Group: END Trial. *Am J Med.* 1999;106:172–178.
12. Cacciabaudo JM, Hachamovitch R. Stress myocardial perfusion SPECT in women: Is it the cornerstone of the noninvasive evaluation? *J Nucl Med.* 1998;39:758–759.
13. Gibbons RJ, Chatterjee K, Daley J, et al. ACC/AHA/ACP-ASIM Guidelines for the management of patients with chronic stable angina: executive summary and recommendations. *J Am Coll Cardiol.* 1999;33:2092–2097.
14. Mieres JH, Shaw LJ, Hendel RC, et al. Consensus statement of the American Society of Nuclear Cardiology: the role of myocardial perfusion imaging in the clinical evaluation of coronary artery disease in women. *J Nucl Cardiol.* 2003;10:95–101.
15. Chou TC. Left bundle branch block in electrocardiography. In Chou TC (ed). *Electrocardiography in Clinical Practice, Adult and Pediatric,* 4th ed. Philadelphia: WB Saunders Company; 1996:75–87.
16. Depuey EG, Krawczynska EG, Robbins WL. Thallium-201 SPECT in coronary artery disease patients with left bundle branch block. *J Nucl Med.* 1988;29:1479–1485.
17. Burns RJ, Galligan L, Wright LM, et al. Improved specificity of myocardial thallium-201 single photon emission computed tomography in patients with left bundle branch block by dipyridamole. *Am J Cardiol.* 1991;68:504–508.
18. Depuey EG. Artifacts in SPECT in cardiac SPECT imaging. In Depuey EG, Garcia EV, Berman DS (Eds). *Cardiac SPECT Imaging* 2nd ed. Philadelphia: Lippincott Williams & Wilkins; 2001:231–262.
19. Hirzel HO, Senn M, Nuesch K, et al. Thallium-201 scintigraphy in complete left bundle branch block. *Am J Cardiol.* 1984;53:764–769.
20. O'Keefe HH, Bateman TM, Silveotri R. Safety and diagnostic accuracy of adenosine ^{201}Tl scintigraphy in patients unable to exercise and those with left bundle branch block. *Am Heart J.* 1992;124:614–621.
21. Ebersole DG, Heironimu J, Toney MO. Comparison of exercise and adenosine Technetium 99m sestamibi myocardial scintigraphy for diagnosis of coronary artery disease in patients with left bundle branch block. *Am J Cardiol.* 1993;71:450–453.
22. Rockett JF, Wood WC, Mouinuddin M, et al. Intravenous dipyridamole thallium-201 SPECT imaging in patients with left bundle branch block. *Clin Nucl Med.* 1990;15:401–407.
23. Larcos G, Brown ML, Gibbons RF. Role of dipyridamole thallium-201 imaging in left bundle branch block. *Am J Cardiol.* 1991;68:1097–1098.
24. Grundy SM, Benjamin IJ, Burke GL, et al. Diabetes mellitus: A major risk factor for cardiovascular disease: a joint editorial statement by the American Diabetes Association; the National Heart, Lung, and Blood Institute; the Juvenile Diabetes Foundation International; the National Institute of Diabetes and Digestive and Kidney Disease and the American Heart Association. *Circulation.* 1999;100:1134–1146.
25. Hachamovitch R, Hayes S, Friedman JD, et al. Determinants of risk and its temporal variation in patients with normal stress myocardial perfusion scans: what is the warranty period

of a normal? *J Am Coll Cardiol.* 2003;41: 1329–1340.
26. Kang X, Berman DS, Lewin H, et al. Comparative ability of myocardial perfusion single-photon emission computed tomography to detect coronary artery disease in patients with and without diabetes mellitus. *Am Heart J.* 1999;137:949–957.
27. Giri S, Shaw LJ, Murthy DR, et al. Impact of diabetes on the risk stratification using stress single-photon emission computed tomography myocardial perfusion imaging in patients with symptoms suggestive of coronary artery disease. *Circulation.* 2002;105:32–40.
28. Kang X, Berman DS, Lewin HC, et al. Incremental prognostic value of myocardial perfusion single photon emission computed tomography in patients with diabetes mellitus. *Am Heart J.* 1999;138:1025–1032.
29. Wackers FT, Zaret BL. Editorial: Detection of myocardial ischemia in patients with diabetes mellitus. *Circulation.* 2002;105:5–7.
30. Raisinghani A, Blanchard D, DeMaria AN. Role of cardiac ultrasound in heart failure. *J Nucl Cardiol.* 2002;9:S53–S59.
31. Udelson JE, Shafer CD, Carrio I. Radionuclide imaging in heart failure: assessing etiology and outcomes and implications for management. *J Nucl Cardiol.* 2002;9:S40–S52.
32. Hunt SA, Baker DW Chin MH, et al. ACC/AHA Guidelines for the evaluation and management of chronic heart failure in the adult: executive summary. *J Am Coll Cardiol.* 2001;38:2101–2113.
33. Bounos EP, Mark DB, Pollock BG, et al. Surgical survival benefits for coronary artery disease patients with left ventricular dysfunction. *Circulation.* 1988;78:I151–I157.
34. Alderman EL, Fisher LD, Litwin P, et al. Results of coronary artery surgery in patients with poor left ventricular function (CASS). *Circulation.* 1983;68:785–795.
35. Danias PG, Ahlberg AW, Clark III BA, et al. Combined assessment of myocardial perfusion and ventricular function with exercise technetium-99m sestamibi gated single-photon emission tomography imaging to differentiate ischemic and nonischemic dilated cardiomyopathies. *Am J Cardiol.* 1998;82:1253–1258.
36. Greenland P, Abrams J, Aurigemmi GP, et al. Prevention Conference V. Beyond secondary prevention: identifying the high-risk patient for primary prevention: noninvasive burden. *Circulation.* 2000;101:E12–E15.
37. Ritfkin RD, Hood WB Jr. Bayesian analyses of electrocardiographic exercise stress testing. *N Engl J Med.* 1977;297:681–686.
38. Bruce RA, De Rouen TA, Hossack KF. Value of maximal exercise tests in risk assessment of primary coronary heart disease events in healthy men. *Am J Cardiol.* 1980;46:371–378.
39. Froelicher VF, Maron D. Exercise testing and ancillary techniques to screen for coronary heart disease. *Prog Cardiovasc Dis.* 1981;24: 261–274.
40. Froelicher VF. Special applications: screening apparently healthy individuals. In Froelicher VF (Ed). *Manual of Exercise Testing*, 2nd ed. St. Louis: Mosby; 1994:160–176.
41. Froelicher VF, Thompson AJ, Wolthius R, et al. Angiographic findings in asymptomatic aircrewmen with electrocardiographic abnormalities. *Am J Cardiol.* 1997;39:32–39.
42. Blumenthal RS, Becker DM, Moy TF, et al. Exercise thallium tomography predicts future clinically manifest coronary heart disease in a high-risk asymptomatic population. *Circulation.* 1996;93:915–923.
43. Zaret BL, Beller GA. Wintergreen Panel Summaries Panel III: Risk assessment in stable patients. *J Nucl Cardiol.* 1999;6:93–155.
44. Vita JA, Treasure CB, Yeung AC, et al. Patients with evidence of coronary endothelial dysfunction as assessed by acetylcholine infusion demonstrate marked increase in sensitivity to constrictor effects of catecholamines. *Circulation.* 1992;85:1390–1397.
45. Ritchie JL, Bateman TN, Bonow RO, et al. ACC/AHA Task Force Report: Guideline for clinical use of cardiac radionuclide imaging. *J Am Coll Cardiol.* 1995;25:521–547.
46. Hachamovitch R, Berman DS, Kiat H, et al. Exercise myocardial perfusion SPECT in patients without known coronary artery disease: incremental prognostic value and impact on subsequent patient management. *Circulation.* 1996;93:905–914.

13
Pitfalls and Artifacts in Cardiac Imaging

Ernest V. Garcia, Cesar Santana, Gabriel Grossman, Russell Folks, and Tracy Faber

ECG gated myocardial perfusion single photon emission computerized tomographic (SPECT) studies, properly acquired, processed, displayed, quantified, and interpreted, provide important perfusion and function information that has been shown to have high efficacy in the diagnosis, prognosis, and management of patients with coronary artery disease (CAD). Totally automatic computer processing software packages have been developed and validated for assisting physicians in their assessment of myocardial perfusion and function. These programs help to expedite, standardize, and objectify image processing and interpretation.[1–3]

The accuracy of interpreting these studies, either by subjective visual interpretation or with the assistance of computer programs is dependent on the overall quality of the study and on how consistent and predictable is the tracer distribution for a patient's specific disease state. Consistency is obtained when using standard acquisition and processing protocols that have been documented in imaging guidelines from the American Society of Nuclear Cardiology.[4,5] Variations in imaging protocols result in unexpected variations in the normal distribution of myocardial perfusion and function that can confuse either the physician performing the interpretation or the computer program in one or more aspects of the quantitative process. Because these programs are automated and validated, the users could be lulled into believing that all computer results reported by these packages are correct even in the presence of unexpected variation or imaging artifacts.

Several previous publications have documented the imaging artifacts that occur either due to variations in the patient, equipment, acquisition protocol, processing protocol, quantification program, or image interpretation.[6,7] Quality control measures to prevent these artifacts as well as the basic principles of how images and artifacts are created are well documented.[8,9] This chapter first provides a list of these possible artifacts and then discusses their manifestation and recognition in clinical cases.

ECG Gated SPECT Imaging Artifacts

SPECT imaging artifacts are most often due to inconsistencies between projections. Because the image reconstruction algorithms expect the same object to be imaged or seen by each projection, any inconsistencies between projections cause image artifacts. The most common causes of inconsistencies between projections are due to instrument response, patient anatomy, cardiac position, tracer distribution, or variation in heart rate (HR). It is useful to categorize the artifacts either as conventional, the type that has been recognized for many years and common in other SPECT imaging procedures, or contemporary, the type that has been more recently recognized and caused by ECG-gating or quantitative software problems.

The following list presents conventional artifacts:

1. Instrument related artifacts (discussed in Chapter 2), such as center or rotation errors, flood field nonuniformity, inappropriate collimator type, detector not parallel to axis of rotation.
2. Patient-related variants, such as patient motion, cardiac creep, LBBB, myocardial hypertrophy, unusual heart rotation in the chest, and so forth.
3. Attenuation artifacts, usually caused by the breast in women, the diaphragmatic wall in men, and the lateral chest wall in either; these can often be corrected with second-generation attenuation correction algorithms.[10]
4. Tracer kinetics/distribution artifacts, such as high uptake in abdominal visceral activity adjacent to the myocardium, high uptake in the liver, and change in concentration over the acquisition period (discussed in Chapter 3).
5. Processing related artifacts, such as incorrect selection of oblique axes, inappropriate filter, incorrect identification of LV landmarks.

With the new automated software packages for the quantification of myocardial perfusion and function, many of the artifacts stated previously can also occur. In addition the acquisition and processing associated with the functional analysis can result in new inconsistencies that can lead to reduced accuracy for assessing myocardial perfusion and function.

The contemporary artifacts are presented:

1. Failure of the automatic analysis to perform adequately, either due to acquisition or processing inconsistencies or failure of the automatic algorithm.[11]
2. Gating problems causing inaccurate measurement of not only global and regional function but also of myocardial perfusion due to angular inconsistencies during acquisition.[12]
3. Overestimation of global and regional LV function in small ventricles (<20 ml ESV) due to cross-talk of activity from nearby walls.
4. Underestimation of global and regional LV function from methods that use eight frames per cardiac cycle and no phase and amplitude analysis[11,13] (discussed in Chapter 7).

Careful review of these studies on a computer screen coupled with an understanding of the causes of imaging artifacts will contribute to an increase in the specificity of detecting the absence of CAD. The rest of this chapter uses clinical cases to illustrate the appearance and recognition of the most common imaging artifacts.

Case Presentations

Case 13.1

History

A 46-year-old woman with a medical history of atypical chest pain was referred for myocardial perfusion imaging (MPI) for preoperative assessment of cardiac risk before major abdominal surgery. She had no cardiac risk factors other than mild hypercholesterolemia. A week before the MPI study, an exercise treadmill test (TMT) demonstrated 1.5 mm horizontal inferolateral ST-segment depression without symptoms of angina. This was interpreted as probable ischemia and she was referred for MPI using a rest ^{201}Tl/exercise ^{99m}Tc-MIBI dual isotope protocol. The patient exercised 11 minutes, achieving stage IV of a standard Bruce protocol and reaching 90% of the maximum predicted heart rate (HR). No significant ECG changes or symptoms of chest pain occurred during the exercise.

Figure C13-1A displays the perfusion quantification quality control parameter page. This display shows the stress study on the left side and rest study on the right side. The top row shows midventricular short-axis slice images. These are used to illustrate the location of the radial-search boundaries and left ventricular cavity center. The middle row shows both mid-

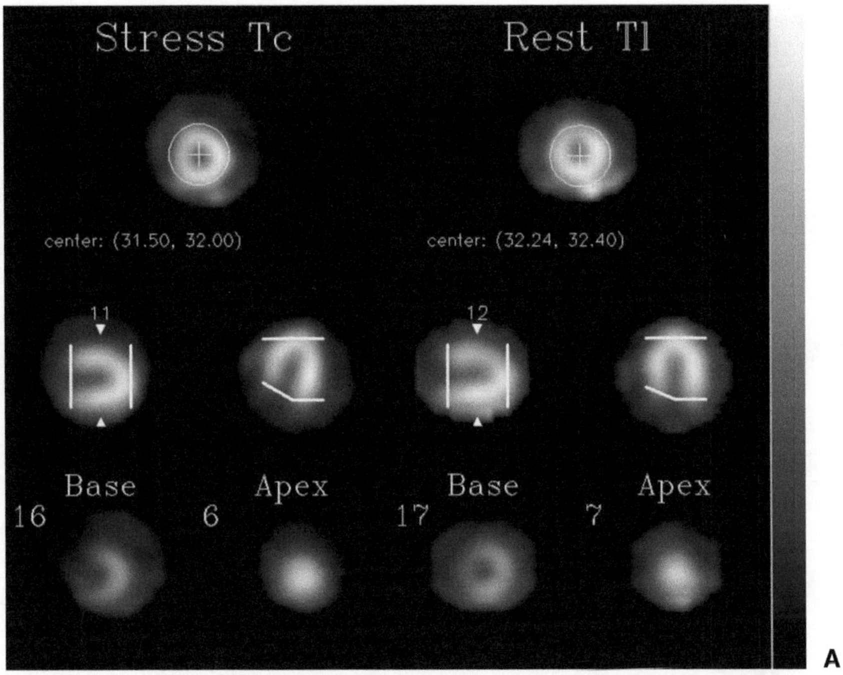

FIGURE C13-1. (A)

ventricular vertical and horizontal long-axis slice images. The vertical long-axis and horizontal long-axis reference images are used to illustrate the placement of the apical and basal slice selections. The bottom row displays short-axis slices, which correspond to the apical and basal slice selections identified in the middle row.

Figure C13-1B shows the optimized display of oblique slices and planar projections. As labeled, this display shows the short axis at stress and rest, the vertical long axis at stress and rest, and the horizontal long axis at stress and rest. The two images in the lower right panel are stress and rest planar steep LAO projections.

Figure C13-1C shows the perfusion quantification polar map display. This display shows the polar map representation where the stress results are in the left column, the rest in the middle column, and the reversibility in the right column. In the top row are the raw polar maps, in the middle row are the extent of the perfusion abnormality as compared with the perfusion database, and the bottom row shows the color-coded severity of the defect and magnitude of reversibility.

Findings

The study showed a moderate-sized reversible perfusion defect in the septal wall, which accounts for approximately 10% of total left ventricular (LV) myocardium and is suggestive of a stenosis in the left anterior descending artery (LAD) territory. A small fixed perfusion defect (3% of the LV myocardium) was also noted in the lateral wall. The study could incorrectly be interpreted as abnormal myocardial perfusion, with ischemia in the LAD territory. Nevertheless, the expert readers realized that the perfusion defects were spuriously caused by the heart misalignment as shown (Figures C13-1A and C13-1B). Therefore, the original data were reprocessed and selection of the LV's oblique axis was performed under physician supervision. Reprocessed data are displayed in Figures C13-1D, C13-1E, and C13-1F. The reprocessed oblique slices show homogeneous distribution of the perfusion tracer at stress and rest, interpreted as normal perfusion. The patient was categorized as a low likelihood for CAD. The abdominal surgery was performed without complications and 4 years later she remained asymptomatic for CAD.

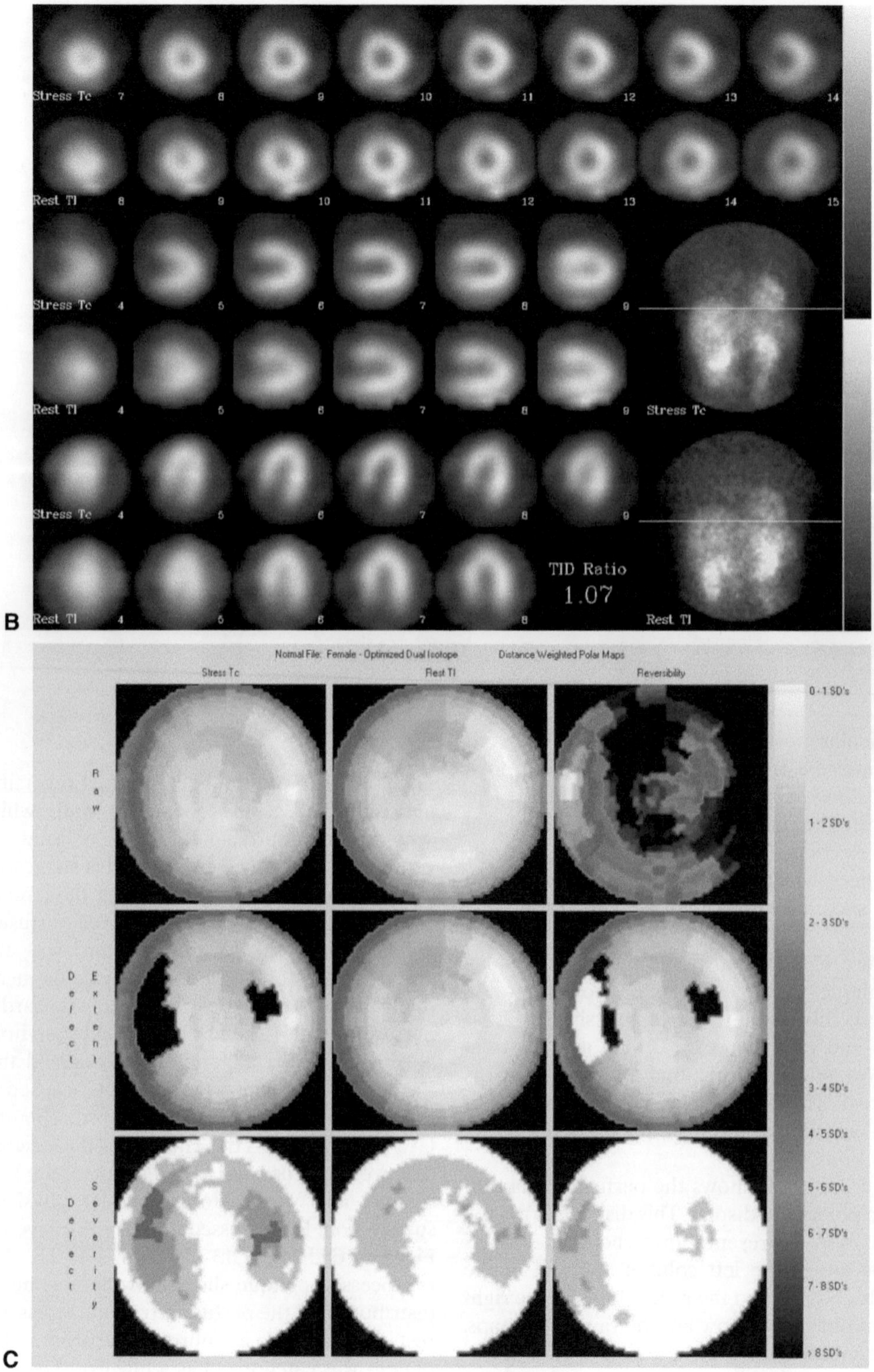

FIGURE C13-1. (B and C)

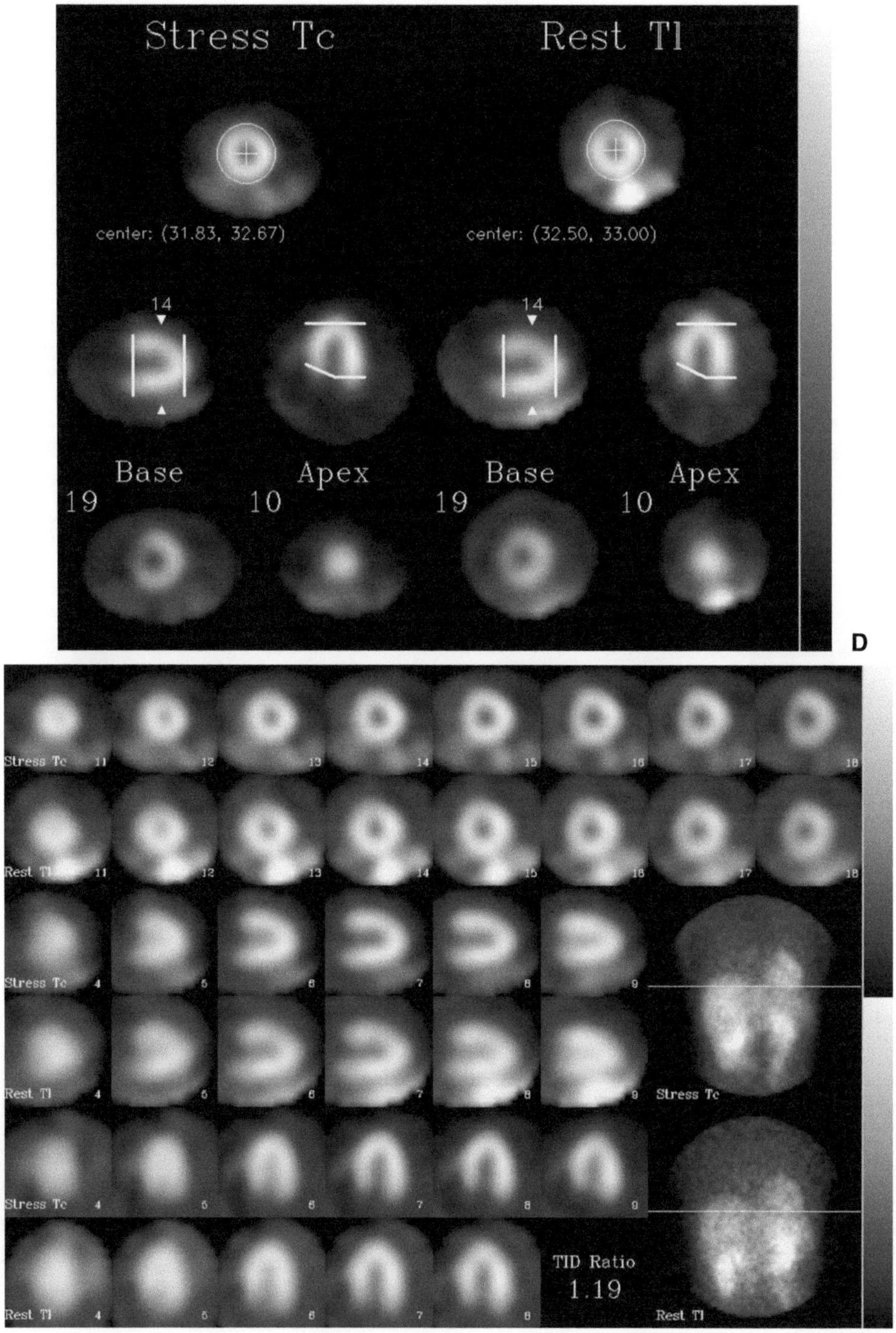

FIGURE C13-1. (D and E)

Discussion

It is important to recognize that diagnostically accurate images can be obtained only if careful quality control is performed during acquisition, reconstruction, and processing of the image data. The position of the heart within the chest can vary significantly from person to person,

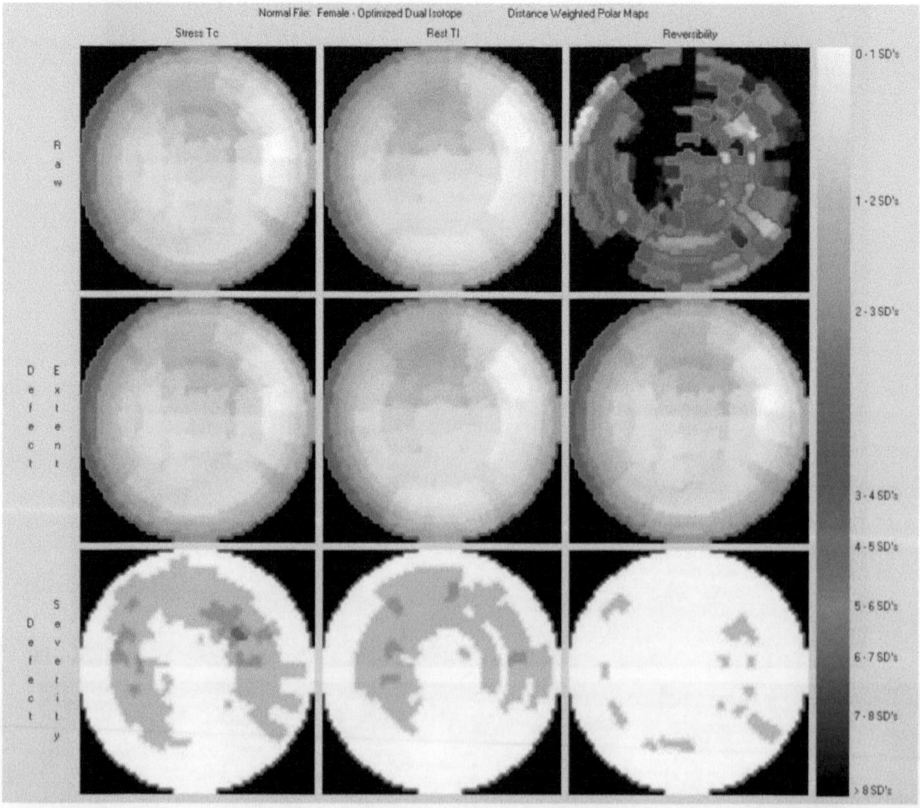

F

FIGURE C13-1. (F)

and so the appearance of the LV in a transaxial tomographic section can vary greatly as well. For that reason, oblique reformatting is used to reslice the heart into three planes perpendicular to the axes of the heart to standardize LV display and analysis.

Errors in the placement of the long axis of the LV result in improper display of the slices and may lead to erroneous interpretation. Depending on the plane where the placement of the axis is erroneous, artifactual defects may appear in different regions of the myocardium on the erroneous display of the vertical, horizontal, or short-axis views. These errors consequently result in apparent alteration of myocardial perfusion seen on both of the slices displayed and in the polar maps.

Specifically, this patient's artifact was generated during the reconstruction of the vertical long axis; minus 15-degree rotation was applied to the stress raw images. The effect of this heart misalignment is more evident in the vertical long axis in this case, but affect the lateral wall.

To avoid these artifacts the midpoint of the valve plane and the exact apex location should be carefully selected. The axes selected should be identical for stress and rest studies. These errors can be detected by reviewing both the parameter page and slices display (Figures C13-1E and C13-1F). Such quality-control screens are available in all of the major commercial systems. This type of error tends to be more common when there is a severe perfusion defect at the apex, which makes selection of the exact location of the apex more difficult.

Interpretation

1. Incorrect oblique axis selection leading to artifactual perfusion defects.
2. Normal myocardial perfusion seen after reprocessing.

Case 13.2

History

A 54-year-old business woman presented with atypical chest pain and was referred for MPI to assess cardiac risk before plastic surgery. Her father died at age 55 of MI. She has a sedentary lifestyle, hypercholesterolemia, and a smoking history. Myocardial perfusion SPECT study was performed following a conventional resting ^{201}Tl/exercise ^{99m}Tc-MIBI dual isotope protocol. The patient exercised for 3 minutes without experiencing angina, reaching 95% of her maximum predicted HR. Her stress EKG demonstrated 1 mm of horizontal, lateral ST-segment depression.

Figure C13-2A displays the perfusion quantification quality control parameter page as described for Figure C13-1A. Figure C13-2B shows the optimized display of oblique slices and planar projections as described for Figure C13-1B. The two images displayed in the lower right panel are stress and rest planar RAO projections. Figure C13-2C shows the perfusion quantification polar map display, as described for Figure C13-1C.

Findings

The quality-control images from the parameter display showed that the automatic base selection algorithm during the reconstruction process has improperly selected the base of the heart in the rest study (Figure C13-2A). On closer inspection it was evident that during the reconstruction and reorientation process the operator incorrectly cut off a portion of the LV base at rest. Display of the oblique slices in this patient showed homogeneous distribution of the perfusion at stress and rest, which was interpreted as normal (Figure C13-2B). Nevertheless, the transient ischemic dilatation (TID) index of 1.37 is higher than the normal 1.22 value.[14–16]

The myocardial perfusion distribution in this patient was normal as seen in the raw polar maps (Figure C13-2C). In addition, the comparison with the reference database did not show any perfusion segment under the lower limit of normal. Nevertheless, the difference polar maps located in the rightmost column showed a red-yellow circular *rim*. This rim

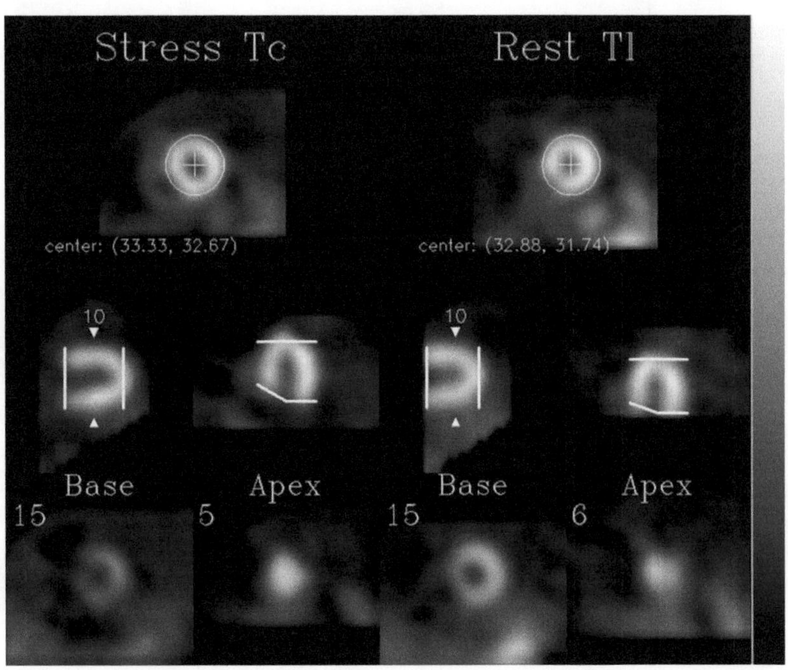

FIGURE C13-2. (A)

A

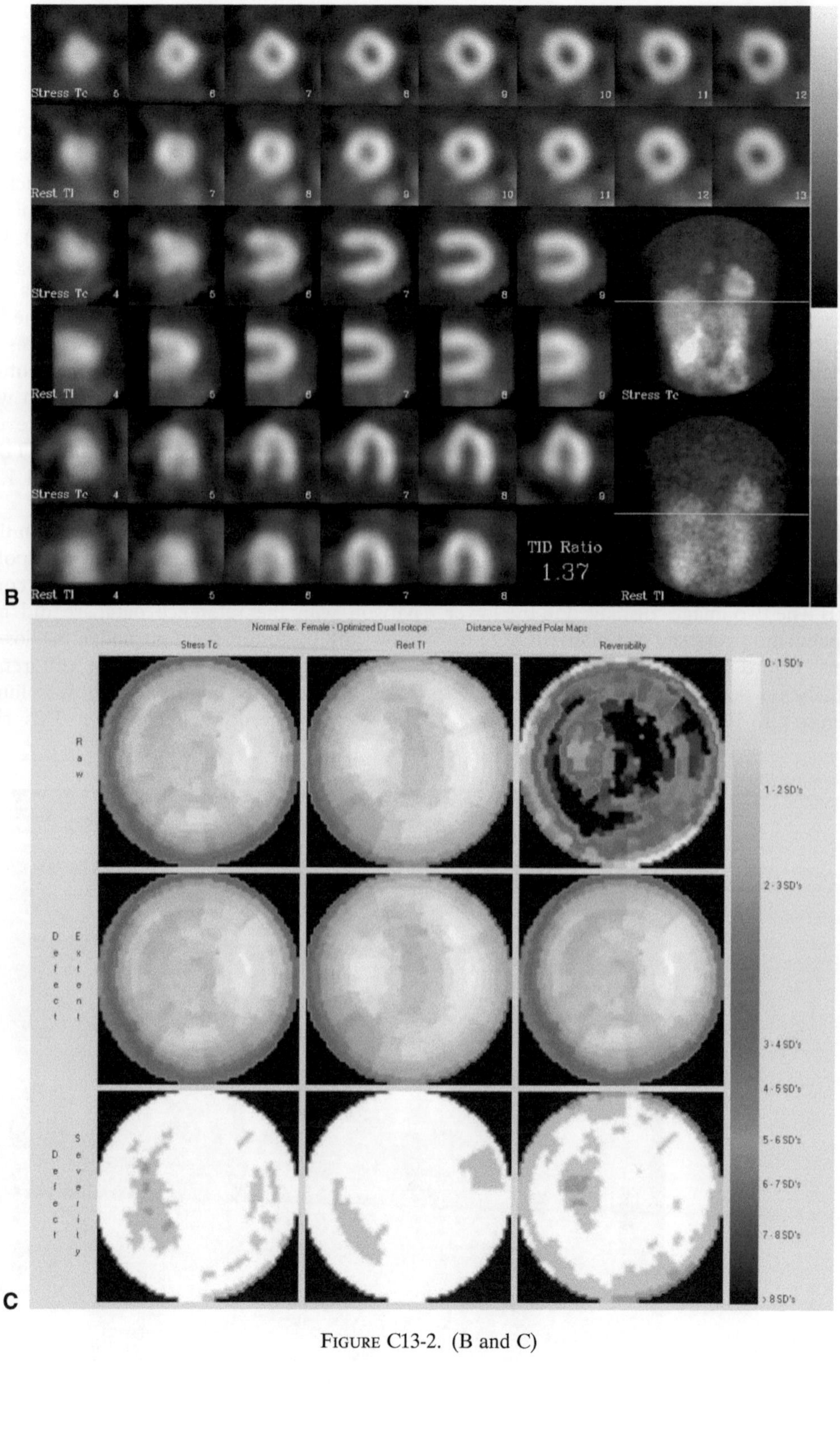

FIGURE C13-2. (B and C)

indicates erroneously that the rest myocardial perfusion was higher than the stress perfusion. This finding was due to the cut off of the base of the heart during the reconstruction process.

Figures C13-2D, C13-2E, and C13-2F display images similar to Figures C13-2A, C13-2B, and C13-2C after corrected reconstruction. After corrected reconstruction, the TID was now normal at 1.08, and the red-yellow rim on the polar maps had disappeared. Therefore, after corrected reconstruction the patient was categorized as having a low likelihood for CAD. The plastic surgery was performed without complications and 7 years after surgery, the patient continues to be asymptomatic from the cardiac point of view.

Discussion

This is an example of a middle-aged woman with multiple risk factors for CAD who was referred for risk stratification before plastic surgery. She has a normal MPI study but in the first set of images the reconstruction artifact created a falsely high TID and a rim artifact in the polar maps. In this example, it is easy to identify the artifacts in the display of the SPECT slices (Figure C13-2B), where we can see that the base of the resting study was cut improperly. The parameter page (Figure C13-2A) helped to define whether the mistake was done during image reconstruction or in the quantification process. In this case the mistake was made during reconstruction with improper selection of the base of the heart. It is important to know that all of the currently available processing software automatically selects the limits of the heart; this process requires verification routinely by both the technologist and the interpreting physician for accurate interpretation. The TID ratio expresses the ratio between the LV volume post-stress and at rest. The normal limits for TID may change according to the protocol used. For example, a

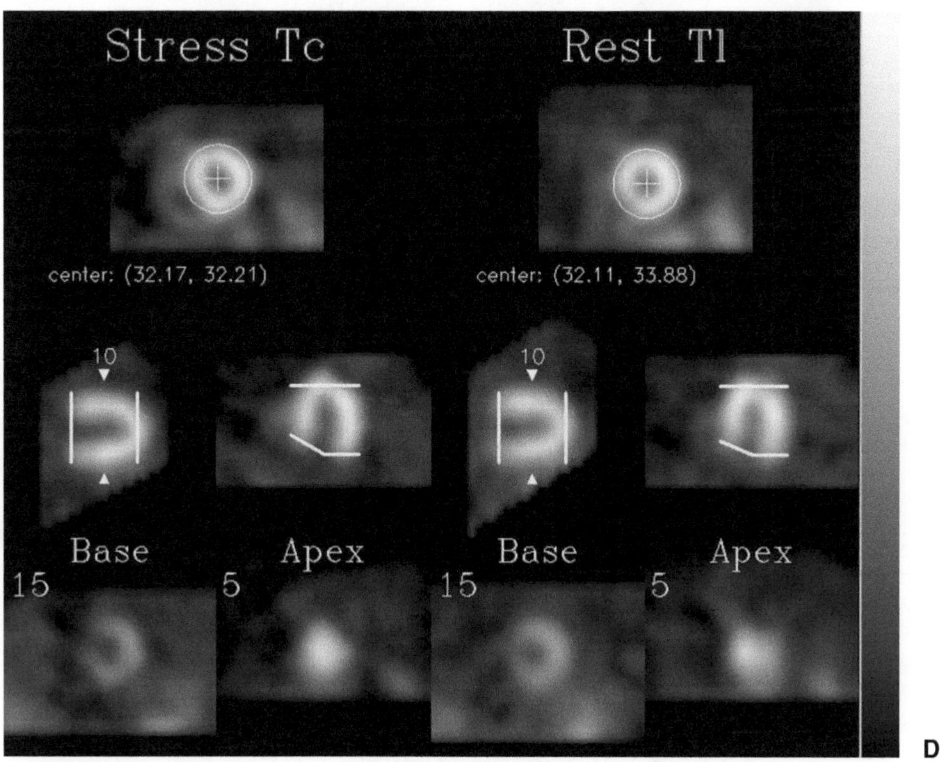

FIGURE C13-2. (D)

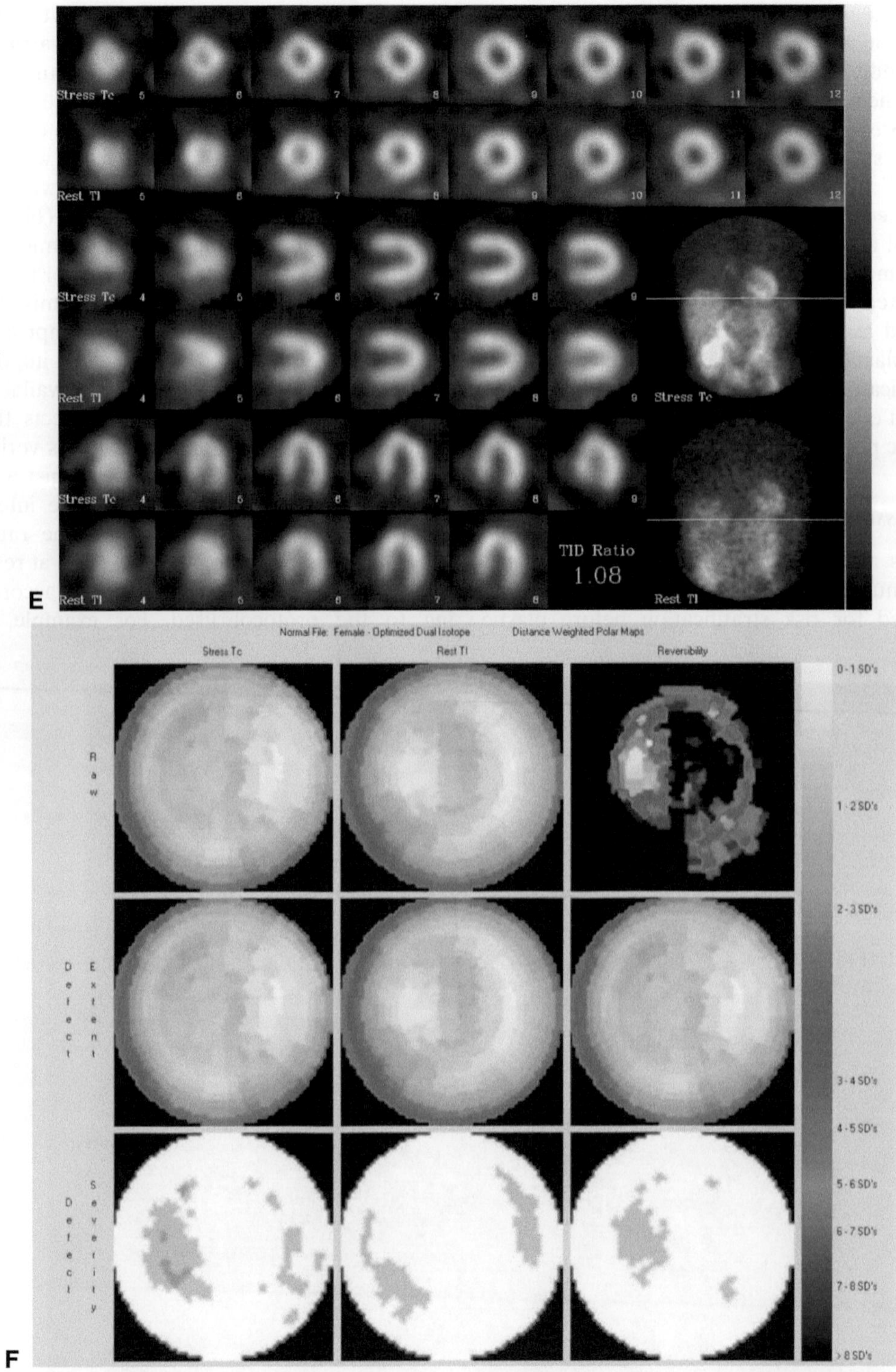

FIGURE C13-2. (E and F)

TID ratio greater than 1.21 using a dual isotope protocol has been defined as abnormal. This quantitative parameter represents a post-stress dilatation of the LV and has been reported to be a marker of severe and extensive CAD. An elevated TID ratio is particularly helpful as an indicator of multivessel disease and balanced reduction of myocardial blood flow in patients in whom the myocardial perfusion distribution may appear relatively homogenous. If the apical or basal limit is incorrectly placed on the stress or resting images, the computer algorithm may calculate an erroneous TID.

Incorrect selection of the base or apex of the LV can generate false perfusion defects when the apex or the base limits are placed outside the limits of the LV myocardium, or false reversibility in patients with fixed perfusion defects and these errors are displayed on the polar plots.

Interpretation

1. Incorrect selection of the base of the heart on the resting images leading to erroneous TID and a rim artifact on the polar plot display.
2. Normal myocardial perfusion and function seen after reprocessing.

Case 13.3

History

A 91-year-old man with known CAD was referred for a resting ^{201}Tl/dipyridamole stress ^{99m}Tc-MIBI dual isotope gated SPECT study before peripheral vascular surgery. During dipyridamole infusion, the blood pressure (BP) decreased from 142/61 to 120/50 mmHg. No symptoms or ECG changes occurred. The rest and stress studies were acquired in the supine position using a dual-head SPECT system equipped with a high-resolution collimator (Figure C13-3A). The post-stress acquisition on the dipyridamole study was performed during

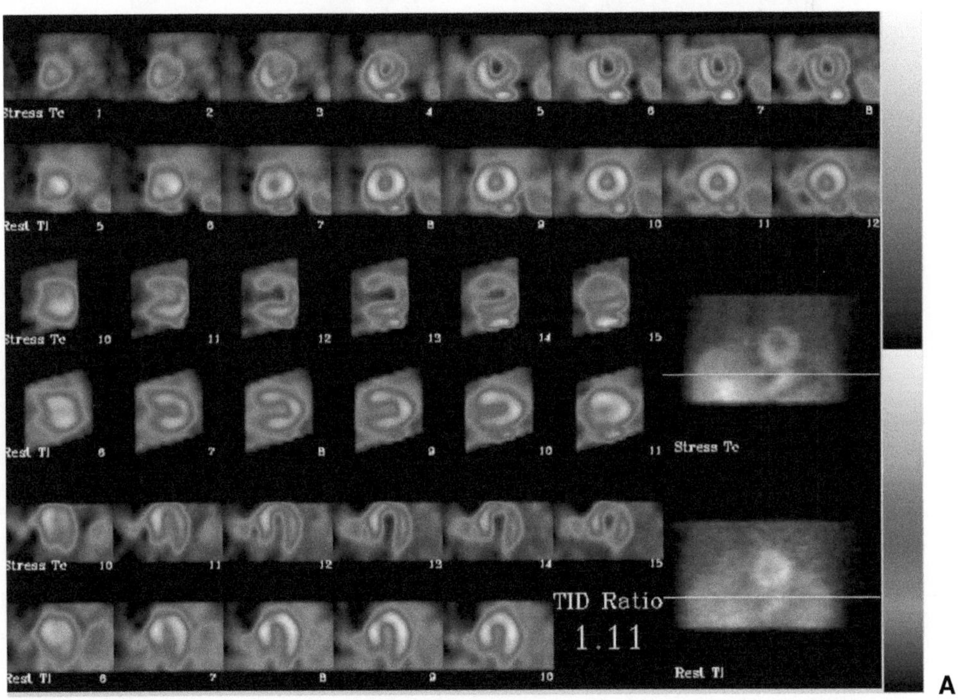

FIGURE C13-3. (A)

ECG-gating using eight frames per cardiac cycle. Quantification of myocardial perfusion was performed using the Emory Cardiac Toolbox by comparing the LV tracer distribution with a dual-isotope normal database and the results are represented in a polar map configuration (Figure C13-3B).

Findings

The stress perfusion images demonstrated a severe defect involving a large portion of the anterior wall and moderate-sized portion of the left circumflex artery (LCX) and/or right coronary artery (RCA)/posterior descending artery (PDA) vascular territory that were normal at rest, indicative of severe ischemia (Figure C13-2A). The defect extent polar map (blackout map) showed a blacked-out region from approximately 10 o'clock to 4 o'clock and from apex to base involving the LAD and LCX region but sparing the septum and RCA/PDA vascular territory. There was a discrepancy in the septal and inferior walls between the uptake (color intensity) seen in the short-axis slices and that illustrated in the polar maps, with the short-axis slices appearing to show significantly less uptake. Displaying the images so that the maximum color intensity was assigned to the maximum count *in the entire image* artificially created this discrepancy. When the image normalization was changed to assign the maximum color intensity to the maximum *counts in the LV*, the discrepancy was resolved and the color intensity demonstrated in the septal and inferior walls from the short-axis slices (Figure C13-3C) exactly matched those seen on the polar maps (Figure C13-3B).

Discussion

This case illustrates the problems that arise when images are normalized differently and demonstrates the need to always automatically normalize all the MPI slices and polar maps to the maximum counts over the LV. The most practical approach to ensure proper normalization is to use totally integrated software pack-

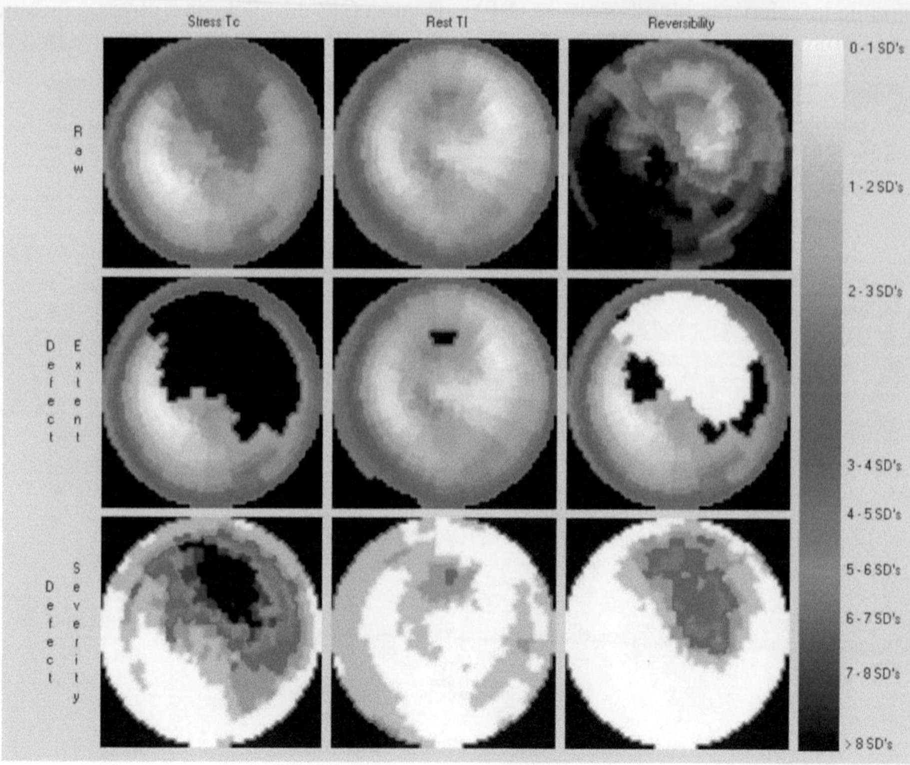

B

FIGURE C13-3. (B)

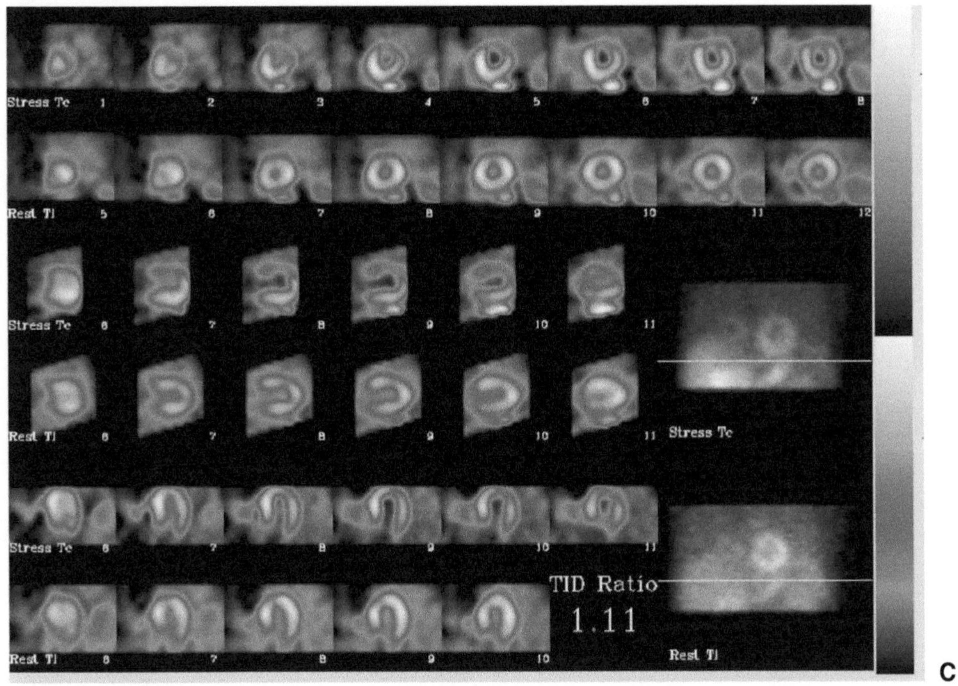

FIGURE C13-3. (C)

ages that first automatically isolate the LV from the rest of the image and extract the maximum counts over the LV to generate consistent displays. These integrated programs also have the benefit of providing all of the information necessary for interpreting an ECG-gated MPI SPECT study, usually at the click of a button. The most important available information includes (1) quality assurance images of the automatically determined parameters, (2) properly normalized rotating planar projections, (3) properly normalized short, vertical, and horizontal long-axis slices, (4) quantitative myocardial perfusion polar maps, (5) dynamic displays of the gated short, vertical, and horizontal long-axis slices, and (6) a quantitative report of LV global function including LV ejection fraction (LVEF) and end-diastolic (EDV) and end-systolic volumes (ESV).

Interpretation

1. Suboptimal display.
2. Reversible stress-induced perfusion defect in the LAD and LCX vascular territory, indicative of significant ischemia.

Case 13.4

History

A 40-year-old man undergoing evaluation for renal transplantation was referred for a 1-day low-dose rest/high-dose exercise stress ^{99m}Tc-MIBI SPECT study. The patient had a past history of pericardiectomy. Both the rest and exercise studies were acquired in the supine position using a single-head SPECT system and a high-resolution collimator.

Figures C13-4A and C13-4B show the optimized display of oblique slices and planar projections. Note the dynamic display of planar projections showing the LV in the RAO projection above the line cursor in Figure C13-4A and in the LPO projection below the line cursor in Figure C13-4B.

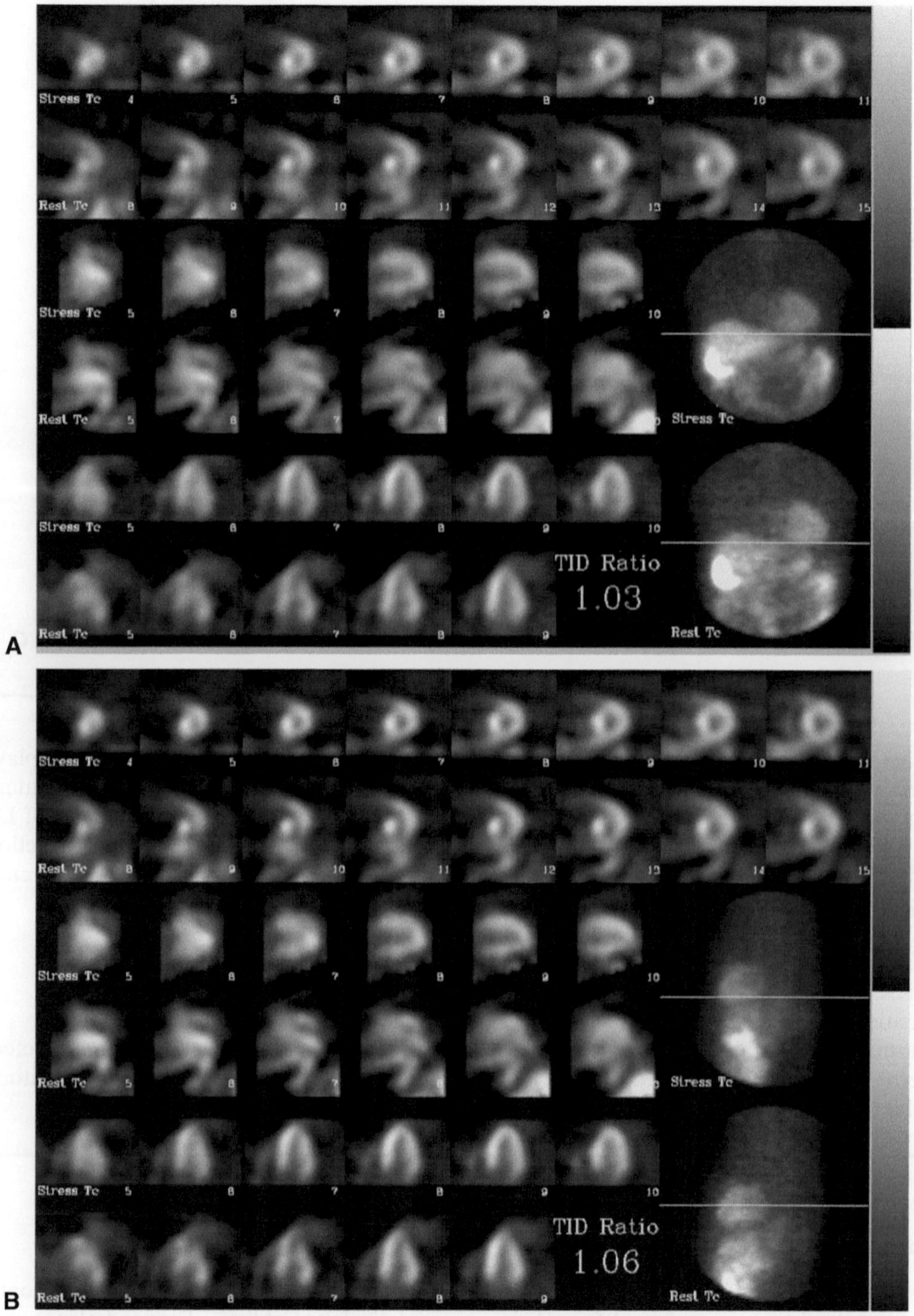

FIGURE C13-4. (A and B)

Findings

Both the stress and particularly the rest short-axis oblique slices demonstrated rays of intensity or streaks emanating from regions in the LV myocardium next to regions of apparent hypoperfusion in the anterior and inferior walls. Visual inspection of the rotating planar projections of both the stress and the rest acquisitions demonstrated that the LV is located above a line cursor in the RAO projection (Figure C13-4A) and well below the same line during display of the LPO projections (Figure C13-4B). This shift in LV position observed during dynamic cine display of the planar projections was indicative of vertical patient motion during the SPECT acquisition. After application of motion correction algorithms,[17] the shift in the LV position in both the stress and rest studies was shown to be significantly reduced between the corrected RAO projection (Figure C13-4C) and the corrected LPO projection (Figure C13-4D). The rest and stress short-axis slices reconstructed from the corrected projections (Figures C13-4C and C13-4D) showed that the streaks seen in the uncorrected studies have mostly disappeared, and the anterior and inferior defects were no longer seen.

Discussion

The anterior and inferior perfusion defects as well as the streaks seen in the initial processing are not present in the motion-corrected study. This finding confirms that patient motion during imaging acquisitions caused the streaks and the hypoperfusion artifacts. These artifacts occur during the filtered back projection process anytime that the reconstruction program is presented with projections that are inconsistent. In this study, the inconsistency was the location of the object being reconstructed, i.e., the LV. Motion as small as 3 mm begins to affect the quality of the image, and motion of 6 to 12 mm begins to be associated with artifacts mimicking perfusion defects.[18] Patient motion is best detected by visual inspection of the dynamic display of rotating planar images. Vertical motion is easier to detect than lateral

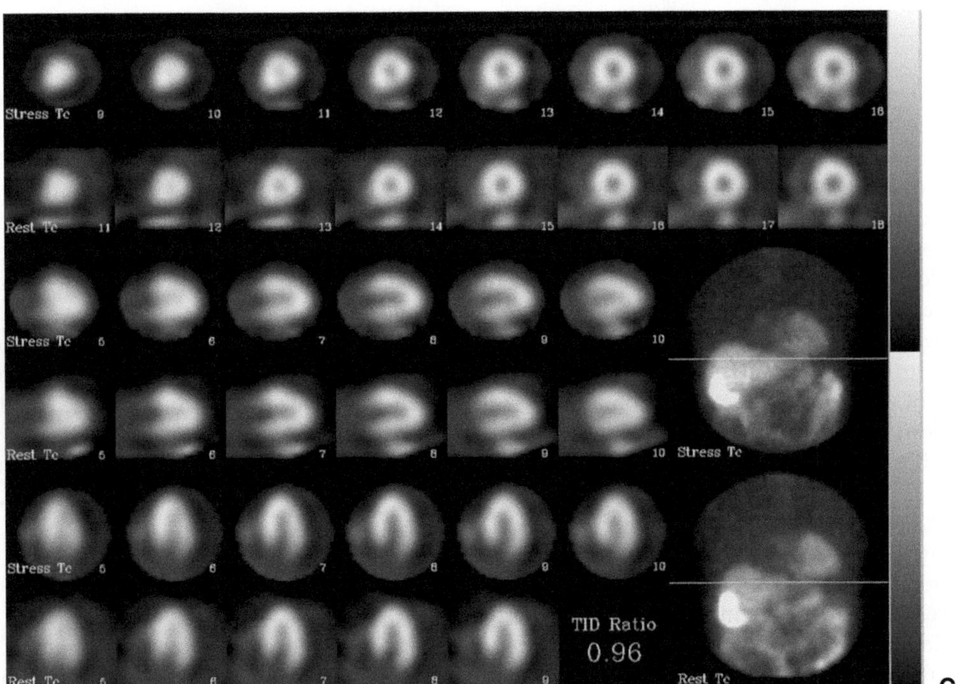

FIGURE C13-4. (C)

D
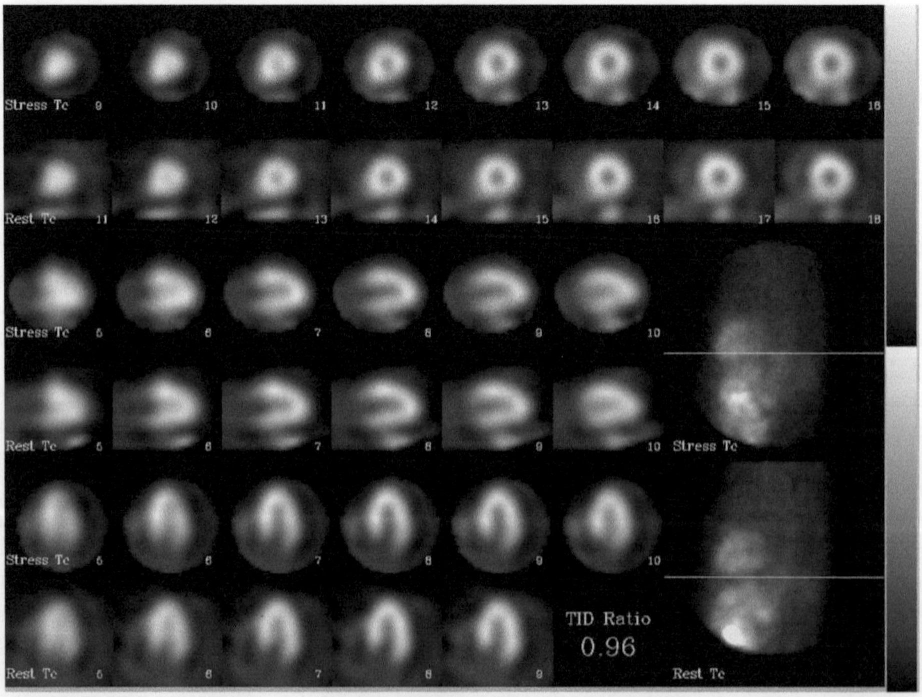

FIGURE C13-4. (D)

motion, although both may result in significant interpretive errors. In this patient, in whom a single-head SPECT system was used, the translation of the LV was seen progressively from the RAO to the LPO projections. In dual-head 90-degree systems, the same LV translation would have been seen as an abrupt movement in the mid-LAO projections. This is the interval between observing the last view of the first detector (after the patient motion) and the first view of the second detector (before the patient motion).

Other inconsistencies between projections, such as photon attenuation, detector misalignment, incorrect center of rotation, or ECG-gating errors, can also create similar artifacts. Although the motion correction program was successful in correcting for this patient's motion, any type of algorithm might fail under certain conditions. It is the responsibility of the interpreter to confirm that corrected studies are indeed corrected or at least improved before rendering an interpretation. Whenever possible, the technologist acquiring the SPECT study should detect the motion and determine whether the acquisition can be repeated without patient motion as a more effective way of eliminating motion artifacts. The interpreter should be informed of this repeated study to take into consideration any potential tracer redistribution. Patient motion is less common when the acquisitions are performed with the patient lying prone on the imaging table. Any measure that makes the patient more comfortable, such as a wedge under the knees, will decrease patient's motion.

Interpretation

1. Artifact caused by patient's motion.
2. Normal myocardial perfusion after correction of motion artifact.

Case 13.5

History

A 48-year-old woman with a history of intermittent chest pain over the last 3 years presented with worsening chest pain. She had no other significant medical history except for a brother who had an MI at age 47. The patient was referred for a resting ^{201}Tl/exercise ^{99m}Tc-MIBI gated SPECT study. She exercised for 7 minutes and 30 seconds using a standard Bruce protocol, reaching a peak HR of 163 bpm, exceeding 85% maximum predicted HR. No symptoms or ECG changes were noted. The rest and stress studies were acquired in the supine position using a single-head SPECT system equipped with a high-resolution collimator. The post-stress acquisition of the exercise study was performed during ECG-gating using eight frames per cardiac cycle.

Figure C13-5A shows the display of oblique slices and planar projections, and Figure C13-5B shows the functional analysis display.

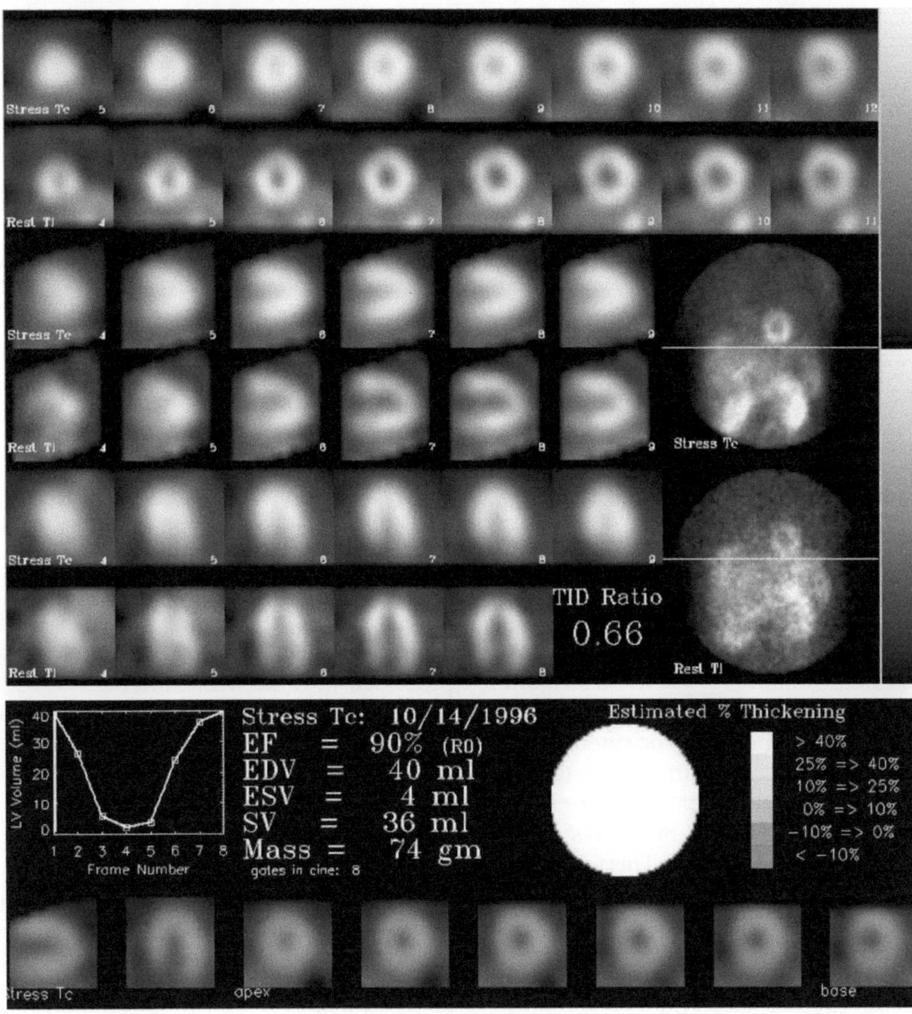

A

B

FIGURE C13-5. (A and B)

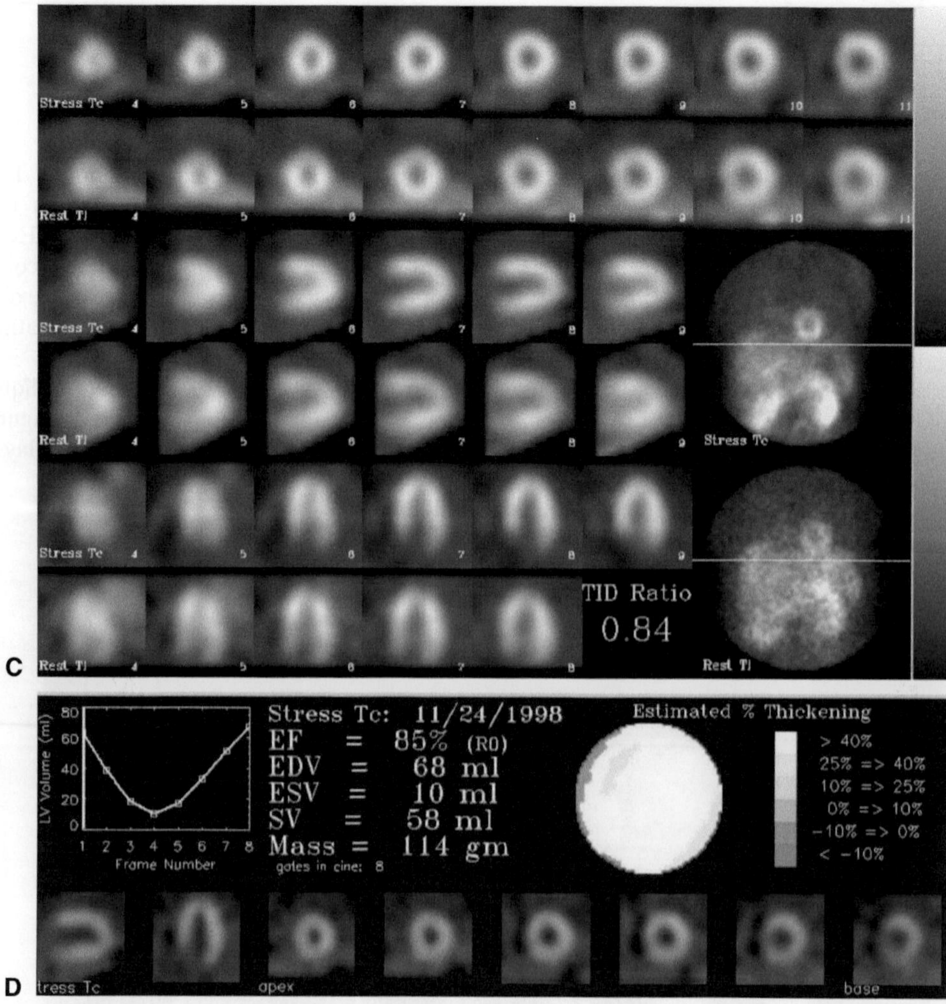

FIGURE C13-5. (C and D)

Findings

Both the stress and rest oblique axis images demonstrated uniform tracer distribution throughout the myocardium (Figure C13-5A). The stress images appeared to be smoother and of lower resolution compared with the rest images. The LV chamber in the images appeared to be smaller in the stress images compared with the rest images. This finding was confirmed by an unusual TID ratio of 0.66. Analysis of LV function reveals an LVEF of 90% and normal thickening of the myocardium (Figure C13-5B). The LV chamber almost totally disappears in the end-systolic images yielding an unrealistic ESV of 4ml. Although this study was interpreted as totally normal, it is clear that the exercise study had been processed with the wrong filter.

Once the stress study was reprocessed with the correct filter, both the stress and the rest study continue to appear normal, but now the stress study demonstrated a similar high image quality compared with rest, including a similar LV chamber size and a significantly larger TID ratio of 0.84 (Figure C13-5C). The LV function analysis using the appropriately filtered study generated images of superior quality, a larger LV chamber with an ESV of 10ml, and an LVEF of 85%.

Discussion

This study illustrates two important technical points that can affect the overall interpretation of the study. The first deals with the importance of using standard acquisition, reconstruction, and processing protocols to obtain images in which the tracer distribution in the myocardium of normal patients follows the normal pattern expected by the interpreter and the normal database found in quantitative analysis programs. These protocols are well documented in society guidelines.[4,5] In this study the stress study was filtered with an incorrect filter that over-smoothed the images, resulting in a thicker myocardial wall with a concomitant smaller LV chamber. This overfiltering resulted in an inaccurate TID ratio of 0.66, a reduced ESV of 4 ml, and an exaggerated LVEF of 90%.

The second technical point to be noted is the effect of small ESV on generating an inaccurately increased LVEF. Due to limited spatial resolution and photon scatter it has been observed that for ventricles with an ESV smaller than 20 ml (more common in women), the LV chamber appears smaller than it should be. The EDV is affected to a lesser extent since EDV is always larger than ESV. Thus, a falsely reduced ESV always generates an LVEF that is spuriously high. The magnitude of the artifactual increase is a function of the small size of the ventricle, i.e., the smaller the LV, the larger the LVEF. In the corrected study (Figures C13-5C and C13-5D), the LV chamber is larger and much better resolved, resulting in an ESV of 10 ml and an LVEF of 85%. Even in the corrected study, the LVEF is artificially increased due to an ESV of less than 20 ml. In these cases LVEF should be reported as normal (or greater than 60%) rather than the incorrectly determined value.

Interpretation

1. Incorrect filtering and small LV giving artifactually low ESV and high LVEF.
2. Normal myocardial perfusion and function.

Case 13.6

History

A 78-year-old woman with a 1-month history of intermittent chest pain was referred for MPI for risk stratification before surgery for repair of thoracic and abdominal aortic aneurysms. The thoracic aneurysm was approximated at 7 cm in diameter and contained a mural thrombus. The abdominal aortic aneurysm measured approximately 8 cm and extended down to the aortic bifurcation. Her cardiac risk factors included hypertension and tobacco use. A resting ^{201}Tl/adenosine stress ^{99m}Tc-MIBI gated SPECT study was performed.

Figure C13-6A shows the display of oblique slices and planar projections. From top to bottom, this display shows the short axis at stress and rest, the vertical long axis at stress and rest, and the horizontal long axis at stress and rest. The planar images in the lower right panel are stress and rest RAO projections.

Figure C13-6B shows the functional analysis display of the post-stress gated study with ^{99m}Tc-MIBI. Specifically, the LV volume-time curve, LV function parameters, and a thickening polar map are shown in the top row. The middle row shows vertical, horizontal, and multiple short axes at end-diastole (ED), which are repeated in the lower row, at end systole (ES).

Findings

These myocardial perfusion images showed homogeneous distribution of the myocardial perfusion tracers in the post-stress and in the corresponding rest study and were interpreted as normal (Figure C13-6A). The LVEF was 25% (Figure C13-6B). This LVEF was derived from an EDV of 42 ml and an ESV of 32 ml. The LV volume/time curves appeared to be normal

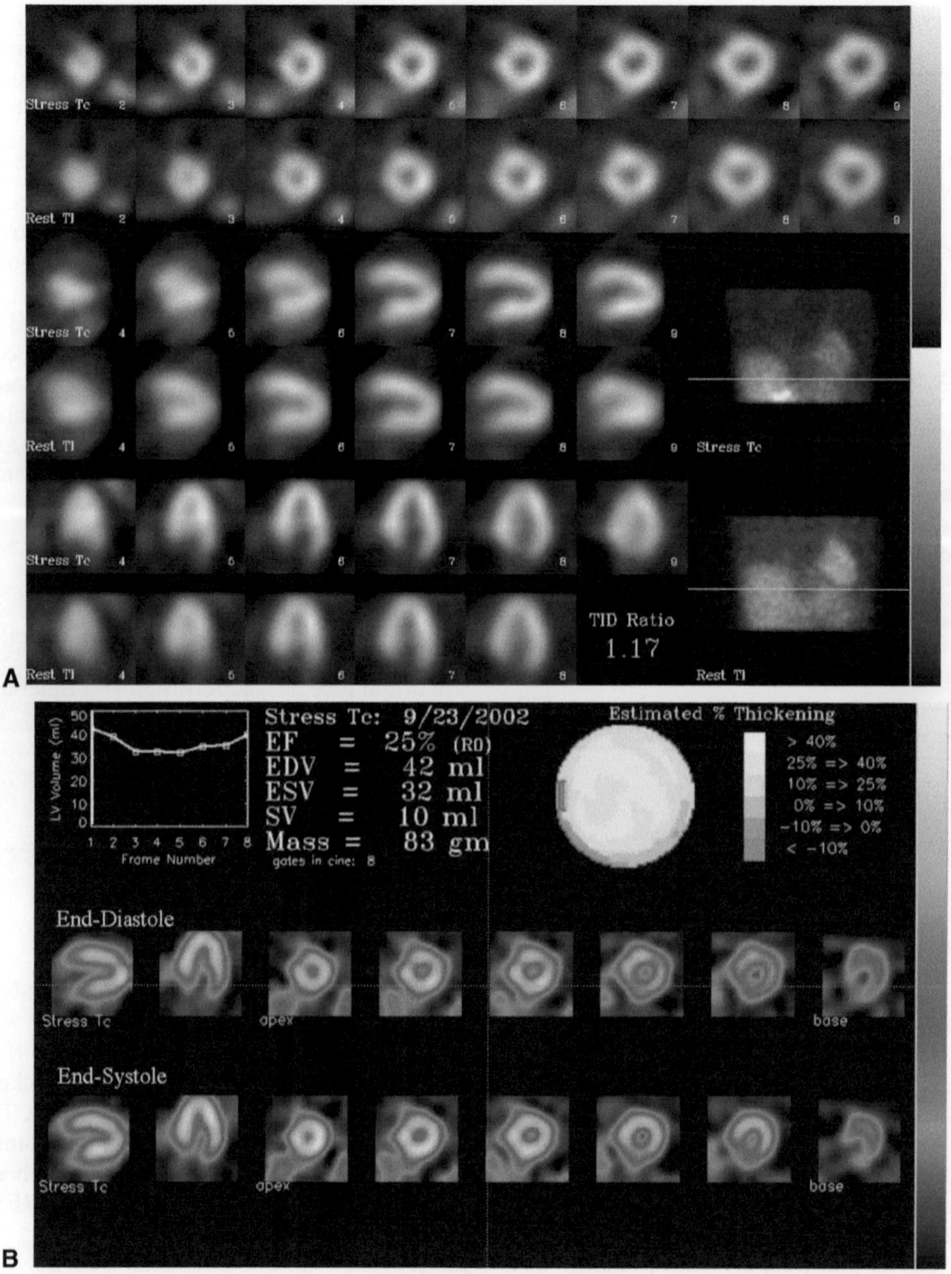

FIGURE C13-6. (A and B)

in shape, interpreted by some as an adequate ECG synchronization. The thickening polar map showed that the percentage of thickening falls below the lower limits for a female patient. It is noted that the end-diastolic slices were brighter than usual. The end-systolic slices were normal in count distribution and brighter than the end-diastolic slices. The wall motion images showed an abnormal contractility pattern with a loss in counts toward the later frames. The

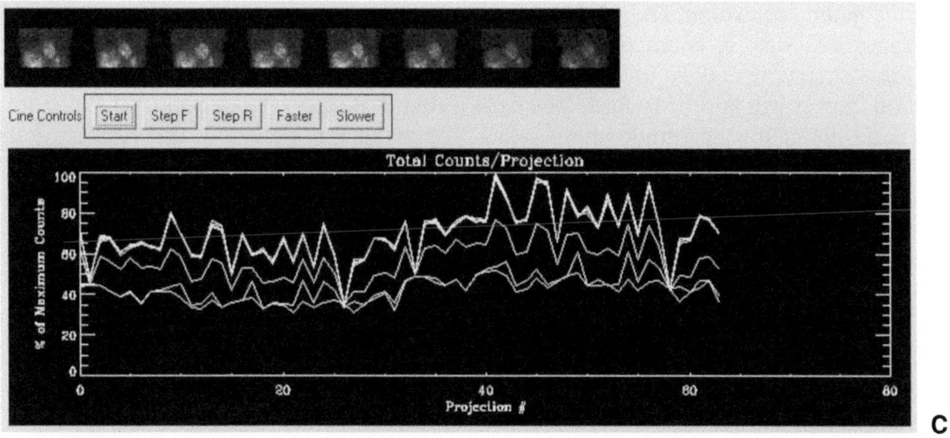

FIGURE C13-6. (C)

dynamic display of these wall motion images resulted in a flash of background intensity, on visual inspection, between the display of the last and the first frame.

Automatic detection of ECG-gating artifact was flagged by the computer algorithm (not shown) and confirmed on display of the ECG-gating quality control results (Figure C13-6C). Figure C13-6C shows the display of quality control of ECG-gated SPECT information. The first set of images corresponds to the raw eight frame gated. Currently, the ECTb program displays the eight-gated projection frames rotating and with the option to stop the rotation for the readers convenience. The graph shows the total counts/projection curves for each of the gated frames. The graph is plotted as the percentage of the maximum counts versus all of the 64 raw projections. A correct graph shows the count curves corresponding to each gated framed having the same number of counts. Curves that deviate from the others are automatically flagged and the interpreter informed.

This study was interpreted as a normal myocardial perfusion scan with inconclusive LV function related to the gating acquisition artifact. The patient was referred for an echocardiogram, which subsequently demonstrated normal LV function.

Discussion

This patient was referred for risk stratification before high-risk surgery. In our day-to-day practice, clinicians frequently refer patients with advanced cardiac or noncardiac disease for an MPI study to decide if a major operative procedure should be performed. This patient had a normal myocardial perfusion scan, but the assessment of the LV function was inaccurate because of a gating artifact. If the low LVEF had been reported, this patient would possibly have been excluded from the operative aneurysm repair because of the high surgical risk of patients with very low LVEF. Fortunately, further evaluation of this patient with two-dimensional echocardiography confirmed that the LV function was normal.

ECG-gated myocardial perfusion SPECT is now routinely used to assess global and regional LV function in addition to myocardial perfusion. This technical development has accelerated the use of MPI for the diagnosis and prognosis of CAD. Gating errors have been reported in as many as 30% of patients in some publications, but only a few of these patients have image artifacts large enough to significantly affect the clinical value of the reported LV function.

Artifacts in ECG gating can be related to the placement of the ECG leads, the stability of the patient's HR, and the adequacy of quantification of the LV function. Most commonly, artifacts are related to the patients' cardiac rhythm. If arrhythmias are present, or if the HR changes during the SPECT acquisition, inordinately short or long cardiac cycles will be rejected during the gated acquisition. Therefore, projection images will vary in count density. When viewed in a cinematic endless loop format, the projection images will appear to flash. The best way of determining the magnitude of the gating problem is using a quality control gating acquisition algorithm (Figure C13-6C). Deciding whether these flashes constitute serious errors can be determined by the quality control curves. If there are no gating errors, all eight projection curves should superimpose nearly perfectly. In this patient at least four separate gated curves are detected. The numbers of total counts are changing in the 64 projections. These images proved that in this particular patient a gated acquisition problem related to the variable R-R interval had occurred. When this type of artifact is detected, the results of the LV function cannot be reported.

Interpretation

1. ECG gating problems.
2. Normal myocardial perfusion but inconclusive LV function due to arrhythmia requiring referral for echocardiography.

Case 13.7

History

A 73-year-old man with a history of lung cancer and right upper lobectomy was evaluated for recurrent atrial fibrillation (AF), refractory to treatment. After his surgery in April 2000, he had AF that resolved after 4 weeks. In July 2002 he presented with shortness of breath and ankle swelling and was diagnosed with recurrent AF. At that time an echocardiogram revealed an LVEF of 50%, mild mitral annular calcification, and moderate to severe mitral regurgitation. He failed medical therapy with antiarrhythmic drugs and cardioversion. The symptoms of congestion improved with furosemide and digoxin. The patient was referred for MPI to evaluate CAD as a cause of refractory AF. Physical examination revealed a patient measuring 73 inches and weighing 190 pounds. The HR was irregular, averaging 73 bpm. A resting low-dose/adenosine stress high-dose ^{99m}Tc-MIBI gated SPECT study was performed. The BP dropped from 148/80 to 132/70 mm Hg. The patient experienced no symptoms, and there were no ECG changes. Attenuation correction (AC) software was applied to both rest and pharmacologic stress studies, using an external source of Americium to acquire transmission data simultaneous to acquisition of the emission data.

Figure C13-7A displays the SPECT images without AC, Figure C13-7B the SPECT images with AC, and Figure C13-7C the functional analysis display.

Findings

The study was of excellent quality, showing a mildly dilated LV. SPECT images and polar map quantification demonstrated a fixed inferior wall perfusion defect on both stress and rest images (Figure C13-7A). These perfusion abnormalities disappeared with AC and therefore are characteristic of diaphragmatic attenuation (Figure C13-7B). The post-stress gated study demonstrated normal wall motion and thickening with an LVEF of 61% (Figure C13-7C). The transmission map demonstrated altered anatomy in the thorax due to previous right upper lobectomy (not shown).

Discussion

In Case 13.7, a gated SPECT myocardial perfusion study of a male patient showed moderately decreased counts in the inferior wall on both the rest and stress images. The functional analysis demonstrated normal global LVEF and normal inferior wall motion, suggestive of diaphragmatic attenuation. AC software was applied and the inferior wall count density normalized, confirming that the fixed defect in the inferior wall was related to diaphragmatic attenuation.

Soft tissue attenuation, Compton scatter, and depth-dependent reduction of spatial resolution degrade myocardial perfusion SPECT image quality, thereby decreasing the test accuracy for the detection of CAD. In addition, soft

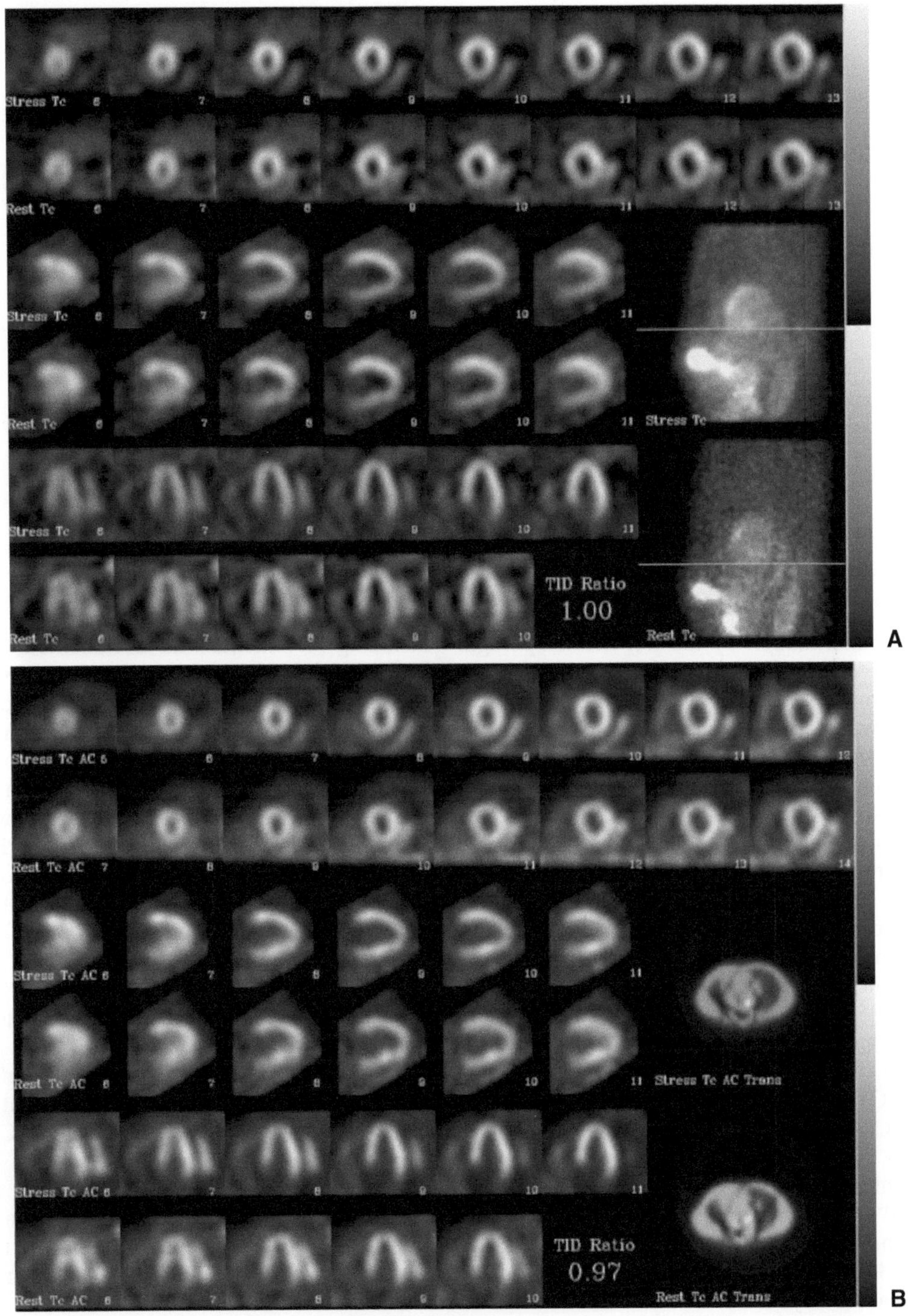

FIGURE C13-7. (A and B)

C
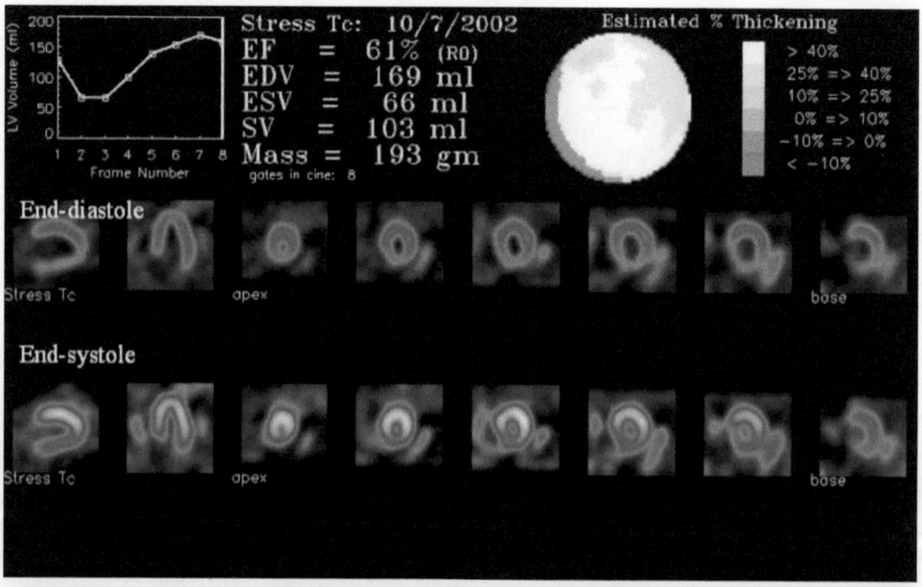

FIGURE C13-7. (C)

tissue attenuation by the left hemidiaphragm may create artifacts that mimic true perfusion abnormalities and decrease the test specificity.[6] One type of diaphragmatic attenuation artifact is *upward creep* of the diaphragm when images are acquired immediately post-exercise for a ^{201}Tl stress study. At the beginning of the acquisition, the patient may still be breathing heavily and the diaphragm lying relatively low due to deep inspiration. Over time, the patient progressively breathes normally and the diaphragm and heart creep upward.

Functional analysis of the LV using ECG-gated SPECT[19] and AC[10] are the most important techniques to differentiate true defects from artifacts, increasing the accuracy of SPECT MPI.

ECG-gated SPECT MPI with ^{99m}Tc-MIBI help in the differentiation of diaphragmatic attenuation artifacts from MI. When an inferior fixed defect is caused by diaphragmatic attenuation, wall motion and thickening of the inferior wall is normal, whereas when the defect is caused by an MI, the inferior wall is hypokinetic or akinetic, with decreased wall thickening.[19,20]

The advantages and limitations of AC for cardiac SPECT imaging have been debated in the literature. A prospective multicenter trial including 96 patients with documented CAD and 88 patients with a low likelihood of disease concluded that AC significantly improved the normalcy rate without a decline in sensitivity but with a reduction in the detection of extensive CAD.[21] Another study concluded there was no difference in interpretation between gated SPECT images and ungated SPECT images corrected for AC.[22] A relatively recent study of 83 patients concluded that AC generates overcorrection for the inferior wall, leading to a lower sensitivity and to false evaluation of myocardial viability in 73% of patients with inferior wall infarctions. In addition, it sometimes generates anteroapical artifacts despite scatter correction.[14,23] Therefore, when AC is applied, it is important to review both images with and without AC for interpretation.

Alternatively, images can be acquired with the patient in the prone position. Prone imaging can be used to try to separate the heart from the diaphragm and reduce diaphragmatic attenuation.

In summary, when MPI demonstrates a fixed defect in the inferior wall, especially in male and obese patients, global and regional wall motion of the myocardium should be evaluated. If the inferior wall motion is normal, the fixed defect is probably due to diaphragmatic attenuation. Prone imaging is helpful by separating the heart from the diaphragm. AC, when available, may increase confidence to report the case as a normal perfusion study, but both images with and without AC need to be reviewed for interpretation.

Interpretation

1. Inferior wall attenuation resolved by ECG-gated SPECT and attenuation correction.
2. Normal myocardial perfusion with diaphragmatic attenuation.

Case 13.8

History

A 63-year-old woman with dyslipidemia, hypertension, and a family history of CAD presented with atypical chest pain related to exercise. She denied shortness of breath, palpitations, or syncope. She was referred for MPI. Physical examination revealed a patient measuring 66 inches and weighing 200 pounds. The HR was 60 bpm and regular and the BP 160/88 mm Hg. A resting low-dose/exercise high-dose ^{99m}Tc-MIBI gated SPECT study was performed. The patient exercised for 4 minutes on a standard Bruce protocol and reached an HR of 143 bpm exceeding 85% of the predicted maximal HR. The patient experienced no symptoms, and there were no ECG changes. Figure C13-8A displays the SPECT images without AC, Figure C13-8B the SPECT images with AC, and Figure C13-8C the functional analysis display.

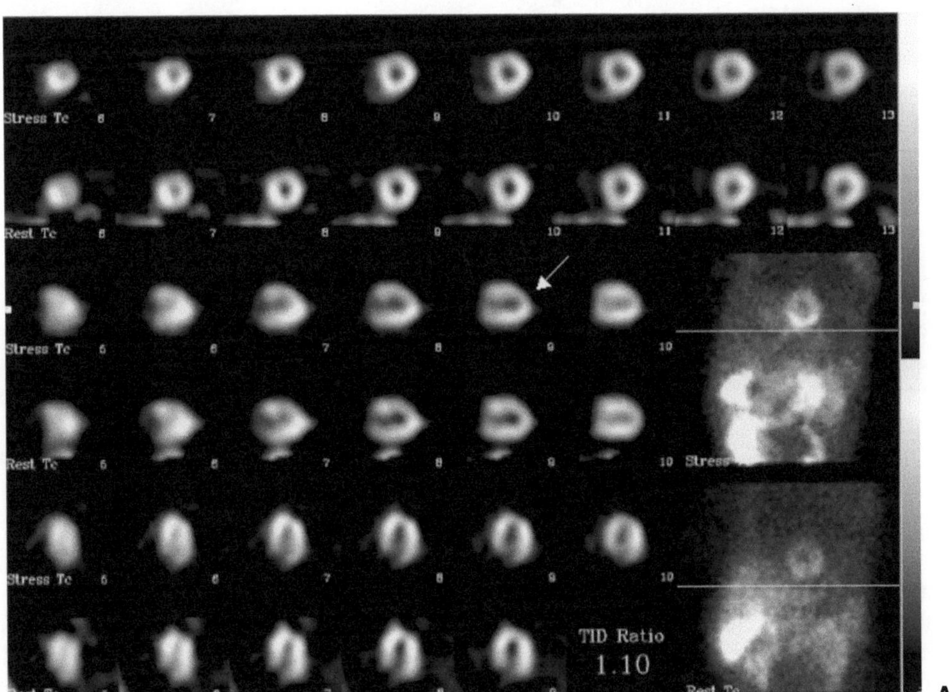

FIGURE C13-8. (A)

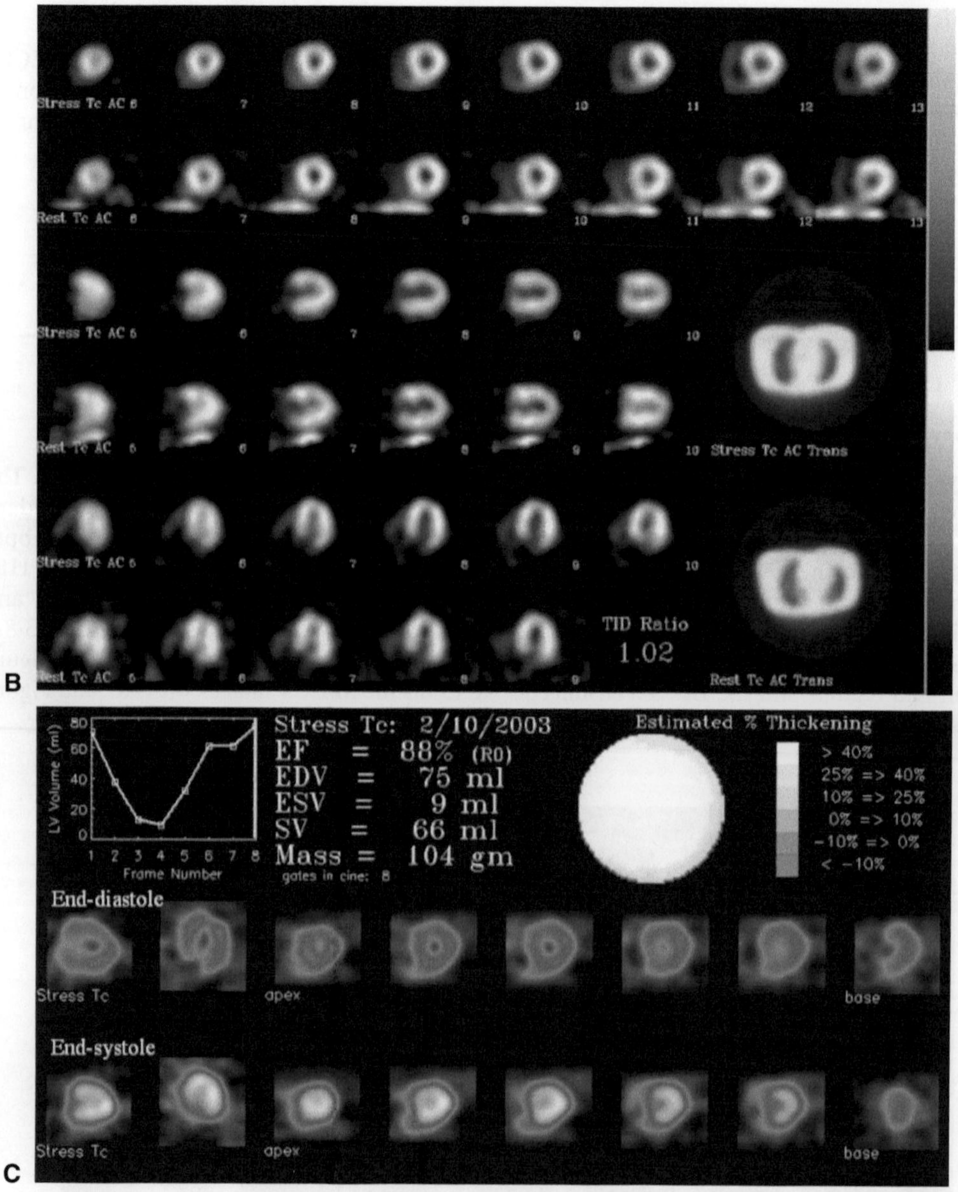

FIGURE C13-8. (B and C)

Findings

The study was of adequate quality and the LV was normal in size. SPECT images demonstrated a mildly reversible defect in the anteroapical segment (Figure C13-8A). After applying AC software, the oblique slices showed normal perfusion (Figure C13-8B). The gated study demonstrated an LVEF of 88% and normal wall motion (Figure C13-8C). The LVEF was artifactually elevated due to the small size of this woman's heart (see Case 13.5). These findings are consistent with breast attenuation artifact.

Discussion

In this case, decreased counts in the anteroapical wall more pronounced at stress could lead the physician to interpret this study as positive for myocardial ischemia. It is important to observe that in the rotating planar images the position of the breast is different during acquisition of the stress and the rest images. After applying AC, this artifact disappears, and the final interpretation is that the perfusion is normal.

Breast attenuation can mimic true perfusion defects, decreasing the specificity of SPECT MPI.[6] When this artifact is more pronounced at stress than at rest, it can lead the to an erroneous interpretation of ischemia. In this situation, functional analysis of the LV using ECG-gated SPECT[19] is not helpful, because even after stress-induced ischemia the global and regional function are often normal. This happens because the ECG-gated images are acquired post-stress (after 30 minutes, or more) and this time interval can be enough for normalization of the LV function. Prolonged myocardial stunning after stress is more common when ischemia is severe and involves a large portion of the myocardium.[24] Therefore, in clinical situations similar to this case, AC is the method of choice to differentiate true defects from artifacts.

AC leads to a more uniform distribution of the radiotracer and decreases the influence of anatomic artifacts (breast and diaphragmatic attenuation). Several publications have demonstrated an increase in specificity and normalcy rate of MPI with AC as compared to without AC, with no significant loss of sensitivity. Because of this strong clinical validation, the position statement of the ASNC and SNM suggests the incorporation of AC in the routine use of nuclear cardiology.[10]

In this case, the quality of the transmission map and the attenuation-corrected study is excellent, and after the correction the myocardial perfusion study became normal.

If AC is not available, keeping the breasts in a similar position for rest and stress studies is critical. Most centers image female patients without bra for both imaging sessions. The breast can also be consistently shifted upward and fixed with tape, for example. Prone imaging is another alternative; the breasts usually lie in a different position in prone and supine position and the defect due to attenuation will either disappear or move in a different location.

Interpretation

1. Breast attenuation artifact resolved after AC using transmission imaging.
2. Normal myocardial perfusion.

Case 13.9

History

A 63-year-old man with hypercholesterolemia and without other cardiac risk factors was diagnosed with left bundle branch block (LBBB) on a routine ECG in August 2001. At that time he was referred for stress echocardiography that revealed a resting LVEF in the 45% range, increasing systolic function during exercise, and no evidence of myocardial ischemia. He was referred for a resting ^{201}Tl/exercise stress ^{99m}Tc-MIBI gated SPECT study to evaluate ischemia. The patient exercised for 7 minutes and 30 seconds on a standard Bruce protocol reaching an HR of 140 bpm exceeding 85% of the predicted maximal HR. The patient experienced no symptoms and the ECG was nondiagnostic due to the LBBB.

Figure C13-9A displays the dual-isotope myocardial SPECT images, Figure C13-9B the polar map representation of stress and rest myocardial perfusion distributions, and Figure C13-9C the functional analysis display.

Findings

The study (Figure C13-9A) was of adequate quality without attenuation artifacts. The LV was normal in size. The oblique slices and the

A

B

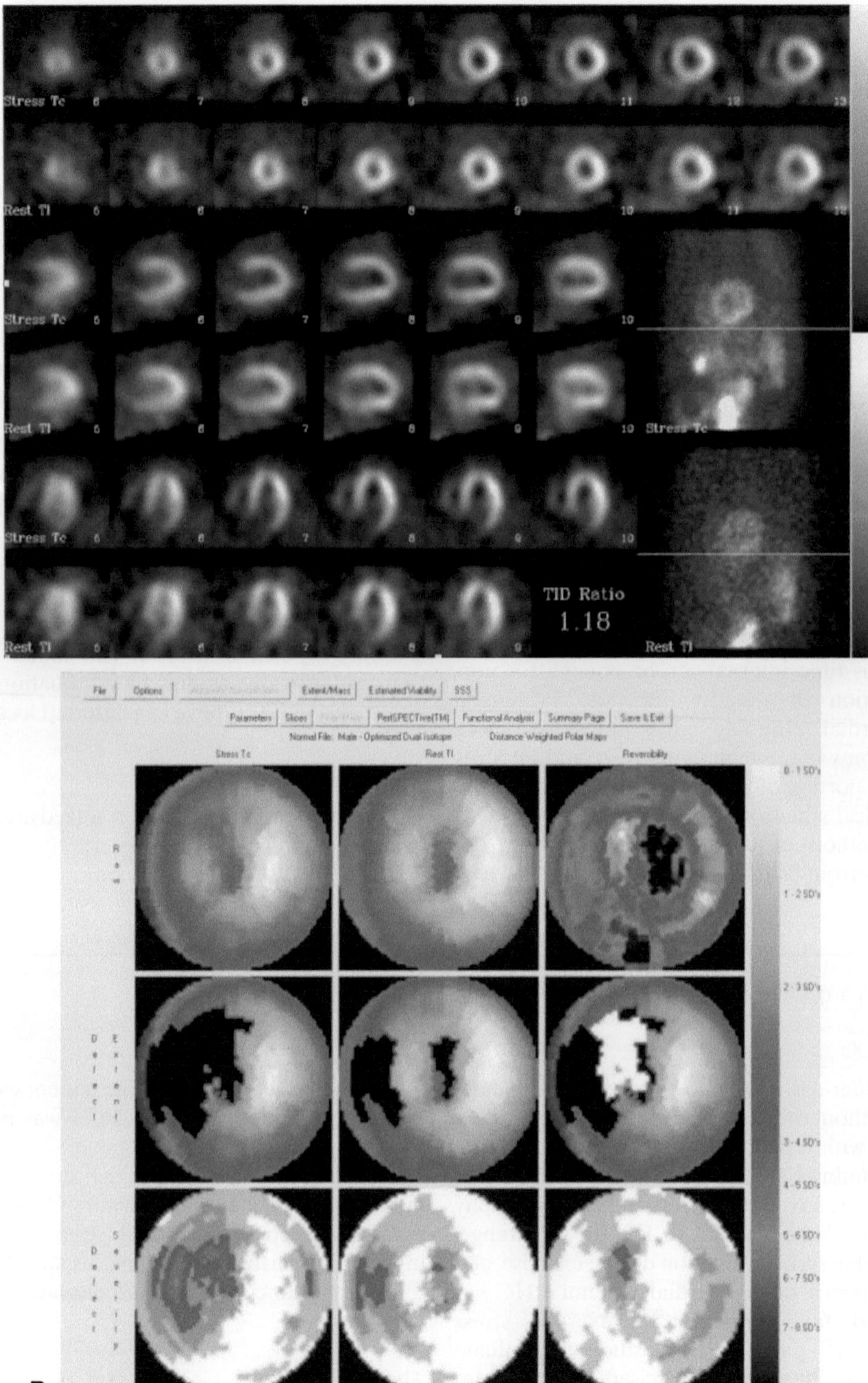

FIGURE C13-9. (A and B)

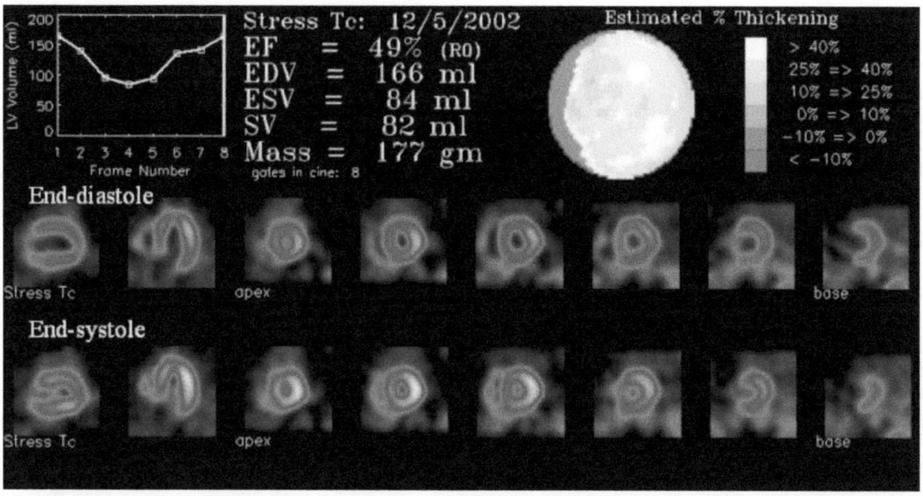

C

FIGURE C13-9. (C)

polar map quantification demonstrated a septal defect at stress with partial reversibility at rest (Figure C13-9B). The gated study revealed an LVEF of 49% and septal dyskinesis (Figure C13-9C).

The study was repeated with pharmacologic stress due to the fact that the perfusion abnormality could be associated with the LBBB. The patient was brought to the nuclear laboratory 24 hours after the exercise test and underwent pharmacologic stress with 50 mg of adenosine. At the beginning of the fourth minute, 22 mCi of ^{99m}Tc-MIBI was administered IV. The patient reported some chest tightness during the adenosine infusion. Myocardial perfusion tomographic images (Figure C13-9D) and the polar map quantification (Figure C13-9E) demonstrated only mild fixed hypoperfusion of the septum and no other abnormalities. The gated study revealed an LVEF of 62% (Figure C13-9F). The reversible perfusion defect within the septal wall that was seen on the first study with exercise represented a functional myocardial perfusion abnormality induced by exercise in a patient with LBBB.

Discussion

In this case, a reversible septal defect was detected on a gated SPECT myocardial perfusion study in a patient with LBBB who was stressed with exercise. When a vasodilator pharmacologic stress was performed in the same patient, this reversible septal defect disappeared and mild fixed reduced uptake of the radiotracer persisted in the septum. The LVEF increased from 49% to 62%.

Hirzel et al.[25] demonstrated reduced uptake of ^{201}Tl and blood flow in the septum of dogs during right ventricular pacing, a situation with conduction abnormalities similar to LBBB. During right atrial pacing, ^{201}Tl activity and blood flow were normal. The authors concluded that perfusion abnormalities in the septum of patients with LBBB may reflect functional ischemia due to asynchronous septal contraction.

Reversible septal perfusion defects can occur in 30% to 90% of patients with LBBB stressed with exercise, mimicking septal ischemia.[26,27] Usually, LBBB causes a defect that is restricted to the septum.[28] If the anterior wall and apex are involved, ischemia in the LAD territory should be suspected. The sensitivity to detect ischemia in territories supplied by the RCA and LCX coronary arteries is not affected by the presence of LBBB. Right bundle branch block and left anterior hemiblock do not cause perfusion artifacts.

Since the decrease in septal blood flow in LBBB seems to be dependent on HR, pharma-

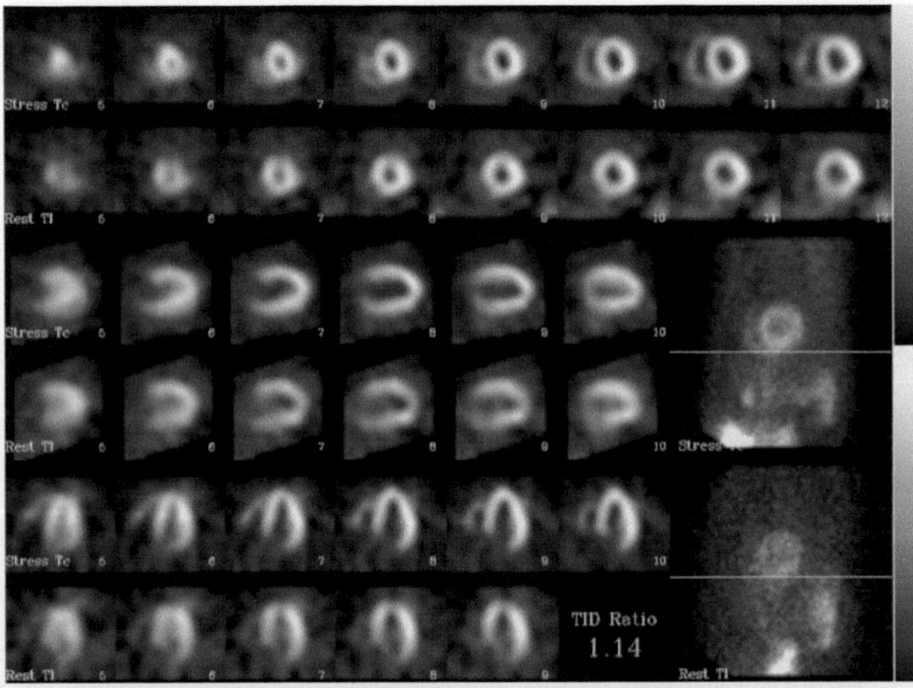

D

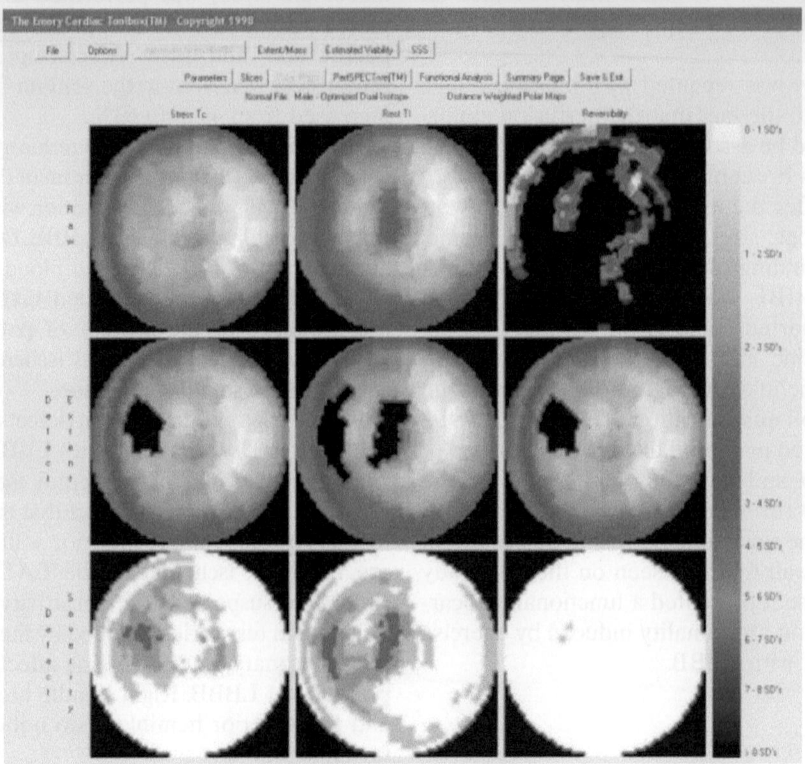

E

FIGURE C13-9. (D and E)

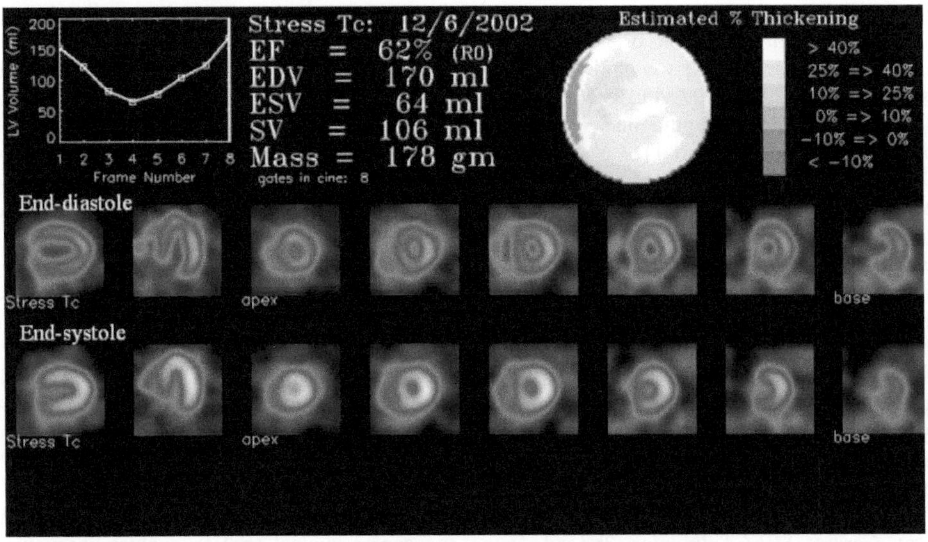

FIGURE C13-9. (F)

cologic stress with vasodilators reduces this physiologic artifact and is indicated in patients with LBBB who are referred for MPI.[29,30] Adenosine and dipyridamole have a mild chronotropic effect and do not provoke an intense septal asynchrony, minimizing the possibility of reversible perfusion septal defects. However, if the patient has a moderate to marked increase in HR after the infusion of the vasodilator, a reversible septal defect can occur. Because of the septal asynchrony, a fixed perfusion septal defect, even with pharmacologic stress, can be expected.

It is important that the interpreting physician be aware of the characteristics of the resting ECG and reports the presence of LBBB as a cause of possible artifact in isolated septal defects. There is also a characteristic contraction pattern on gated SPECT MPI in patients who underwent CABG. This pattern is characterized by septal hypokinesis with preservation of septal wall thickening, apparent increase in endocardial lateral wall motion, and anterior epicardial swing. This pattern of motion is different from that seen in normal patients and patients with previous anterior wall MI.[31] In patients with prior MI, there is decreased wall motion and decreased thickening of the myocardium involved. Because the wall motion analysis by gated SPECT in these patients underestimates septal motion and overestimates lateral wall motion, the wall thickening analysis is critical for interpretation of the images,[32] especially when evaluating improved wall motion after revascularization of ischemic or hibernating myocardium. This topic is also discussed in Cases 5.3 and 12.2.

Interpretation

1. Reversible septal perfusion defect in a patient with LBBB undergoing exercise.
2. Mild fixed hypoperfusion of the septum due to LBBB with vasodilator pharmacologic stress.

References

1. Faber TL, Cooke CD, Folks RD, et al. Left ventricular function and perfusion from gated SPECT perfusion images: an integrated method. *J Nucl Med.* 1999;40:650–659.
2. Germano G, Kiat H, Kavanagh PB, et al. Automatic quantification of ejection fraction from gated myocardial perfusion SPECT. *J Nucl Med.* 1995;36:2138–2147.

3. Ficaro EP, Kritzman JN, Corbett JR. Development and clinical validation of normal ^{99m}Tc sestamibi database: comparison of 3D-MSPECT to Cequal. *J Nucl Med.* 1999;40:125P.
4. Garcia EV (ed). Imaging guidelines for nuclear cardiology procedures (part 1). *J Nucl Cardiol.* 1996;3:G1–G46.
5. DePuey EG, Garcia EV (eds). Updated imaging guidelines for nuclear cardiology procedures (part 1). *J Nucl Cardiol.* 2001;8:G1–G58.
6. DePuey EG, Garcia EV. Optimal specificity of thallium-201 SPECT through recognition of imaging artifacts. *J Nucl Med.* 1989;30:441–449.
7. DePuey, EG. Artifacts in SPECT myocardial perfusion imaging. In DePuey EG, Berman DS, Garcia EV (eds). *Cardiac SPECT Imaging*, 2nd edition. New York: Raven Press; 2001:231–262.
8. Nichols KJ, Galt JR. Quality control in SPECT imaging. In DePuey EG, Berman DS, Garcia EV (eds). *Cardiac SPECT Imaging*, 2nd ed. New York: Lippincott Willians & Wilkins; 2001:17–40.
9. Garcia EV, Galt JR, Cullom SJ, Faber TL. *Principles of Myocardial Perfusion SPECT Imaging.* North Billerica, MA: Du Pont Pharma; 1994:30.
10. Hendel RC, Corbett JR, Cullom SJ, DePuey EG, Garcia EV, Bateman TM. The value and practice of attenuation correction for myocardial perfusion SPECT imaging. *J Nucl Med.* 2002;43: 273–280.
11. Germano G, Nichols KJ, Cullom SJ, Faber TL, Cooke CD. Gated perfusion SPECT: technical considerations. In DePuey EG, Berman DS, Garcia EV (eds). *Cardiac SPECT Imaging*, 2nd ed. New York: Lippincott Willians & Wilkins; 2001:103–116.
12. Nichols K, Dorbala S, DePuey EG, Mieres J, Malhotra S, Rozanski A. Influence of arrhythmias on gated SPECT myocardial perfusion and function quantification. *J Nucl Med.* 1999;40:924–934.
13. Nichols K, Santana CA, Folks R, et al. Comparison between ECTb and QGS for assessment of left ventricular function from gated myocardial perfusion SPECT. *J Nucl Cardiol.* 2002;9:285–293.
14. Weiss T, Berman D, Garcia E, Swan HJC, Waxman A, Maddahi J. Transient ischemic dilatation of the left ventricle on stress-redistribution thallium-201 scintigrams: a marker of severe and extensive coronary artery disease. *Circulation.* 1984;70-2:275.
15. Folks RD, Faber TL, Cooke CD, Krawczynska EG, Vansant JP, Garcia EV. Transient ischemic dilatation index determined automatically from dual isotope myocardial perfusion SPECT. *Clin Nucl Med.* 2001;26(1):86.
16. Transient ischemic dilatation validation. Emory Cardiac Toolbox manual. Syntermed; 2003. Available at www.syntermed.com/emory.htm.
17. Lee KJ, Barber DC. Use of forward projection to correct patient motion during SPECT imaging. *Phys Med Biol.* 1998;43:171–187.
18. Eisner RL. Sensitivity of SPECT thallium-201 myocardial perfusion imaging to patient motion. *J Nucl Med.* 1992;33:1571–1573.
19. DePuey EG, Rozanski A. Using gated technetium-99m-sestamibi SPECT to characterize fixed myocardial defects as infarct or artifact. *J Nucl Med.* 1995;36:952–955.
20. Smanio PE, Watson DD, Segalla DL, Smith WH, Beller GA. Value of gating of technetium-99m-sestamibi single-photon emission computed tomography imaging. *J Am Coll Cardiol.* 1997; 29:69–77.
21. Hendel RC, Berman DS, Cullom SJ, et al. Multicenter clinical trial to evaluate correction for photon attenuation and scatter in SPECT myocardial perfusion imaging. *Circulation.* 1999; 99:2742–2749.
22. Lee DS, So Y, Cheon GJ, et al. Limited incremental diagnostic values of attenuation-noncorrected gating and ungated attenuation correction to rest/stress myocardial perfusion SPECT in patients with an intermediate likelihood of coronary artery disease. *J Nucl Med.* 2000;41:852–859.
23. Harel F, Genin R, Daou D, et al. Clinical impact of combination of scatter, attenuation correction and depth dependent resolution recovery for 201-thallium studies. *J Nucl Med.* 2001;42:4P.
24. Johnson LL, Verdesca SA, Aude WY, et al. Postischemic stunning can affect left ventricular ejection fraction and regional wall motion on post-stress gated sestamibi tomograms. *J Am Coll Cardiol.* 1997;30:1641–1648.
25. Hirzel HO, Senn M, Nuesch K, et al. Thallium-201 scintigraphy in complete left bundle branch block. *Am J Cardiol.* 1984;53:764–769.
26. DePuey EG, Krawczynska EG, Robbins WL. Thallium-201 SPECT in coronary artery disease patients with left bundle branch block. *J Nucl Med.* 1988;29:1479–1485.
27. Burns RJ, Galligan L, Wright LM, Lawand S, Burke RJ, Gladstone PJ. Improved specificity of myocardial Thallium-201 single-photon emission computed tomography in patients with left bundle branch block by dipyridamole. *Am J Cardiol.* 1991;68:504–508.
28. Matzer LA, Kiat H, Friedman JD, Van Train K, Maddahi J, Berman DS. A new approach to the

assessment of tomographic thallium-201 scintigraphy in patients with left bundle branch block. *J Am Coll Cardiol.* 1991;17:1309–1317.
29. Rockett JF, Chadwick W, Moinuddin M, Loveless V, Parrish B. Intravenous dipyridamol thallium-201 SPECT imaging in patients with left bundle branch block. *Clin Nucl Med.* 1990; 6:401–407.
30. Larcos G, Brown ML, Gibbons RJ. Role of dipyridamole thallium-201 imaging in left bundle branch block. *Am J Cardiol.* 1991;68:1097–1098.
31. Yun JH, Block M, Botvinick EH. Unique contraction pattern in patients after coronary bypass graft surgery by gated SPECT myocardial perfusion imaging. *Clin Nucl Med.* 2003;28:18–24.
32. Taki J, Higushi T, Nakajima K, et al. Electrocardiographic gated ^{99m}Tc-MIBI SPECT for functional assessment of patients after coronary artery bypass surgery: comparison of wall thickening and wall motion analysis. *J Nucl Med.* 2002;43:589–595.

14 Correlation of Nuclear Imaging with Cardiac MRI

José Claudio Meneghetti and Carlos Eduardo Rochitte

Magnetic resonance imaging (MRI) is a technique widely applied in musculoskeletal and neurological evaluation. In the past decade there has been increasing interest in applying MRI to also evaluate the heart. Some of the possible applications of cardiac MRI, which are further discussed in this chapter, include evaluation of myocardial infarction, LV function, viability, and ischemia. The MRI techniques for the evaluation of myocardial viability (myocardial delayed enhancement, MDE) and myocardial ischemia (myocardial first-pass perfusion during vasodilator infusion) are described briefly in the following section. The radiopharmaceuticals used for myocardial perfusion imaging (MPI) and gated single photon emission tomography (SPECT) technique and protocols, discussed in the following cases, have already been presented in detail in Chapters 2 and 3.

MRI for the Evaluation of Myocardial Infarction and LV Function

Myocardial viability, perfusion, and contractility undergo dynamic and dramatic changes after acute myocardial infarction (MI). The pathophysiological changes in the myocardium during the first 6 months after acute MI are complex and have not been studied with imaging modalities as extensively as chronic MIs. Moreover, this post MI period (LV remodeling phase) has crucial effects on the clinical course in terms of cardiovascular events and survival. Particularly, direct image comparisons of nuclear imaging and magnetic resonance imaging (MRI) are not commonly available. Myocardial delayed enhancement (MDE) uses a gradient-echo inversion-recovery prepared sequence to image the myocardium 10 to 20 minutes after intravenous (IV) administration of gadolinium (Gd). Further refinements of the original concept described by Lima et al.[1] allow visualization of infarcted tissue with exquisite definition of the edges and excellent correlation with pathology.[2–8] The Gd MDE MRI technique allows detection of small subendocardial infarcts, missed otherwise,[9,10] has excellent agreement with positron emission tomography (PET) for detection of myocardial viability,[11] and compares favorably with SPECT scintigraphy for determination of infarct size.[12]

Basically, this technique takes advantage of the kinetic differences of the Gd-based contrast agents between normal myocardium and myocardial necrosis or fibrosis. Gd-based contrast agents distribute in the extracellular space and does not cross the cellular membrane of normal myocytes. In addition, the extracellular space (vascular and interstitial space) of the myocardium is small (10% to 20% of the total myocardial volume) compared with its intracellular space (80% to 90% of the myocardium total volume). Therefore, the volume of distribution of Gd is small in the normal myocardium, resulting in a rapid wash-in and wash-out. In acute MI, the cellular membrane of the myocytes ruptures and the previously small extracellular space becomes 100% of volume of distribution for Gd. The wash-in and wash-out kinetics of Gd in MI differ significantly from that of normal myocardium. The wash-in is slower to a variable degree, depending on the amount of microvascular obstruction (no-reflow phenomenon) within the infarcted region.[13–15] More importantly, the wash-out is dramatically reduced and allows for a striking difference of Gd concentration between normal and infarcted myocardium at 10 to 20 minutes after IV administration.[1,4]

MRI for the Evaluation of Myocardial Viability

MRI provides the combined information of tissue characterization (Gd MDE) and LV function (cine MRI images at rest and/or during pharmacological induced stress), allowing differentiation of viable myocardium with normal or abnormal (stunned or hibernated myocardium) function and irreversibly damaged or nonviable myocardium.[16,17] As described previously, MDE MRI can delineate well areas of infarcted tissue; however, to determine the amount of viable ischemic tissue at risk, a different MRI technique needs to be used as described in the following section. Certainly the presence and amount of viable tissue has a major impact on a patient's management, helping the physician decide whether to treat clinically or with revascularization.

MRI for the Evaluation of Myocardial Ischemia

During the equilibrium phase in the extracellular space, there is no relationship between the distribution of Gd and perfusion of the myocardium. Therefore, evaluation of myocardial perfusion with Gd requires imaging of the first-pass extraction (less than 20 seconds) and fast imaging techniques with the best temporal and spatial resolution possible.[18] Myocardial first-pass perfusion MRI is a fast MRI technique that acquires one complete image set in approximately 100 to 150ms. Usually, a hybrid gradient-echo and echo-planar imaging technique is used. This very fast acquisition, covering the entire LV with 4 to 8 short-axis slices, in one or two heartbeats, is repeated over time and during IV administration of Gd-based contrast. This provides visualization of the arrival of Gd in the heart chambers and in the myocardium and gives information about myocardial perfusion. There is a progressive and homogenous increase of signal from subepicardium to subendocardium during the first pass of Gd throughout the normal myocardium. In ischemic myocardium, there is a relatively lower Gd concentration compared with normal myocardium. This phenomenon is seen in the first-pass perfusion images as a perfusion defect. The application of this technique at rest and during stress with dipyridamole or adenosine has been reported in pilot studies to detect myocardial ischemia in a similar fashion to radionuclide perfusion imaging.[19–21] One of the main obstacles for a wider use of MR perfusion has been the lack of large clinical outcome data based on standardized protocols and analysis. In addition, despite the wealth of strictly investigational MR perfusion data worldwide,[22] at the time of this writing neither the current contrast agents nor MR perfusion sequences have clinical approval from the Food and Drug Administration (FDA) in the United States. Larger clinical trials will be required to obtain FDA approval and would be a prerequisite for a wider use of this technique in clinical practice.

Case Presentations

The 6 clinical cases presented in this chapter include side-by-side comparison of nuclear imaging and MRIs in the early and late period after MI. Five cases address evaluation with imaging in the acute setting of MI, 4 of them with 6 months' image follow-up with both MRI and nuclear imaging. MIs of different sizes are presented with clinical implications related to variable contractility. The case discussions address early findings on imaging studies that could predict the long-term LV remodeling and function. One of the case presentations addresses evaluation of myocardial ischemia with both nuclear imaging and MRI.

Case 14.1

History

A 58-year-old man with hypertension, hyperlipidemia, and a family history of CAD presented to the emergency department (ED) at 12 hours from the onset of intense chest pain, extending to left arm and associated with nausea, cold sweat, and leading to syncope. His ECG showed ST-segment elevation in the precordial leads (V1 to V6) and the peak CK-MB was elevated more than 40-fold above the upper normal limit. He was transferred to a tertiary hospital with heart failure NYHA class II. His symptoms improved with medical therapy. Coronary angiography demonstrated mid-left anterior descending coronary artery (LAD) occlusion without collateral circulation to anterior wall. An echocardiogram revealed a large LV thrombus and compromised function with an LV ejection fraction (LVEF) of 32% but no LV dilation. A dipyridamole stress/reinjection ^{201}Tl gated SPECT study and rest cardiac MRI were performed 9 to 10 days later to evaluate the extent of infarction and the volume of remaining viable myocardium (Figure C14-1).

Findings

The stress ^{201}Tl SPECT myocardial perfusion images showed absence of perfusion in the apex, apical anterior and apical inferior segments with moderately decreased perfusion in the septal region. The reinjection images remained unchanged, suggesting no regional

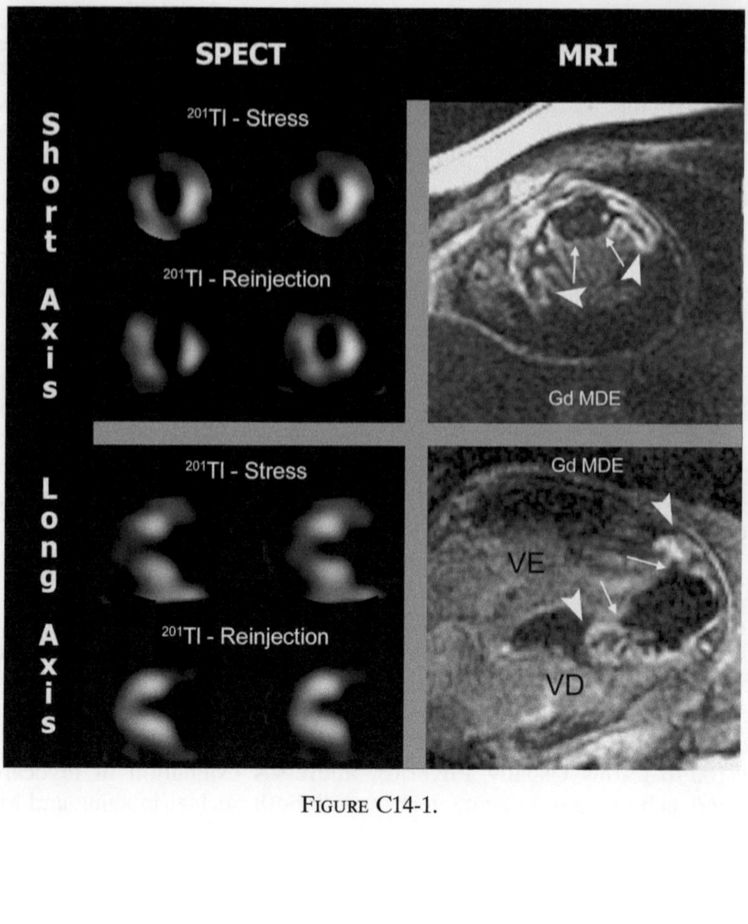

FIGURE C14-1.

myocardial viability. The gated images revealed dyskinesis of the apex and the LVEF, end-diastolic volume (EDV), and end-systolic volume (ESV) were 25%, 123 ml and 93 ml, respectively.

Resting cardiac MRI with Gd MDE showed transmural myocardial hyperenhancement (Figure C14-1, between arrowheads) in the apex, distal inferior, distal anterior, and septal LV segments, and nontransmural enhancement in the mid-inferior segment. A large LV thrombus is seen on both views contiguous to the distal anterior and distal septal segments (between arrows), and filling most of the apical portion of LV cavity. There is also a focal region with hypoenhancement within the infarct compatible microvascular obstruction, also known as *no-reflow phenomenon*. The cine MR images (not shown) demonstrated apical dyskinesia characterizing an LV aneurysm. Despite the large anterior MI and LV aneurysm, the remaining walls had increased contractility on the cine MRIs, mainly in the basal segments, resulting in a relatively preserved global LV function with LVEF of 50%.

He was discharged asymptomatic on appropriate medical management. One month after the acute MI, the patient presented with a recurrent episode of chest pain followed by irreversible cardiac arrest. Rupture of the anterior wall of the LV was demonstrated at autopsy.

Discussion

On the SPECT images, the LV apex is not visualized and the reinjection images showed no signs of myocardial viability. The nonperfused distal walls of the myocardium lead to LV remodeling, causing an increase in the normal angulation of the preserved basal walls. This can also precipitate cardiac heart failure.[23–26] The MRI was able to demonstrate an anterior MI (high signal myocardium between arrowheads) and associated large LV thrombus, as seen on the short- and long axis images acquired using the Gd MDE technique.

Although both gated SPECT and cine MRI demonstrated an apical aneurysm, there was a discrepancy in the estimate of the LVEF: 50% by MRI and 25% by scintigraphy. On gated SPECT, an LVEF less than 45% with and ESV higher than 70 ml is highly predictive of increased mortality.[27] The apparent discrepancy between MRI and gated SPECT is due to the presence of large LV thrombus filling almost the entire LV apical portion. The LV thrombus was included in the region of interest (ROI) surrounding the LV cavity to measure the LVEF by gated SPECT, whereas it was excluded from the LV cavity ROI on the MRIs. When the thrombus was included in the LV cavity ROI on MRI, the LVEF fell to 33%. The presence of microvascular obstruction could be seen in close relationship with the LV thrombus and has been described to be associated with worse prognosis and worse LV remodeling.[28–31]

The combined information of both imaging modalities demonstrating distal anterior wall thinning associated with a large thrombus suggest the possibility of underlying LV wall rupture. These findings on imaging studies have a major clinical impact and should lead to evaluation of potential rupture of the LV wall and consideration of surgical repair of the LV aneurysm.

Interpretations

1. Large anterior MI due to LAD occlusion with absent viability demonstrated both by stress/rest ^{201}Tl and MDE MRI.
2. Large LV thrombus detected by MRI, and issue to be considered while drawing the ROIs to calculate LVEF calculations using this technique.
3. Medical therapy and LV rupture and death 1 month after MI.

Case 14.2

History

A 57-year-old man with hypertension and tobacco use presented to the ED with chest pain. The ECG was indicative of an anterior MI and the serum CK-MB levels increased to eightfold above upper normal limit. Coronary angiography demonstrated occlusion of proximal LAD and moderate stenosis of the distal right coronary artery (RCA). There was grade II collateral circulation from marginal branches of the left circumflex coronary artery (LCX) to the LAD and a suggestion of an apical thrombus on LV ventriculography. The patient was not revascularized and was discharged without symptoms of heart failure on medical therapy with aspirin, angiotensin converting enzyme (ACE) inhibitor, and beta-blocker, remaining stable for the next 6 months after MI. He underwent resting cardiac MRI with Gd MDE and dipyridamole stress/reinjection ^{201}Tl gated SPECT during admission for the acute episode and 6 months later. The images obtained during admission are displayed in Figures C14-2A and C14-2B.

Findings

The stress ^{201}Tl SPECT images showed decreased uptake in mid- and apical anterior walls, mostly fixed, with only subtle improvement on reinjection images indicating little viable myocardium at risk. The post-stress gated images revealed an LVEF of 27% that increased to 41% at 6 months follow-up. This interesting finding may represent a component

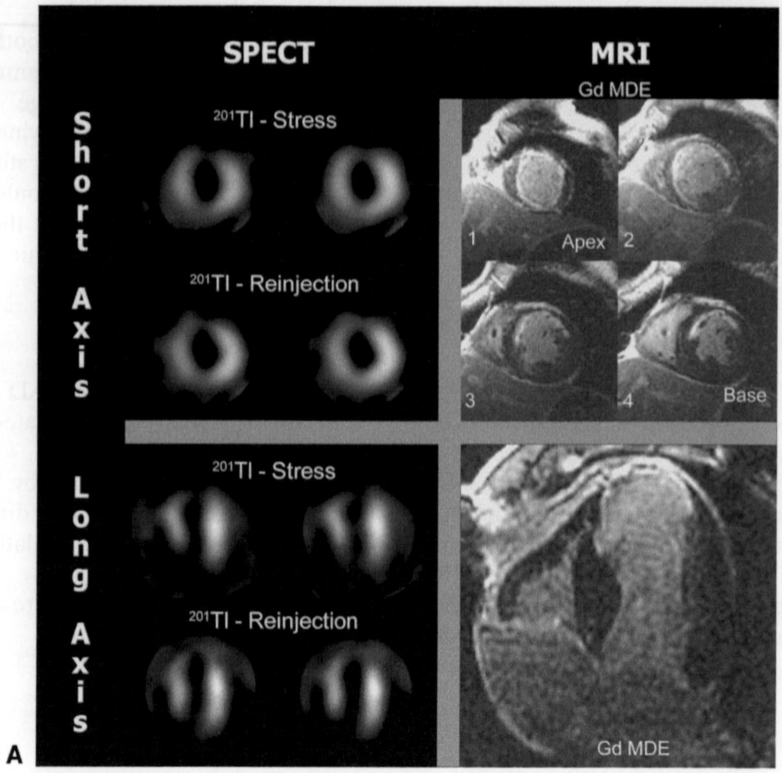

FIGURE C14-2. (A)

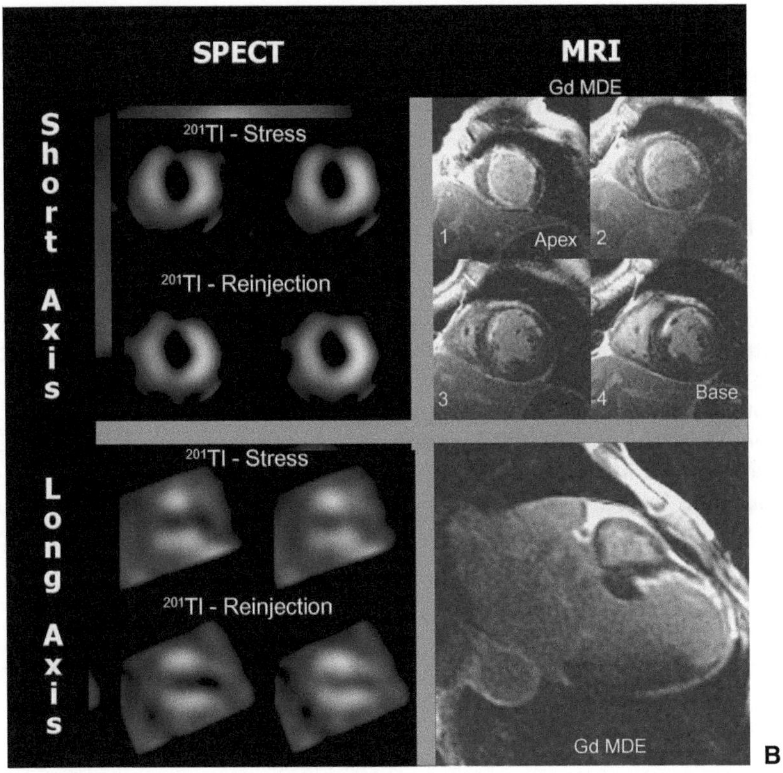

FIGURE C14-2. (B)

of myocardial stunning following the acute event, partially recovering on medical therapy alone. Resting cardiac MRI with Gd MDE immediately after MI and at 6 months follow-up showed a moderate sized anterior MI (infarct size = 15% of LV mass). Although this MI is almost transmural at the apex, there was a small epicardial layer of preserved myocardium in the anteroapical segment, which was concordant with the ^{201}Tl reinjection image at this same region and also concordant with the presence of collateral circulation coming from the LCX. Therefore, it was concluded that the anterior MI is nontransmural (less than 50% of transmural extent) at the mid-ventricle level. By cine MRI criteria, there were no significant changes in LV function at rest over the next 6 months. Immediately after the MI, the LVEF was 53%, EDV 85 ml, ESV 40 ml, and after 6 months follow-up the LVEF was 50%, EDV 82 ml, and ESV 40 ml.

Discussion

Both MPI and MRI showed a moderate sized MI. No evidence existed of a significant amount of viable myocardium at risk by stress/reinjection ^{201}Tl. The patient had preserved LV function and shape 6 months later without revascularization, which indicates that the collateral vessels partially protected the mid-anterior wall. The apical region showed less recovery, which is common due to its distal location and terminal perfusion. Stress/reinjection ^{201}Tl MPI allows evaluation of viability in areas of myocardium at risk and therefore identification of viable ischemic myocardium that could potentially recover function following revascularization. Patients without evidence of significant ischemic viable myocardium should be managed clinically, as a worse outcome may occur when revascularization is attempted.[32]

MDE MRI allows identification of dead myocardium and because of the exquisite spatial resolution of this imaging technique, MDE MRI is being recognized as the best modality to quantify the extent of MI. One limitation of performing only MDE MRI is its inability to differentiate normal viable myocardium from viable ischemic myocardium at risk. Another MRI study, including the myocardial first-pass perfusion technique would be necessary to specifically evaluate rest/vasodilator stress perfusion and to be able to determine whether myocardium at risk is present or not (as shown in Case 14.6). Despite this limitation, the extent of MI defined on MDE MRI after acute MI is inversely correlated with outcome in terms of LV function and remodeling.[30] In the case of the patient presented, after 6 months follow-up, the imaging studies demonstrated that the LV had suffered little remodeling with only mild compromised LV function (LVEF 41% by gated SPECT), even though the apex had become akinetic.

Interpretations

1. Moderate sized, nontransmural anterior MI due to LAD occlusion, demonstrated by both MDE MRI and SPECT.
2. No significant viable ischemic myocardium demonstrated with stress/reinjection ^{201}Tl.
3. After 6 months, stable LV function and remodeling without revascularization.

Case 14.3

History

A 50-year-old man with multiple risk factors presented to the ED with chest pain associated with nausea. His ECG showed minimal ST-segment changes but clearly inverted T waves in leads V1 to V3. The peak serum CK-MB was twofold above upper limit of normal, and he was diagnosed as having a non-ST elevation MI. He was initially treated medically without thrombolytic therapy. His clinical course was unremarkable. Coronary angiography revealed distal LAD occlusion and 50% stenoses of both the proximal LCX and proximal RCA. A stent was successfully placed in the LAD. He was discharged on medical therapy with aspirin, ACE inhibitor, ticlopidine, and a beta-blocker.

He underwent resting cardiac MRI with Gd MDE and viability evaluation using rest ^{201}Tl gated SPECT after the acute episode (but before the PTCA) and 6 months later to evaluate the extent of MI and the corresponding regional function. The rest SPECT images and MDE MRI images are displayed in Figure C14-3.

Findings

The rest ^{201}Tl SPECT after the acute event showed a small perfusion defect at the apex and distal inferoseptal segments. On the SPECT images obtained 6 months later, the small perfusion defect has improved slightly.

Resting cardiac MRI using Gd MDE after the acute phase showed a small infarction in the apical inferior and apical septal segments (Figure C14-3, arrows). The pattern of delayed enhancement was typical but heterogeneous with several islets of normal myocardium within the necrotic area (Figure C14-3, arrowheads in the bottom right detail). Cine MRI showed very slight hypokinesia of these segments.

Discussion

The small size of the perfusion defect on rest SPECT images is indicative of a good prognosis for preserved function due to the amount of viable tissue. This was confirmed on the SPECT images obtained 6 months later revealing near normal perfusion. This improvement is often

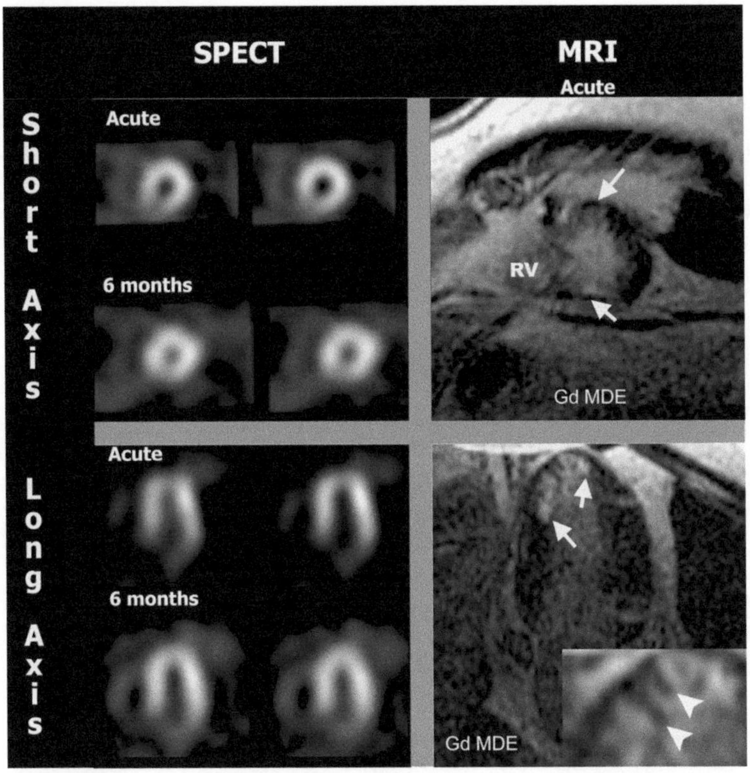

FIGURE C14-3.

seen in patients with small and nontransmural perfusion defects several months after the acute event, even when revascularization is not performed.[33,34]

Although cardiac MRI with Gd MDE demonstrated almost complete transmural enhancement in the apex and distal inferoseptal segments (around 75% of the segment) predictive of no contractile recovery, the small size of the infarct (5.7% of LV mass) and the heterogeneous pattern of delayed enhancement (with visible islands of normal myocardium within the necrotic myocardium) were indicative of a high probability for eventual improvement of contractile function. This was confirmed on the 6-month follow-up cardiac MRI study demonstrating complete recovery of function. Therefore, in this case the near transmural extent of the MI on MRI was misleading in predicting segmental contractile recovery.[35] Close attention to the pattern of enhancement on MRI, such as circumferential extent, heterogeneous pattern, presence of islets of normal myocardium within the infarcted area, and the total infarct size, should improve the accuracy of MRI with Gd MDE for prediction of segmental contractile recovery. Additionally, this case illustrates that patients with implanted stents can be safely evaluated using MRI, which is not true for patients with pacemakers, considering the strong magnetic field present.

Interpretations

1. Small apical and distal inferoseptal MI with little contractile dysfunction due to distal LAD occlusion and demonstrated with both stress/reinjection ^{201}Tl and MDE MRI.

2. Improvement of perfusion and function 6 months after stent placement in the LAD predicted by the small size of the MI and heterogeneous pattern of enhancement on MDE MRI.

Case 14.4

History

A 59-year-old woman with hypertension presented to the ED with a 9-hour history of oppressive chest pain, radiating to the left arm and associated with diaphoresis and nausea. The ECG showed absence of R waves on leads V1 to V3 and ST-segment elevation. The peak CK-MB was elevated to fivefold above normal values. Coronary angiography revealed occlusion of the mid-LAD and the descending posterior branch of the RCA, as well as an 80% stenosis at the ostium of a relatively small LCX. There was collateral circulation to the LAD territory with grade III flow. She underwent angioplasty and stenting of the LAD. On echocardiography, the LV diastolic and systolic diameters were 51 and 38 mm, respectively, and the LVEF was 50%. She was treated with propranolol, aspirin, simvastatin, and enalapril during her hospitalization. She underwent dipyridamole stress/reinjection ^{201}Tl gated SPECT study and resting cardiac MRI to evaluate anterior wall viability before the PTCA procedure (Figure C14-4A) and 6 months later (Figure C14-4B).

Findings

In the acute phase, the stress ^{201}Tl SPECT images demonstrated hypoperfusion in the mid- and apical anteroseptal walls, partial reversibility on the reinjection images (Figure C14-4A). The LVEF, EDV, and ESV were 46%, 92 ml, and 50 ml, respectively.

After 6 months, the size of the apical and anteroseptal defect decreased with near normalization (Figure C14-4B). The LV function

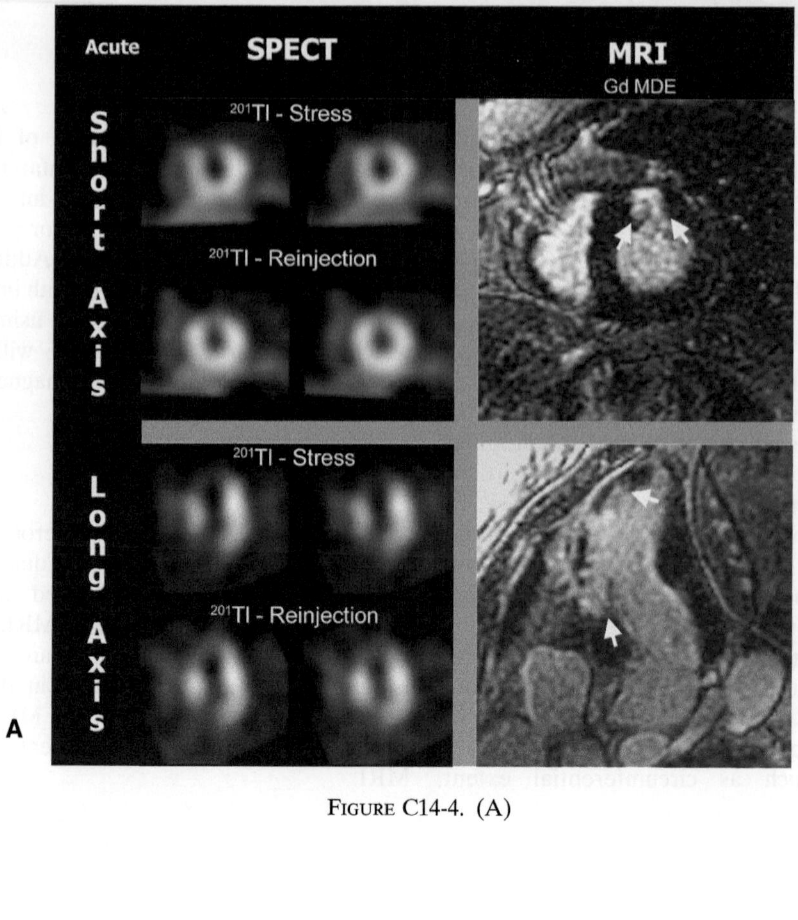

FIGURE C14-4. (A)

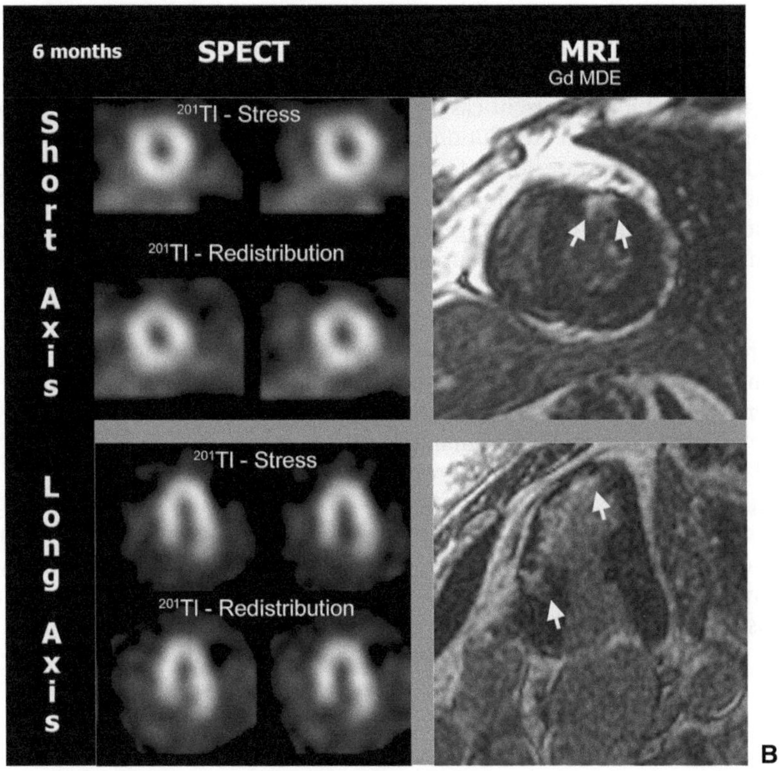

FIGURE C14-4. (B)

also improved with the LVEF, EDV, and ESV at 57%, 83 ml, and 36 ml, respectively.

Resting cardiac MRI with Gd MDE demonstrated hyperenhancement in the mid-anterior and apical anterior and septal walls. The hyperenhancement was mostly transmural in the mid-anterior and apical septal walls and nontransmural in the apical anterior segment (Figures C14-4A and C14-4B). However, in mid-anterior segment the circumferential extent of the infarct was small (Figures C14-4A and C14-4B, short-axis MRI). Cine MRI revealed hypokinesia in the same segments in the acute phase. However, the 6-month follow-up study revealed almost complete recovery of segmental function. The LVEF by MRI improved significantly from 43% at presentation to 53% at 6-month follow-up in agreement with the gated SPECT findings.

Discussion

The gated SPECT ^{201}Tl images showed a partially reversible perfusion defect compatible with myocardial viability predictive of improvement of the LV function that was mildly impaired. In fact, there was an almost complete recovery of function and perfusion at the 6-month follow-up. Nuclear imaging has been used to predict recovery of LV function and myocardial perfusion over time, sometimes independently of a revascularization procedure.[36–39] This case demonstrated one limitation of resting MDE MRI, which can detect and accurately quantify small areas of MI but cannot predict if the adjacent viable myocardium is normal (and will not improve) or ischemic (and can potentially improve).[40] Although the viable ischemic and nonischemic myocardium can be detected accurately by stress MRI perfusion using dipyridamole, as described in the introduction of this chapter, this was not performed in the current case. On the other hand, the limited resolution of nuclear imaging is less accurate for detection of small areas of MI. These imaging modalities are complementary and may be used together, especially in cases of borderline surgical indication.

From the knowledge accumulated in the MRI literature, this barely transmural infarct in some segments would have little or no functional recovery over time. However, due to the small circumferential extent, the segmental function had a surprising degree of recovery after 6-month follow-up. Some preliminary results from our laboratory indicate that the circumferential extent can play an important role on the contractile prognosis of an infarcted segment. This case illustrates that the sole information of infarct transmurality can be misleading regarding the prediction of recovery of segmental contractile function. The small size of the circumferential extent (this case) and heterogeneous pattern of hyperenhancement (Case 14.3) should be considered when predicting recovery of contractile function especially on images of the acute phase of MI. Accepted standardized criteria for these characteristics of myocardial hyperenhancement have yet to be formulated. In this patient, partial reversibility on the ^{201}Tl reinjection images accurately predicted recovery of function post-revascularization.

Interpretations

1. Small MI due to occlusion of the mid-LAD.
2. Good recovery of function post-revascularization predicted by significant amount of viable myocardium on stress/reinjection ^{201}Tl SPECT and small circumferential extent of MI on MDE MRI.

Case 14.5

History

A 49-year-old woman with multiple risk factors presented to the ED with intense precordial pain, associated with nausea, diaphoresis, shortness of breath, and palpitations of 3 hours' duration. Her ECG showed absence of R wave from lead V1 to V4 and ST-segment elevation from V1 to V5. Serum CK-MB remained within normal limits and troponin I was 4.8 ng/ml (normal <0.5 ng/ml). She was diagnosed with an anterior MI, treated medically, and developed symptoms of heart failure. Coronary angiography revealed occlusion of the proximal LAD and moderate stenosis of the proximal RCA with collateral circulation from the RCA to the LAD territory. No attempt to perform angioplasty of the occluded LAD was made. She was discharged in functional class II (NYHA) and was medicated with aspirin, nitrate, ACE inhibitor, beta-blocker, and diuretic. During the 6 months ensuing, her medical treatment was optimized without improvement of symptoms.

Dipyridamole stress/reinjection ^{201}Tl gated SPECT and resting cardiac MRI were performed during the acute phase (Figure C14-5A) and after 6 months follow-up (Figure C14-5B).

Findings

After the acute phase, the stress ^{201}Tl SPECT images showed absence of apical inferior perfusion and hypoperfusion in the anteroseptal wall with no changes on the redistribution images. The gated SPECT ventriculography showed an LVEF of 15%, EDV of 216 ml, and ESV of 184 ml.

Resting cardiac MRI with Gd MDE in the acute phase revealed hyperenhancement in the mid-anteroseptal, mid-inferoseptal, mid-inferior, apical inferior, and septal segments with a transmural pattern (Figure C14-5A; the arrows show the borders of the MI with delayed enhancement). These findings are compatible

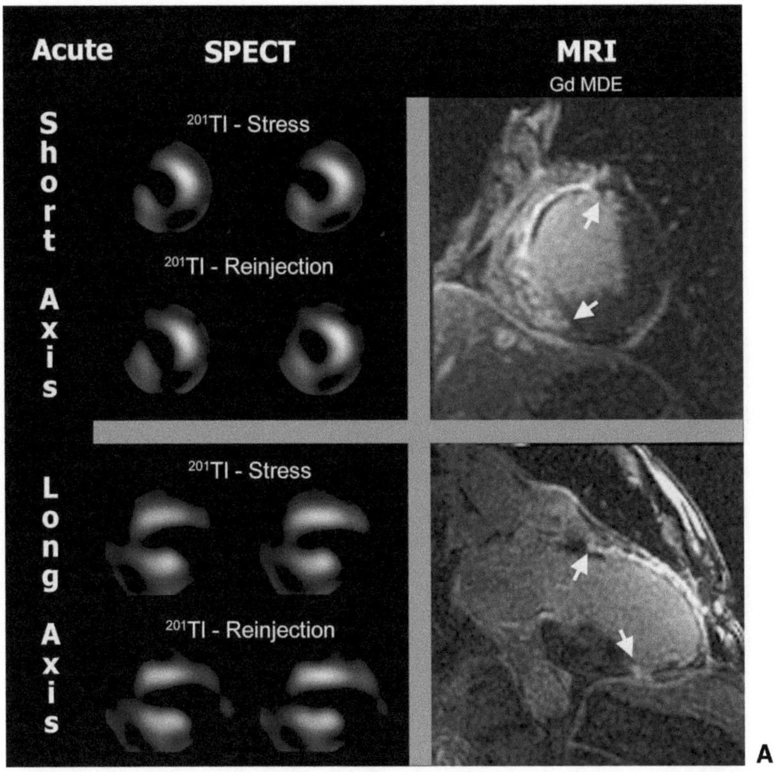

FIGURE C14-5. (A)

with a transmural MI and absence of myocardial viability in those segments. Significant wall thinning is associated with the hyperenhanced areas, mainly on the mid-anteroseptal and apical segments, which is surprising considering the early phase of this acute MI. There was no evidence of aneurysm on the study performed early after the acute phase. Cine MRI revealed an LVEF of 28%, EDV of 120 ml, and ESV of 86 ml. The discrepancy between the volume measurements on the SPECT and MRI studies may be related to an automatic (QGS software package for the SPECT image analysis) versus manual (MRI) method to draw the regions of interest.

After 6 months follow-up (Figure C14-5B), the myocardial perfusion SPECT images confirmed the absence of myocardial viability on the same regions. Gated SPECT ventriculography demonstrated progressive LV dilation and poor LV function with an LVEF of 14%, EDV and ESV of 261 ml and 225 ml, respectively. In addition, there was an LV apical inferior aneurysm and mid-apical anterior wall akinesis. After 6 months follow-up, cine MRI showed an apical inferior LV aneurysm with important wall thinning and possible LV apical thrombus. The global LVEF, EDV, and ESV were 22%, 193 ml, and 151 ml, respectively.

She underwent surgical repair of LV (aneurysmectomy and LV geometric reconstruction) with improvement of symptoms. After aneurysmal repair, the LV global function on MRI, 10 days after surgery, improved dramatically with an LVEF of 37%, EDV of 116 ml, and ESV of 84 ml.

Discussion

The initial scintigraphic images predicted no functional or perfusional recovery based on

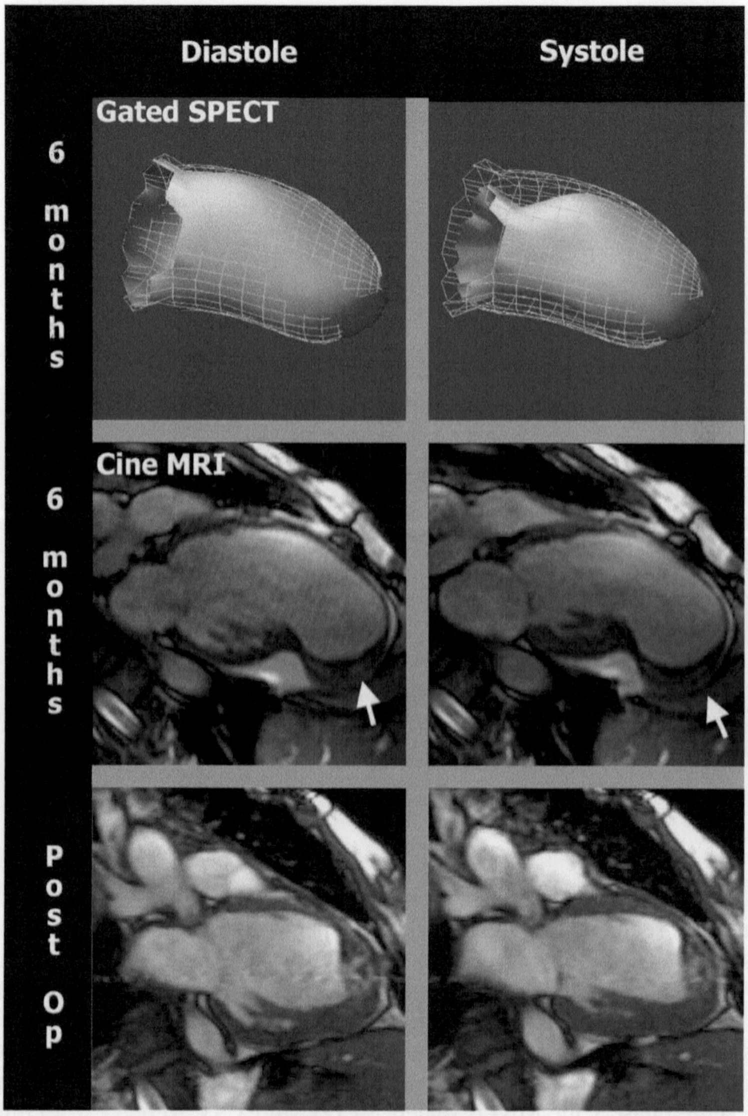

FIGURE C14-5. (B)

the absence of demonstrable viability by ^{201}Tl SPECT. The ^{201}Tl gated SPECT images demonstrated worsening of LV function and no improvement of myocardial perfusion over the follow-up period of 6 months. There was a clear development of dyskinetic motion at the LV apex, contributing to the clinical symptoms of congestive heart failure.[41–43]

Images from the cardiac MRI added the information of an LV aneurysm, with severe wall thinning in the apical inferior wall, which led to a gross deformation of LV chamber. The severe wall thinning in the acute phase raised the possibility of a previous silent MI that has recently extended as suggested by the slightly elevated serum troponin levels, whereas the serum levels of CK-MB were within normal but with absent R waves on precordial leads. The findings described on the imaging studies could predict progressive clinical worsening and a high mortality for this patient if an aneurysmal repair was not planned.

Another question that could be raised is the possibility of having performed angioplasty of the occluded LAD. Is angioplasty indicated in a patient without evidence of myocardial viability? This is still a question not answered by the literature addressing the *open-artery hypothesis* proposed in the past.[44] The benefit of opening an infarct-related artery after 12 hours of the acute onset is still unknown. The open-artery hypothesis is related to possible benefit of opening an infarct-related artery after 12 hours of the acute onset in terms of better remodeling of the LV, less arrhythmia, less apoptosis, and salvage of hibernating myocardium. Would an open artery influence the LV remodeling beyond the myocardial salvage? Although the answer to this question remains unknown, preliminary studies suggest that the answer is yes.[45] In this patient, MRI with delayed enhancement detected a transmural infarct with unusual wall thinning in the acute phase of the MI that may be predictive of late LV remodeling. A combined effort with multimodality imaging may help to better predict the long-term clinical course of an MI.

Interpretations

1. Large transmural anterior, apical, and inferoapical MI due to proximal LAD occlusion and demonstrated by ^{201}Tl SPECT and MDE MRI.
2. Severe wall thinning in the acute phase suggestive of an episode of remote silent MI.
3. After 6 months of medical therapy, severe LV remodeling and deformation by aneurysm.
4. Improvement of the LV function after aneurysmectomy.

Case 14.6

History

A 61-year-old man with multiple risk factors for CAD presented with chest pain associated with intense physical activity and improving after exercise cessation. Dobutamine echocardiography demonstrated inferior wall akinesia and apical dyskinesia at peak stress indicating ischemia, and the patient complained of chest pain at peak dobutamine dose. An adenosine stress/redistribution ^{201}Tl gated SPECT study and stress MRI first-pass perfusion with dipyridamole are displayed in Figure C14-6.

Findings

The adenosine ^{201}Tl SPECT images demonstrated hypoperfusion in the inferior, midlateral, and apical walls, with normalization on the redistribution images. Additionally, there is a mild anteroseptal reversible defect. This scintigraphic pattern is compatible with multivessel CAD. The gated study demonstrated normal LV function.

The MRI first-pass perfusion images during stress with dipyridamole demonstrated a perfusion defect in the entire inferior segment (Figure C14-6, from 1 to 4, right upper panel, the arrow points to the perfusion defect in the inferior wall) with extension to the mid-inferolateral and apical lateral segments. On the resting MRI perfusion images, no significant hypoperfusion was noted (Figure C14-6, from 1 to 3, the arrow point to the inferior wall without perfusion defect). Additionally, MRI with Gd MDE did not show any hyperenhancement indicating preserved myocardial viability (Figure C14-6, bottom right panel, number 4, the arrow points to the inferior wall without enhancement). The combined information provided by the previous images indicates significant myocardial ischemia in a viable myocardial territory.

Coronary angiography revealed 95% stenosis of the distal RCA, occlusion of the PDA, 90% stenosis of the distal LAD, 70% stenosis

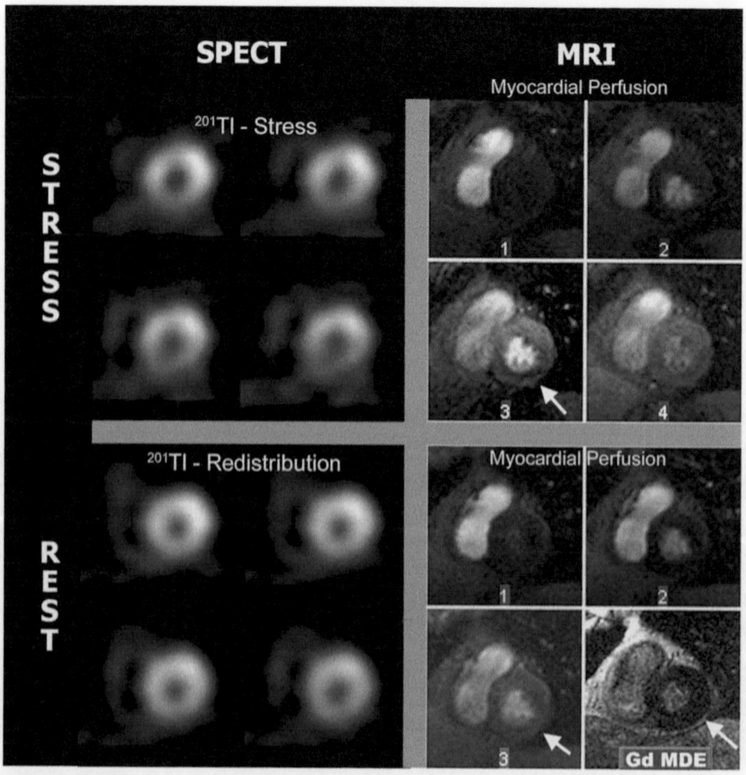

FIGURE C14-6.

of the first and second diagonal branches, multiple high-grade stenoses in the LCX, and 95% stenosis of the first obtuse marginal branch. The patient underwent surgical coronary artery revascularization and had an excellent clinical course with disappearance of symptoms and normalization of imaging test results.

Discussion

Scintigraphically, this is a classical example of myocardial ischemia in multiple territories, with preserved viability. The most severe transient hypoperfusion is located in the inferior wall. A corresponding perfusion defect is seen on the MRI first-pass perfusion images during dipyridamole infusion. In addition, there was no myocardial hyperenhancement after Gd, not even small or micro infarcts in those ischemic segments.

As expected from the imaging findings, the clinical course of the patient after revascularization was excellent. Although the data are still preliminary on a small number of patients, several comparative studies between MRI and nuclear imaging showed a good agreement of both methodologies, suggesting that MRI may be a suitable alternative to scintigraphy in the evaluation of myocardial ischemia. Results from large trials, showing outcome data based on standardized protocols and analysis, will be necessary and a prerequisite for a wider use of this new technology in clinical practice.

Interpretation

Multivessel myocardial ischemia detected by rest/vasodilator first-pass perfusion MRI and MPI and successfully treated with revascularization.

References

1. Lima JA, Judd RM, Bazille A, et al. Regional heterogeneity of human myocardial infarcts demonstrated by contrast-enhanced MRI: potential mechanisms. *Circulation.* 1995;92:1117–1125.
2. Kim RJ, Fieno DS, Parrish TB, et al. Relationship of MRI delayed contrast enhancement to irreversible injury, infarct age, and contractile function. *Circulation.* 1999;100:1992–2002.
3. Kim RJ, Chen EL, Lima JA, et al. Myocardial Gd-DTPA kinetics determine MRI contrast enhancement and reflect the extent and severity of myocardial injury after acute reperfused infarction. *Circulation.* 1996;94:3318–3326.
4. Judd RM, Lugo-Olivieri CH, Arai M, et al. Physiological basis of myocardial contrast enhancement in fast magnetic resonance images of 2-day-old reperfused canine infarcts. *Circulation.* 1995;92:1902–1910.
5. Kim RJ, Wu E, Rafael A, et al. The use of contrast-enhanced magnetic resonance imaging to identify reversible myocardial dysfunction. *N Engl J Med.* 2000;343:1445–1453.
6. Simonetti OP, Kim RJ, Fieno DS, et al. An improved MR imaging technique for the visualization of myocardial infarction. *Radiology.* 2001;218:215–223.
7. Wu E, Judd RM, Vargas JD, et al. Visualisation of presence, location, and transmural extent of healed Q-wave and non-Q-wave myocardial infarction. *Lancet.* 2001;357:21–28.
8. Hillenbrand HB, Kim RJ, Parker MA, et al. Early assessment of myocardial salvage by contrast-enhanced magnetic resonance imaging. *Circulation.* 2000;102:1678–1683.
9. Wagner A, Mahrholdt H, Holly TA, et al. Contrast-enhanced MRI and routine single photon emission computed tomography (SPECT) perfusion imaging for detection of subendocardial myocardial infarcts: an imaging study. *Lancet.* 2003;361:374–379.
10. Ricciardi MJ, Wu E, Davidson CJ, et al. Visualization of discrete microinfarction after percutaneous coronary intervention associated with mild creatine kinase-MB elevation. *Circulation.* 2001;103:2780–2783.
11. Klein C, Nekolla SG, Bengel FM, et al. Assessment of myocardial viability with contrast-enhanced magnetic resonance imaging: comparison with positron emission tomography. *Circulation.* 2002;105:162–167.
12. Mahrholdt H, Wagner A, Holly TA, et al. Reproducibility of chronic infarct size measurement by contrast-enhanced magnetic resonance imaging. *Circulation.* 2002;106:2322–2327.
13. Rochitte CE, Lima JA, Bluemke DA, et al. Magnitude and time course of microvascular obstruction and tissue injury after acute myocardial infarction. *Circulation.* 1998;98:1006–1014.
14. Wu KC, Kim RJ, Bluemke DA, et al. Quantification and time course of microvascular obstruction by contrast-enhanced echocardiography and magnetic resonance imaging following acute myocardial infarction and reperfusion. *J Am Coll Cardiol.* 1998;32:1756–1764.
15. Wu KC, Zerhouni EA, Judd RM, et al. Prognostic significance of microvascular obstruction by magnetic resonance imaging in patients with acute myocardial infarction. *Circulation.* 1998; 97:765–772.
16. Gunning MG, Kaprielian RR, Pepper J, et al. The histology of viable and hibernating myocardium in relation to imaging characteristics. *J Am Coll Cardiol.* 2002;39:428–435.
17. Underwood R. Magnetic resonance imaging compared with thallium myocardial perfusion tomography after acute myocardial infarction. *Magn Reson Imaging.* 1994;12:827.
18. Wilke NM, Jerosch-Herold M, Zenovich A, et al. Magnetic resonance first-pass myocardial perfusion imaging: clinical validation and future applications. *J Magn Reson Imaging.* 1999;10:676–685.
19. Muhling OM, Dickson ME, Zenovich A, et al. Quantitative magnetic resonance first-pass perfusion analysis: inter- and intraobserver agreement. *J Cardiovasc Magn Reson.* 2001;3:247–256.
20. Al Saadi N, Nagel E, Gross M, et al. Improvement of myocardial perfusion reserve early after coronary intervention: assessment with cardiac magnetic resonance imaging. *J Am Coll Cardiol.* 2000;36:1557–1564.
21. Al Saadi N, Nagel E, Gross M, et al. Noninvasive detection of myocardial ischemia from perfusion reserve based on cardiovascular magnetic resonance. *Circulation.* 2000;101:1379–1383.
22. Wilke NM, Jerosch-Herold M, Zenovich A, et al. Magnetic resonance first-pass myocardial perfusion imaging: clinical validation and future applications. *J Magn Reson Imaging.* 1999;10: 676–685.
23. Ho KT, Miller TD, Christian TF, et al. Prediction of severe coronary artery disease and long-term outcome in patients undergoing vasodilator SPECT. *J Nucl Cardiol.* 2001;8:438–444.
24. Galassi AR, Azzarelli S, Tomaselli A, et al. Incremental prognostic value of technetium-99m-tetrofosmin exercise myocardial perfusion

imaging for predicting outcomes in patients with suspected or known coronary artery disease. *Am J Cardiol.* 2001;88:101–106.
25. Ho KT, Miller TD, Christian TF, et al. Prediction of severe coronary artery disease and long-term outcome in patients undergoing vasodilator SPECT. *J Nucl Cardiol.* 2001;8:438–444.
26. Galassi AR, Azzarelli S, Tomaselli A, et al. Incremental prognostic value of technetium-99m-tetrofosmin exercise myocardial perfusion imaging for predicting outcomes in patients with suspected or known coronary artery disease. *Am J Cardiol.* 2001;88:101–106.
27. Sharir T, Germano G, Kavanagh PB, et al. Incremental prognostic value of post-stress left ventricular ejection fraction and volume by gated myocardial perfusion single photon emission computed tomography. *Circulation.* 1999;100:1035–1042.
28. Gerber BL, Rochitte CE, Melin JA, et al. Microvascular obstruction and left ventricular remodeling early after acute myocardial infarction. *Circulation.* 2000;101:2734–2741.
29. Gerber BL, Rochitte CE, Bluemke DA, et al. Relation between Gd-DTPA contrast enhancement and regional inotropic response in the periphery and center of myocardial infarction. *Circulation.* 2001;104:998–1004.
30. Gerber BL, Garot J, Bluemke DA, et al. Accuracy of contrast-enhanced magnetic resonance imaging in predicting improvement of regional myocardial function in patients after acute myocardial infarction. *Circulation.* 2002;106:1083–1089.
31. Hachamovitch R, Berman DS, Shaw LJ, et al. Incremental prognostic value of myocardial perfusion single photon emission computed tomography for the prediction of cardiac death: differential stratification for risk of cardiac death and myocardial infarction. *Circulation.* 1998;97:535–543.
32. Allman KC, Shaw LJ, Hachamovitch R, et al. Myocardial viability testing and impact of revascularization on prognosis in patient with coronary artery disease and left ventricular dysfunction: a metaanalysis. *J Am Coll Cardiol.* 2002;39:1151–1158.
33. Di Carli MF. Assessment of myocardial viability after myocardial infarction. *J Nucl Cardiol.* 2002;9:229–235.
34. Petrasinovic Z, Ostojic M, Beleslin B, et al. Prognostic value of myocardial viability determined by a ^{201}Tl SPECT study in patients with previous myocardial infarction and mild-to-moderate myocardial dysfunction. *Nucl Med Commun.* 2003;24:175–181.
35. Rochitte CE, Silva JC, Ávila LF, et al. Late recanalization of infarct related artery improves circumferential shortening of infarct related left ventricular segment at 6 months follow-up. *J Cardiovasc Magn Reson.* 2000;4(abstract):21.
36. Bonow RO. Myocardial hibernation: a noninvasive physician's point of view. *Ital Heart J.* 2002;3:285–290.
37. Mari C, Strauss WH. Detection and characterization of hibernating myocardium. *Nucl Med Commun.* 2002;23:311–322.
38. Acampa W, Cuocolo A, Petretta M, et al. Tetrofosmin imaging in the detection of myocardial viability in patients with previous myocardial infarction: comparison with sestamibi and ^{201}Tl scintigraphy. *J Nucl Cardiol.* 2002;9:33–40.
39. Chalela WA, Moffa PJ, Ramires JA, et al. Detection of the viable myocardium. A perfusion scintigraphic study, before and after coronary bypass surgery in myocardial infarction patients. *Arq Bras Cardiol.* 1999;72:523–545.
40. Klein C, Nekolla SG, Bengel FM, et al. Assessment of myocardial viability with contrast-enhanced magnetic resonance imaging: comparison with positron emission tomography. *Circulation.* 2002;105:162–167.
41. Sciagra R, Pellegri M, Pupi A, et al. Prognostic implications of ^{99m}Tc sestamibi viability imaging and subsequent therapeutic strategy in patients with chronic coronary artery disease and left ventricular dysfunction. *J Am Coll Cardiol.* 2000;36:739–745.
42. Borges-Neto S, Shaw LK. The added value of simultaneous myocardial perfusion and left ventricular function. *Curr Opin Cardiol.* 1999;14:460–463.
43. Stollfuss JC, Haas F, Matsunari I, et al. ^{99m}Tc-tetrofosmin SPECT for prediction of functional recovery defined by MRI in patients with severe left ventricular dysfunction: additional value of gated SPECT. *J Nucl Med.* 1999;40:1824–1831.
44. Kim CB, Braunwald E. Potential benefits of late reperfusion of infarcted myocardium. The open artery hypothesis. *Circulation.* 1993;88:2426–2436.
45. Silva JC, Rochitte CE, Ávila LF, et al. Effects of late recanalization for acute myocardial infarction on left ventricular remodelling: a prospective randomized study preliminary data. *Eur Heart J.* 2002; 23(abstract):348.

15
Cardiac Applications of Multislice Computed Tomography

Jaydip Datta

There has been remarkable progress in imaging technology in recent years. This is especially true in the field of computed tomography (CT), in which the introduction of multidetector CT and continuing improvement in image reconstruction capabilities have strengthened the role of CT in diagnostic radiology.

The introduction of the latest generation of multi–detector row CT systems allows continuous acquisition of data by using 16 parallel detectors with rotation times of up to 400 msec. By being able to acquire up to 0.5-mm slices, one can maximize spatial resolution and also cover the entire heart in a very reasonable breath hold of less than 20 seconds. When combined with retrospective ECG gating, reconstruction of cross-sectional images of the heart in any defined phase of the heart cycle has become possible. Along with improvement in spatial resolution, improvements in reconstruction algorithms have increased the temporal resolution to between 60 and 250 msec. The short data acquisition window of multi-detector row CT results in a significant reduction of heartbeat-related motion artifacts, permitting detailed visualization of the cardiac anatomy.[1]

Cardiac CT is a noninvasive modality well accepted by patients. Cardiac CT is performed in a single breath hold and has very few contraindications. The study can be performed in seriously ill patients and in those with pacemakers and defibrillators. The lower cost, reliability, low risk profile, quick throughput, and availability in an outpatient setting put cardiac CT on the threshold of being a major imaging modality in the evaluation of cardiac disease. The detailed morphological data obtained by CT are unsurpassed by any other cross-sectional modalities and can supplement the functional information provided by nuclear imaging.

Cardiac CT is now beginning to play a role in coronary artery imaging. By being able to detect and quantitate vessel stenosis as well as characterize coronary plaque, we are at a new and exciting phase in the development of coronary artery evaluation. In a recent study conducted by Ropers et al.,[2] CT angiography had an excellent correlation with conventional angiography. They reported a sensitivity of 92% and a specificity of 93% in being able to accurately diagnose significant stenosis in 77 patients. At the time of this writing, multicenter trials are underway to compare CT angiography and conventional angiography in larger patient groups. Another area of increased cardiac CT use is likely to be in the evaluation of coronary artery bypass graft patency. Patent graft vessels are often incidentally noted on CT done for other indications. Tello et al.[3] demonstrated that CT was able to identify patent bypass grafts with a sensitivity of 93% and specificity of 100%. Their study compared a single detector row CT with coronary angiography and obtained these impressive results. With the present availability of 16-row multidetector CT, the results could only get better.

The following case studies demonstrate the emerging role and new clinical applications of cardiac CT.

Case Presentations

Case 15.1

History

A 65-year-old man was referred to coronary arteriography for atypical chest pain. The right coronary artery (RCA) was opacified at the time of the left coronary artery (LCA) injection. The exact anatomical course of the RCA and its relationship with the pulmonary artery could not be accurately visualized by contrast angiography (Figure C15-1A). The patient was then referred for a cardiac CT to confirm the presence of the anomaly and to precisely trace the course of the anomalous RCA.

A retrospectively gated cardiac CT was performed on an MX 8000 IDT system (Phillips Medical Systems, Andover, MA). Using a gantry rotation time of 0.42 second, collimation of 0.75 mm, 16 parallel detectors, field of view of 250, pitch of 0.3, and biphasic injection of 140 ml of iodinated contrast agent, the scan was performed with a breath hold duration of 25 seconds. Images were then analyzed using the raw axial data; volume rendered and reformatted images are shown in Figure C15-1B.

Findings

Figure C15-1A is an RAO view during coronary angiography demonstrating an anomalous RCA that filled during an LCA injection. The course of the vessel could not be accurately depicted on this study. Figure C15-1B is an oblique sagittal volume rendered image demonstrating the origin of the anomalous RCA from the very proximal LCA. The anomalous vessel courses between the ascending aorta and the main pulmonary artery to descend into the right atrioventricular groove.

Figures C15-1C and C15-1D are of another patient with a single right coronary ostia, showing an anomalous left circumflex (LCX) that arises from the right coronary cusp and courses inferiorly and posteriorly to the aortic root and crosses over to the left to enter the atrioventricular groove. In Figure C15-1D, the left anterior descending coronary artery (LAD) is shown to be arising from the right coronary cusp, which then coursed between the aortic root and the pulmonary trunk.

A

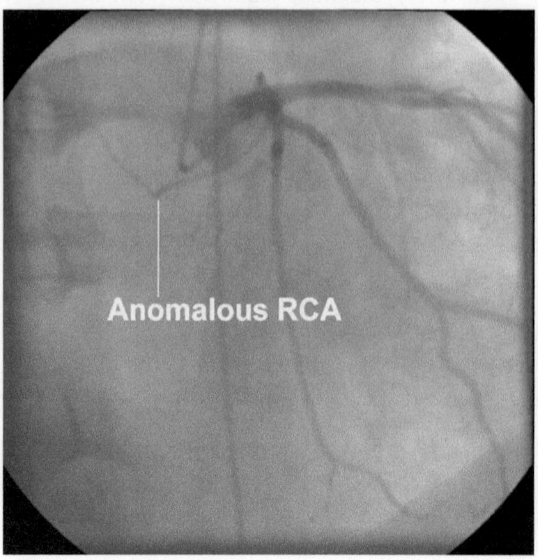

FIGURE C15-1. (A)

FIGURE C15-1. (B and C)

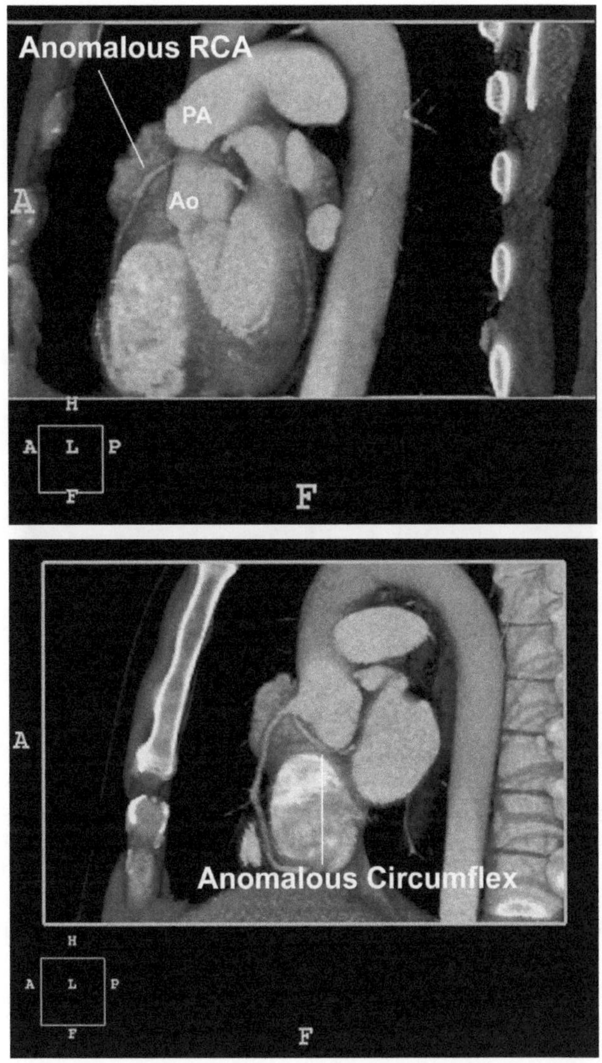

Discussion

Primary congenital anomalies of the coronary vessels are observed in approximately 1% of patients who undergo coronary angiography.[4] While the majority of congenital anomalies are hemodynamically insignificant, others cause abnormal myocardial perfusion and may lead to ischemia and sudden death. Coronary anomalies may be responsible for 19% of deaths in competitive athletes according to the Sudden Death Committee of the American Heart Association (AHA).[5] Currently, invasive coronary angiography is the modality most often used to analyze aberrant coronary anatomy. However, coronary angiography is suboptimal to visualize the course of the anomalous vessel. It is therefore important to identify an alternate modality that can reliably identify and document the anatomical course of anomalous coronary vessels to assess their significance. With the advent of 16-row multidetector CT with retrospective cardiac gating, CT coronary angiography can be an effective tool in the

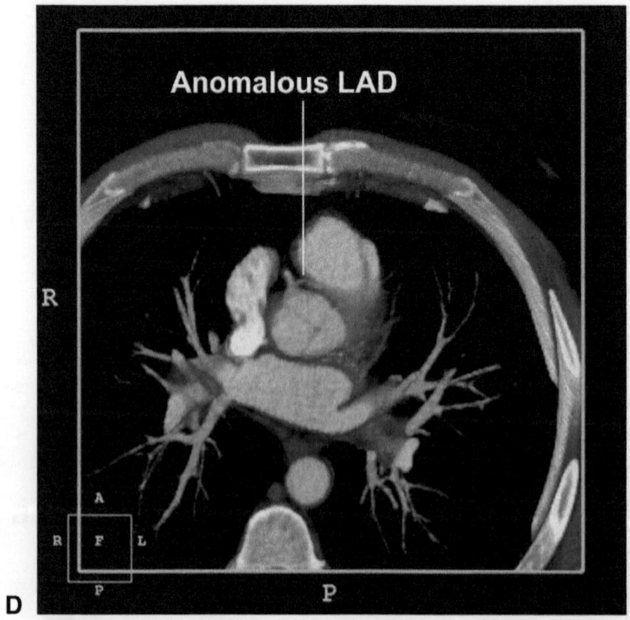

FIGURE C15-1. (D)

management of patients with coronary artery anomalies.

With the risk of sudden death in certain congenital anomalies, it is important to describe the aberrant coronary anatomy so as to consider surgical intervention in an otherwise asymptomatic patient. One proposed classification[6] is based on the location of a single coronary ostium, the presence or absence of an aberrant coursing vessel, and the course taken by the aberrant vessel. The anomaly is documented type L if originating from the left aortic sinus and type R if originating from the right aortic sinus. Subtype is derived from the course of the anomalous vessel, in which groups I to III correspond to the relationship of the vessel with the aorta and the pulmonary trunk. The patient represented in Figures C15-1A and C15-1B belongs in the R II B group in which there is a single LCA giving rise to an anomalous RCA that passes between the aorta and the right ventricular infundibulum. The patient shown in Figure C15-1C belongs in group R III. There is a single RCA with the LCX originating from the proximal RCA and passing behind the root of the aorta on its way toward the left atrioventricular groove. The LAD also originates from the proximal RCA and passes in between the right ventricular infundibulum and aorta on its way to the anterior interventricular groove.

Numerous mechanisms of myocardial ischemia in these anomalies have been advanced and likely occur secondary to acute angulation and the slit-like ostium often associated with anomalous anatomy.[7] During intense physical activity, the aortic wall stretches and dilates to support the increased cardiac output, thus further compressing the slit-like ostium and anomalous vessel between the pulmonary outflow track.[8] If the anomalous vessel lies intramurally, further compression would result during periods of increased cardiac output.[7,9]

Because invasive coronary angiography provides a 2-dimensional view of the complex course of aberrant coronary anatomy, an alternate modality is required to precisely discern the anatomic course of vessels in relation to the myocardium, aorta, and pulmonary outflow track. CT angiography is a new, noninvasive, and well-tolerated imaging modality that can evaluate the three-dimensional course of the anomalous vessel. The superior spatial resolution and the ability to post process the volumetric data makes CT a useful imaging option in the management of these difficult patients. This topic is also discussed in Cases 5.8 and 5.9.

Interpretation

Anomalous origin and course of the RCA in an elderly patient.

Case 15.2

History

A 63-year-old woman with a history of paroxysmal atrial fibrillation was referred for a cardiac CT to evaluate the morphology of the pulmonary venous ostia. This was a component of a preprocedure workup before having a radiofrequency ablation procedure for the treatment of atrial fibrillation.

A retrospectively gated cardiac CT was performed on an MX 8000 IDT system. Using a gantry rotation time of 0.42 second, collimation of 1.5 mm, 16 parallel detectors, field of view of 250, pitch of 0.3, and injection of 140 ml of iodinated contrast agent at 4 ml/second, the scan was performed with a breath hold duration of 11 seconds. Images were then analyzed using the raw axial data; volume rendered and reformatted images and displayed in Figures C15-2A and C15-2B.

Findings

Figure C15-2A is a coronal volume rendered display of an enlarged left atrium with the draining pulmonary veins. In Figure C15-2B, the proximal segment of the left superior pulmonary vein (a-b) is selected for true cross-sectional reconstruction. The bottom right corner of this image demonstrates the circumferential area of the cross section of the left superior pulmonary vein at the ostium. Figure C15-2C is a virtual angioscopic view of the right wall of the left atrium, demonstrating the ostia of the main and the accessory right-sided pulmonary veins.

Discussion

A revolution has occurred in the treatment of patients with atrial fibrillation since the description by Haisaguerre et al.[10] that 90% of ectopic beats that lead to atrial fibrillation originate in the pulmonary veins. These ectopic foci arise from left atrial myocardial sleeves, which have been shown to extend into the pulmonary veins for 2 to 17 mm.[11]

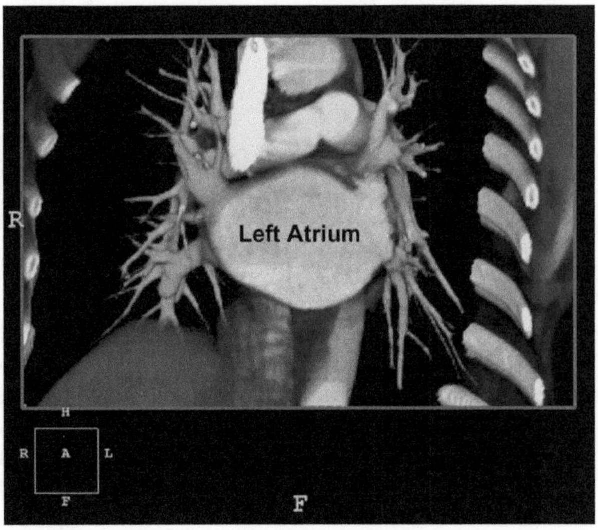

A

FIGURE C15-2. (A)

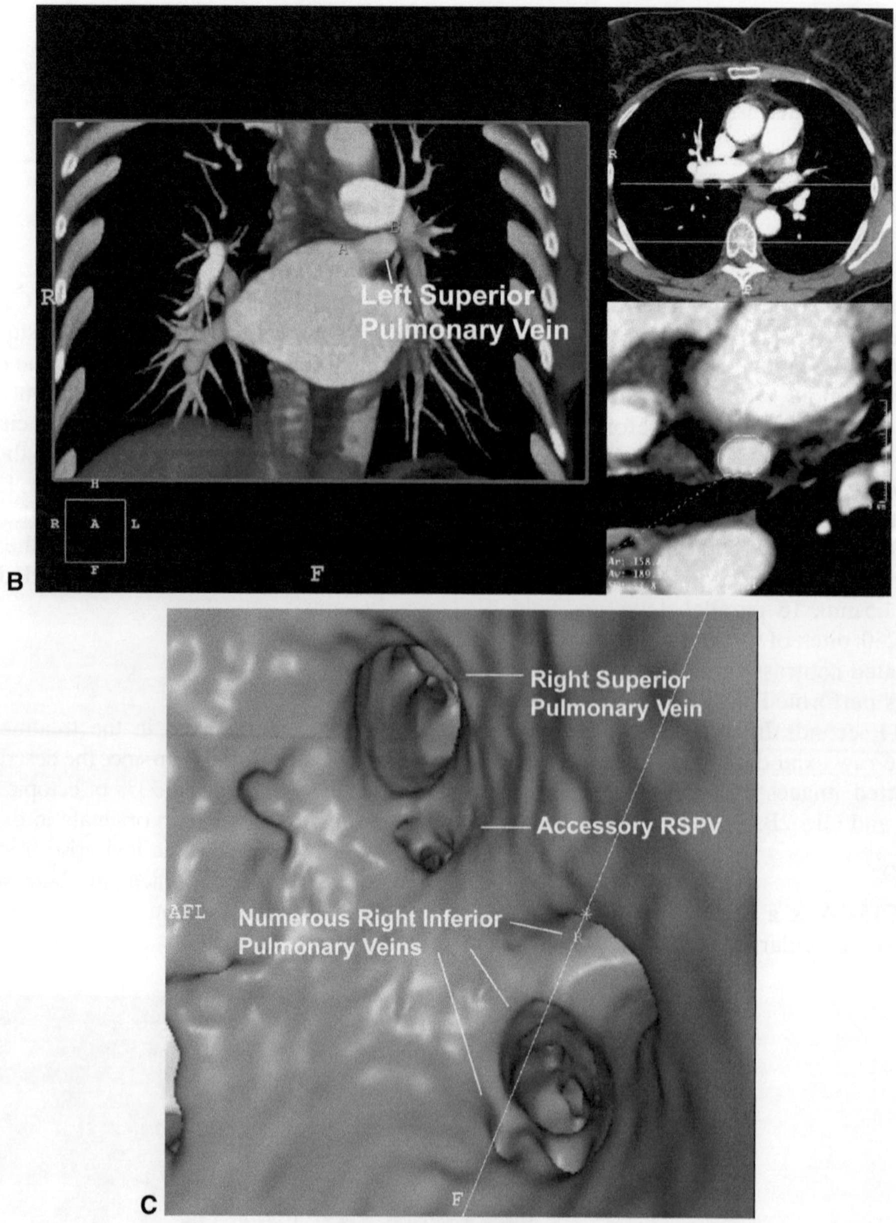

FIGURE C15-2. (B and C)

A new treatment approach involves fluoroscopic isolation of the pulmonary venous ostia and radiofrequency ablation around its circumference to abolish the arrhythmogenic foci. This has been shown to eliminate atrial fibrillation in a majority of patients and provides symptomatic relief in the remainder. The potential complications of this procedure include pulmonary vein stenosis, which can be severe and lead to pulmonary venous hypertension, venous infarction, and pulmonary veno-occlusive disease. Other complications include radiation-related effects, pericardial and/or pleural effusions, stroke, and mediastinitis.[12]

Preablation evaluation with a gated cardiac CT is now being used to measure the diameter, circumference, number, and anomalies of the pulmonary veins. In the same study, mediastinal structures are also evaluated to exclude mass, lymphadenopathy, or vascular anomalies that may complicate the procedure. The cardiac chambers, especially the left atrial appendage (LAA), are studied for excluding thrombus. The three-dimensional representation of the cardiac structures greatly aids the electrophysiologist in planning and preparing for the procedure.

Although there is a wide variation in the size and morphology of the pulmonary venous ostia, a few generalizations can be made based on observational studies. Most of the ectopic foci that lead to atrial fibrillation arise from the superior pulmonary veins, which have a longer and better developed myocardial sleeves than the inferior pulmonary veins.[12] The left-sided pulmonary venous ostia are oval with the short axis oriented in the anteroposterior direction, whereas the right-sided pulmonary veins are more circular.[13] A postablation procedure CT is routinely performed at 3 months to evaluate for possible stenosis. If the patient needed a repeat ablation procedure, the 3-month CT would serve as a new baseline.

Interpretation

Accessory right-sided pulmonary venous ostia in a patient with paroxysmal atrial fibrillation.

Case 15.3

History

A 52-year-old man with a history of deep venous thrombosis, atrial fibrillation, and chest pain was referred for a chest CT angiography to rule out pulmonary embolism. A nongated, breath held, thin section chest CT was performed after intravenous injection of 150 ml of iodinated contrast agent and is displayed in Figures C15-3A and C15-3B.

Findings

Figure C15-3A is an axial section through the left atrium demonstrating a filling defect in the LAA consistent with a thrombus. Figure C15-3B is at a slightly caudal level showing the extension of the thrombus into the left atrial chamber. Figures C15-3C and C15-3D are from a patient with a normal heart. Figure C15-3C is a volume-rendered oblique depiction of a

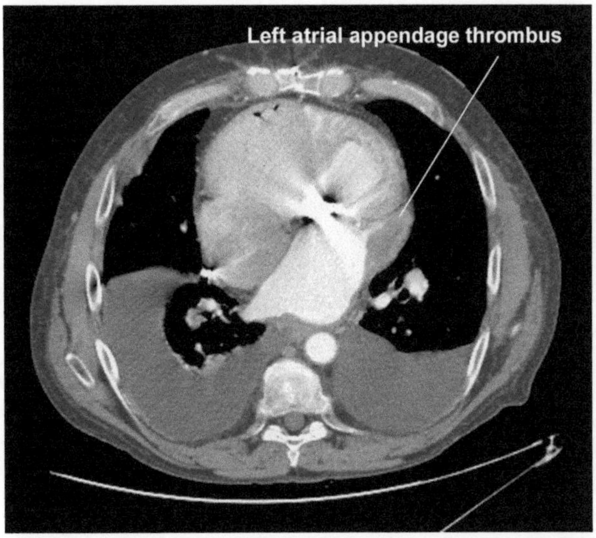

A

FIGURE C15-3. (A)

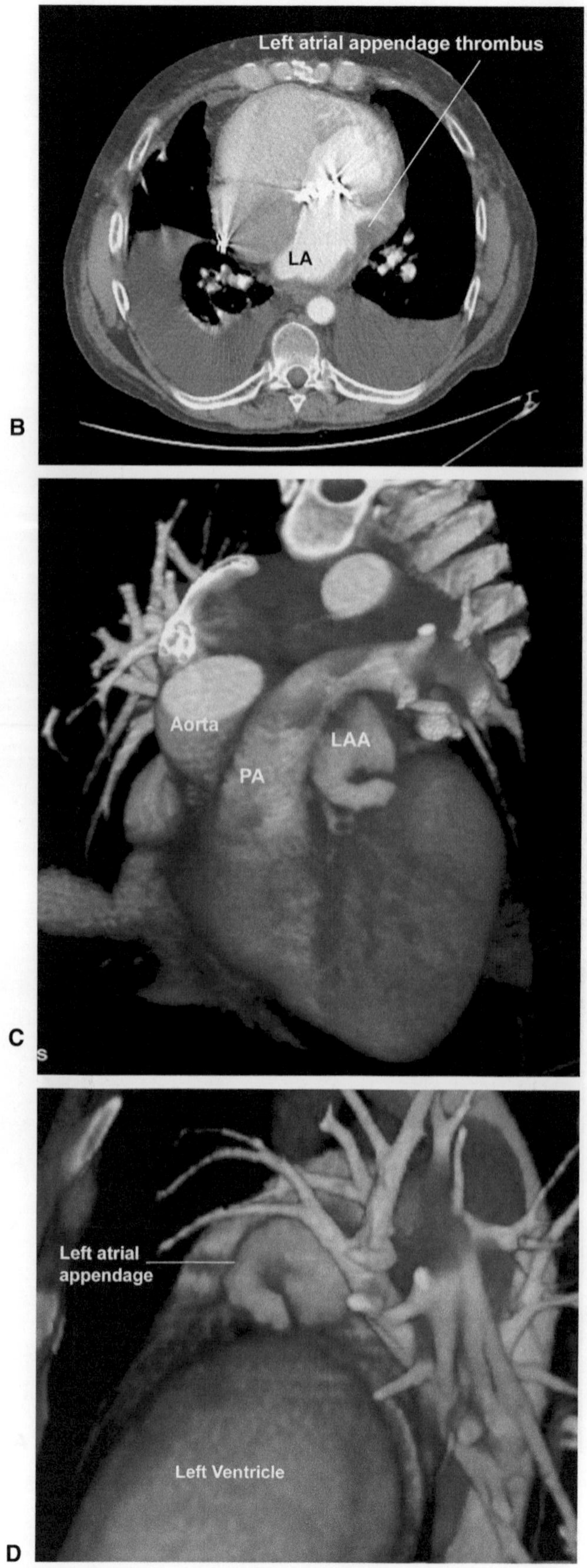

FIGURE C15-3. (B–D)

FIGURE C15-3. (E and F)

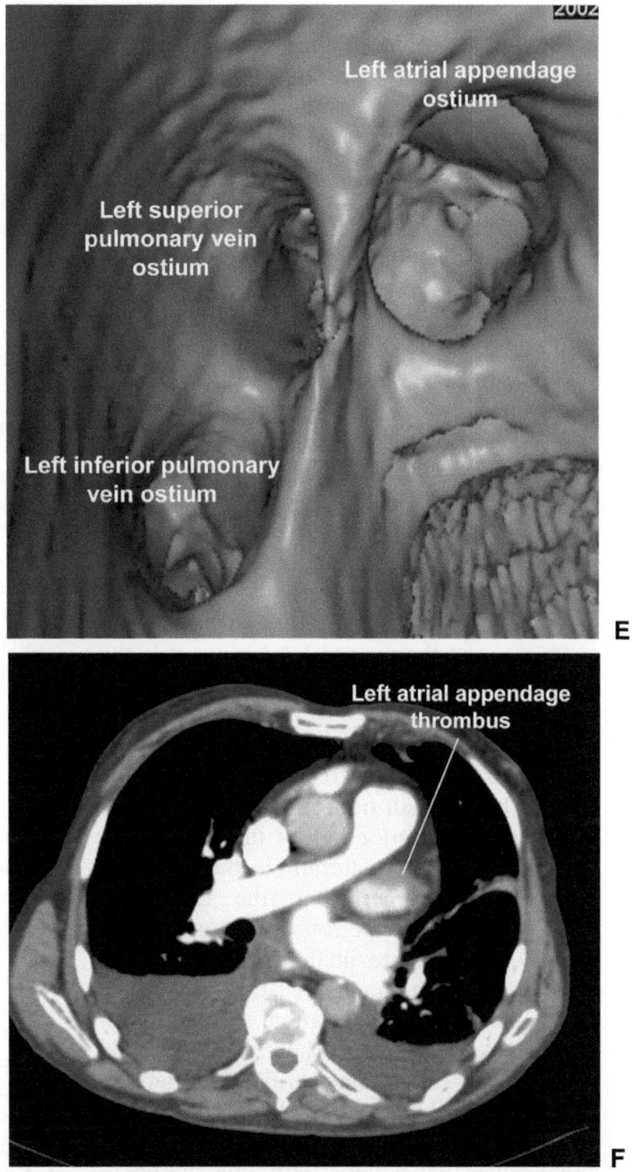

normal heart showing a prominent LAA. Figure C15-3D demonstrates the LAA and the left-sided heart structures in a sagittal view.

Figure C15-3E illustrates a virtual angioscopic depiction of the left wall of the left atrium, the anterosuperior relationship of the ostium of the LAA to that of the left superior pulmonary vein. Figure C15-3F (different patient) is an axial section at the level of the pulmonary artery demonstrating a filling defect in the LAA secondary to a thrombus.

Discussion

Atrial fibrillation is the most common sustained arrhythmia in adults with a prevalence reaching 3% to 5% in people older than 65 years.[14] The LAA is a significant source of cerebral and systemic emboli in these patients. Any thrombus in the left atrium or appendage can potentially have major implications, but the risk of thromboembolism is related to the size and mobility with pedunculated thrombi more than 1.5 cm in length, implying a greater risk.[15] Thrombi may even form after successful electrical or pharmacological cardioversion with prior anticoagulation. The mechanism is known as *stunning* and has been observed with spontaneous, electrical, and pharmacological cardioversion.[16]

Transesophageal echocardiography (TEE) is well established in detecting thrombus in the LAA and evaluating its function, but CT and magnetic resonance imaging (MRI) are often used in patient evaluation and management both before and after diagnosis of the condition. Gated and contrasted CT scans of the chest routinely demonstrate the LAA. It is important to recognize the location and appearance of the normal LAA since it is the site of thrombus formation and potentially devastating emboli.

The LAA is a blind-ended tubular structure continuous with the left atrium but distinguished by its small trabeculations in contrast to the smooth interior wall of the left atrium. The LAA lies anterolaterally in the atrioventricular sulcus superior to the LCX and between the left superior and inferior pulmonary veins. Approximately 55% of LAAs have 2 lobes, with a range of 1 to 4.[17]

The size and configuration of the blind-ending LAA is quite variable, with marked variability in the volume, orifice size, length, shape, and number of lobes. Patients with atrial fibrillation have a larger LAA volume and a larger orifice than patients with sinus rhythm in a postmortem study.[18] The blind end of the appendage and the disordered contraction of the structure during atrial fibrillation predispose patients to thrombus formation.[19]

LAA thrombus on axial contrasted CT images is recognized as a filling defect in the appendage as the clot does not enhance. The filling defect is manifested as a low-density structure within the LAA, outlined by the higher density contrast. The thrombus may be localized in the appendage or extend into the left atrium. The thrombus may also line the wall of the appendage and give the appearance of an abnormally short or truncated appendage. The acquisition of the gated CT is started when the contrast bolus has reached the ascending aorta. This gives adequate time for the mixing of contrasted and noncontrasted blood and therefore accurately characterizes a filling defect as a thrombus.

Interpretation

Left atrial appendage thrombus.

References

1. Ohnesorge B, Fohr T, Becker C, et al. Cardiac imaging by means of electrocardiographically gated multisection spiral CT: initial experience. *Radiology.* 2000;217:564–571.
2. Ropers D, Baum U, Pohle K, et al. Detection of coronary artery stenoses with thin-slice multi-detector row spiral computed tomography and multiplanar reconstruction. *Circulation.* 2003; 107:664–666.
3. Tello R, Hartnell GG, Costello P, Ecker CP. Coronary artery bypass graft flow: qualitative evaluation with cine single detector row CT and comparison with findings at angiography. *Radiology.* 2002;224:913–918.
4. Yamanaka O, Hobbs RE. Coronary artery anomalies in 126,595 patients undergoing coronary angiography. *Cathet Cardiovasc Diagn.* 1990;21:28–40.
5. Maron BJ, Thompson PD, Puffer JC, et al. Cardiovascular preparticipation screening of competitive athletes. *Circulation.* 1996;94:850–856.
6. Lipton MJ, Barry WH, Obrez I, Silverman JF, Wexler L. Isolated single coronary artery: diagnosis, angiographic classification and clinical significance. *Radiology.* 1979;130:39.
7. Cheitlin MD, De Castro CM, McAllister HA. Sudden death as a complication of anomalous left coronary origin from the anterior sinus of Valsalva: a not-so-minor congenital anomaly. *Circulation.* 1974;50:780–787.
8. Robert CW III, Robert WC. Left main coronary artery originating from the right sinus of Valsalva and coursing between aorta and pulmonary trunk. *J Am Coll Cardiol.* 1986;7:366–368.
9. Taylor AJ, Bers JP, Cheitlin MD, et al. Anomalous right or left coronary artery from the contralateral coronary sinus: "high-risk" abnormalities in the initial coronary artery course and

heterogeneous clinical outcomes. *Am Heart J.* 1997;133:428–435.
10. Haisaguerre M, Jais P, Shah DC, et al. Spontaneous initiation of atrial fibrillation by ectopic beats originating in the pulmonary veins. *N Engl J Med.* 1998;339:659–666.
11. Ho SY, Sanchez-Quintana D, Cabrera JA, et al. Anatomy of the left atrium: implications for radiofrequency ablation of atrial fibrillation. *J Cardiovasc Electrophysiol.* 1999;10:1525–1533.
12. Chen SA, Hsieh MH, Tai CT, et al. Initiation of atrial fibrillation by ectopic beats originating from the pulmonary veins: electrophysiological characteristics, pharmacological responses, and effects of radiofrequency ablation. *Circulation.* 1999;100:1879–1886.
13. Wittkamf FH, Vonken EJ, Derksen R, et al. Pulmonary vein ostium geometry—Analysis by magnetic resonance angiography. *Circulation.* 2003;107:21–23.
14. Furberg CD, Psaty BM, Manolio TA, Gardin JM, Smith VE, Rautaharju PM. Prevalence of atrial fibrillation in elderly subjects. *Am J Cardiol.* 1994;74:236–241.
15. Leung DY, Davidson PM, Cranney GB, et al. Thromboembolic risks of left atrial appendage detected by transesophageal echocardiogram. *Am J Cardiol.* 1997;79:626–629.
16. Agmon Y, Khandheria BK, Gentile F, Seward JB. Echocardiographic assessment of the left atrial appendage. *J Am Coll Cardiol.* 1999;34: 1867–1877.
17. Veinot JP, Harrity PJ, Gentile F, et al. Anatomy of the normal left atrial appendage: a quantitative study of age-related changes in 500 autopsy hearts: implications for echocardiographic examination. *Circulation.* 1997;96:3112–3115.
18. Ernst G, Stollberger C, Abzieher F, et al. Morphology of the left atrial appendage. *The Anatomical Record.* 1995;242:553–561.
19. Al-Saady NM, Obel OA, Camm, AJ. Left atrial appendage: structure, function, and role in thromboembolism. *Heart.* 1999 Nov;82(5):547–554.

16
Correlation of Nuclear Cardiology with Stress Echocardiography

João V. Vitola, Wilson Mathias, Jr., José Claudio Meneghetti, and Dominique Delbeke

In the last two decades there has been extensive discussion about the advantages and limitations of nuclear imaging using stress myocardial perfusion imaging (MPI) single photon emission computed tomography (SPECT) compared with stress echocardiography. Since their early descriptions, the quality of the images and diagnostic accuracy of both modalities improved significantly with still evolving technological developments. Both imaging modalities have been extensively investigated as noninvasive tools to diagnose and estimate prognosis in coronary artery disease (CAD) and to evaluate myocardial viability.

Nuclear imaging allows evaluation of myocardial perfusion with SPECT during rest and stress as well as evaluation of wall motion with the gated technique at rest and in the post-stress period. The nuclear imaging literature and to a lesser degree the echocardiographic literature contain data on all patient populations including men, women, patients of different age groups, patients with hypertension, left bundle block, diabetes, different exercise tolerance, different pretest likelihood of disease, single or multivessel disease, post revascularization, and post myocardial infarction (MI). Outcome data on thousands of patients over many years of follow-up have been analyzed using qualitative, semiquantitative and quantitative analysis.

The combination of stress and 2-D echocardiography allows evaluation of the contractility of myocardial segment at rest and during stress. A review of stress echocardiography has recently been published.[1] To understand the basis of this technique it is imperative to remember the ischemic cascade, in which myocardial ischemia starts with an impairment in coronary flow reserve under stress, followed by alterations of cell metabolism, then impaired diastolic function, and finally, wall motion abnormalities that can be detected on echocardiography. Recent advances in equipment, including the second harmonic and the use of myocardial ultrasonic contrast agents, have increased the accuracy of echocardiography, allowing a better definition of LV borders and providing additional information on myocardial perfusion.[2] Echocardiography has advanced into the use of sophisticated equipments, allowing 3-D evaluation of the heart although the application of 3-D echocardiography is still investigational at the time of this writing.[3]

Stress Modalities and Protocols for Echocardiography

Physical exercise, dipyridamole (plus atropine), dobutamine (plus atropine), and transesophageal atrial pacing have all been applied as stressors for echocardiography. These modalities have different mechanisms of actions, as discussed in Chapter 4. The two most widely used forms of stress are physical exercise and dobutamine. Exercise echocardiography is in fact usually performed in the early post-exercise period when the image quality is better. Since recovery of LV function may occur rapidly after exercise, exercise should be reserved for those able to achieve 100% of maximum predicted heart rate (HR) to avoid missing the ischemic period at the time of imaging. Compared with nuclear imaging, this is a limitation of exercise echocardiography. Radiopharmaceuticals (especially ^{99m}Tc-based agents) are injected and distribute at peak stress and the images can be acquired later, with no compromise of diagnostic accuracy.

However, when properly performed, exercise and dobutamine stress echocardiography yield similar diagnostic accuracy.[4–6] On the other hand, dipyridamole stress has a lower sensitivity. This difference may be related to a lower sensitivity of dipyridamole echocardiography to detect single vessel disease. In a study of 100 patients who underwent stress echocardiography with the three stress methods, the overall sensitivity to detect CAD was 52% for dipyridamole compared with 72% for dobutamine and 76% for exercise.[5] In a metaanalysis pooling studies addressing the methodology, feasibility, safety, and diagnostic accuracy of dobutamine stress echocardiography, the overall sensitivity of dobutamine stress echocardiography was 80%.[6]

The mechanism of action of dobutamine and the contraindications have been discussed in Chapter 4. In this chapter the emphasis is on the application of dobutamine stress to echocardiography. Dobutamine is a fast-acting drug with the effect starting 2 minutes into infusion. Drug clearance occurs predominantly by the liver, with a short plasma half-life of approximately 2 minutes.[7,8] It activates beta-1 receptors in the heart causing increased HR and myocardial contractility, with hemodynamic effects depending highly on the dose infused.[9] At low doses (5 to 10 mcg·kg·min^{-1}) dobutamine activates beta-1 and alpha-1 receptors, increasing myocardial contractility without significant effects on HR. At doses greater than 10 to 20 mcg·kg·min^{-1}, dobutamine activates beta-1 and beta-2 receptors, increasing HR, contractility, and myocardial blood flow. At doses greater than 30 mcg·kg·min^{-1}, dobutamine increases the development of ventricular arrhythmias in approximately 30% of cases. Dobutamine also causes a reduction of systemic vascular resistance mediated by activation of the beta-2 receptors and may cause a vasovagal reaction. Both of these effects may cause the blood pressure (BP) to drop in approximately 10% of the cases. Early administration of atropine during infusion of dobutamine (at the dose of 20 mcg·kg·min^{-1}) allows it to reach the target HR earlier, minimizing the vasovagal effects and hypotension.[10,11] Recent data support the administration of beta-blockers at the end of the dobutamine infusion (given as an intravenous [IV] bolus), improving the detection of CAD in some patients.[12] An example of a dobutamine/atropine/metoprolol protocol is shown in Figure 16-1.[12]

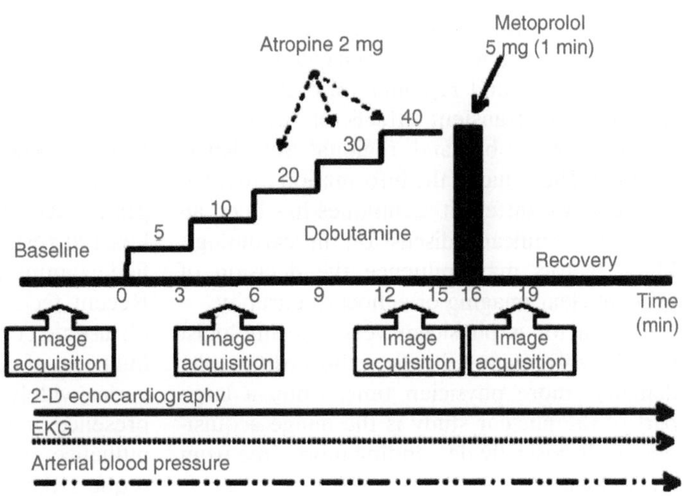

FIGURE 16-1. Dobutamine-atropine stress echocardiography-metoprolol protocol. EKG = electrocardiogram. (From Mathias Jr W, Tsusui JM, Andrade JL et al. [12], by permission of *J Am Coll Cardiol.*)

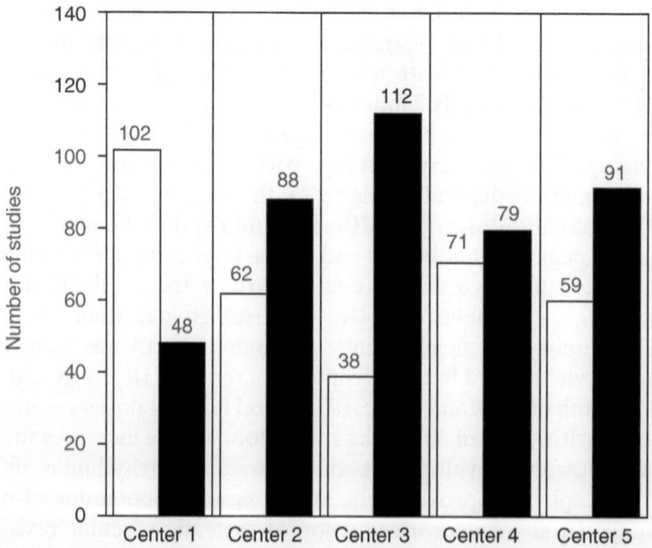

FIGURE 16-2. Observer variability: Evaluation of negativity (solid bars) versus positivity (open bars) for 150 dobutamine stress echocardiograms by institution. Number above bars = number of patients. (From Hoffmann R, Lethen H, Marwick T, et al. [13], by permission from *J Am Coll Cardiol.*)

Comparison of Stress Nuclear Imaging and Stress Echocardiography

Stress nuclear imaging and stress echocardiography differ with each other, considering the parameters evaluated to diagnose and establish prognosis in CAD. Nuclear imaging evaluates myocardial perfusion during maximal or near maximal vasodilatation, testing coronary artery blood flow reserve (CBFR) and evaluating LV function with the gated technique following stress. Echocardiography evaluates real-time resting and exercise or pharmacologic stress-induced global and regional ventricular function and the transient effects of myocardial ischemia on global and regional ventricular function. The value of the information provided by these two different techniques has been an issue of significant discussion in cardiology. Many factors may influence the decision of using nuclear imaging or echocardiography.

One factor is physician versus technologist time involvement. Stress echocardiography demands more physician time, while a large part of the nuclear study is the image acquisition itself, basically demanding more time from technologists.

The second factor is the issue of interobserver and intraobserver variability with echocardiography (Figure 16-2),[13] which is a subject of ongoing debate, but seems to have improved with better equipment and the use of ultrasonic contrast agents (Figure 16-3).[14]

The third factor is the issue of cost depending highly on the health care system, cost of equipment and personnel in different countries, and whether or not a comprehensive morphological examination of the heart is performed at rest, generating a separate bill. Echocardiography offers the advantage of the possibility of a comprehensive morphological evaluation of the heart at rest, providing, for example, detailed information on valves, chamber diameters and volumes, and myocardial wall thickness. However, sometimes stress echocardiography does not include a comprehensive morphological examination of the heart at rest. What is usually done is a simplified examination of ventricular function at rest. Recent technological developments, including ultrasonic contrast agents, certainly add to the final cost of echocardiography. Reimbursement varies widely from country to country and the presence or absence of financial incentives may influence the numbers and the type of tests requested.

The fourth factor is availability. Echocardiography is more widely available than nuclear imaging, and the equipment can be used for other diagnostic applications, which is attractive in terms of cost-benefit. State-of-the-art nuclear imaging today requires equipment with tomographic capabilities built with complex technology to detect ionizing radiation. The use of radioisotopes with nuclear imaging carries several implications from the regulatory and technical standpoint, which can be limiting factors.

Each of these imaging modalities suffers from limitations related to patients themselves. The acoustic window has to be adequate to visualize well all myocardial segments with echocardiography, which can be a significant limitation in patients with chronic obstructive pulmonary disease (COPD) and obesity. Acoustic window, of course, is not an issue with nuclear imaging, but soft tissue attenuation may be a problem in the obese or those with large breasts, limiting the specificity. Patients with LV hypertrophy seem to be at an increased risk of having a false-negative stress echocardiography result,[15] especially when significant concentric remodeling and small LV cavity size are present.[16] Small ventricles pose a problem for nuclear imaging as well, since small perfusion defects can be missed due to scatter between myocardial segments and LV ejection fraction may be overestimated.

Comparing test accuracy several issues should be considered. First, technological advances occur rapidly. The advances in nuclear imaging include SPECT versus planar imaging, the use of ^{99m}Tc-perfusion agents versus ^{201}Tl, semiquantitative versus visual analysis, and gated versus nongated imaging techniques. The advances in echocardiography include the use of different signal harmonics and the use or not of ultrasonic contrast agents to better define LV borders and to evaluate myocardial perfusion in addition to wall motion abnormalities. Few studies are available in the literature comparing the two imaging modalities in the same patient population to avoid biases in patient selection and technical factors.[17] This issue

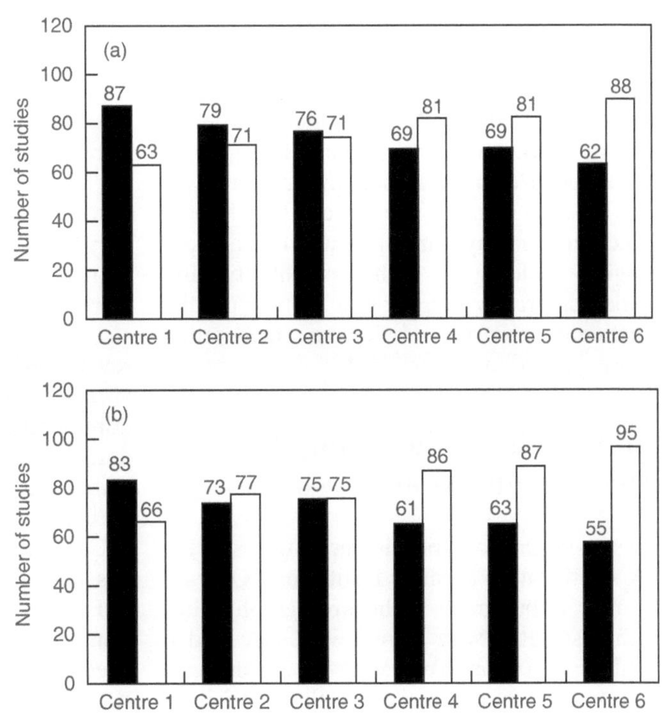

FIGURE 16-3. Observer variability: Evaluation of positivity (solid bars) versus negativity (open bars) for 150 dobutamine stress echocardiograms by institution. Number above bars = number of patients. The upper panel (a) relates to assessment using harmonic imaging, the lower panel (b) relates to fundamental imaging. (From Hoffman R, Marwick TH, Poldermans D, et al. [14], by permission of *Eur Heart J.*)

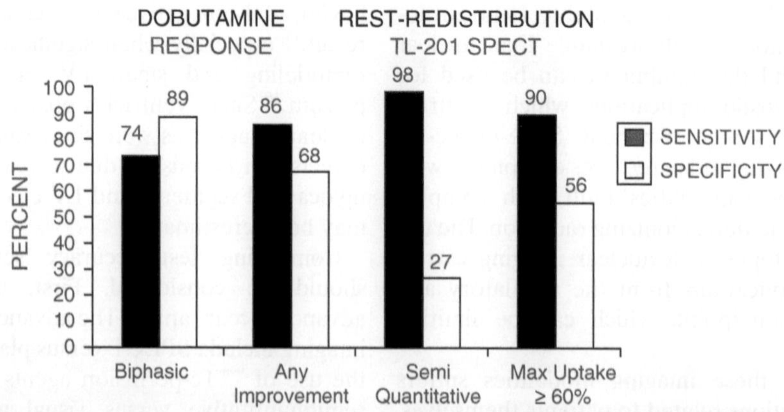

FIGURE 16-4. Sensitivity and specificity of dobutamine echocardiography and rest-redistribution thallium tomography for recovery of segmental function. Any improvement indicates biphasic response or sustained improvement response. SPECT = single photon emission tomography; Max = maximum at rest or during redistribution. (From Qureshi U, Nagueh S, Afridi I, et al. [28], by permission of *Circulation*.)

becomes even more important when attempting to pool data from different studies or performing meta-analyses, as it becomes extremely complex to control for all these factors. Considering these limitations, several comparative studies have been published in the literature over the past two decades.[18–27] Most of these studies concluded that nuclear imaging techniques are more sensitive (more true-positive and/or fewer false-negative results) for detection of CAD, whereas echocardiography is more specific (more true-negative and/or fewer false-positive results). The same is true for the detection of myocardial viability, nuclear imaging yielding a higher sensitivity and echocardiography a higher specificity to predict functional recovery following myocardial revascularization (Figure 16-4).[28]

Stress Echocardiography for Risk Stratification

Stress echocardiography is currently used for risk stratification at many institutions. Overall, normal dobutamine echocardiography has been associated with a low event rate and a death rate of approximately 1% per year. Elderly patients, and patients with heart failure and significant LV remodeling following MI are at a higher risk, even in the presence of a nonischemic stress echocardiogram.[29] Similar prognostic data are available with other forms of stress applied to echocardiography, such as exercise[30] and dipyridamole.[31]

The pattern of ischemic findings on both MPI SPECT and echocardiography can be used for risk stratification. With echocardiography, the pattern of contractility in response to dobutamine (indicating scar, ischemia, or both), the number of vascular territories (1, 2, or 3), and the time to ischemia (ischemic threshold) may be used for risk assessment.[29] The presence of resting wall motion abnormalities, such as in patients with a prior MI, is a limitation in stress echocardiography. The presence of severe dysfunction due to large MI may prevent visualization of the full inotropic effects of dobutamine resulting in a lower sensitivity to detect ischemia in the territory containing some viable and ischemic tissue mixed with large amounts of scar tissue.

Cardiac risk stratification using MPI SPECT has been discussed in Chapter 9. With MPI SPECT, the degree and extent of hypoperfusion, the pattern of hypoperfusion (reversible, fixed, or mixed), the location, the degree of stress-induced LV dysfunction, and the presence of lung tracer uptake can be used for risk assessment.

Evaluation of Myocardial Viability

The issue of myocardial viability, including nuclear imaging, echocardiography, and magnetic resonance imaging, has been discussed in details in Chapter 8. In the current chapter we emphasize the aspects that are pertinent to stress echocardiography in correlation with nuclear imaging.

The contribution of various myocardial layers to myocardial contractility, from the inner (subendocardium) to the outer (subepicardium), is not uniform. At rest, more than 60% of the contractility occurs from thickening of the inner 30% of the myocardium (the subendocardial region).[32,33] This issue is illustrated in Figure 16-5.[32] One situation in which this may become an important issue is in a patient with a prior MI. In a nontransmural MI, involving, for example, 20% of the myocardial thickness (the subendocardial layer), the resting echocardiogram may demonstrate an akinetic wall, which cannot be differentiated from a transmural MI.[33] This explains why many patients with evidence of myocardial viability by nuclear imaging do not have significant wall motion recovery following revascularization, despite a significant improvement in functional capacity.[34] This fact may also explain why echocardiography is less sensitive to detect myocardial viability compared with the nuclear techniques, despite having a higher specificity [28,35] (see Figure 16-4).

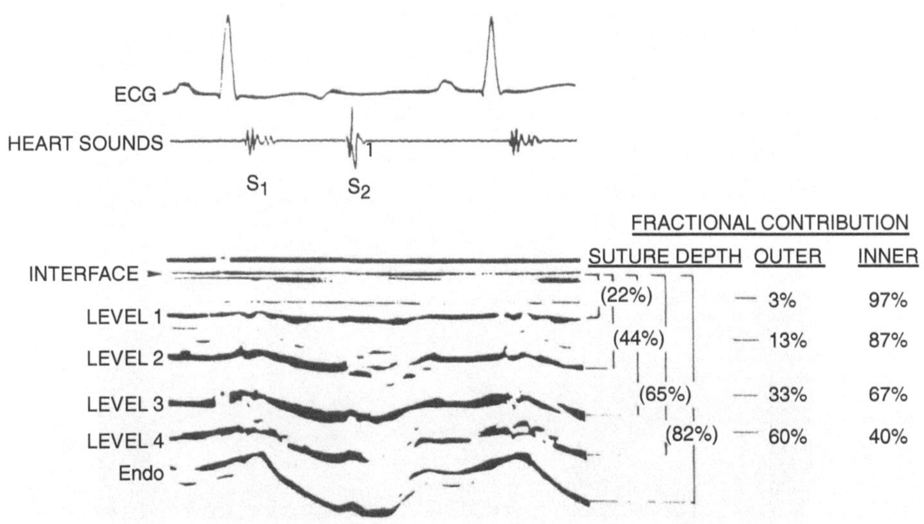

FIGURE 16-5. Example of echocardiographic tracings from one experiment in which four sutures were placed in the myocardial wall to serve as echo targets. The demonstration was feasible in this animal (dog) because of its large size (36 kg) and, frankly, the serendipitous placement of the sutures with minimal myocardial trauma. The fractional contributions (to total thickening) of the inner and outer wall, defined at different depths by the four sutures, are illustrated on the right side of the figure. A gradient of wall thickening is evident, increasing from the epicardium to the endocardium, in close agreement with the combined results from all the experiments. The term INTERFACE refers to the epicardium and ENDO refers to the endocardial surface. (From Lieberman AN, Weiss JL, Jugdutt BI, et al. [33], by permission of *Circulation*.)

Case Presentations

Case 16.1

History

An elderly man is evaluated for atypical chest pain, and as part of a research protocol underwent both an adenosine/redistribution ^{201}Tl SPECT gated study and a dobutamine stress echocardiography (quad screen format of an apical four-chamber view at end-systole) as displayed in Figure C16-1.

Findings

The adenosine ^{201}Tl SPECT images demonstrated decreased uptake in the inferior wall, anteroseptal region, and apex, which improves after redistribution consistent with myocardial ischemia. The poststress gated study revealed inferior and apical hypokinesis.

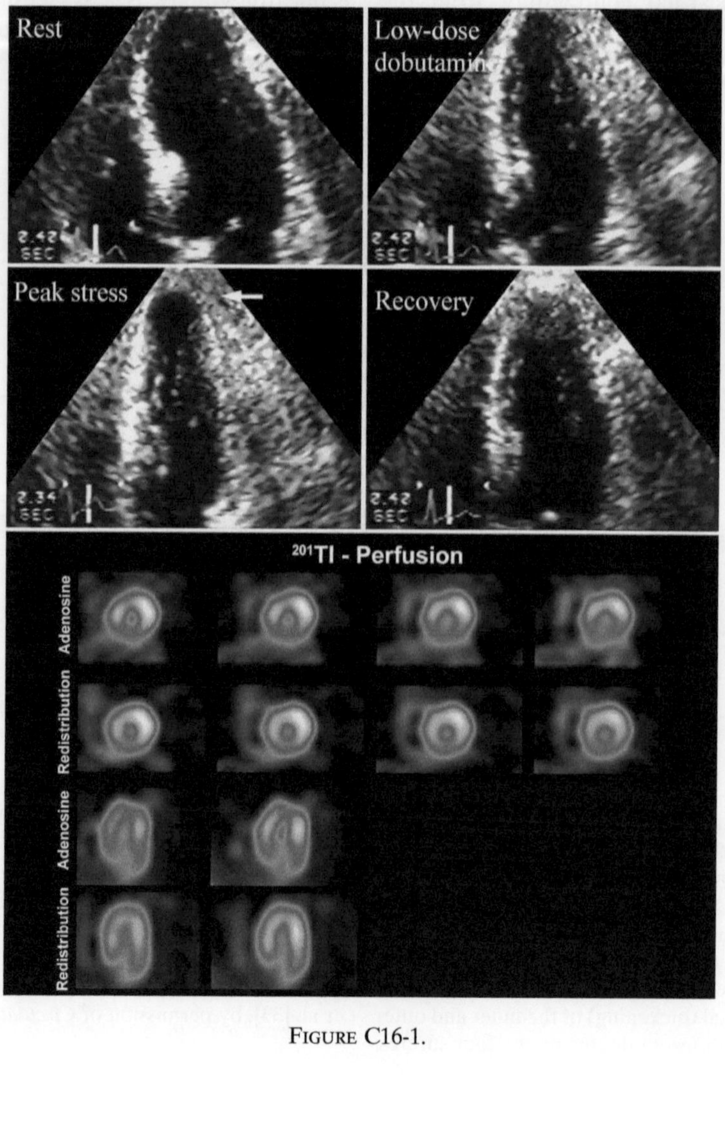

FIGURE C16-1.

Dobutamine stress echocardiography (quad screen format of an apical 4-chamber view at end systole) demonstrated normal LV function at rest (upper left quadrant) and with low-dose dobutamine (upper right quadrant). At peak stress (left lower quadrant) there was apical dyskinesis (arrow), which normalized during the recovery phase (right lower quadrant). Coronary angiography demonstrated 90% stenosis in the left anterior descending coronary artery (LAD) and 75% stenosis in the right coronary artery (RCA).

Discussion

This patient presented with atypical chest pain and was referred for evaluation of the presence of CAD. Both the stress/rest SPECT gated study and dobutamine stress echocardiography revealed multivessel ischemia. Dobutamine echocardiography demonstrated severe ischemic changes in apex with dyskinesis at 7:30 minutes into dobutamine infusion with an HR of 120 bpm, which implies severe ischemic changes in the LAD distribution. The echocardiographic study also demonstrated minor signs of ischemia in the inferior wall with dobutamine-induced hypokinesis (not shown). The severe new wall motion abnormality at low ischemic threshold has a prognostic significance associated with high risk for adverse cardiac events.

Interpretation

Myocardial ischemia in two-vessel territories (LAD and RCA) identified with stress/rest gated SPECT and dobutamine stress echocardiography.

Case 16.2

History

A 50-year-old asymptomatic woman presented for preoperative evaluation before renal transplantation. A 12-lead resting ECG revealed LV repolarization abnormalities. A dipyridamole/rest ^{99m}Tc-MIBI gated SPECT study and dobutamine stress echocardiography (quad screen format of an apical four-chamber view at end-systole) are displayed in Figure C16-2.

Findings

The dipyridamole/rest SPECT images demonstrated a moderate severity and small size partially reversible perfusion defect in the distal inferolateral region. The gated study revealed an LVEF of 43% and distal inferolateral hypokinesis. Dobutamine stress echocardiography demonstrated (quad screen format of an apical four-chamber view at and end-systole) normal LV function at rest (upper left quadrant) and during low-dose dobutamine (upper right quadrant). At peak stress (left lower quadrant), there was a hyperdynamic response to dobutamine that was within normal range.

Discussion

In myocardial ischemia, perfusion abnormalities occur before contractile dysfunction. As myocardial ischemia becomes more severe, wall motion abnormalities develop that can be detected with stress echocardiography. In addition, a hyperdynamic response at peak dobutamine infusion may make regional contractile dysfunction difficult to identify, especially if the ischemic region with contractile dysfunction is small, such as in the present case. A bolus dose of metoprolol at the end of the dobutamine infusion has been shown to increase the sensitivity of stress echocardiography.[12]

Interpretation

Myocardial ischemia in a small myocardial region identified with dipyridamole/rest SPECT gated study but masked by a hyperdynamic response of the LV to dobutamine with echocardiography.

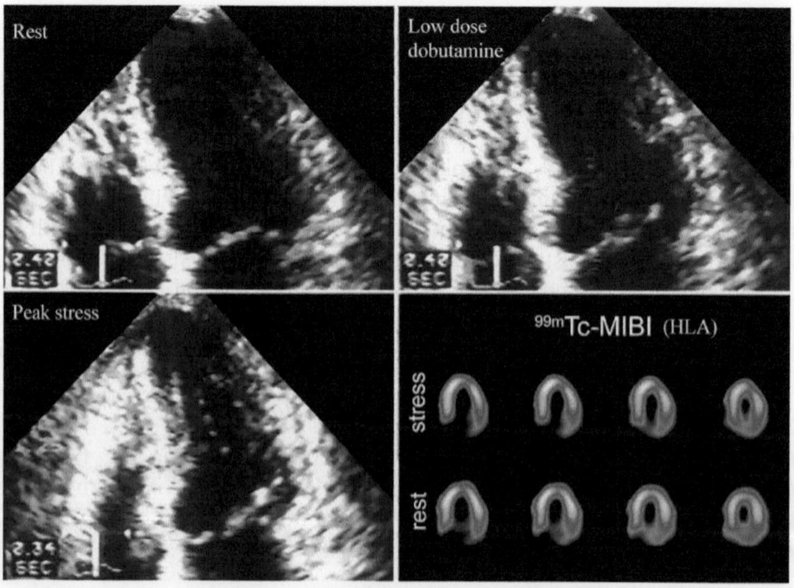

FIGURE C16-2.

Case 16.3

History

A 54-year-old man presented for preoperative evaluation before carotid surgery. His past medical history included hypertension, hypercholesterolemia, smoking, surgical correction of an abdominal aorta aneurysm 5 years earlier, and coronary artery bypass graft (CABG) surgery 2 years earlier. He underwent placement of a left internal mammary artery (LIMA) to the LAD and a saphenous graft to the RCA. Clinically, he was asymptomatic. He underwent adenosine stress echocardiography with microbubbles as the ultrasonic contrast agent (Figure C16-3A) at an outside facility and a rest/exercise gated SPECT ^{99m}Tc-MIBI study (Figure C16-3B). He exercised on the treadmill using a standard Bruce protocol for 11 minutes, reaching 83% of MPHR at peak exercise. He denied chest pain and his ECG showed new 3-mm downsloping ST-segment depression in leads V5–6, II, III, and AVF. His ECG was still positive 6 minutes into recovery.

Findings

The adenosine echocardiogram showed stress-induced hypoperfusion of the middle and basal anterior wall (Figure C16-3A, arrow). The inferior wall appeared normally perfused. There was no report on wall motion abnormalities.

The exercise/rest MPI SPECT showed a moderate to severe perfusion defect in the inferior wall and inferolateral region that was partially reversible on the resting images consistent with inferior nontransmural MI and peri-infarct ischemia (Figure C16-3B). In addition, there was mild to moderate anteroseptal, septal, and apical partially reversible defect consistent with ischemia. The gated SPECT images (not shown) revealed an LVEF of 35% with global hypokinesia worse in the inferior wall, and LV dilatation with an end-diastolic volume (EDV) of 175 ml and end-systolic volume (ESV) of 113 ml.

The coronary angiography revealed a patent graft to the LAD but a severe obstruction

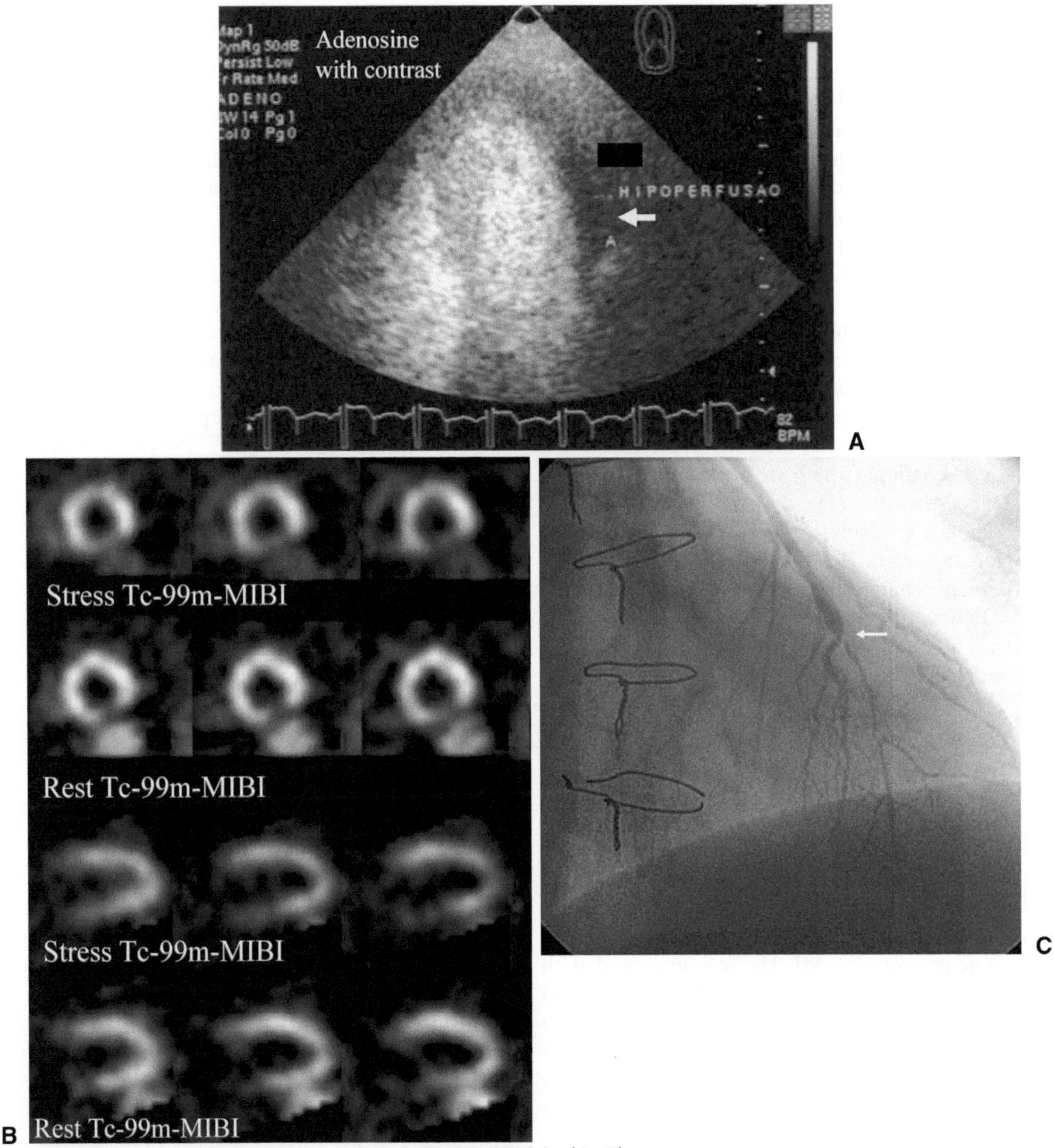

FIGURE C16-3. (A–C)

distal to the anastomosis (Figure C16-3C, arrow). The RCA was occluded and the saphenous graft to the RCA was patent but supplying only the distal inferior wall. The ventriculogram revealed akinesia of the basal and mid inferior wall.

Discussion

One of the most valuable contributions of nuclear cardiology relates to its ability to accurately stratify cardiac risk. This is especially true when all the available information is taken into consideration, such as the clinical history (risk factors and co-morbidities) and the results from the treadmill exercise test and MPI SPECT study. The SPECT, in the case presented, images provided several findings consistent with increased risk for adverse cardiac events: (1) large perfusion defects, (2) hypoperfusion in more than one coronary artery territory, (3) the presence of both fixed and reversible defects, (4) increased LV volume, especially end-systolic volume, and (5) a depressed LVEF. These are all independent indicators of increased risk for cardiac death or MI. The Duke treadmill score was minus 9, indicating intermediate risk for cardiac events. However, there are other factors that indicate an increased risk for this patient (which are not considered in the Duke score): (1) depressed chronotropic response to exercise, (2) ST-segment depression in several leads, and (3) prolonged ST-segment changes into recovery (>6 minutes).

Echocardiography with microbubbles contrast is a new diagnostic imaging modality, still under investigation, which consists of injecting adenosine intravenously to promote vasodilation, while sonicated microbubbles are continuously infused intravenously to serve as a contrast agent, attempting to evaluate myocardial perfusion and define LV borders. Areas of ischemia should appear darker than the normally perfused myocardium, as shown in Figure C16-3A.

In the present case, MPI SPECT revealed several predictors of increased risk for cardiac events (including ischemia in more than one vascular territory) that were not evident by echocardiography. Additionally, the exercise test performed during MPI added some additional information known to predict increased risk for cardiac events.

Interpretation

Multivessel (LAD and RCA) ischemia detected with exercise/rest gated SPECT and LAD ischemia detected with contrast-enhanced adenosine echocardiography.

Case 16.4

History

A 79-year-old man with known CAD and remote inferior MI presented with a 6-hour onset of chest pain and was diagnosed as having an acute anterior MI. He was managed with thrombolytics. His rest ECG demonstrated Q waves inferiorly and anteriorly. His rest echocardiogram showed global severe ventricular dysfunction with akinesia of the inferior wall as well as the apical, septal, and anterior wall. The LVEF was estimated to be 29%. The stress/ rest SPECT images and rest echocardiography with ultrasonic contrast (apical two-chamber view) are displayed in Figure C16-4.

Findings

The stress/rest SPECT images demonstrated a dilated LV with a severe fixed perfusion defect in the anterior wall and apex consistent with the acute anterior wall MI. There is also a moderate fixed decreased perfusion in the inferoseptal region consistent with the remote MI.

The echocardiographic study was performed within the first 24 hours after acute MI and the image demonstrated the ultrasonic contrast agent in the left ventricular cavity and a large area of severe hypoperfusion in the anterior wall consistent with a *no-reflow* phenomenon (Figure C16-4, arrow). There is also a small area of thinning in the inferobasal segment related to the old MI. This patient has developed LV remodeling and his LVEF was 24% at 6 months follow-up.

Discussion

This case illustrates the application of echocardiography during the acute phase of MI in determining not only LV function, but also the possibility of early diagnosis of the no-reflow

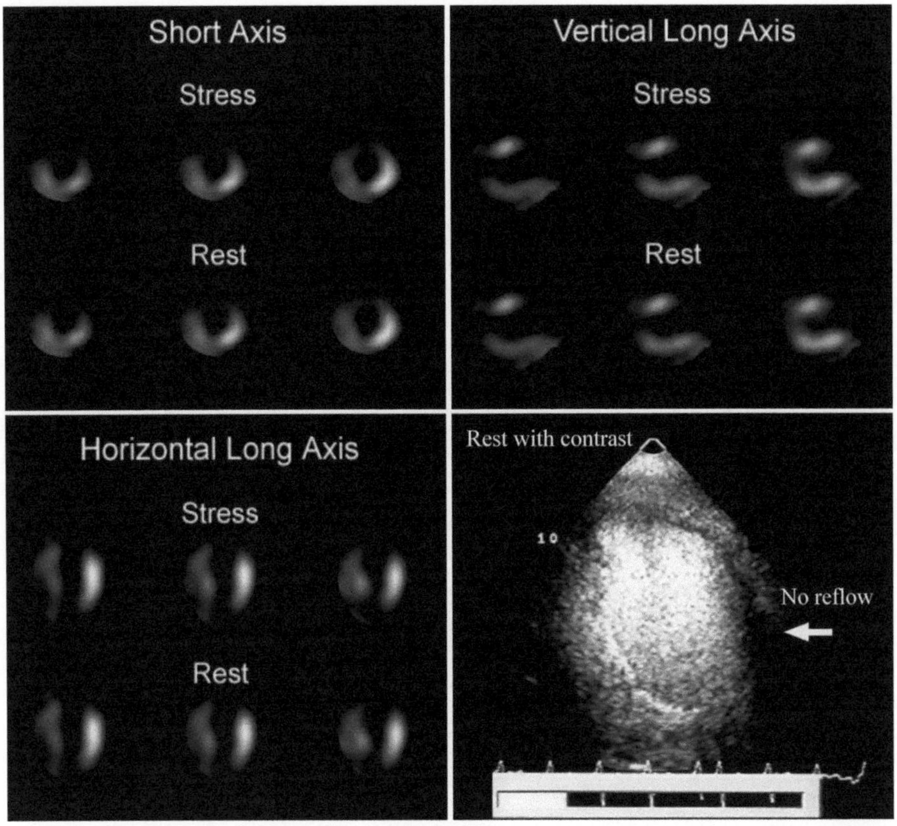

FIGURE C16-4.

phenomenon after revascularization by a qualitative analysis of microvascular integrity provided by microbubble contrast agent. During acute MI, the immediate therapeutic goal is to restore blood flow by reestablishing the patency of the culprit vessel. However, this does not mean that nutritive flow is provided to the myocardium because structural microvascular disruption can occur (no-reflow phenomenon). The extent no-reflow usually parallels the extent of necrosis and therefore can predict the degree of myocardial salvage after treatment. The no-reflow phenomenon has significant implications regarding recovery of function and clinical outcome.[36,37] In a study of 199 patients with anterior wall MI who underwent successful coronary reperfusion within 24 hours after the onset of acute MI, the development of no-reflow phenomenon evaluated with myocardial contrast echocardiography was related to the severity of myocardial damage, the size of the risk area, and the occlusion status of the infarct-related artery.[38] The no-reflow phenomenon can also be evaluated using myocardial perfusion SPECT.[39]

Interpretation

Extensive acute anterior wall MI with no-reflow phenomenon demonstrated with myocardial contrast echocardiography and SPECT.

Case 16.5

History

A 60-year-old woman with a history of smoking, diabetes mellitus, hypertension, and hyperlipidemia presented with recent onset of chest pain. She underwent a dipyridamole/rest SPECT ^{99m}Tc-MIBI study and an adenosine stress echocardiography with ultrasonic contrast displayed in Figures C16-5A and C16-5B (apical two-chamber view), respectively.

Findings

The dipyridamole/rest SPECT ^{99m}Tc-MIBI images (Figure C16-10A) demonstrated moderate inferior wall and apical hypoperfusion after dipyridamole infusion that improves on the resting images. The apical 2-chamber view of real-time myocardial perfusion echocardiogram (low mechanical index) demonstrated normal perfusion in all myocardial walls at rest and adenosine-induced hypoperfusion in the inferior wall and in a focal area of the anteroapical segment (Figure C16-5B, upper left: black subendocardial line). Coronary angiography revealed a 70 % stenosis in LAD and 100% stenosis in RCA with collaterals from the LAD.

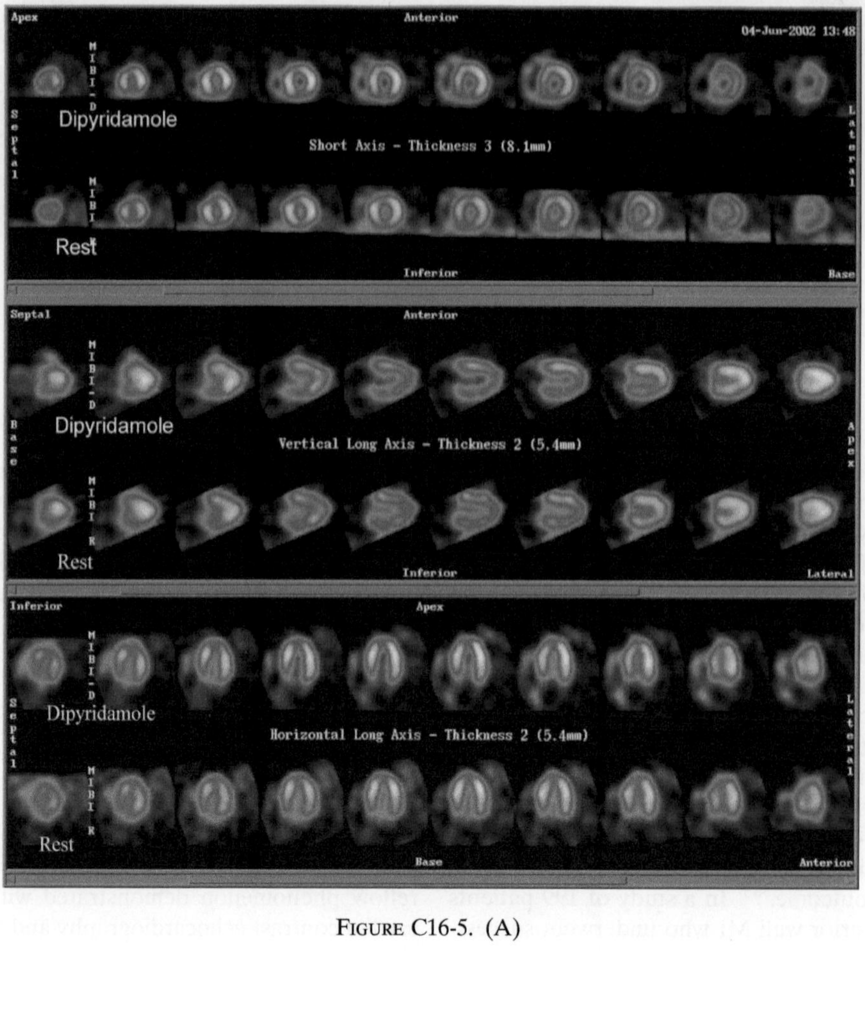

A

FIGURE C16-5. (A)

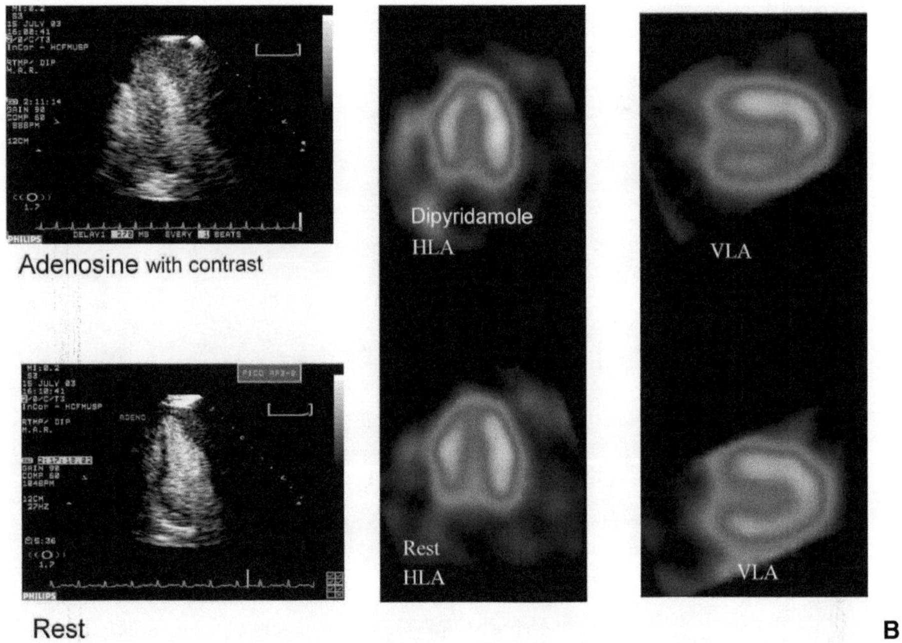

FIGURE C16-5. (B)

Discussion

This case illustrates how qualitative myocardial perfusion echocardiography using adenosine stress with ultrasonic contrast can enhance the ability to detect CAD. In this particular case, the patient had no adenosine-induced wall motion abnormality, but adenosine-induced hypoperfusion could be seen in inferior wall (RCA distribution) and in apical wall (LAD distribution) on the echocardiographic images with ultrasonic contrast as well as on the dipyridamole SPECT images.

Interpretation

Two-vessel CAD detected with both dipyridamole/rest SPECT and adenosine stress echocardiography with ultrasonic contrast, whereas there was no stress-induced wall motion abnormality on echocardiography.

Case 16.6

History

A 75-year-old man with history of smoking presented with chest pain at low level exercise in the past 2 months. He underwent a dipyridamole/rest SPECT ^{99m}Tc-MIBI study and an adenosine stress echocardiography with ultrasonic contrast displayed in Figures 16-6A and 16-6B (apical four-chamber view), respectively. Parametric images of perfusion during echocardiography were generated (Figure C16-6B, middle panel).

Findings

The dipyridamole/rest SPECT images (Figure C16-6A) demonstrated normal myocardial perfusion in anterior wall and moderate hypoper-

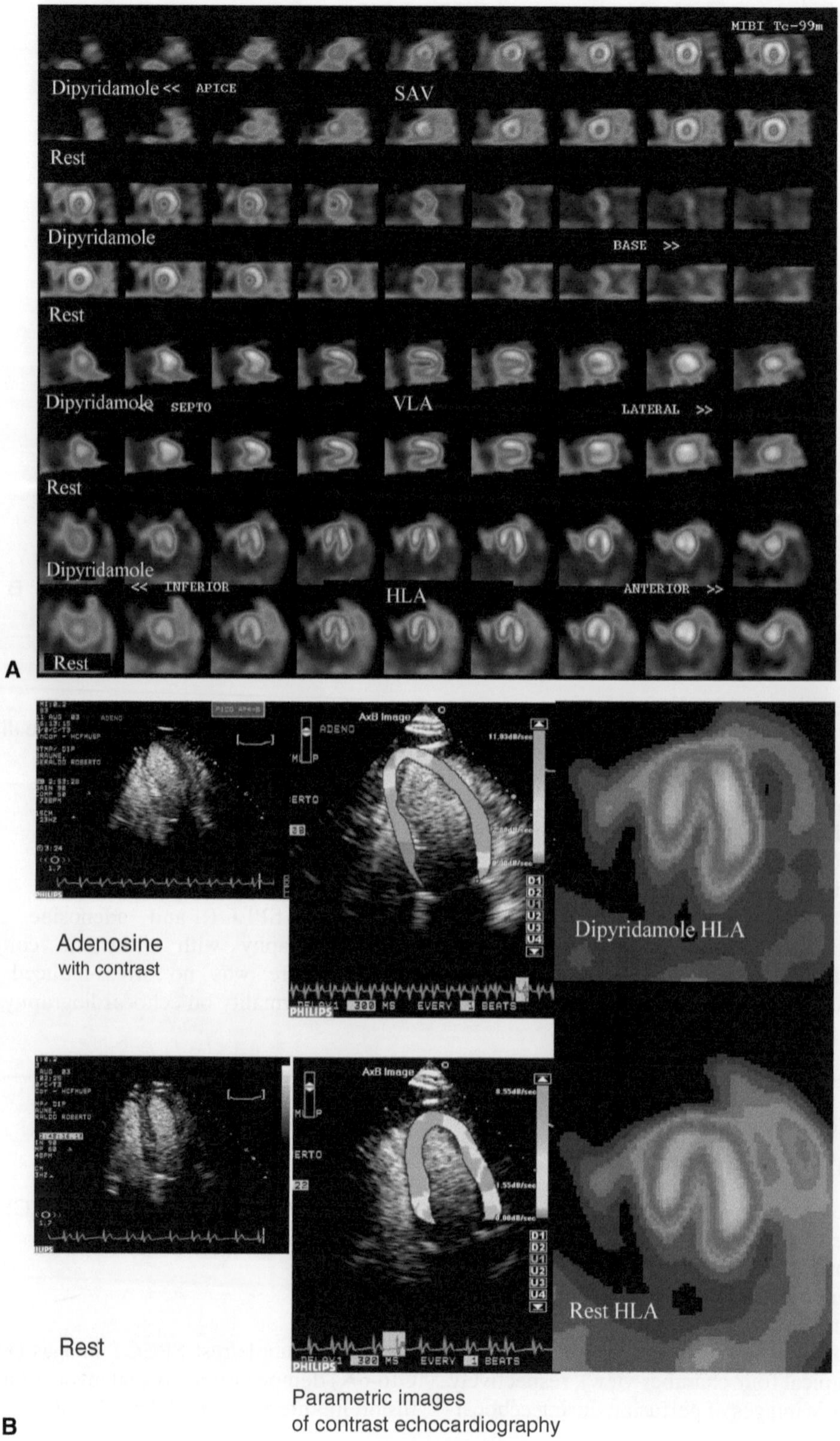

FIGURE C16-6. (A and B)

fusion in the inferoseptal region and apex on the dipyridamole images that normalized on the rest images indicating ischemia.

The apical 4-chamber view of real-time myocardial perfusion two-dimensional echocardiogram (low mechanical index) demonstrated normal perfusion in all myocardial walls at rest and adenosine-induced hypoperfusion in inferior septum and apex. In addition, there was lack of apical thickening during adenosine infusion (Figure C16-6B, left panels).

Parametric images of perfusion during echocardiography (Figure C16-6B, middle panel) demonstrated normal perfusion at rest (green and yellow) and adenosine-induced hypoperfusion not only in the inferior septum and apex (red and yellow) but also in the basal septum (red). Coronary angiography demonstrated 90% stenosis in the LAD, 100% stenosis in the RCA, 70% stenosis in the left circumflex, and 90% stenosis in the first obtuse marginal branch.

Discussion

This case illustrates how parametric images of myocardial perfusion during echocardiography can enhance the ability to detect multivessel disease. In this particular case, the patient had adenosine-induced wall motion abnormality only in the LAD distribution, but additional regions of reduced myocardial perfusion could be identified on the parametric images despite the absence of induced wall motion abnormality. The additional defects in basal septum and in basal lateral wall can be attributed to another coronary artery territory (RCA). Therefore, parametric imaging associated with contrast-enhanced adenosine echocardiography may improve the overall diagnostic accuracy of vasodilator stress echocardiography.

Interpretation

Multivessel CAD demonstrated with parametric imaging associated with contrast-enhanced adenosine echocardiography, whereas single-vessel CAD was detected with wall motion evaluation on echocardiography and dipyridamole/rest SPECT ^{99m}Tc-MIBI.

References

1. Marwick TH. Stress echocardiography. *Heart.* 2003;89:113–118.
2. Amyot R, Morales MA, Rovai D. Contrast echocardiography for myocardial perfusion imaging using intravenous agents: progress and promises. *Eur J Echocardiogr.* 2000;4:233–243.
3. Ahmad M, Xie T, McCulloch M, et al. Real-time three-dimensional dobutamine stress echocardiography in assessment of ischemia: comparison with two-dimensional dobutamine stress echocardiography. *J Am Coll Cardiol.* 2001; 37:1303–1309.
4. Beleslin B, Ostojic M, Stepanovic J, et al. Stress echocardiography in the detection of myocardial ischemia. Head-to-head comparison of exercise, dobutamine and dipyridamole tests. *Circulation.* 1994;90:1168–1176.
5. Dagianti A, Penco M, Agati L, et al. Stress echocardiography: comparison of exercise, dipyridamole and dobutamine in detecting and predicting the extent of coronary artery disease. *J Am Coll Cardiol.* 1995;26:18–25.
6. Geleijnse ML, Fioretti PM, Roelandt JR. Methodology, feasibility, safety and diagnostic accuracy of dobutamine stress echocardiography. *J Am Coll Cardiol.* 1997;30(3):595–606.
7. Leier CV, Unverferth DV. Drugs five years later: dobutamine. *Ann Intern Med.* 1983;99:490–496.
8. Kates RE, Leier CV. Dobutamine pharmacokinetics in severe heart failure. *Clin Pharmacol Ther.* 1978;24:537–541.
9. Geleijnse ML, Elhendy A, Fioretii PM, Roelandt JR. Dobutamine stress myocardial perfusion imaging. *J Am Coll Cardiol.* 2000;36:2017–2020.
10. Tsutsui JM, Osorio AFF, Fernandes DRA, et al. Efficacy of early use of atropine during dobutamine stress echocardiography—a comparative study with standard protocol. *Circulation.* 2004 (in press).
11. Picano E, Mathias W Jr, Pingitore A, Bigi R. Safety and tolerability of dobutamine-atropine stress echocardiography: a prospective, multicentre study. *Lancet.* 1994;344:1190–1192.
12. Mathias W Jr, Tsutsui JM, Andrade JL, et al. Value of rapid beta-blocker injection at peak dobutamine-atropine stress echocardiography for detection of coronary artery disease. *J Am Coll Cardiol.* 2003;41:1583–1589.
13. Hoffmann R, Lethen H, Marwick T, et al. Analysis of interinstitutional observer agreement in interpretation of dobutamine stress echocardiograms. *J Am Coll Cardiol.* 1996;27:330–336.

14. Hoffman R, Marwick TH, Poldermans D, et al. Refinements in stress echocardiographic techniques improve inter-institutional agreement in interpretation of dobutamine stress echocardiograms. *Eur Heart J*. 2002;23:821–829.
15. McCully RB, Roger VL, Mahoney DW, et al. Outcome after normal exercise echocardiography and predictors of subsequent cardiac events: follow-up of 1325 patients. *J Am Coll Cardiol*. 1998;31:144–149.
16. Smart S, Knickelbine T, Malik F, et al. Dobutamine atropine stress echocardiography for the detection of coronary artery disease in patients with left ventricular hypertrophy: importance of chamber size and systolic wall stress. *Circulation*. 2000:101(3):258–263.
17. Kymes SM, Bruns DE, Shaw LJ, et al. Anatomy of a meta-analysis: a critical review of exercise echocardiography or exercise SPECT imaging? a meta-analysis of diagnostic test performance. *J Nucl Cardiol*. 2000;7:599–615.
18. Maurer G, Nanda NC. Two dimensional echocardiographic evaluation of exercise-induced left and right asynergy: correlation with thallium scanning. *Am J Cardiol*. 1981;48:720–727.
19. Quinones MA, Verani MS, Haichin RM, et al. Exercise echocardiography versus thallium-201 single-photon emission computed tomography in evaluation of coronary artery disease. Analysis of 291 patients. *Circulation*. 1992;85:1026–1031.
20. Hecht HS, Debord L, Shaw R, et al. Supine bicycle stress echocardiography versus tomographic thallium-201 exercise imaging for the detection of coronary artery disease. *J Am Soc Echocardiogr*. 1993;6:177–185.
21. Pozzoli MM, Fioretti PM, Salustri A, et al. Exercise echocardiography and technetium-99m MIBI single-photon emission computed tomography in the detection of coronary artery disease. *Am J Cardiol*. 1991;67:350–355.
22. Galanti G, Sciagra R, Comaglio M, et al. Diagnostic accuracy of peak exercise echocardiography in coronary artery disease: comparison with thallium-201 myocardial scintigraphy. *Am Heart J*. 1991;122:1609–1616.
23. Salustri A, Pozzoli MM, Hermans W, et al. Relation between exercise echocardiography and perfusion single-photon emission computed tomography in patients with single-vessel coronary artery disease. *Am Heart J*. 1992;124:75–83.
24. Gunalp B, Dokumaci B, Uyan C, et al. Value of dobutamine technetium-99mm-sestamibi SPECT and echocardiography in the detection of coronary artery disease compared with coronary angiography. *J Nucl Med*. 1993;34:889–894.
25. Marwick TH, D'Hondt AM, Baudhuin T, et al. Optimal use of dobutamine stress for the detection and evaluation of coronary artery disease: combination with echocardiography, scintigraphy or both? *J Am Coll Cardiol*. 1993;22:159–167.
26. Forster T, MacNeill AJ, Salustri A, et al. Simultaneous dobutamine stress echocardiography and 99m-technetium isonitrile single photon emission computed tomography in patients with suspected coronary artery disease. *J Am Coll Cardiol*. 1993;21:1591–1596.
27. Senior R, Sridhara BS, Anagnostou E, et al. Synergistic value of simultaneous stress dobutamine sestamibi single-photon emission computerized tomography and echocardiography in the detection of coronary artery disease. *Am Heart J*. 1994;128:713–718.
28. Qureshi U, Nagueh S, Afridi I, et al. Dobutamine echocardiography and quantitative rest-redistribution ^{201}Tl tomography in myocardial hibernation: relation of contractile reserve of ^{201}Tl uptake and comparative prediction of recovery of function. *Circulation*. 1997;95:626–635.
29. Marwick TH, Case C, Sawada S, et al. Prediction of mortality using dobutamine echocardiography. *J Am Coll Cardiol*. 2001;37:754–760.
30. Arruda AM, Das MK, Roger VL, et al. Prognostic value of exercise echocardiography in 2632 patients >65 years of age. *J Am Coll Cardiol*. 2001;37:1036–1041.
31. Cortigiani L, Picano E, Landi P, et al. Value of pharmacologic stress echocardiography in risk stratification of patients with single-vessel disease: a report from the echo-persantine and echo-dobutamine international cooperative studies. *J Am Coll Cardiol*. 1998;32:69–74.
32. Myers JH, Stirling MC, Choy M, et al. Direct measurement of inner and outer wall thickening dynamics with epicardial echocardiography. *Circulation*. 1986;74:164–172.
33. Lieberman AN, Weiss JL, Jugdutt BI, et al. Two dimensional echocardiography and infarct size: relationship of regional wall motion and thickening to the extent of myocardial infraction in the dog. *Circulation*. 1981;63:739–746.
34. Picano E, Sicari R, Landi P, et al. Prognostic value of myocardial viability in medically treated patients with global left ventricular dysfunction

early after an acute uncomplicated myocardial infarction. A dobutamine stress echocardiographic study. *Circulation.* 1998;98(11):1078–1084.
35. Bax JJ, Wijns W, Cornel JH, et al. Accuracy of current available techniques for prediction of functional recovery after revascularization in patients with left ventricular dysfunction due to chronic coronary artery disease: comparison of pooled data. *J Am Coll Cardiol.* 1997;30:1451–1460.
36. Zoghbi WA. Evaluation of myocardial viability with contrast echocardiography. *Am J Cardiol.* 2002;90:65J–71J.
37. Villanueva FS. Myocardial contrast echocardiography in acute myocardial infarction. *Am J Cardiol.* 2002;90:38J–47J.
38. Iwakura K, Ito H, Kawano S, et al. Predictive factors for development of the no-reflow phenomenon in patients with reperfused anterior wall acute myocardial infarction. *J Am Coll Cardiol.* 2001;38:472–477.
39. Hamada S, Nakamura S, Sugiura T, et al. Early detection of the no-reflow phenomenon in reperfused acute myocardial infarction using technetium-99m tetrofosmin imaging. *Eur J Nucl Med.* 1999;26:208–214.

17
Advances in Cardiac Applications for PET and PET/CT

Dominique Delbeke, Thomas H. Schindler, David Townsend,
Philipp A. Kaufmann, Gustav K. von Schulthess, and Heinrich R. Schelbert

The rapid advances in imaging technologies are a challenge for both imaging experts and clinicians who must integrate these technologies for optimal patient care and outcomes at minimal cost. Multiple indications for molecular imaging using ^{18}F-fluorodeoxyglucose (FDG) are now well accepted in the fields of neurology, cardiology, and oncology.[1] The widespread oncologic applications, including differentiation of benign from malignant lesions, staging malignant lesions, detection of malignant recurrence, and monitoring therapy, have contributed to the establishment of positron emission tomography (PET) technology in many medical centers in the United States, Europe, and progressively throughout the world, making PET systems available for less common clinical indications such as in cardiology.

Both myocardial perfusion and metabolic imaging can be performed with PET. Three positron emitters have been approved for reimbursement by Medicare for cardiac applications, ^{82}Rb and ^{13}N-ammonia for evaluation of myocardial perfusion, and FDG for evaluation of myocardial viability.

Evaluation of Metabolism with PET

FDG PET has become the gold standard for evaluation of myocardial viability, although other imaging modalities and SPECT radiopharmaceuticals have a good accuracy to detect dysfunctional viable myocardium. Evaluation of myocardial viability with FDG has been extensively reviewed in Chapter 8. Measurements of LVEF from ECG-gated FDG studies have also been validated.

Other PET radiopharmaceuticals can be used to evaluate myocardial viability including ^{11}C-acetate and ^{11}C-palmitate. ^{11}C-palmitate is taken up by the myocardium with an extraction fraction of 50%. Clearance from the myocardium occurs in a bi-exponential pattern that is dependent on the availability of cardiac substrate. The early clearance depends essentially on the relative contribution of beta-oxidation to long-chain fatty acid metabolism and correlates with myocardial oxygen consumption.[2–4] The major limitation of ^{11}C-palmitate for evaluation of mitochondrial function and viability is its dependence of plasma substrate levels. ^{11}C-acetate allows evaluation of the oxidative metabolism by being converted to ^{11}C acetyl-CoA into the mitochondria and then entering into the tricarboxylic acid cycle (TCA). ^{11}C is then incorporated into TCA intermediates and clears from the myocardium as $^{11}CO_2$. ^{11}C-acetate kinetics can be assessed with dynamic PET imaging, correlates closely with myocardial oxygen consumption, and does not depend that much on plasma substrate level.[5–7] Kinetic models have been developed to quantitate ^{11}C-acetate metabolism,[8,9] but a simple determination of clearance rates using curve fitting of regional ^{11}C myocardial time-activity curve is commonly used for clinical purposes.[10]

In addition to evaluation of myocardial viability, FDG imaging may have a role in imaging inflammation. Inflammation is associated with increased glucose utilization that can be identified on FDG images.[11,12] The increased glucose metabolism in inflammation is related to the respiratory burst of macrophages in the process of activation and phagocytosis. The inflammatory infiltrate that is present early after myocardial infarction (MI) has limited the use of FDG in the setting of acute MI.[13]

Early in the development of atherosclerosis, there is endothelial injury leading to release of lipids and an inflammatory response. At this stage, the lumen of the vessel is rarely compromised and perfusion changes are minimal and difficult to detect, although there is impairment of vasoreactivity. Early lipid-lowering therapy may reduce inflammation and restore normal vasoreactivity.

Detection of inflammatory changes in early atheromas with FDG is a promising imaging modality for detection of early CAD. Preliminary studies have demonstrated the feasibility of FDG vascular imaging in the aorta and carotid arteries.[14,15] This has been discussed in Chapter 1 and Case 1.1. For FDG imaging of the coronary arteries, several problems have to be resolved. For example, cardiac motion can be minimized with gating and myocardial FDG uptake can be reduced with infusion of fatty acids.

Another potential clinical application of cardiac FDG imaging, in conjunction with resting ^{13}N-ammonia, is the evaluation of cardiac involvement with sarcoidosis. Granulomatous lesions are well known to accumulate FDG because of the presence of macrophages. FDG has to be administered in the fasting state to prevent accumulation by normal myocardium.

A recent study demonstrated that cardiac involvement with sarcoidosis presents as photopenic defects on the perfusion images and to FDG accumulation on the metabolic images (mismatch perfusion/metabolism in the fasting state).[16] These mismatch defects were seen more commonly in the anteroseptal, anterior, and anterolateral wall of the LV.

Myocardial Perfusion with PET

Semiquantitative Evaluation of Myocardial Perfusion with PET Tracers

Protocols and established clinical applications of PET perfusion radiopharmaceuticals have been addressed in Chapter 3. Advantages of PET over SPECT perfusion radiopharmaceuticals are faster protocols because of the shorter half-lives, lower radiation exposure, higher resolution, and superior attenuation correction (particularly important in women and obese patients). Normal databases of myocardial blood flow with ^{82}Rb and ^{13}N-ammonia have been generated and are available commercially. These software packages also include tools for quantitative determination of matched and mismatched defects.

Absolute Quantitation of Coronary Blood Flow and Blood Flow Reserve with PET

Noninvasive approaches for measurements of myocardial blood flow (MBF) entail intravenous administration of positron emitting flow tracers such as ^{13}N-ammonia and ^{15}O-water and imaging of the radiotracer transit through the central circulation and its retention in the myocardium.[17] Absolute quantification of radioactivity from the PET images requires accurate attenuation correction and calibration of the detectors to determine the radioactivity in a region of interest (myocardium or blood pool) in microCi/ml. From the serially acquired PET images, the arterial tracer input function and its uptake into myocardium are determined through regions of interest assigned to the myocardium and the left ventricular (LV) blood pool. The resulting time activity curves are fitted with tracer kinetic models and estimates of MBF are obtained in units of ml/min/g.[17] The short physical half-life of the flow tracers used for such measurements permits repeat studies of MBF during the same study session and thus, determination of flow responses to for example exercise or pharmacological stimulation.[17]

^{15}O-water is the perfect tracer for measurement of perfusion because it freely diffuses across capillary membranes and is metabolically inert. Its extraction fraction is nearly 100%, is not flow-dependent, and its short half-life of 2 minutes allows repetitive measurements. However, it also remains in the blood pool, contaminating the images, and therefore blood-pool scan with ^{15}O CO needs to be obtained as well.[18]

^{82}Rb is available from an ^{82}Strontium generator system, avoiding the need for a cyclotron on-site. However, the ^{82}Strontium generator is expensive and needs to be replaced on a monthly basis. The extraction of ^{82}Rb is flow-related at high flow rates and therefore a correction for extraction at high flow rates is necessary. The half-life of ^{82}Rb is 75 seconds, resulting in relatively low count-rate images. In addition, the energy of the positrons emitted is higher than that of ^{13}N, for example, and the distance traversed by ^{82}Rb positrons is longer than that of ^{13}N before the annihilation process. Therefore, the quality of the ^{82}Rb images is limited compared with ^{13}N. These factors explain the technical limitations of ^{82}Rb for quantification of myocardial perfusion.

^{13}N-ammonia is the PET tracer of choice for quantitative measurement of coronary blood flow (CBF) and coronary blood flow reserve (CBFR) using compartment modeling and kinetic analysis but requires a complex technical protocol and image analysis.[19–22] ^{13}N-ammonia is rapidly cleared from the blood pool, diffuses intracellularly, and is trapped into the myocardium as glutamate. Two- and three-compartmental models have been described for quantification of MBF. Correction needs to be made for some metabolites remaining in the blood pool and for its flow-dependent extraction fraction at high flow rates. Measurements of quantitative MBF can be performed at rest or during stress. However, because dynamic imaging needs to be performed during administration of the radiopharmaceutical to obtain the arterial input function, pharmacologic stress or cold pressor testing are the stress modalities of choice.

The possibility of evaluation of absolute CBF and CBFR using pharmacologic stress or cold pressor testing offers a means of investigating endothelial function and vascular smooth muscle relaxation and detecting early atherosclerosis.

Clinical Applications for Quantitative Myocardial Perfusion Imaging

The possibility of measuring MBF and its responses to physiological and pharmacological interventions offers the opportunity of exploring and characterizing the function of the coronary circulation in the human heart. Such measurements of blood flow expand the diagnostic scope of radionuclide approaches beyond that of conventional SPECT perfusion imaging or even coronary angiography. Functional alterations may affect the coronary circulation uniformly so that the relative distribution of myocardial blood flow remains homogenous and cannot be identified through traditional myocardial perfusion imaging. Functional abnormalities may also exist in the absence of structural changes of the coronary arteries and therefore remain undetected on coronary angiography. However, functional alterations of the coronary circulation are associated with abnormal flow responses to physiological and pharmacological stimuli and thus can be identified through measurements of coronary or MBF.

Probes of coronary circulatory function include measurements of flow responses to adenosine or dipyridamole stimulation or to cold pressor testing.[17,23] The magnitude of hyperemic blood flows achieved with direct vascular smooth muscle dilators such as adenosine or dipyridamole reflects the vasodilator capacity of the entire system including resistance and epicardial conduit vessels. Although the flow increase is predominantly vascular smooth muscle dependent, endothelium-dependent factors contribute so that the hyperemic flow estimate serves as a measure of the integrated coronary circulatory function.[24] Flow responses to sympathetic stimulation with cold pressor testing contain more specific information on the endothelium-dependent regulation.[25] Exposure to cold prompts a rise in heart rate (HR) and systolic blood pressure (BP) and thus an increase in cardiac work. The corresponding increase in demand leads to a metabolically regulated flow increase through dilation of the arteriolar resistance vessels, presumably mediated through release of adenosine. Upstream of the resistance vessels, the flow increase leads to a flow-mediated most likely endothelium-dependent vasodilation that further augments the flow increase. Thus, under normal conditions, an increase in cardiac work is accompanied by a proportionate increase in MBF. If, however, endothelial function is altered or impaired, then the vasoconstrictor effect of the sympathetically mediated-adrenergic stimulation of the vascular smooth muscle cell prevails. The flow response to cold pressor testing then becomes attenuated, is absent, or even is paradoxical. Thus, diminished, absent, or paradoxical responses of MBF to cold pressor testing signifies the presence of endothelial dysfunction.[25,26]

Integrated PET/CT Imaging

For oncologic application, although FDG PET imaging is more accurate than CT for staging and restaging various malignancies, one limitation of molecular imaging with FDG PET is the lack of anatomical landmarks for accurate localization of FDG-avid lesions. For many years, optimal interpretation was provided by interpreting PET and CT images in conjunction with each other by visual correlation, or where required, software could be used to align the functional and anatomical images. While software approaches work well for the brain, in the rest of the body difficulties with patient positioning and movement of internal organs potentially makes the software technique less successful. More recently, integrated PET/CT systems became available providing PET, CT, and fusion images acquired with state-of-the-art multislice (2 to 16 slices) CT units and state-of-the-art, high-resolution PET systems side-by-side in a common gantry and with a common imaging table. The fusion of anatomical and molecular images obtained with integrated PET/CT systems, sequentially in time but without moving the patient from the imaging table, allows optimal co-registration of anatomic and molecular images, leading to accurate attenuation correction and precise anatomic localization of lesions with increased metabolism. The recent development in multislice CT technology with 16-slice CT allows fast acquisition of CT angiographic images and permits detailed visualization of the cardiac anatomy.[27]

Design Concepts for PET/CT Scanners

While anatomical and functional imaging devices have historically developed along separate paths, the concept to physically integrate the imaging of anatomy and function into a single device originated with the pioneering work of Hasegawa in the early nineties.[28] Hasegawa and coworkers addressed the problem of combining CT with single photon imaging (SPECT) and were successful in showing the benefits of anatomy and function imaged together. In the mid-1990s, the development of the first CT scanner with integrated dedicated PET by Beyer et al.[29] represented a further evolution in combined imaging technology. The first patients were scanned on a combined PET/CT prototype at the University of Pittsburgh in mid-1998, and the positive results from the studies [30–34] stimulated commercial interest in the concept of combined CT and PET imaging.

The first combined device to become commercially available was a dual-head coincidence system with anatomical imaging capability[35] developed by General Electric as the Hawkeye and now marketed as the Discovery VH (Figure 17-1a). Functional imaging with this device is inferior to dedicated PET scanners even though it is a useful CT/SPECT imaging system. For PET/CT, a number of design alternatives were considered and reviewed by the different vendors before appropriate configurations began to emerge. Important design decisions that have to be addressed include the performance require-

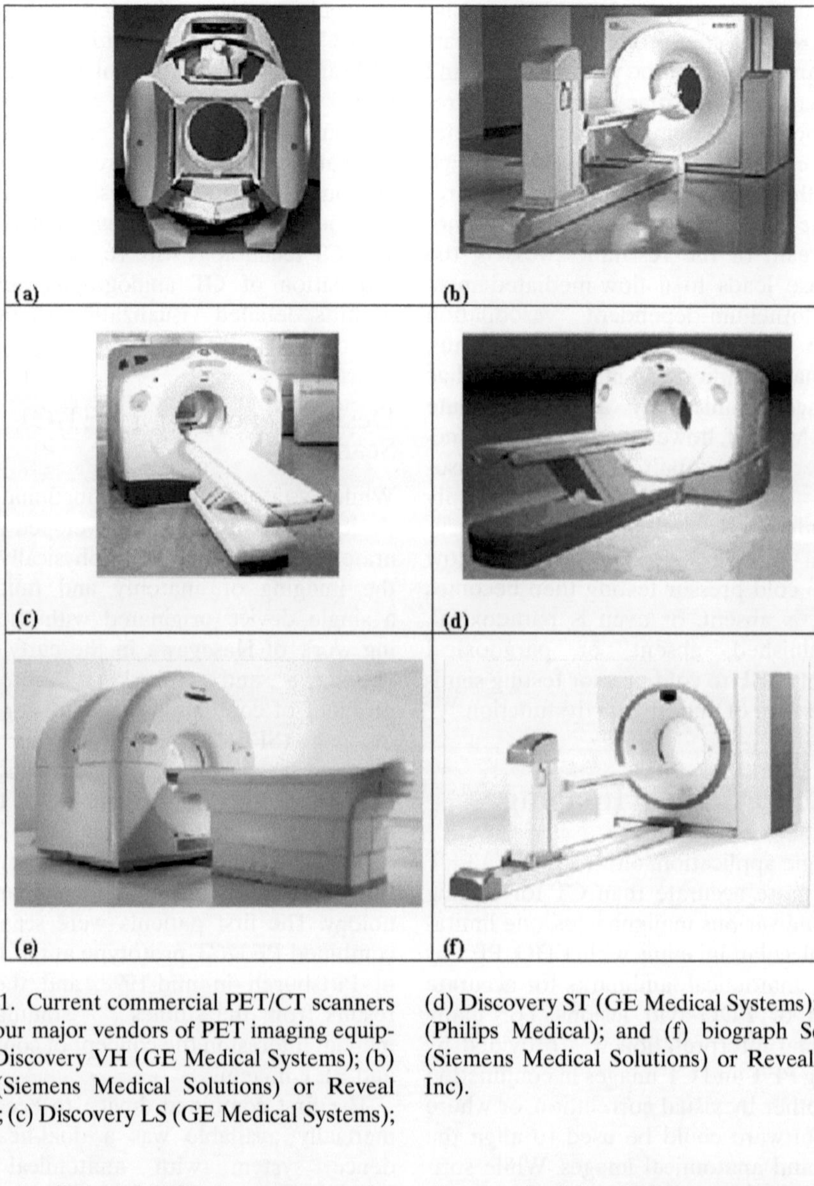

FIGURE 17-1. Current commercial PET/CT scanners from the four major vendors of PET imaging equipment: (a) Discovery VH (GE Medical Systems); (b) biograph (Siemens Medical Solutions) or Reveal (CTI, Inc.); (c) Discovery LS (GE Medical Systems); (d) Discovery ST (GE Medical Systems); (e) Gemini (Philips Medical); and (f) biograph Sensation 16 (Siemens Medical Solutions) or Reveal XVI (CTI, Inc).

ments of the CT and PET components, the extent of integration, the flexibility of the configuration and protocols, the potential for upgrades, the targeted users and applications, and of course, the cost.[36]

One typical commercial PET/CT design, distributed by Siemens as the biograph and by CTI as the Reveal, is shown schematically in Figure 17-2. The scanner comprises a Siemens Somatom Emotion dual-slice spiral CT (Siemens Medical Solutions, Forchheim, Germany) with a CPS Innovations ECAT PET scanner (Knoxville, TN). The PET scanner can be either a BGO-based ECAT HR+ or an LSO-based ECAT ACCEL (CPS Innovations, Knoxville, TN). Both the BGO and LSO versions are without septa and operate entirely in 3-D acquisition mode. Also, since no PET transmissions sources are incorporated into the design, CT-based attenuation correction is standard on these systems. Of note in this design is the minimal level of actual hardware integra-

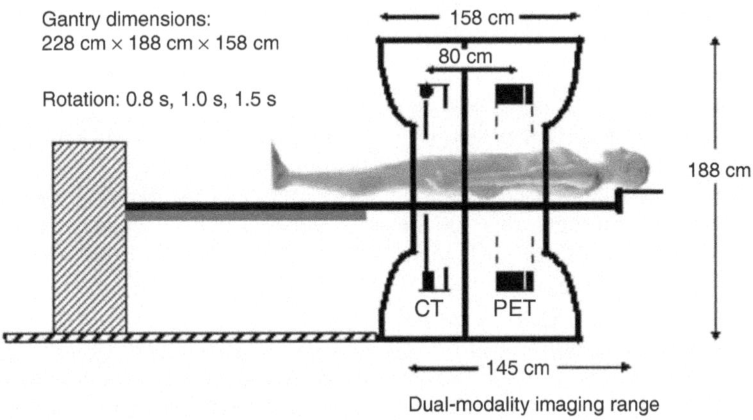

FIGURE 17-2. A schematic of the biograph PET/CT scanner. The axial separation of the two imaging fields is 80cm. The co-scan range for acquiring both PET and CT is 145cm maximum.

tion. The two scanners are essentially placed in tandem within the gantry housing. The gantry is 188cm high and 228cm in width. The overall length is 158cm, although with the front and rear contouring, the effective tunnel length is 110cm. The axial separation of the centers of the CT and PET fields-of-view is approximately 80cm. The patient port diameter is 70cm throughout the length of the tunnel, which is an important feature when scanning patients for radiation therapy, and which also reduces claustrophobic effects despite the 110-cm tunnel length. An example of the scanner that first received FDA 510(k) clearance in October 2000 is shown in Figure 17-1b.

The Discovery LS CT/PET design from GE Medical Systems was announced at the Radiology Society of North America (RSNA) in December 2000, a design (Figure 17-1c) that comprises a Lightspeed Plus HiLite MDCT scanner with either 4 or 8 slices and an Advance NXi BGO-based PET scanner. The Advance scanner in the CT/PET is essentially unchanged from the stand-alone version, incorporating both retractable septa and standard PET transmission sources. The Discovery LS can therefore acquire either 2-D or 3-D PET emission data and perform a standard PET transmission scan with germanium rod sources as an alternative to CT-based correction factors. The patient port is 70cm for the CT, and then tapered to 60cm for the PET portion, somewhat limiting the application of the device for radiation therapy treatment planning where a large patient port is to be preferred.

The third PET/CT design in addition to the biograph/Reveal and the Discovery series is the Gemini, manufactured and marketed by Philips Medical. This is a more open design than others with the CT and PET scanners kept separate to allow access to the space between the two devices (Figure 17-1e). The Gemini comprises a Philips MX 8000D dual-slice CT scanner with a GSO-based ALLEGRO PET scanner. The PET scanner has no septa and operates entirely in 3-D. The patient port diameter is also 70cm throughout, facilitating the scanning of radiation therapy patients in the treatment position.

Finally, the most recent additions to the range of commercial PET/CT scanners were presented at the RSNA in December 2002. General Electric announced the introduction of the Discovery ST, a PET/CT device with a redesigned BGO-based PET scanner that incorporates finer axial sampling, an increased number of detector rings, shorter septa, and a 70-cm patient port throughout the entire length (Figure 17-1d). The CT scanner in the Discovery ST is again a Lightspeed Plus HiLite MDCT with an option of 4, 8, or 16 slices. The exterior gantry dimensions of the redesigned

PET scanner now match those of the Lightspeed CT, as can be seen in Figure 17-1d. At the same RSNA meeting, Siemens also announced the biograph Sensation 16, a PET scanner developed by CPS Innovations (Knoxville, TN) that comprises a 16-slice, high-performance CT scanner in-line with an LSO-based ACCEL PET scanner. CTI Inc. markets this as the Reveal XVI. The incorporation of such high-level CT performance into combined PET/CT scanner technology now opens up potential cardiac applications in addition to those in oncology.

The required level of CT and PET performance obviously depends on the applications envisaged for the device. Since the PET scanner performance is the limiting factor in terms of statistical image quality, spatial resolution, and scan duration, the highest possible PET performance is generally indicated. The appropriate choice for the CT performance has been more controversial, ranging from mid to top-of-the-line. The main differences are in the number of axial detectors (CT slices) and the rotation speed. In CT, the current trend is to multislice detectors and sub second rotation times. The most rapid CT scan protocols are obviously targeted primarily at cardiac applications, although from the perspective of the patient a short scan time is always to be preferred when breath-holding is required. For oncology purposes, such high-performance CT may not necessarily be required, particularly when the patient is allowed to breathe shallowly throughout the CT scan to more closely match the PET acquisition protocol for which breath-holding is not an option.

The importance of matching the CT and PET scan protocols is not only to ensure precise registration between anatomy and function, but also to generate accurate CT-based attenuation correction factors. Any mismatch could result in incorrect attenuation factors that will propagate errors into the reconstructed PET emission scan.[37] The potential to use the CT images for attenuation correction of the PET emission data obviously eliminates the need for a separate, lengthy PET transmission scan. The use of the CT scan for attenuation correction not only reduces whole-body scan times by at least 40%, but provides essentially noiseless attenuation correction factors compared with those from a standard PET transmission scan. The attenuation values are, however, energy dependent, and hence the correction factors derived from a CT scan at a mean photon energy of 70 keV must be scaled to the PET energy of 511 keV, for which a hybrid scaling algorithm has been developed.[38] The algorithm scales bone and soft tissue using different factors after applying a simple threshold to classify the CT pixel values. Recent modifications to the algorithm now allow the CT to be acquired with intravenous and oral contrast present in the patient[39] without generating artifacts in the reconstructed PET images. The modified algorithm can also minimize the effect of artifacts due to metallic objects in the patient.[40]

While not all vendors have followed the same design choices, nevertheless all have in common that their top-of-the-line design comprises a high-performance CT scanner in tandem with a high-performance PET scanner. The use of CT-based attenuation correction and faster scintillators such as GSO or LSO for PET detectors has resulted in a significant reduction in whole-body imaging times to below 10 minutes, compared with an hour or more just a few years ago. In the future, as the technology matures, specific design configurations will target different application areas such as neurology, cardiology, and oncology. Very high-performance CT that is essential for cardiac studies may be of less interest in oncology, for example, where lower performance (and lower cost) CT will still be more than adequate for clinical studies. The future of this evolution in imaging technology will be significant in the management of disease.

Potential Clinical Applications for Integrated PET/CT

The recent technological advances in integrated multimodality imaging with PET/CT systems offer the possibility for simultaneous evaluation of anatomy and function and are one of the most exciting new developments in imaging technology. In these systems, the use of an x-ray tube-based transmission scan provides attenuation-corrected emission images of high quality due to the high photon flux inherent with this technique. One advantage over the radioactive sources (Germanium 68) typically used in standalone PET systems is the short duration for the transmission scan, which is less than 20 seconds for one bed position compared with 10 to 20 minutes with radioactive sources. This allows a transmission CT scan to be performed for each emission PET acquisition as necessary. Adequate CT transmission map can actually be obtained with very low current (10 mA) that limits radiation exposure (approximately 0.1 rem).[41] In addition, optimal co-registration between attenuation maps and emission images is possible using integrated PET/CT systems when the CT attenuation maps and FDG PET emission images are obtained sequentially in time without moving the patient from the imaging table. Because the FDG emission images must be acquired during normal breathing, there is still a debate as to whether optimal attenuation maps are provided by attenuation maps obtained with the breath-hold technique or during normal breathing when performing oncologic studies.[42,43] Normal respiratory movements have an impact on the emission images corrected for attenuation, depending on whether the CT images are obtained during normal respiration or the breath-hold technique because the acquisition time for the CT images over the area of the diaphragm is in the order of less than 30 seconds with the diaphragm in a more defined position than on the emission images. Preliminary results show that myocardial blood flow quantitation is independent of the CT beam intensity and that ECG gating of the CT transmission scan seems not to be necessary.[44]

Advanced cardiac applications are possible with integration of 16-slice CT and PET systems. Noninvasive visualization of the coronary tree has been investigated for a long time. MR angiography was promising in that regard but in a multicenter trial, only 84% of the vessels segments could be evaluated and the evaluation was limited to the proximal 3 to 5 cm of the major coronary arteries. In addition, the examination time was over 1 hour, which is a limitation in clinical practice.[45] The multi-slice, especially 16-slice, CT technology allows the performance of CT coronary angiography (CTCA) and visualization of the major branches of the coronary tree and definition of luminal narrowing.[46] This subject has been discussed in Chapter 15. There is some discussion in the literature that noninvasive angiography may be acceptable to evaluate patients with low clinical probability for CAD, considering that between 20% to 40% of all diagnostic invasive angiograms are normal.[47]

The cardiac PET/CT technology can potentially allow evaluation in one imaging setting of (1) calcium scoring with multislice CT, (2) coronary artery anatomy with contrast-enhanced CTCA, (3) rest/stress myocardial perfusion with the possibility of quantitative measurement of coronary blood flow (CBF) and coronary blood flow reserve (CBFR) and localization of the hypoperfused regions to specific coronary arteries, (4) evaluation of myocardial viability with FDG and precise anatomical localization, and (5) localization of atheromatous plaques with inflammation using FDG.

Preliminary data have demonstrated the feasibility of obtaining fusion images with such a PET-CT system superimposing perfusion ^{13}N-ammonia images to CT angiographic images displaying coronary anatomy.[48]

With the introduction of the 16-slice integrated PET/CT systems, the PET/CT technology may become the long waited *one-stop shop* in cardiology, where algorithm will be elaborated incorporating calcium scoring, for example, to further select patients for appropriate tests. For example, low-risk patients could be referred for calcium scoring and PET MPI and high-risk patients for PET MPI and CTCA. In addition, patients could be just referred for MPI with CT attenuation correction for the diagnosis or prognostic implications of CAD. The group of patients with poor LV function evaluated for viability can be referred for PET FDG viability and CTCA.

Case Presentations

Case 17.1

History

A 36-year-old man was referred for evaluation of angina-like chest pain during exercise and during mental stress. The patient presented a family history of CAD and long-term smoking. At peak exercise on the treadmill (Bruce protocol), horizontal ST-segment depression of 1.5mm was noted on ECG in the inferolateral leads and angina-like chest pain occurred. Coronary angiography revealed normal epicardial coronary vessels with smooth luminal surfaces and without evidence of luminal narrowing (Figures C17-1A and C17-1B). For evaluation of myocardial perfusion, the patient underwent a ^{201}Tl bicycle stress-redistribution SPECT myocardial perfusion study. Regional myocardial blood flow at rest and its response to cold pressor testing was measured with intravenous ^{13}N-ammonia and serial PET imaging. The three-dimensional (3-D) display of myocardial perfusion reconstructed from ^{201}Tl SPECT images, fused with the 3-D display of the coronary angiogram, are shown in Figure C17-1C. The ^{13}N-ammonia PET time activity curves derived from the serially acquired PET images (input = blood pool, response = myocardium) at rest (left) and during cold pressor testing (right) for estimating regional MBF in the left anterior descending coronary artery (LAD) territory are displayed in Figure C17-1D.

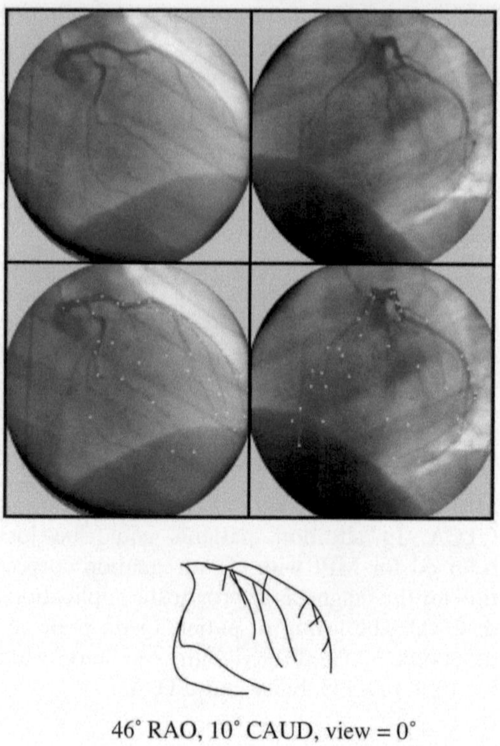

A

46° RAO, 10° CAUD, view = 0°

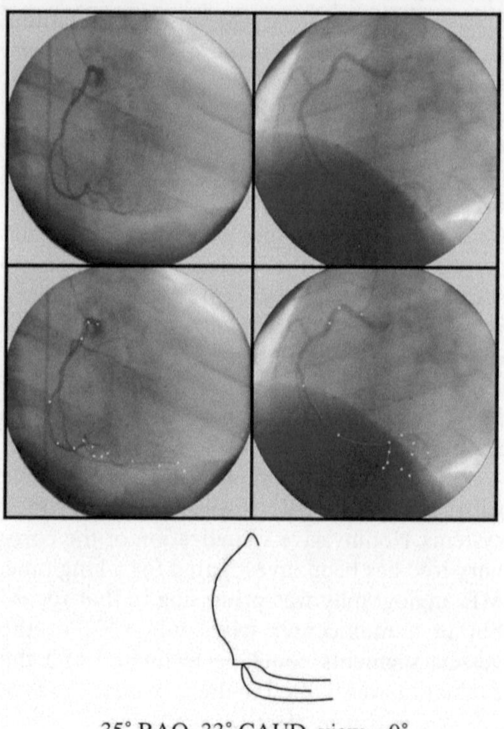

35° RAO, 33° CAUD, view = 0°

B

FIGURE C17-1. (A and B, from Schindler, Nitzsche, Magosaki, et al. [49], by permission of *Heart.*)

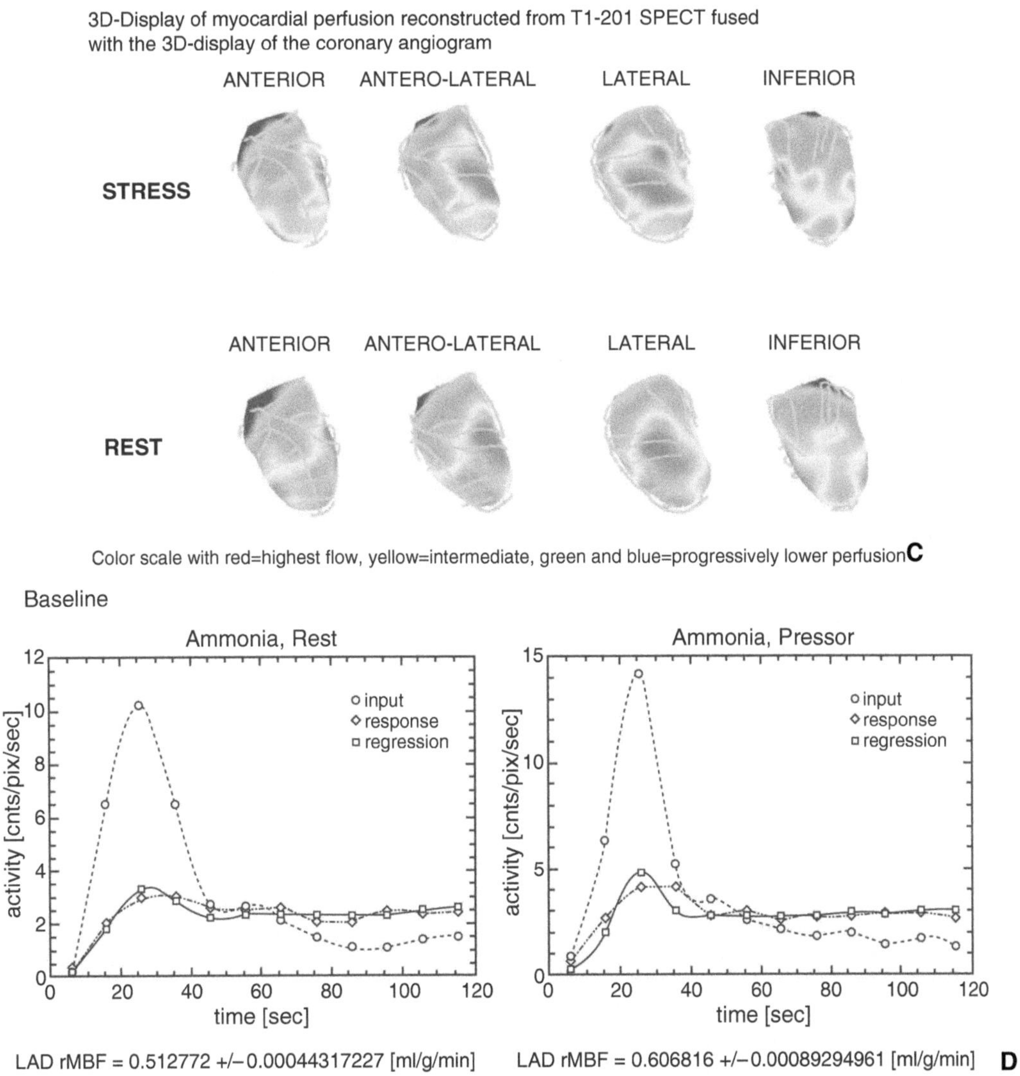

FIGURE C17-1. (C and D, from Schindler, Nitzsche, Magosaki, et al. [49], by permission of *Heart.*)

Findings

Figure C17-1A displays the left coronary angiogram (right and left anterior oblique views, RAO and LAO) in a patient without significant obstructive coronary artery disease (CAD). Both projections were used for construction of the 3-D display of the coronary tree as shown in the bottom panel. The middle panel shows RAO and LAO superimposition of the re-projected 3-D models onto the angiograms from the same views. The lower panels show views of the computed 3-D structure of the left and right coronary trees.

Figure C17-1B displays the right coronary angiogram in the same patient without significant obstructive coronary artery disease. Again, the two projections were used for construction of the 3-D display of the coronary artery. The middle panel shows RAO and LAO superimposition of the re-projected 3-D models onto the angiograms from the same views. The lower panel depicts the computed 3-D structure of the right coronary tree.

Figure C17-1C demonstrates an example of the overall approach of merging coronary artery anatomy (coronary angiogram) with myocardial perfusion (^{201}Tl SPECT) in a 3-D format viewed from four different angles during stress (upper panel) and rest (lower panel). On the anterior view the 3-D fusion image revealed a markedly reduced tracer uptake from the mid-ventricular to apical of the anterior wall during stress (upper panel, green) as compared with corresponding images at rest (lower panel, red), indicative for an exercise-induced regional scintigraphic perfusion defect. This stress-induced perfusion defect corresponds in location to the LAD. In contrast, there is a similar tracer uptake in the anterolateral, lateral, and inferior myocardial regions during stress and rest demonstrating normal myocardial perfusion in these areas. Because no attenuation correction was performed on the ^{201}Tl SPECT images, reduced but similar tracer uptake during stress and rest are found in the inferior wall. The normally perfused myocardium was supplied by an obtuse marginal branch (OM) of the left circumflex coronary artery (LCX) and the right coronary artery (RCA) was normal.

The ^{13}N-ammonia PET images revealed homogeneously distributed MBF both at rest and during cold pressor testing. Myocardial blood flow at rest was 0.51 ml/min/g in the LAD (Figure C17-1D) and 0.52 ml/min/g in the LCX and RCA territories. With cold pressor testing, myocardial blood flow increased by only 20% (to 0.61 ml/min/g) in the LAD (Figure C17-1D) and by only 31% (to 0.68 ml/min/g) in the LCX and RCA territory. Both responses were markedly attenuated and suggested an alteration in the flow-mediated and presumably endothelial-dependent coronary vasomotor function. Thus, disturbance of flow-mediated coronary vasomotor response appeared to more homogenously affect the coronary circulation during cold pressor testing in this patient with a normal coronary angiogram. In contrast, the ^{201}Tl SPECT myocardial perfusion images revealed a stress-induced defect. This implied a greater spatial heterogeneity of the abnormal flow-mediated, endothelial-dependent vascular reactivity in response to greater flow during bicycle exercise.

The attenuated flow response to cold pressor testing together with a stress-induced perfusion defect in the presence of a normal coronary angiogram implicated an endothelium-dependent coronary vasomotor abnormality as the possible cause of the patient's clinical symptoms. The patient was therefore placed on 3-month treatment with vitamin C (2 g/day orally) as antioxidant to improve coronary vasomotor function.

At follow-up after 3 months, treadmill exercise again revealed ST-segment depression at the same exercise level, but less than 0.5 mm and thus no longer significant; no typical chest pain occurred during peak exercise. Repeat measurements of MBF with PET revealed a markedly improved flow response to cold pressor testing. Myocardial blood flow increased by 74% in the LAD territory (from 0.78 ml/min/g at rest to 1.36 ml/min/g; Figure C17-1E) and by 72% in the LCX and RCA territories (from 0.77 ml/min/g to 1.33 ml/min/g).

Discussion

The vascular endothelium plays an active and pivotal role in maintaining the functional integrity of the vascular wall, including its structure and permeability, vasomotor tone, and hemostasis.[25,26] It regulates the vasomotor tone through release of substances such as prostacycline, endothelin-1, hyperpolarizing factor, and, importantly, nitric oxide (NO). In the functionally intact endothelium, physiological stimuli such as physical exercise induce an increase in flow-mediated shear stress that prompts release of endothelium-derived NO, which in turn induces vasodilation. Reduced bioavailability of NO or of prostaglandin together with enhanced activity of vasoconstrictors such as endothelin or angiotensin II may be responsible for an impairment of the coronary vasodilator capacity that may cause ischemia even in the absence of significant obstructive CAD.[49,50]

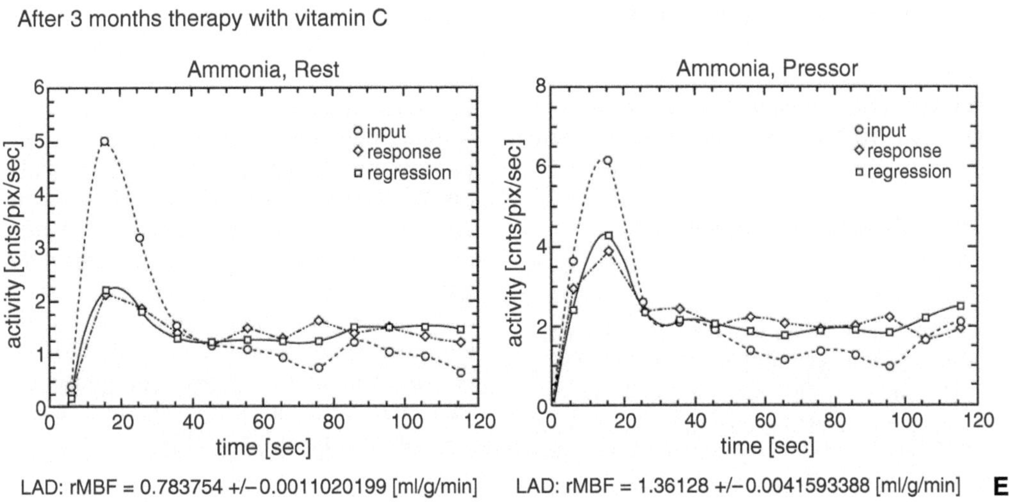

FIGURE C17-1. (E)

Conventionally, a fluid-dynamically significant stenosis of the epicardial coronary artery has been considered as cause and determinant of a diminished coronary flow reserve.[51] This concept has been uniformly accepted as the cause of stress-induced myocardial ischemia because the obstructive CAD precludes an adequate increase in blood flow that matches an increase in metabolic demand.[51] However, multiple factors are involved in the regulation of MBF including metabolic and neurohumoral factors as well as physical determinants such as changes in intraluminal pressure or flow-mediated shear stress on endothelial vasomotion.[25] The importance of these functional determinants of CBF lead to the formulation of a new concept of endothelial dysfunction as contributor or cause of clinically manifest ischemia and myocardial perfusion defects.[49,50] The concept entails a critical role of the endothelium for ensuring appropriate levels of blood flow in response to increases in demand.[25,26] Consequently, the dysfunctional endothelium may be an important determinant of exercise-induced myocardial perfusion defects in patients with angiographically normal coronary arteries. Indeed, the patient in this case report revealed an impaired flow response to cold pressor testing as evident on the PET examination that implied an alteration of endothelium-dependent coronary vasomotion and thus most likely accounted for the exercise-induced myocardial perfusion defect in the anterior wall. This is in keeping with recent findings in patients with normal coronary angiograms. These studies observed a correlation between the impairment of endothelium-dependent regional myocardial blood flow responses to cold pressor testing and the severity of exercise-induced scintigraphic regional myocardial perfusion-defects, and implicated an abnormal endothelium-dependent vasoreactivity as the cause of myocardial perfusion defects.[49,50] These observations emphasize the important role of the endothelium-dependent vasomotor tone that, in addition to obstructive coronary artery lesions, contributes to the clinically manifest regional myocardial perfusion defects.

Apart from regulating endothelium-dependent vasodilation, NO has several fundamental protective cardiovascular effects including control of leukocyte adhesion, platelet aggregation, expression of adhesion molecules and endothelin-1, and inhibition of vascular growth and inflammation.[26] Consequently, endothelial dysfunction is associated with an increased risk factor for coronary events.[52,53] Improvement of the bioavailability of endothelium-derived NO has therefore become the goal of therapeutic interventions in patients with impaired endothelium-dependent coronary vasomotion to prevent future cardiovascular events such as an acute coronary syndrome, nonfatal MI, and sudden cardiac death.

Possible Therapeutic Interventions

Approaches for improving or restoring endothelial function and, thus, for preventing coronary events include cardiovascular conditioning and lifestyle modification as well as use of HMG-CoA reductase inhibitors (statins), angiotensin-converting enzyme (ACE) inhibition, L-arginine, folic acid, and antioxidants.[25,26] The patient in this case study was treated for 3 months with the antioxidant vitamin C.

Endothelial Dysfunction and Statin Treatment. The beneficial effects of HMG-CoA reductase inhibitors on coronary vascular function may be related to their ability to lower levels of low-density lipoproteins (LDL) cholesterol by enhancing hepatic receptor-mediated clearance of apolipoprotein-B-containing particles, since oxidized LDL has also been shown to selectively target G-protein-dependent signal transduction, leading to a decrease of receptor-mediated stimulation of endothelial NO production.[54] In hypercholesterolemic patients, HMG-CoA reductase inhibitors have been shown to improve endothelial function of the coronary resistance vessels.[55] The improvement appears to be independent of the extent of the achieved cholesterol reduction. Thus, in addition to lowering plasma cholesterol levels, HMG-CoA reductase inhibitors exert other beneficial effects on endothelial function during long-term therapy such as an induction of endothelial NOS.[56] Moreover, HMG-CoA reductase inhibitors may also reduce angiotensin II type-1 receptor expression and activity that is associated with a reduction of angiotensin II-induced radical formation.[57] These findings imply that HMG-CoA reductase inhibitors increase NO bioavailability in vivo in part by mechanism unrelated to their effects on cholesterol plasma concentrations (that is, by increasing the synthesis of NO and by reducing inactivation of NO by superoxides). The improvement of the vasodilator capacity in patients with hypercholesterolemia and CAD has also been shown to result in a clinically relevant benefit, because it was also associated with a reduction of angina pectoris and an improvement in stress-induced myocardial perfusion defects as assessed by PET imaging.[58] The latter benefits again emphasize the notion of coronary vasomotion as an important determinant for myocardial perfusion and myocardial perfusion abnormalities. In addition, long-term therapy of patients with HMG-CoA reductase inhibitor improves prognosis and is associated with an early reduction of cardiovascular events and mortality.[26]

Oxidative Stress and Antioxidant Treatment. Oxidative stress within the vessel wall plays an important role for an impaired vasomotor regulatory tone. Mechanisms underlying an abnormal endothelium-dependent vascular tone in patients with traditional coronary risk factor such as hypercholesterolemia, hypertension, and smoking are likely to be multifactorial. Yet, there is growing evidence to suggest that increased vascular production of reactive oxygen species (ROS) derived from the superoxide producing endothelial enzymes, such as NAD(P)H oxidase, xanthine oxidase, and uncoupled NO synthase, reduce the bioavailability of endothelium-derived NO, and thus diminish the vasodilator function.[25,26] Antioxidants, such as vitamin C, acutely improve endothelial function in patients with diabetes mellitus, CAD, smoking, hypertension, and hypercholesterolemia.[25,26,59] Further, coronary microcirculatory dysfunction in long-term smokers has been shown to improve after intravenous vitamin C administration in response to adenosine.[60] Different from the beneficial effect of acute vitamin C supplementation, long-term supplementation of 1g of vitamin C or 600IU of alpha-tocopherol daily failed to demonstrate a sustained beneficial effect on endothelial function of arm vessels in smokers, suggesting the operation of intracellular and/or extracellular adaptive mechanisms.[61,62] To complicate matters, others[63] reported a beneficial effect of alpha-tocopherol supplementation on endothelial dysfunction of forearm vessels only in long-term smokers with hypercholesterolemia, but not in those with either risk factor alone. These apparently discordant results may be related to differences in patient characteristics, antioxidant dose, and/or differential responses of arm and coronary vessels. Regarding the appropriate dosage, supraphysiological vitamin C concentrations may be required to effectively scavenge reactive oxygen species.[64] In addition, some evidence suggests that vascular responses in the large conduit vessels of the peripheral and the coronary circulation do not necessarily extend into the microcirculation.[65]

In hypercholesterolemic patients, regular intake of vitamin C yielded contradictory results.[25,26] Failure of vitamin C to improve endothelial dysfunction in hypercholesterolemia may be related to mechanisms other than increased oxidative stress. In hypercholesterolemia, oxidized LDL has been shown to activate protein kinase C, leading to interruption of G-protein-dependent signal transduction and, thereby, to a decrease of receptor-mediated stimulation of endothelial NO production.[54] Despite these observations, a beneficial effect of vitamin C treatment in hypercholesterolemic patients may be present but remain undetected in the more complex clinical setting.

Finally, beneficial effects of long-term vitamin C supplementation on endothelial dysfunction have been reported for arm vessels in patients with CAD and congestive heart failure.[66,67] Apart from its scavenging effect on oxygen reactive species, vitamin C might also improve NO activity by sparing intracellular glutathione, which together with vitamin C is primarily involved in the regulation of the intracellular redox state (for review see reference 68). Reduced thiols stabilize NO by reaction to form 5-nitrosothiol species. Vitamin C also acts synergistically with alpha-tocopherol, promoting its regeneration and resulting in enhanced intracellular antioxidant capacity. Furthermore, in vitro studies suggest important additional effects of vitamin C in endothelial cells such as increased NO generation through enhanced bioavailability of tetrahydrobiopterin to NO synthase and/or increase nitric-oxide-synthase gene expression. Of note, the latter effect of vitamin C to enhance cellular NO formation indicates that endothelial cell NO bioactivity is sensitive to intracellular vitamin C.

Clinical Relevance of Therapeutic Approaches to Improve Endothelial Function. Impaired NO bioactivity leads to unopposed paradoxical vasoconstriction of the coronary circulation to a physiological stimuli such as sympathetic activation.[25,26,59] Therefore, endothelial dysfunction contributes to the ischemic manifestation of CAD. Even when significant obstructive CAD is absent, abnormal endothelial vasomotion may be responsible for exercise-induced scintigraphic myocardial perfusion defects.[49,50] Paradoxical vasoconstriction and loss of endothelial antithrombotic properties might unfavorably modulate the course of acute coronary syndromes. Thus, the ultimate aim of therapeutic interventions is to increase NO bioavailability by either increasing NO production or decreasing superoxide formation in the endothelium. This aim can be achieved, for example, by ACE inhibitors, HMG-CoA reductase inhibitors, increased shear-stress by physical exercise, estrogens, antioxidants, and L-arginine.[25,26] All have been shown to improve endothelium-dependent vasodilator function and myocardial perfusion. Nevertheless, whether improvements in endothelial function will indeed, as suggested recently, contribute to an improved clinical prognosis remains to be more firmly established.

Interpretation

Endothelial dysfunction demonstrated with quantitative rest/cold pressor stress ^{13}N-ammonia.

Case 17.2

History

A patient who had suffered from a minor lateral myocardial infarction was enrolled in a research protocol designed to evaluate the image quality of an integrated PET/CT system for combined acquisition of coronary anatomy and function. He underwent a contrast-enhanced CTCA with retrospective ECG gating followed by a rest/ adenosine stress ^{13}N-ammonia PET study on the integrated PET/CT system (GE Discovery LS, General Electric Medical Systems, Milwaukee, WI). Figure C17-2A displays short axis views (SAV) of the 2-D fusion display of the stress images. Figure C17-2B displays one representative slice of the SAV, vertical long axis (VLA) and horizontal long axis (HLA) views of the 2D fusion display of both the rest and stress images.

Findings

The short-axis images of the 2-D fusion display (Figure C17-2A) demonstrated a lateral perfusion defect. Using the fusion the defect can be assigned more precisely to the segment with the defect corresponding to a high-grade stenosis of the LCX.

In Figure C17-2B, a small lateral perfusion defect was seen on the rest images indicating a small scar and the perfusion defect is much larger on the stress images indicating adenosine-induced ischemia.

Discussion

The case presented is from a pilot feasibility study of four patients performed with an integrated PET/CT system in which the CT unit is a 4-slice CT scanner.[48]

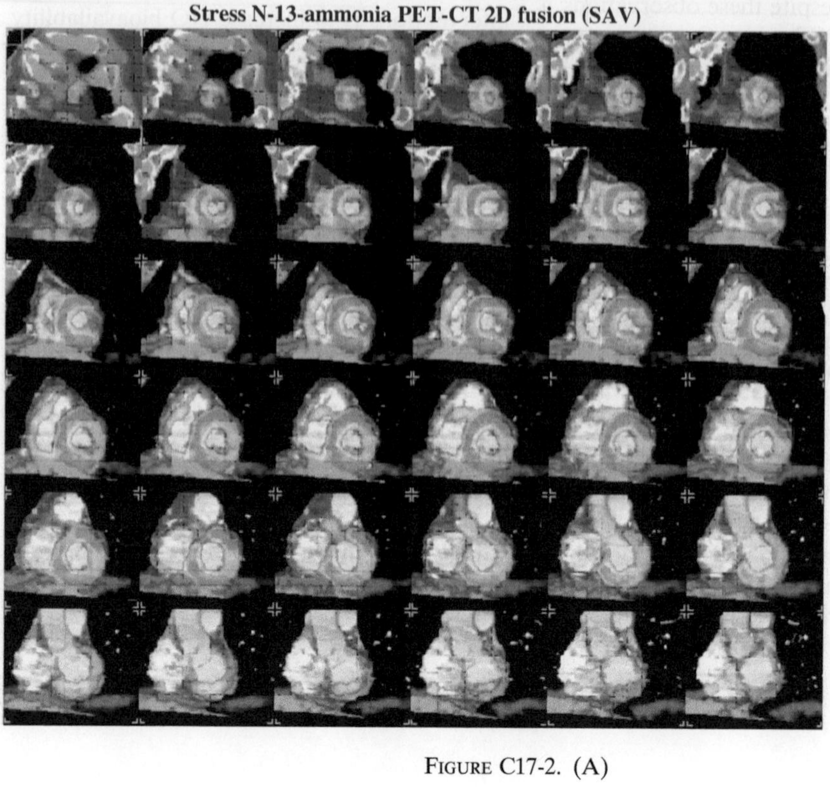

A

FIGURE C17-2. (A)

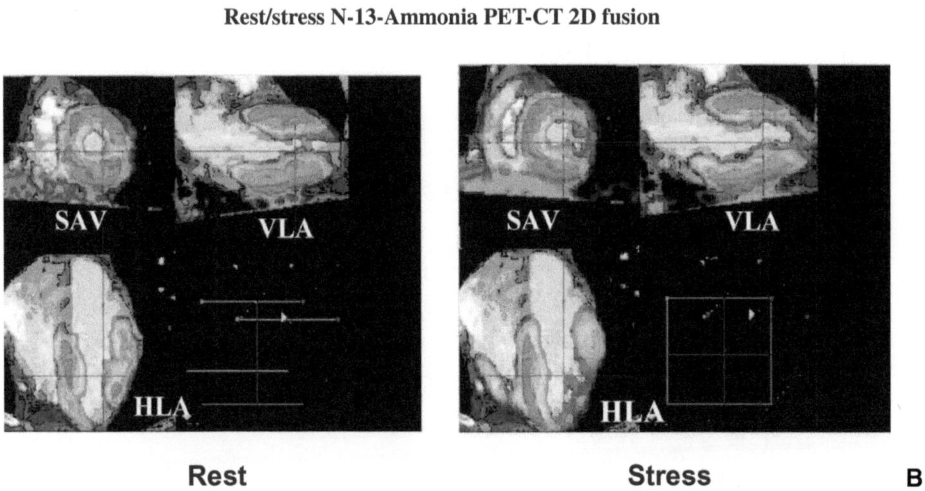

FIGURE C17-2. (B)

Interpretation

2-D-fusion PET perfusion/CTCA images obtained with an integrated PET/CT (4-slice) system demonstrated the feasibility of the technique in a patient with ischemia and scar in the LCX territory.

Case 17.3

History

A 64-year-old patient suffered from anginal pain and underwent coronary angiography revealing a proximal calcified LAD plaque with high-grade stenoses of the diagonal branches, high-grade stenoses of all posterolateral branches of the LCX, and generalized narrowing of the RCA with high-grade stenosis of the right interventricular posterior branch.

Despite these findings and clinical symptoms, the patient refused to undergo any intervention for revascularization. To assess the extent of jeopardized myocardium, the patient underwent a contrast-enhanced CTCA with retrospective ECG gating followed by a rest/adenosine stress ^{13}N-ammonia PET perfusion study. The PET scan was performed in an integrated PET/CT system according to the same research protocol as in Figure C17-2A, designed to evaluate the feasibility of combined acquisition of coronary anatomy and function. Anterior and left lateral views of the 3-D fusion PET/CT image of this patient are given in Figures C17-3A and C17-3B, respectively.

Findings

During adenosine stress ST-segment depression of up to 5 mm were documented, indicating coronary steal phenomena with decrease in absolute flow. Resting perfusion imaging shows a fixed anterior defect (scaring) in the LAD territory. During adenosine stress the defect is more pronounced and slightly more extended, indicating adenosine-induced ischemia predominantly in the LAD territory. The Houndsfield units for the coronary artery tree have been chosen to show predominantly calcifications, explaining why most side branches are not visualized.

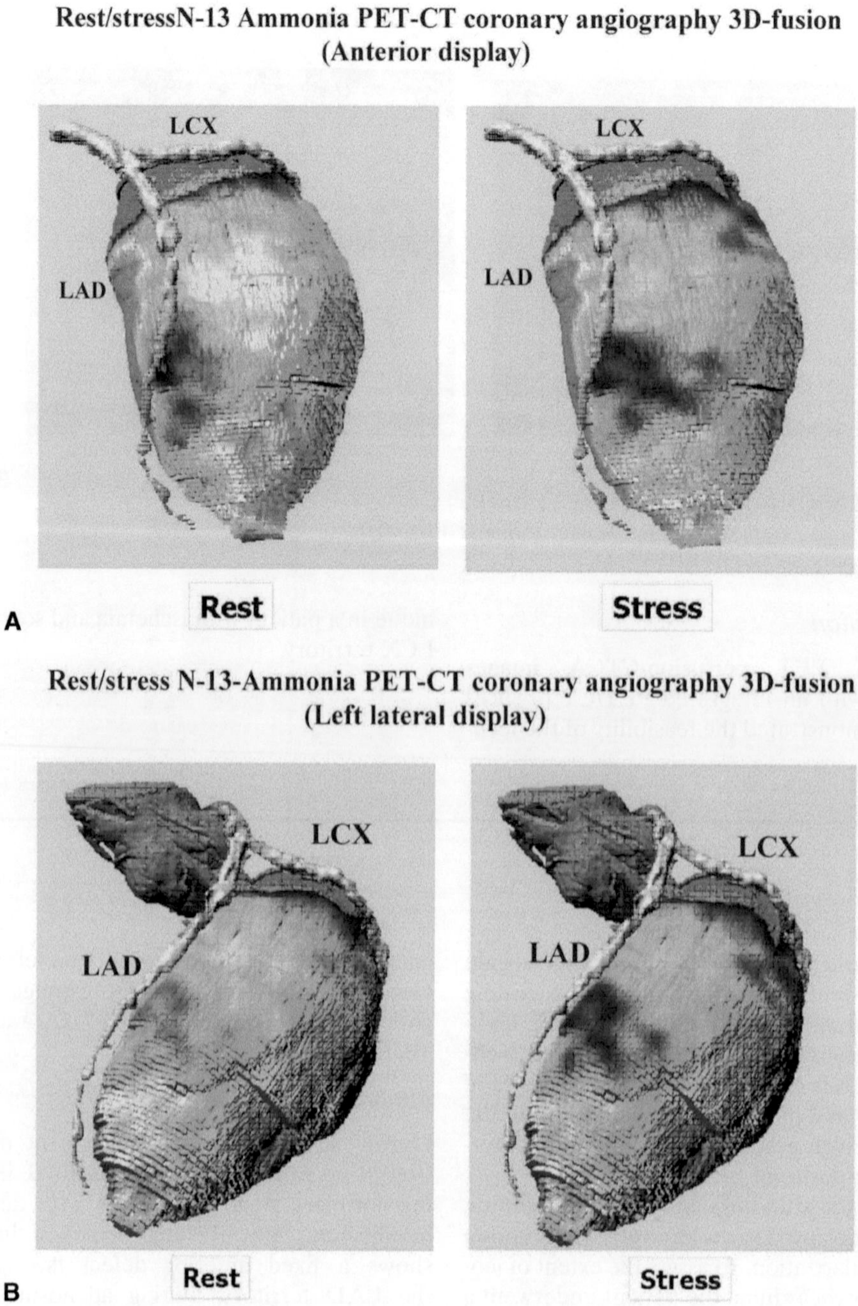

FIGURE 17-3. (A and B)

Discussion

The case presented is also from the pilot feasibility study of four patients performed with an integrated PET/CT system in which the CT unit is a 4-slice CT scanner.[48] The coronary arteries show relatively low image quality. This is not due to low quality of the CT scan, but rather at this time to the lack of appropriate software solutions for adequate post-processing and fusion. At present, this makes interpretation of images very difficult. In fact, it is preferable to judge coronary arteries separately using the dedicated software for CTCA. However, as the combined assessment of coronary anatomy and perfusion has been shown to be technically feasible, software solutions will soon be available.

Interpretation

3-D-fusion PET perfusion/CTCA images obtained with an integrated PET/CT (4-slice) system demonstrating the feasibility of the technique in a patient with ischemia and scar in the LAD territory.

References

1. Delbeke D, Martin WH, Patton JA, Sandler MP (eds). *Practical FDG Imaging: A Teaching File.* New York: Springer Verlag; 2002.
2. Schelbert H, Henze E, Schon H, et al. ^{11}C palmitic acid for the non-invasive evaluation of regional myocardial fatty acid metabolism with positron computed tomography, IV: in vivo demonstration of impaired fatty acid oxidation in acute myocardial ischemia. *Am Heart J.* 1983;106:736–750.
3. Bergmann S, Nomura H, Rand A, et al. Externally detectable changes in fatty utilization by perfused hearts from rabbits to alcohol. *Circulation.* 1982;66-2:109 (Abstract).
4. Schoen HR, Schelbert HR, Robinson G, et al. ^{11}C labeled palmitic acid for the non-invasive evaluation of regional myocardial fatty acid metabolism with positron emission tomography, I: kinetics of C-111 palmitic acid in normal myocardium. *Am Heart J.* 1982;103:532–546.
5. Buxton DB, Schwaiger M, Nguyen A, et al. Radiolabeled acetate as a tracer of myocardial tricarboxylic acid flux. *Circ Res.* 1988;63:628–634.
6. Brown MA, Marshall DR, Sobel BE, et al. Delineation of myocardial oxygen utilization with carbon-11 labeled acetate. *Circulation.* 1987;76:687–696.
7. Brown MA, Myears DW, Bergmann SR. Validity of estimates of myocardial oxidative metabolism with carbon-11 acetate and positron emission tomography despite altered patterns of substrate utilization. *J Nucl Med.* 1989;30:187–193.
8. Buck A, Wolpers HG, Hutchins GD, et al. Effect of carbon-11-acetate recirculation on estimates of myocardial oxygen consumption by PET. *J Nucl Med.* 1991;32:1950–1957.
9. Buxton DB, Nienaber CA, Luxen A, et al. Non-invasive quantitation of regional myocardial oxygen consumption in vivo with [1–11C]acetate and dynamic positron emission tomography. *Circulation.* 1989;79:134–142.
10. Kotzerke J, Hicks RJ, Wolfe E, et al. Three-dimensional assessment of myocardial oxidative metabolism: a new approach for regional determination of PET-derived carbon-11-acetate kinetics. *J Nucl Med.* 1990;31:1876–1883.
11. Zhao S, Kuge Y, Tsukamoto E, et al. Fluorodeoxyglucose uptake and glucose transporter expression in experimental inflammatory lesions and malignant tumors: effects of insulin and glucose loading. *Nucl Med Commun.* 2002;23: 545–550.
12. Mochizuki T, Tsukamoto E, Kuge Y, et al. FDG uptake and glucose transporter subtype expressions in experimental tumor and inflammation models. *J Nucl Med.* 2001;42:1551–1555.
13. Bianco JA, Hammes R, Sebree L, Wilson M. Imaging of acute myocardial infarction and reperfusion. *Cardiology.* 1995;86:189–196.
14. Yun M, Jang S, Cucchiara A, et al. ^{18}F-FDG uptake in the large arteries: a correlation study with the atherogenic risk factors. *Semin Nucl Med.* 2002;32:70–76.
15. Rudd JH, Warburton EA, Fryer TD, et al. Imaging atherosclerotic plaque inflammation with ^{18}F-fluorodeoxyglucose positron emission tomography. *Circulation.* 2002;105:2708–2711.
16. Yamagishi H, Shirai N, Yoshiyama M, et al. Identification of cardiac sarcoidosis with ^{13}N-NH3/^{18}F-FDG PET. *J Nucl Med.* 2003;44: 1030–1036.
17. Schelbert HR. Positron emission tomography and the changing paradigm in coronary artery disease. *Z Kardiol.* 2000;89(Suppl 4): IV55–60.
18. Bergmann SR, Fox KA, Rand AL, et al. Quantification of regional myocardial blood flow in vivo with H_2 ^{15}O. *Circulation.* 1984;70:724–733.
19. Kuhle WG, Porenta G, Huang SC, et al. Quantification of regional myocardial blood flow using ^{13}N-ammonia and reoriented dynamic positron emission tomography imaging. *Circulation.* 1992;86:1004–1017.
20. Schelbert HR, Phelps ME, Huang SC, et al. ^{13}N-ammonia as an indicator of myocardial blood flow. *Circulation.* 1981;63:1259–1272.
21. Nitzsche EU, Choi Y, Czernin J, Hoh CK, Huang SC, Schelbert HR. Noninvasive quantification of

myocardial blood flow in humans. A direct comparison of the ^{13}N ammonia and the ^{15}O water techniques. *Circulation.* 1996;93:2000–2006.
22. Krivokapich J, Smith GT, Huang SC, et al. ^{13}N-ammonia myocardial imaging at rest and with exercise in normal volunteers. Quantification of absolute myocardial perfusion with dynamic positron emission tomography. *Circulation.* 1989; 80(5):1328–1337.
23. Campisi R, Czernin J, Schoder H, Sayre JW, Schelbert HR. L-Arginine normalizes coronary vasomotion in long-term smokers. *Circulation.* 1999;99:491–497.
24. Buus NH, Bottcher M, Hermansen F, Sander M, Nielsen TT, Mulvany MJ. Influence of nitric oxide synthase and adrenergic inhibition on adenosine-induced myocardial hyperemia. *Circulation.* 2001;104:2305–2310.
25. Drexler H. Endothelial dysfunction: clinical implications. *Prog Cardiovasc Dis.* 1997;39: 287–324.
26. Hornig B, Drexler H. Reversal of endothelial dysfunction in humans. *Coron Artery Dis.* 2001; 12:463–473.
27. Ohnesorge B, Flohr T, Becker C, et al. Cardiac imaging by means of electrocardiographically gated multisection spiral CT: initial experience. *Radiology.* 2000;217:564–572.
28. Lang TF, Hasegawa BH, Soo Chin L, et al. Description of a prototype emission-transmission computed tomography imaging system. *J Nucl Med.* 1992;33:1881–1887.
29. Beyer T, Townsend DW, Brun T, et al. A combined PET/CT scanner for clinical oncology. *J Nucl Med.* 2000;41:1369–1379.
30. Charron M, Beyer T, Bohnen N, et al. Image analysis in patients with cancer studies with a combined PET and CT scanner. *Clin Nucl Med.* 2000;25(11):905–910.
31. Townsend DW, Beyer T, Kinahan PE, et al. Recent studies with a combined PET/CT scanner: a synergistic approach to patient management. In Tamaki N, Tsukamoto E, Kuge Y, et al (eds). *Positron Emission Tomography in the Millenium: Proceedings of the International PET Symposium.* Hokkaido, Japan: Elsevier 2000;229–244.
32. Kluetz PG, Meltzer CC, Villemagne MD, et al. Combined PET/CT imaging in oncology: impact on patient management. *Clin Posit Imaging.* 2001;3(3):1–8.
33. Meltzer CC, Martinelli MA, Beyer T, et al. Whole-body FDG PET imaging in the abdomen: value of combined PET/CT. *J Nucl. Med.* 2001; 42:35P.
34. Meltzer CC, Snyderman CH, Fukui MB, et al. Combined FDG PET/CT imaging in head and neck cancer: impact on patient management. *J Nucl Med.* 2001;42:36P.
35. Patton JA, Delbeke D, Sandler MP. Image fusion using an integrated, dual-head coincidence camera with x-ray tube-based attenuation maps. *J Nucl Med.* 2000;41:1364–1368.
36. Townsend DW. A combined PET/CT scanner: the choices. *J Nucl Med.* 2001;43(3):533–534.
37. Osman MM, Cohade C, Nakamoto Y, Marshall LT, Leal JP, Wahl RJ. Clinically significant inaccurate localization of lesions with PET/CT: frequency in 300 patients. *J Nucl Med.* 2003; 44:240–243.
38. Kinahan PE, Townsend DW, Beyer T, Sashin D. Attenuation correction for a combined 3D PET/CT scanner. *Med Phys.* 1998;25:2046–2053.
39. Carney JP, Beyer T, Brasse D, Yap JT, Townsend DW. Clinical PET/CT scanning using oral CT contrast agents. *J Nucl Med.* 2002;45(3):57P.
40. Cohade C, Osman M, Marshall L, Wahl RL. Metallic object artifacts on PET-CT: clinical and phantom studies. *J Nucl Med.* 2002;43:308P.
41. Kamel E, Hany TF, Burger C, et al. CT vs 68GE attenuation correction in a combined PET/CT system: evaluation of the effect of lowering the CT current. *Eur J Nucl Med Mol Imaging.* 2002; 29:346–350.
42. Goerres GW, Burger C, Schwitter MW, et al. PET/CT of the abdomen: optimizing the patient breathing pattern. *Eur Radiol.* 2003;13:734–739.
43. Goerres GW, Burger C, Kamel E, et al. Respiration-induced attenuation artifact at PET/CT: technical considerations. *Radiology.* 2003;226:906–910.
44. Koepfli P, Wyss CA, Hany T, et al. CT-transmission for attenuation correction in quantitative myocardial perfusion measurements using a combined CT-PET scanner: a pilot dose-finding study for different CT energies. *Circulation.* 2001;104-Supl 2:587.
45. Kim WY, Daniass PG, Stuber M, et al. Coronary magnetic resonance angiography for detection of coronary stenoses. *N Engl J Med.* 2001;345: 1863–1869.
46. Gerber TC, Kuzo RS, Karstaedt N, et al. Current results and new developments of coronary angiography with the use of contrast-enhanced computed tomography of the heart. *Mayo Clin Proc.* 2002;77:55–71.
47. Achenbach S, Daniel WG. Noninvasive coronary angiography: an acceptable alternative. *N Engl J Med.* 2001;345:1909–1910.

48. Namdar MM, Hany TF, Burger C, von Schulthess GK, Kaufman PA. Combined CT-angiogram and PET perfusion imaging for assessment of CAD in a novel PET/CT: a pilot study. *J Nucl Cardiol.* 2003;2(10):1(abstract 11.12):577.
49. Schindler TH, Nitzsche E, Magosaki N, et al. Regional myocardial perfusion defects during exercise, as assessed by three dimensional integration of morphology and function, in relation to abnormal endothelium dependent vasoreactivity of the coronary microcirculation. *Heart.* 2003;89:517–526.
50. Zeiher AM, Krause T, Schachinger V, Minners J, Moser E. Impaired endothelium-dependent vasodilation of coronary resistance vessels is associated with exercise-induced myocardial ischemia. *Circulation.* 1995;91:2345–2352.
51. Gould KL, Lipscomb K, Hamilton GW. Physiologic basis for assessing critical coronary stenosis. Instantaneous flow response and regional distribution during coronary hyperemia as measures of coronary flow reserve. *Am J Cardiol.* 1974;33:87–94.
52. Schachinger V, Britten MB, Zeiher AM. Prognostic impact of coronary vasodilator dysfunction on adverse long-term outcome of coronary heart disease. *Circulation.* 2000;101:1899–1906.
53. Schindler TH, Hornig B, Buser PT, Olschewski M, et al. Prognostic value of abnormal vasoreactivity of epicardial coronary arteries to sympathetic stimulation in patients with normal coronary angiograms. *Arterioscler Thromb Vasc Biol.* 2003;23:495–501.
54. Ohgushi M, Kugiyama K, Fukunaga K, et al. Protein kinase C inhibitors prevent impairment of endothelium-dependent relaxation by oxidatively modified LDL. *Arterioscler Thromb.* 1993; 13:1525–1532.
55. Egashira K, Hirooka Y, Kai H, Sugimachi M, et al. Reduction in serum cholesterol with pravastatin improves endothelium-dependent coronary vasomotion in patients with hypercholesterolemia. *Circulation.* 1994;89:2519–2524.
56. Laufs U, La Fata V, Plutzky J, Liao JK. Upregulation of endothelial nitric oxide synthase by HMG CoA reductase inhibitors. *Circulation.* 1998;97:1129–1135.
57. Nickenig G, Baumer AT, Temur Y, Kebben D, Jockenhovel F, Bohm M. Statin-sensitive dysregulated AT1 receptor function and density in hypercholesterolemic men. *Circulation.* 1999; 100:2131–2134.
58. Gould KL, Martucci JP, Goldberg DI, et al. Short-term cholesterol lowering decreases size and severity of perfusion abnormalities by positron emission tomography after dipyridamole in patients with coronary artery disease. A potential noninvasive marker of healing coronary endothelium. *Circulation.* 1994;89: 1530–1538.
59. Schindler TH, Magosaki N, Jeserich M, et al. Effect of ascorbic acid on endothelial dysfunction of epicardial coronary arteries in chronic smokers assessed by cold pressor testing. *Cardiology.* 2000;94:239–246.
60. Kaufmann PA, Gnecchi-Ruscone T, di Terlizzi M, Schafers KP, Luscher TF, Camici PG. Coronary heart disease in smokers: vitamin C restores coronary microcirculatory function. *Circulation.* 2000;102:1233–1238.
61. Raitakari OT, Adams MR, McCredie RJ, Griffiths KA, Stocker R, Celermajer DS. Oral vitamin C and endothelial function in smokers: short-term improvement, but no sustained beneficial effect. *J Am Coll Cardiol.* 2000;35: 1616–1621.
62. Neunteufl T, Priglinger U, Heher S, et al. Effects of vitamin E on chronic and acute endothelial dysfunction in smokers. *J Am Coll Cardiol.* 2000;35:277–283.
63. Heitzer T, Yla Herttuala S, Wild E, Luoma J, Drexler H. Effect of vitamin E on endothelial vasodilator function in patients with hypercholesterolemia, chronic smoking or both. *J Am Coll Cardiol.* 1999;33:499–505.
64. Jackson TS, Xu A, Vita JA, Keaney JF, Jr. Ascorbate prevents the interaction of superoxide and nitric oxide only at very high physiological concentrations. *Circ Res.* 1998;83:916–922.
65. Bottcher M, Madsen MM, Refsgaard J, et al. Peripheral flow response to transient arterial forearm occlusion does not reflect myocardial perfusion reserve. *Circulation.* 2001;103: 1109–1114.
66. Gokce N, Keaney JF, Jr., Frei B, et al. Long-term ascorbic acid administration reverses endothelial vasomotor dysfunction in patients with coronary artery disease. *Circulation.* 1999;99:3234–3240.
67. Ellis GR, Anderson RA, Lang D, et al. Neutrophil superoxide anion-generating capacity, endothelial function and oxidative stress in chronic heart failure: effects of short- and long-term vitamin C therapy. *J Am Coll Cardiol.* 2000; 36:1474–1482.
68. May JM. How does ascorbic acid prevent endothelial dysfunction? *Free Radic Biol Med.* 2000;28:1421–1429.

18 Future Directions in Nuclear Cardiology

Raed Al-Dallow and Robert C. Hendel

The cases presented in this chapter have been selected to illustrate emerging techniques in nuclear cardiology for the care of patients with cardiovascular diseases. Promising radiopharmaceuticals, stress agents, and imaging procedures offer valuable tools in the diagnosis and risk stratification of such patients and play a significant role in patient selection and follow-up of current and emerging surgical and medical therapies. The basic principles of imaging with some of the unique radiopharmaceuticals mentioned in this chapter (^{99m}Tc-teboroxime, ^{99m}Tc-N-NOET, ^{99m}Tc-annexin, ^{99m}Tc-glucarate, ^{67}Ga, ^{123}I-MIBG, ^{123}I-BMIPP) have also been addressed to some extent in Chapter 3; new stress agents have been discussed in Chapter 4; and alternative imaging modalities other than nuclear methods in Chapters 14 (MRI), 15 (multislice CT), and 16 (contrast echocardiography).

Case Presentations

Case 18.1

History

A 58-year-old man with a history of a prior inferior wall myocardial infarction (MI) and coronary artery bypass graft (CABG) surgery presented with chest pain. His cardiac risk factors include hypertension, hyperlipidemia, diabetes mellitus, and a 20 pack-year smoking history. He underwent a dual isotope myocardial perfusion study. ^{201}Tl (4.0 mCi) was administered at rest and image acquisition required approximately 19 minutes with a dual-detector gamma camera. ^{99m}Tc-teboroxime (53.9 mCi) was administered at 4 minutes into a 6-minute adenosine infusion and acquisition of the images was begun 108 seconds after tracer injection, using a fast fanning method. Each 180-degree orbit (scan) was completed in 36 seconds; the final images were reconstructed with the summation of 6 scans. The adenosine ^{99m}Tc-teboroxime/rest ^{201}Tl SPECT images are displayed in Figure C18-1A.

Findings

The images demonstrated a moderate- to large-sized perfusion abnormality of moderate severity in the inferior wall and more severe in the inferolateral region. Some reversibility (ischemia) is noted in the inferoseptal and inferior regions, with the inferolateral wall essentially fixed. Figure C18-1A was obtained with a dual isotope protocol using ^{99m}Tc-teboroxime as noted previously.

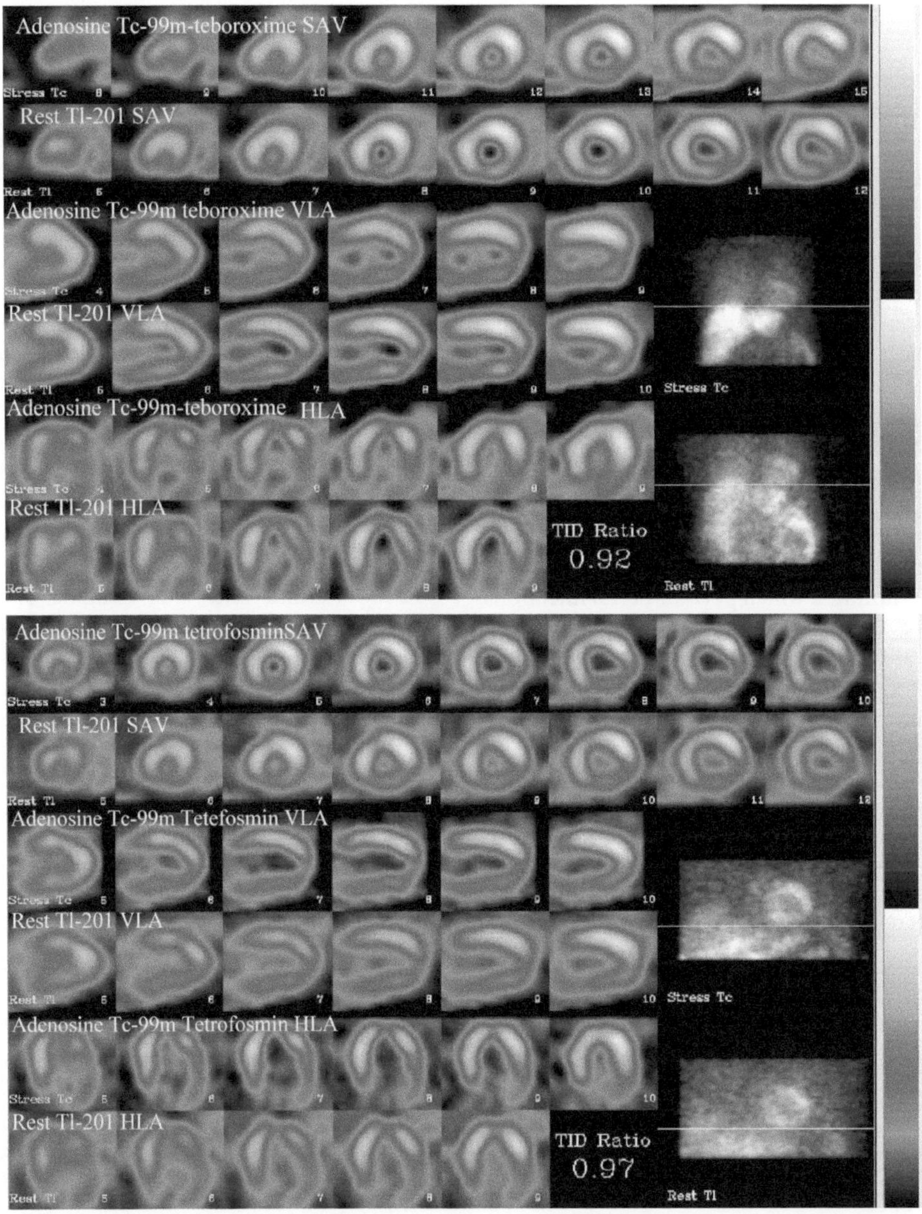

FIGURE C18-1. (A and B, courtesy of E.G. Krawcznski, Emory University, Atlanta, GA.)

For comparison, Figure C18-1B displays a dual isotope study obtained using ^{99m}Tc-tetrofosmin for the poststress images. Substantial concordance is noted between the 2 imaging agents. Additionally, the overall quality of the ^{99m}Tc-teboroxime images (Figure C18-1A) is comparable with that of the ^{99m}Tc-tetrofosmin ones (Figure C18-1B).

Discussion

^{99m}Tc-teboroxime is a boronic acid adduct of technetium dioxime (BATO), which is a neutral and highly lipophilic tracer. Its use for clinical application remains difficult due to the technical limitations related to its unique pharmacodynamic characteristics. ^{99m}Tc-teboroxime has the highest extraction fraction among the single photon tracers (over 3.4% of the injected dose) and has a linear correlation with coronary blood flow over a wide range of flow rates ranging from ischemic to hyperemic (see Figure 3-1).

Although myocardial uptake is rapid and excellent visualization is achieved within 1 to 2 minutes postinjection, the clearance of this agent is also rapid, requiring a short interval between injection and the onset of imaging. Residual myocardial activity is negligible after 60 to 90 minutes, which permits serial injections within a short period of time. Hepatic uptake peaks at 5 to 6 minutes and is related to the patient's position, splanchnic blood flow, and left ventricular (LV) function. Due to the reasons mentioned previously, imaging should start within 2 minutes postinjection and should be quickly completed within 6 to 9 minutes.[1]

Due to the need for rapid patient positioning, the use of pharmacological stress is preferred with ^{99m}Tc-teboroxime. Both planar and SPECT imaging have been described in clinical studies. Image acquisition in a seated position allows for inferior displacement of the liver, thereby reducing the hepatic interference with the inferior wall.[2] Imaging with multi-detector gamma cameras allows completion of the SPECT image acquisition in less than 5 minutes. As hepatic activity is often a significant problem with this agent, imaging with new approaches have been tried; least-squares factor analysis of dynamic structures (FADS) method was used successfully to remove the liver activity that partially overlapped the inferior wall.[3] Additionally, the method of *fast fanning* has shown promises. In this method, dynamic SPECT acquisition is obtained while the gamma camera detectors are fanned 180 degrees every 30 seconds for 3 to 4 minutes; postacquisition frames may then be selected to ensure consistent tracer distribution and reduce hepatic activity.[4,5]

The results of multicenter clinical trials on planar and SPECT ^{99m}Tc-teboroxime imaging reported a sensitivity and specificity of 83% and 92%, respectively.[6] Agreement between ^{99m}Tc-teboroxime and ^{201}Tl imaging is high; 89% agreement for normal vs. abnormal studies, and 86% for infarction vs. ischemia patterns.[2] Applying the previously mentioned fast fanning method in clinical studies yielded promising preliminary results as demonstrated by Garcia et al.[4] The overall accuracy of ^{99m}Tc-teboroxime imaging in the detection of coronary artery disease (CAD) was 89%.[4]

Interpretation

Adenosine stress/rest ^{99m}Tc-teboroxime/rest ^{201}Tl SPECT images demonstrating a fixed defect in the inferior and inferolateral wall and partial reversibility in the inferoseptal region.

Case 18.2

History

A 62-year-old man presented with typical effort angina. He underwent a ^{99m}Tc-N-NOET myocardial perfusion imaging study for further evaluation of his chest discomfort. Poststress imaging was performed 20 minutes following the intravenous injection of 25 mCi of ^{99m}Tc-N-NOET at peak heart rate (HR). Resting images were obtained 4 hours later. The stress/rest ^{99m}Tc-N-NOET SPECT images are displayed in Figure C18-2A and stress/rest ^{99m}Tc-MIBI SPECT images in Figure C18-2B for comparison.

Findings

The ^{99m}Tc-N-NOET SPECT postexercise images (top row) demonstrated a moderate sized, rather severe anterior and apical defect, which is almost completely reversible on the rest images

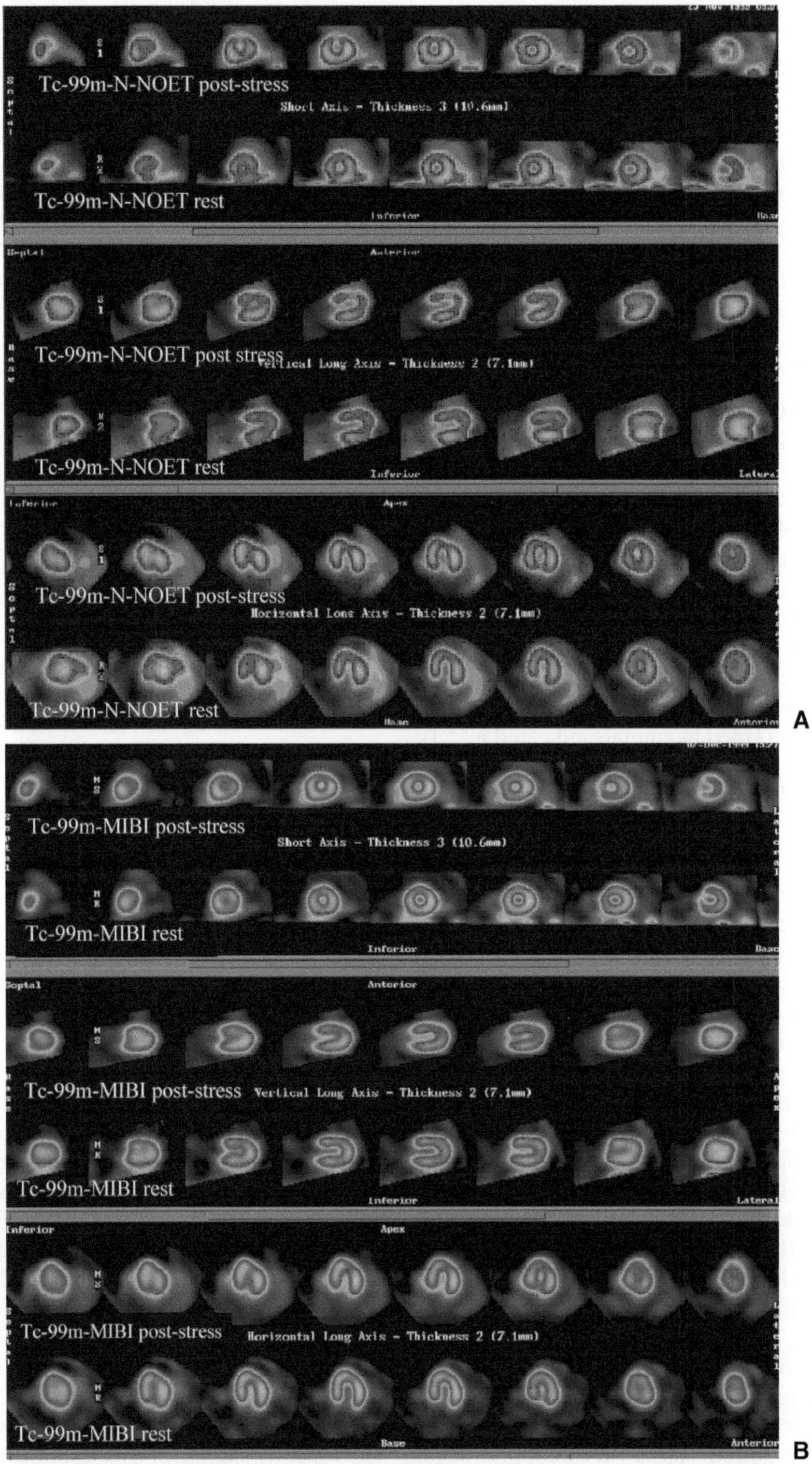

FIGURE C18-2. (A and B, courtesy of R. Taillefer, Centre Hospitalier de l'Universite de Montreal, Montreal, Canada.)

(second row). The ^{99m}Tc-MIBI SPECT images from the same patient as in Figure C18-2A also demonstrated a reversible anterior and apical defect, which appears much less prominent on these images. He then underwent selective coronary arteriography, which revealed a 90% stenosis in the left anterior descending coronary artery (LAD) and a 60% stenosis in the left circumflex coronary artery (LCX).

Discussion

^{99m}Tc-N-NOET is a new single photon tracer that combines the photon energy of ^{99m}Tc and ^{201}Tl-like redistribution properties, which makes it a promising new tracer for stress myocardial perfusion imaging (MPI). ^{99m}Tc-N-NOET is a neutral lipophilic compound that belongs to the ^{99m}Tc-nitridodithiocarbamate family. The clearance of ^{99m}Tc-N-NOET from the blood is rapid, with less than 5% of the injected activity present 5 minutes after injection.[7] Reperfusion studies and low flow delayed studies performed in animals indicated a ^{99m}Tc-N-NOET redistribution phenomenon similar to that of ^{201}Tl. Early clinical studies in humans confirmed the similarity in behavior between ^{99m}Tc-N-NOET and ^{201}Tl.

Close correlation between the myocardial retention of ^{99m}Tc-N-NOET and coronary blood flow exists over a wide range of flow rates.[8] The myocardial uptake of ^{99m}Tc-N-NOET is closely proportional to blood flow during both adenosine and dobutamine stress with no evidence of alteration of ^{99m}Tc N-NOET extraction by dobutamine,[9] such an effect was noted when dobutamine is used as a stressor for ^{99m}Tc-MIBI myocardial perfusion studies compared with adenosine.

^{99m}Tc-N-NOET SPECT imaging has been shown to have a sensitivity of 79% and a specificity of 82% in detecting significant coronary lesions defined as 70% or more reduction in the luminal diameter of the coronary vessel.[10] Phase III clinical trial has recently been completed, but the results have not yet been published at the time of this writing.

Interpretation

Anterior ischemia demonstrated by stress/rest ^{99m}Tc-N-NOET SPECT.

Case 18.3

History

A 43-year-old man who awakened with chest pain presented at the hospital approximately 2 hours after the onset of symptoms. He subsequently sustained a cardiac arrest but was successfully resuscitated. His ECG was consistent with an acute ST-segment elevation anterior wall MI. His cardiac risk factors included cigarette smoking, hypertension, diabetes mellitus, and hyperlipidemia.

Three days after presentation, the patient underwent dual isotope ^{201}Tl/^{99m}Tc-annexin imaging. The ^{99m}Tc-annexin images were obtained first, approximately 90 minutes after the injection of 25.3 mCi. He was subsequently injected with ^{201}Tl (1.2 mCi), and the images were reacquired using a dual-photopeak window. The ^{99m}Tc-annexin images were re-oriented as the ^{201}Tl images. The ^{99m}Tc-annexin/^{201}Tl SPECT images are displayed in Figure C18-3.

Findings

In Figure C18-3, the top row in each set of reoriented images displays the ^{201}Tl images. The prominent perfusion abnormality is noted in the distal anterior and distal inferior walls as well as involving the entire apex. The bottom row of each axis depicts the ^{99m}Tc-annexin images and reveals prominent apical activity, which also involves the distal portion of the septum, anterior wall, and inferior wall. Overall, the ^{99m}Tc-annexin SPECT images demonstrated a large area of necrosis/apoptosis, which is similar in size and location to the perfusion abnormality noted on the ^{201}Tl SPECT images.

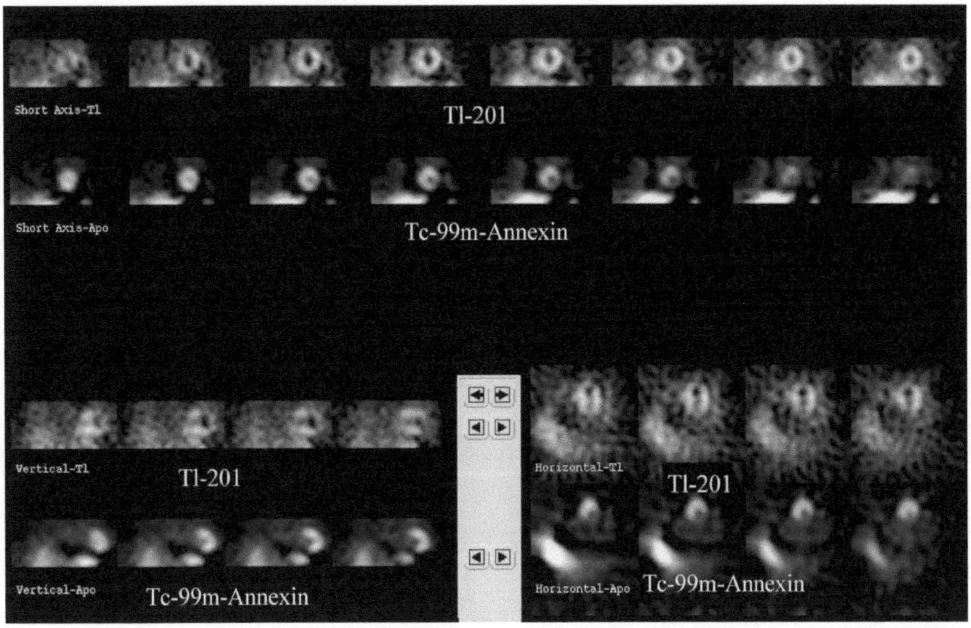

FIGURE C18-3.

Subsequent coronary angiography revealed a completely occluded proximal left anterior descending coronary artery (LAD), which was successfully revascularized with stent implantation.

Discussion

Annexin V has a high affinity for phosphatidylserine, a negatively charged membrane phospholipid expressed on the surface of apoptotic cells. This phosphatidylserine expression is one of the first events occurring during programmed cell death that persists until the final degradation of the cell.[11] Recombinant human annexin V has been radiolabeled with ^{99m}Tc and used for in vitro and in vivo detection of apoptosis.

Recent studies[12,13] demonstrated that ^{99m}Tc-annexin V imaging can accurately localize in vivo increased programmed cell death (apoptosis) in the area at risk of patients with acute MI. In the subacute phase of MI, there is absent ^{99m}Tc-annexin uptake and a decrease in the size of the ^{99m}Tc-MIBI defect, suggesting that reversible myocardial damage rather than necrosis is present in cardiomyocytes of the area at risk. Other studies performed in a rabbit model of severe ischemia suggested that phosphatidylserine expression does not necessarily indicate irreversible damage.[14]

^{99m}Tc-annexin V has been used to detect myocyte apoptosis in heart transplant rejection. In a study of 18 patients, the 5 patients who had positive myocardial uptake of ^{99m}Tc-annexin V demonstrated at least moderate transplant rejection and caspase-3 staining in their biopsy specimens suggesting apoptosis.[15]

^{99m}Tc-annexin V imaging may allow the study of reperfusion-induced cell death and may also prove useful in the evaluation of new therapeutic strategies that intervene in myocardial cell death, the so-called cell death inhibitors. In summary, there may be applications for ^{99m}Tc-annexin in the setting of ischemic heart disease, heart failure, acute MI, myocarditis, and transplant rejection.

Interpretation

Apoptosis demonstrated by ^{99m}Tc-annexin.

Case 18.4

History

A 62-year-old man with a history of remote MI presented with severe chest pain and was treated 2½ hours later with thrombolysis. The electrocardiogram (ECG) demonstrated ST-segment elevation in V1–V6 and AVL. His serum levels of creatine kinase (CK) peaked at 5509 IU/L approximately 5 hours after the onset of chest pain.

^{99m}Tc-glucarate (25 mCi) was administered IV approximately 1 hour after the infusion of the thrombolytic agent. Two hours later, planar images were obtained in the anterior and left anterior oblique projections recording a peak of 2 million counts in each view. Myocardial perfusion imaging with ^{99m}Tc-MIBI was performed several days later. The ^{99m}Tc-glucarate images are displayed in Figure C18-4A, an anterior view of the ^{99m}Tc-glucarate and ^{99m}Tc-MIBI images in Figure C18-4B, and a similar set of images from another patient is displayed in Figure C18-4C.

Findings

There was intense ^{99m}Tc-glucarate uptake in the anterolateral (left panel of Figure C18-4A) and lateral (right panel) walls of the LV. These findings are consistent with acute myocardial necrosis. The left panel was obtained in an anterior planar projection with the right-hand panel being obtained in a best septal LAO view. There was a corresponding perfusion defect on the ^{99m}Tc-MIBI images (right panel in Figure C18-4B). In Figure C18-4C (different patient), the left panel depicts intense uptake in the inferior wall consistent with an inferior MI, which was supported by ST-segment elevation in the inferior leads. The right-hand panel demonstrates a prominent perfusion abnormality, using ^{99m}Tc-MIBI, in the same distribution.

Discussion

A number of agents have been used to image myocardial necrosis. ^{99m}Tc-pyrophosphate has been used to establish the diagnosis of acute MI when conventional work-up is unreliable, due to a delay in presentation or when there is conflicting data. However, ^{99m}Tc-pyrophosphate imaging does not become positive until 12 hours and often until 48 hours after acute infarction because it is targeting sequestered calcium. ^{111}In-antimyosin has also been used for detection and localization of MI and this agent requires a 12- to 24-hour delay after injection due to the slow clearance from the blood pool.

^{99m}Tc-glucaric acid is a 6-carbon dicarboxcylic acid that can detect necrosis early in the process of MI in experimental models and clinical studies.[16,17] ^{99m}Tc-glucarate provides information regarding the location and extent of necrosis based on the ability of this agent to bind avidly the nuclear fraction of the cell following irreversible injury. There is up to a 12-fold increase in uptake compared with background in the setting of nonreperfused infarction.[16] Visualization is apparent within 30 minutes following injection, the elimination half-time is only 36 minutes, and uptake is present for up to 72 hours.[16] One of the principal advantages of ^{99m}Tc-glucarate is that the imaging of hyperacute injury may allow for alteration in management and the use of aggressive therapy, such as thrombolysis or percutaneous coronary intervention (PCI). The ability to detect injury early in the course of an infarction, as well as ability to image ^{99m}Tc-glucarate very early after injection makes this an almost ideal agent for this purpose. Additionally, the high affinity of ^{99m}Tc-glucarate for necrotic tissue provides a strong imaging signal. Although increased retention may be uncommonly seen in the setting of ischemia,[18,19] the signal is very low (1.5 times) and is likely due to the reduced washout of the agent rather than retention in hypoxic tissue.[19] Therefore, most studies have not demonstrated an ability of glucaric acid to detect ischemia in the absence of necrosis.[16–18]

Clinical trials have clearly demonstrated the potential of ^{99m}Tc-glucarate for the definitive identification of acute MI, even when other clinical data are equivocal. Mariani et al.[18]

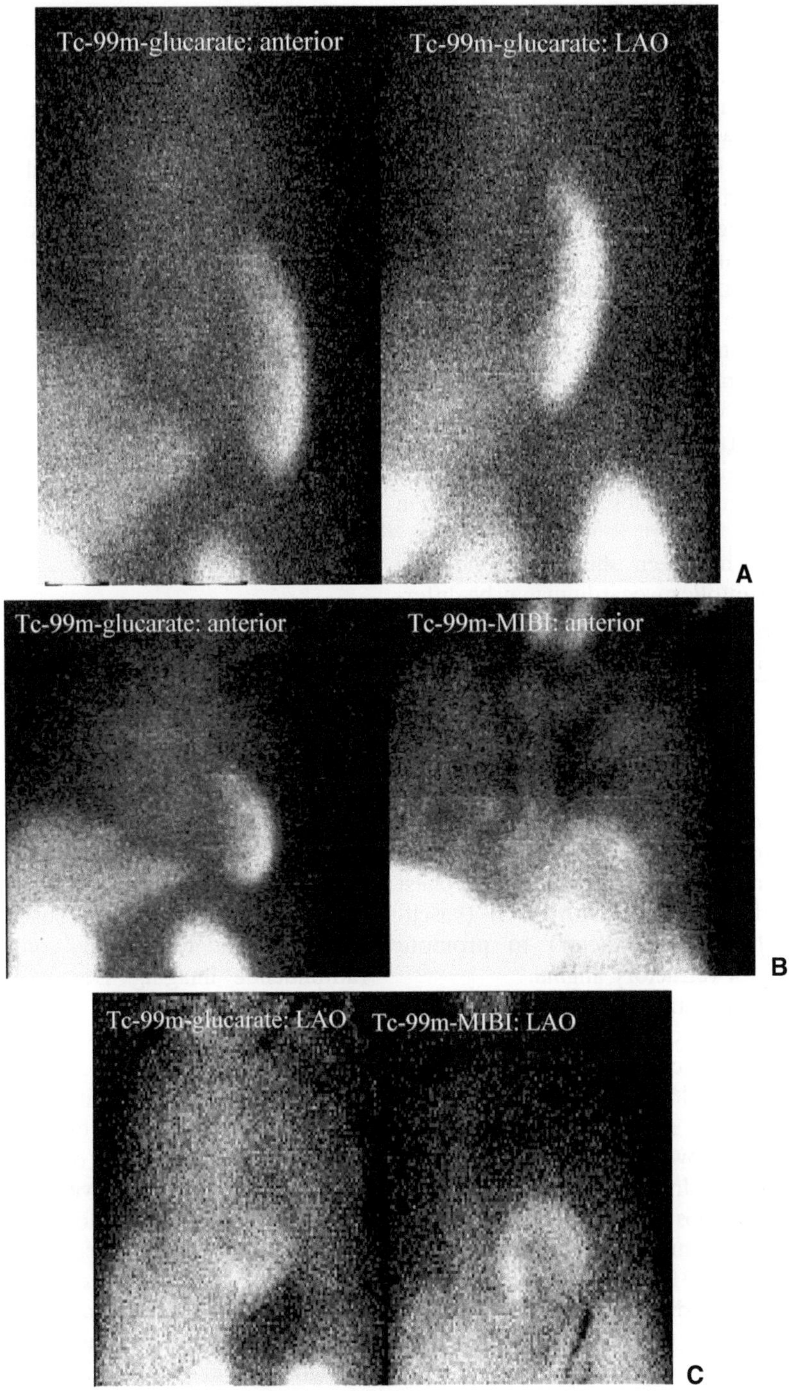

FIGURE C18-4. (A–C, courtesy of G. Mariani, University of Pisa Medical School, Pisa, Italy.)

studied 28 patients admitted from the emergency department with a suspected acute MI. The subjects were injected with ^{99m}Tc-glucarate shortly after arrival and imaged within 3 hours. All 14 patients who were studied within 9 hours of the onset of symptoms had markedly positive ^{99m}Tc-glucarate studies. Five of the 14 patients with negative study results had no confirmation of infarction and were diagnosed with unstable angina. The remaining 9 patients all presented more than 9 hours after symptom onset. Repeat imaging 4 to 6 weeks after the initial admission revealed that all patients had negative study results. Therefore, preliminary data demonstrate that ^{99m}Tc-glucaric acid appears well suited for the detection of early infarction and makes subsequent intervention feasible.

Recently, it has been shown that necrotic (oncotic) and aptotic myocardium may be differentiated noninvasively by the combined use of ^{99m}Tc-glucarate and ^{111}In-antimyosin.[20] There may be significant clinical benefit from such characterization. Previously, this distinction was possible only by biopsy or postmortem examination. ^{99m}Tc-glucaric acid fixes only in necrotic myocardium, whereas ^{111}In-antimyosin demonstrates uptake for both apoptosis and oncolysis. The differences in uptake between ^{99m}Tc-glucaric acid and ^{111}In-antimyosin likely result from glucaric acid's requirement for a nuclear target, which is absent in apoptosis.

Interpretation

Acute myocardial necrosis in the anterolateral region of the LV demonstrated by ^{99m}Tc-glucarate.

Case 18.5

History

A 63-year-old woman with a history of CAD, including prior MI, CABG, and PCI, presented with recurrence of her usual exertional chest pain. She had been treated with VEGF (vascular endothelial growth factor) to promote angiogenesis for refractory angina.

A dual isotope stress ^{99m}Tc-MIBI/rest ^{201}Tl study was performed and the patient was stressed using a selective A_{2A} adenosine receptor agonist, CVT-3146. CVT-3146 (400 mcg) was administered as a single bolus intravenous injection (IV) followed by a saline flush and the immediate IV administration of ^{99m}Tc-MIBI (34.2 mCi). The poststress images were obtained about 75 minutes after tracer administration. The CVT-3146 ^{99m}Tc-MIBI/rest ^{201}Tl SPECT images are displayed in Figure C18-5.

Findings

There was moderately decreased uptake on the poststress SPECT images in the anterior wall and apex (Figure C18-5). The rest images were normal, findings consistent with a lesion in the LAD.

Discussion

Adenosine and dipyridamole are potent vasodilators capable of creating heterogeneous blood flow in the setting of a significant coronary stenosis, serving as the basis of pharmacological stress testing in conjunction with radionuclide imaging. Despite their efficacy as vasodilators, patients receiving adenosine or dipyridamole experience a high prevalence of side effects such as chest pain, flushing, dyspnea, headache, gastrointestinal discomfort, and dizziness. These side effects are mediated by subtypes of receptors other than A_{2A} (see Chapter 4). The coronary vasodilatory effect of adenosine and dipyridamole is mediated primarily by A_{2A} receptors present in the vascular wall. Agents that selectively or preferentially stimulate A_{2A} receptors have the advantage of improved patient safety and comfort. A number of highly potent and selective A_{2A}-receptor agonists have now been synthesized and are in various stages of clinical development.[21]

Binodenoson (MRE-0470)

Binodenoson (MRE-0470, formerly WRC-0470) is a highly selective A_{2A}-receptor agonist

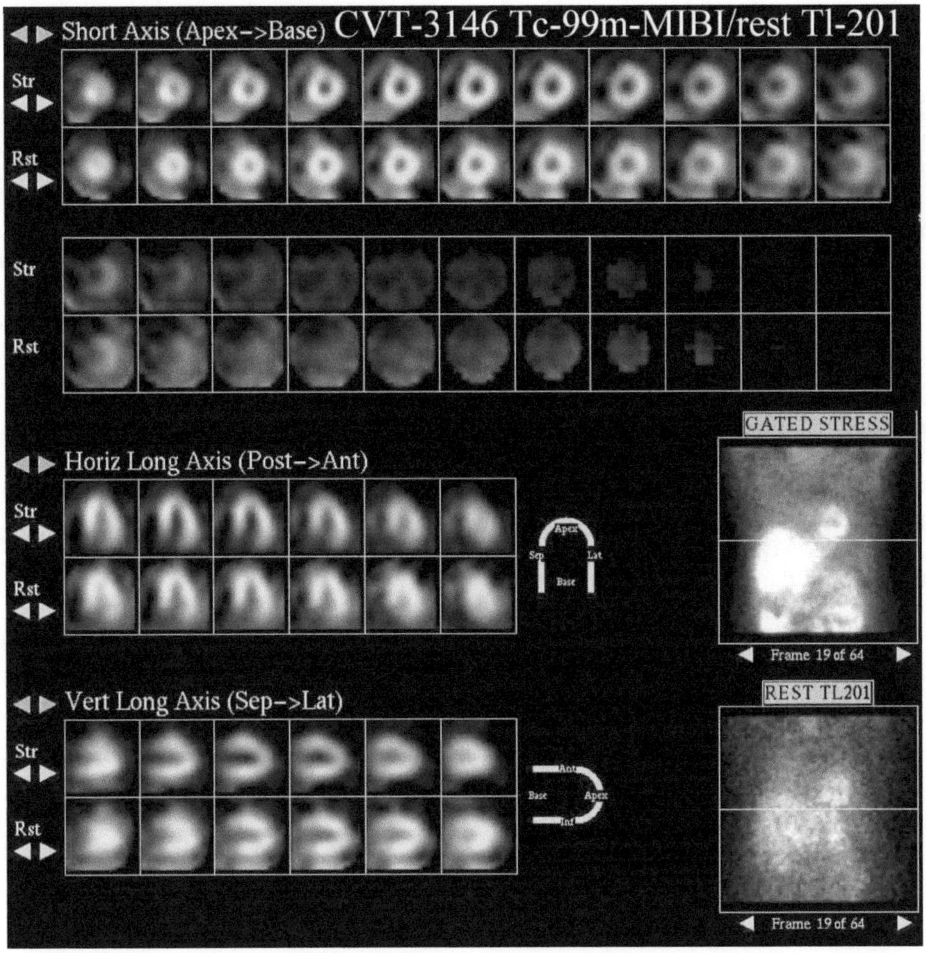

FIGURE C18-5. (Courtesy of J. J. Mahmarian, Baylor University School of Medicine, Waco, TX.)

that is 200 times more potent than adenosine and has high affinity for adenosine A_{2A}-receptors. Glover et al.[22] demonstrated that MRE-0470 produced greater vasodilation at its peak pharmacological infused dose than did adenosine, and without significant hypotension.

The hemodynamic properties and experimental studies suggest that MRE-0470 has the potential to provide comparable or enhanced diagnostic accuracy as adenosine with markedly reduced side effects. Phase II trials with this agent have now been completed, and phase III are planned in the near future.

CVT-3146

The advantages of CVT have been shown in a recent study by Trochu et al.[23] and are illustrated in the current case. CVT was administered as IV bolus and produced a potent, and short-duration, dose-dependent coronary vasodilation with limited peripheral hemodynamic effects. In comparison with adenosine, CVT, in dogs, was more potent, but equally effective.[23] The effects of CVT on coronary blood flow were fully and rapidly reversible within 258 to 317 seconds after an injection dose of 25 mcg/kg. One advantage of this agent is the ability to administer it as a single intravenous bolus injection. Clinical trials using CVT-3146 in conjunction with MPI are now underway.

ATL-193 and ATL-146e

ATL-193 and ATL-146e represent a new class of highly potent and selective adenosine A_{2A}-

receptor agonists. These new ester compounds are more selective for the A_{2A} receptor than the other selective A_{2A} agonists. In animal studies, ATL-146e was given as a bolus injection and produced an increase in coronary blood flow in a dose-dependent manner without producing significant hypotension,[24] with coronary blood flow returning completely to baseline in 20 minutes.

ATP

Like adenosine, ATP is a potent coronary vasodilator with a short half-life (2 seconds for adenosine, and <20 seconds for ATP). Once in the plasma, ATP is gradually degraded into ADP, AMP, and adenosine, which in turn produces coronary vasodilation through its action on A_{2A} receptors. ADP excites the P1 and P2Y1 receptors on endothelial cells producing further vasodilation. ATP administration produces significant changes in coronary flow reserve that returns to baseline within 1.4 minutes.[25]

ATP has been studied in humans by several investigators[25–27] in conjunction with multiple MPI tracers including ^{201}Tl, ^{99m}Tc-tetrofosmin, and ^{99m}Tc-MIBI. Watanabe et al.[25] demonstrated in a study of 140 patients that ATP stress ^{201}Tl SPECT is equivalent to dipyridamole stress ^{201}Tl SPECT in the detection of CAD. Using a one-day protocol, Takeishi et al.[26] demonstrated that ATP stress ^{99m}Tc-tetrofosmin SPECT has a sensitivity of 89% and a specificity of 86% in the detection of CAD compared with coronary angiography. Also compared with coronary angiography, the sensitivity and specificity of ^{99m}Tc-MIBI MPI with intravenous infusion of ATP in the diagnosis of CAD is 97% and 82%, respectively.[27]

Interpretation

Ischemia in the LAD territory demonstrated with a selective adenosine A_{2A} receptor stress ^{99m}Tc-MIBI/rest ^{201}Tl.

Case 18.6

History and Findings

For history, figures, and findings, see Chapter 4, Case 4.5.

Discussion

Dobutamine is a synthetic catecholamine with strong beta-1 receptor and mild beta-2 and alpha-1 receptor agonist activity. At low dose (10 mcg·kg·min^{-1}), dobutamine has a marked inotropic effect mediated by beta-1 and alpha-1 receptors; while at high dose (40 mcg·kg·min^{-1}) it causes a marked chronotropic effect mediated mainly by beta-1 receptors. The beta-2 mediated vasodilatory effect overwhelms the alpha-1 mediated vasoconstriction, leading to a minimal net increase in blood pressure despite the marked increase in HR and cardiac output. Dobutamine is metabolized in the liver and has a half-life of approximately 2 minutes. Although dobutamine may have a minor direct coronary vasodilator effect, the secondary dilation of coronary vessels in response to the increase in myocardial oxygen demand serves as the basis of its use as a stressor for MPI. The most commonly used protocol of dobutamine stress MPI (DSMPI) uses a continuous infusion of dobutamine with increasing doses (10 to 40 mcg·kg·min^{-1}) every 3 minutes with or without an additional atropine injection; the radiotracer is injected at peak HR and dobutamine infusion is maintained for 1 minute after the injection. Target heart rate may be achieved by this protocol in more than 90% of all patients.[28]

The safety of dobutamine use for MPI has been demonstrated in several studies. In a review that combined safety studies involving more than 2500 patients, no patient suffered death, MI, or ventricular fibrillation.[28] The rate of supraventricular and nonsustained ventricular tachycardias ranged from 0.9% to 6.0%.[28]

The diagnostic accuracy of DSMPI is high, although it varies among different studies due to differences in patient population, stress protocols, and imaging techniques. The overall sensitivity, specificity, and accuracy of DSMPI in a total of 1014 patients are 88%, 74%, and 84%, respectively.[28] The inclusion of atropine in the protocol has been reported to increase the sensitivity (90% vs. 82%) without loss in specificity.[29] Studies that compared DSMPI with DSE (dobutamine stress echocardiography) in the same patients demonstrated a higher sensitivity (86% vs. 80%) and a lower specificity (73% vs. 86%) of DSMPI.[28] Since perfusion abnormalities precede wall motion abnormalities in the ischemic cascade, the higher sensitivity of DSMPI is expected. It is also expected that DSMPI is less sensitive than MPI using direct vasodilators such as adenosine and dipyridamole; this was demonstrated in a study that compared dipyridamole with dobutamine MPI in 60 patients, the sensitivity of dipyridamole and dobutamine MPI was 97% and 91%, respectively.[30]

Short- and long-term prognostic value of DSMPI has been demonstrated in several studies. In a long-term follow-up study (average, 8 years) of approximately 500 patients with suspected CAD, a normal DSMPI was associated with a very low rate of cardiac death (0.9%) as opposed to an abnormal study (2.7%).[31] Both abnormal findings and increased summed stress score provided incremental prognostic information over clinical data.[31] In another prospective study of 156 patients undergoing elective vascular surgery, a normal dobutamine stress ^{99m}Tc-MIBI study was characterized by a high negative predictive value (97%) for perioperative cardiac events. An abnormal DSMPI provided additional prognostic information and optimized risk stratification in patients with clinical or electrocardiographic evidence of ischemic heart disease.[32]

Case 18.7

History

A 49-year-old man underwent cardiac transplantation and presented for evaluation of acute rejection a few months after heart transplantation. Anterior and posterior planar images were obtained 48 hours following administration of 3 mCi of ^{67}Ga citrate using a conventional gamma camera with a high-energy collimator and a 25% window on the 93 KeV photon photopeak.

Findings

^{67}Ga images showed faint uptake by the transplanted heart with ill-defined cardiac silhouette graded as mild rejection (Figure C18-7). Endomyocardial biopsy showed mild lymphocytic interstitial infiltrate consistent with mild acute rejection.

Discussion

^{67}Ga has long been used to detect acute and chronic inflammatory lesions. It has been used

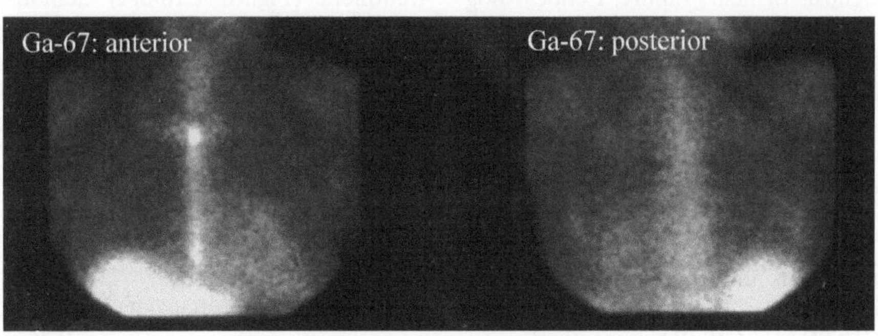

FIGURE C18-7. (Courtesy of J.C. Meneguetti, University of Sao Paulo Medical School, Sao Paulo, Brazil.)

previously to detect inflammation in cardiac diseases such as bacterial endocarditis, myocardial abscess, myocardial sarcoidosis, and pericardial disease.

In the era of heart transplantation, the cardiac applications of ^{67}Ga imaging have been expanded to include the noninvasive detection of acute rejection of the transplanted heart. In an early study by Meneguetti et al.[33] ^{67}Ga imaging was compared with endomyocardial biopsy (which is considered the most accurate method for diagnosis and follow-up of acute rejection of the transplanted heart) in 7 patients who underwent 46 ^{67}Ga scintigrams and 46 endomyocardial biopsies between 1 week and 8 months after transplantation. The overall sensitivity of ^{67}Ga imaging for transplant rejection was 83%. Five studies showed moderately acute rejection and a decline in ^{67}Ga uptake was seen after therapy that correlated with resolving rejection on biopsy.

^{67}Ga imaging in heart transplantation has its limitations. Early after transplantation, there is marked accumulation of the radionuclide in the sternum due to surgical trauma, and this overlaps the cardiac silhouette. Moreover, 48-hour delayed imaging is generally performed that precludes its use for an emergency evaluation of these patients. However, ^{67}Ga imaging is noninvasive and allows evaluation of the entire heart, whereas a biopsy specimen is subject to sampling error; therefore, ^{67}Ga imaging may be used as a sensitive screening method for cardiac rejection instead of sequential endomyocardial biopsies in the follow-up of heart transplant patients.

Another cardiac application of ^{67}Ga imaging is the detection of myocarditis in patients with dilated cardiomyopathy,[34,35] myocarditis has been identified in 8% to 25% of these patients. In a study of 68 patients with dilated cardiomyopathy, O'Connell et al.[35] correlated 72-hour delayed ^{67}Ga imaging with endomyocardial biopsy. In their study, evidence of myocarditis on endomyocardial biopsy was four times as frequent in patients with positive ^{67}Ga images. Conversely, less than 2% of patients had myocarditis on biopsy if the ^{67}Ga scan was negative. Once the correlation between ^{67}Ga images and biopsy is established in an individual patient, ^{67}Ga imaging may be a useful technique in the serial evaluation of these patients, obviating the necessity for frequent invasive procedures.

Interpretation

Cardiac transplant rejection demonstrated with ^{67}Ga.

Case 18.8

History

A 58-year-old man was admitted with dyspnea and a diagnosis of heart failure. Echocardiography demonstrated LV dilation and an LVEF of 20%. Coronary angiography revealed normal coronary arteries and an endomyocardial biopsy was performed. The diagnosis was idiopathic dilated cardiomyopathy. After treatment with enalapril, furosemide, and spironolactone, the patient became essentially asymptomatic. SPECT ^{123}I-MIBG images performed at the start of treatment and 6 months later are displayed in Figures C18-8A and C18-8C and Figures C18-8B and C18-8D, respectively.

Findings

The SPECT images obtained at the start of treatment (Figure C18-8A) demonstrated a large area of reduced activity in the inferior and apical region. Six months later, there was great improvement (Figure C18-8B). The heart/mediastinum (H/M) ratio also improved with therapy (Figures C18-8C and C18-8D), as did the washout rates, declining from 49% to 33%.

Discussion

MIBG (metaiodobenzylguanidine) is an emerging neuroimaging tracer. It is an analog

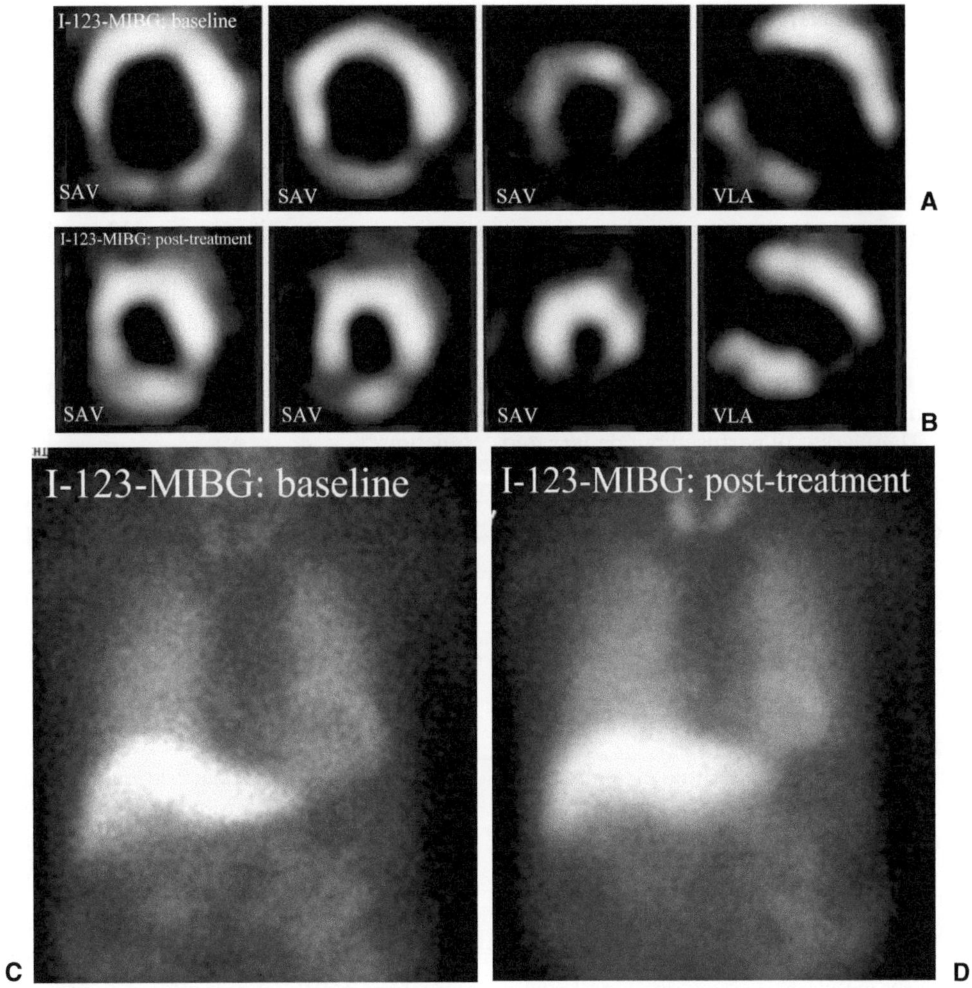

FIGURE C18-8. (A–D) (C and D, images and case history courtesy of S. Kasama, Gumna University, Japan.)

of guanethidine that is taken up by adrenergic neurons in similar fashion to norepinephrine. When labeled with ^{123}I, cardiac adrenergic receptors may be imaged using both SPECT and planar imaging techniques. The usual protocol involves injecting 4 mCi of ^{123}I-MIBG IV at rest, planar imaging followed by SPECT imaging is performed after 15 minutes, delayed planar imaging is done 4 hours later, and conventional SPECT with a perfusion tracer such as ^{99m}Tc-MIBI or tetrofosmin can be done at the same time.[36] On planar imaging, the heart-to-mediastinum ratio (H/M ratio) and myocardial washout rate are determined, normal hearts have a high H/M ratio; decreased ratio indicates reduced adrenergic receptor density as seen after MI. Immediately after heart transplantation, no activity is detected in the myocardium reflecting total denervation. A high washout rate indicates increased adrenergic activity in the heart as seen in patients with dilated cardiomyopathy, for example. MIBG SPECT can be compared with the perfusion tracer SPECT images to reveal matched or unmatched defects. A mismatched pattern indicates an area of denervated perfused viable myocardium, a pattern seen after Q wave MI.

The application of ^{123}I-MIBG imaging can provide useful information in a variety of cardiovascular disease states including ischemic heart disease, heart failure and cardiomyopathies, diabetic autonomic neuropathy, arrhythmias, and parkinsonism.

Sympathetic nerves penetrate the myocardium from the epicardial to the endocardial surface alongside the coronary vessels. In a non-Q-wave infarction, the area of denervation corresponds to the infarct zone and produces matched defects when MIBG SPECT images are compared with a perfusion tracer SPECT. In a Q-wave infarction, the downstream areas of the myocardium are also denervated when the proximal fibers are injured, producing a mismatched defect on SPECT images. These areas of perfused but denervated myocardium have been shown in experimental studies to be arrhythmogenic;[37] the degree of denervation also correlated to the LVEF in some studies.[38] Ischemia without infarction may also cause denervation, and MIBG abnormalities can be detected hours to days after an ischemic insult; MIBG imaging may prove useful in patients who arrive at the emergency room after their ischemic episode has abated.[39]

MIBG imaging has a potential diagnostic and prognostic role in patients with heart failure and cardiomyopathies. Patients with dilated cardiomyopathy have reduced MIBG uptake and increased washout rate compared with healthy subjects. The abnormalities in these patients are typically diffuse as compared with the patients with ischemic cardiomyopathy who display patchy abnormalities that correlate to the necrotic segments. In some studies, MIBG abnormalities correlated to LVEF, plasma norepinephrine levels, NYHA class, and histopathologic abnormalities. The prognostic value of MIBG imaging parameters in patients with mild to moderate chronic heart failure is being investigated. In a recent study, cardiac MIBG washout rate and H/M ratio correlated to cardiac death and hospitalization for worsening heart failure.[40] MIBG washout rate has a higher prognostic value than heart rate variability parameters, and the combination of abnormal washout rate and n-VLFP (normalized very low frequency power, the traditional parameter for measurement of heart rate variability on Holter monitoring) may identify a higher risk subset for cardiac events in chronic heart failure.[40]

MIBG imaging can also be used to predict response to beta-blocker therapy, as several studies showed an increase in H/M ratio and a decrease in the washout rate during the follow-up of patients treated with beta-blockers;[41] overall, 68% of heart failure patients treated with beta-blockers showed improved sympathetic function that could be detected by MIBG imaging before the improvement in LV function.[36]

Early detection of declining adrenergic function in patients receiving doxorubicin is also possible using MIBG imaging, and this deterioration precedes the decline in LV systolic function, which makes MIBG an important tool since LV dysfunction, once established, may not reverse despite discontinuation of anthracycline therapy.[42]

In the early period after heart transplantation, MIBG imaging reveals no uptake in the heart, reflecting total denervation. Evidence of total denervation seems to persist for at least 12 months; thereafter, partial reinnervation may be observed in some patients as patchy MIBG uptake.[43]

Other applications of MIBG imaging include the detection of diabetic autonomic neuropathy, where MIBG abnormalities appear earlier than the clinically detectable neuropathy, and may correlate to overt or latent LV dysfunction.[44]

Abnormal MIBG pattern was also noted in arrhythmogenic areas in patients with arrhythmogenic right ventricular disease, which correlated to the site of origin of ventricular tachycardia demonstrated on electrophysiological studies.[45]

Interpretation

Treatment of heart failure monitored with ^{123}I-MIBG.

Case 18.9

History

A 65-year-old man presented with exertional chest pain. At the time of admission his chest pain was resolved and there was no serologic or electrographic evidence of acute MI. Myocardial perfusion SPECT images with ^{99m}Tc-tetrofosmin were obtained at the time of hospital admission, when the patient was at rest and without pain. Approximately 24 hours after the onset of chest pain, ^{123}I-BMIPP SPECT imaging was performed using a 180-degree orbit with 32 stops at 20 seconds per stop (Figure C18-9).

Findings

Resting SPECT ^{99m}Tc-tetrofosmin images showed no significant myocardial perfusion defects (apical thinning is noted). SPECT ^{123}I-BMIPP images obtained the next day showed severely reduced uptake in the apex and anteroapical regions. Severe stenosis in the LAD was seen on coronary arteriogram.

Discussion

In the normal heart, beta-oxidization of fatty acids provides 70% to 80% of the energy source for myocardial metabolism. In conditions such as ischemia and heart failure, beta-oxidization is reduced, and alterations in the metabolism and utilization of fatty acids may persist in the postischemic dysfunctional segments of the myocardium as *ischemic memory*.[46] Radioiodinated fatty acids have been developed to probe fatty acid utilization using SPECT imaging.

Two groups of iodinated fatty acids are available for imaging purposes: straight chain and modified branched fatty acids. Straight chain fatty acids are metabolized through beta-oxidation, then released from the heart. Assessing the washout kinetics of these tracers reflects the use of fatty acid. However, this requires fast dynamic acquisition of images, which may be difficult in clinical practice. Modified branched fatty acids undergo *storage* in the heart through myocardial retention from metabolic trapping;[47] images can be obtained with long acquisition times. However, the uptake of these tracers may reflect more the uptake and turnover rate of fatty acids rather than their beta-oxidation. Therefore, combined perfusion tracer and fatty acid SPECT is often required to show perfusion-metabolism mismatch and to characterize fatty acid use.

BMIPP, 15-(p-[^{123}I] iodophenyl) methyl-pentadecanoic acid, is the most commonly used branched fatty acid tracer. It has a high myocardial extraction and retention with low background activity and low uptake in the liver and lungs 60 minutes after injection. In clinical studies, less ^{123}I-BMIPP uptake than ^{99m}Tc-MIBI or ^{201}Tl (discordant ^{123}I-BMIPP uptake) has been shown in patients in the subacute phase of MI. Several investigators[48,49] suggested that this finding reflects myocardial stunning, or delayed recovery of metabolism after recovery of perfusion. In patients with successful revascularization after acute MI, Kawai et al.[50] suggested that this discordant ^{123}I-BMIPP uptake reflects prior severe ischemia after recovery of perfusion, or the so-called ischemic memory; follow-up studies proved that these areas show delayed improvement in wall motion, suggesting that they represent stunned myocardium.

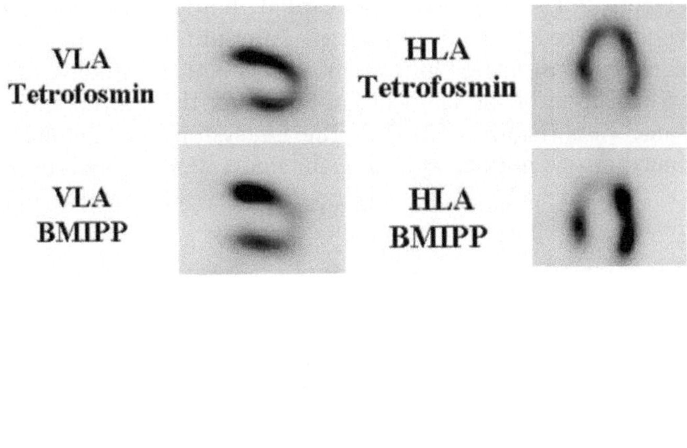

FIGURE C18-9. (Courtesy of N. Tamaki, Hokkaido University, Japan.)

Applying the concept of ischemic memory, ^{123}I-BMIPP imaging at rest has been used to identify myocardial ischemia. In a study of 111 patients with acute chest pain,[51] ^{123}I-BMIPP SPECT imaging was performed at rest less than 24 hours from the last episode of chest pain, and compared with ^{99m}Tc-tetrofosmin SPECT and coronary angiography. Abnormal ^{123}I-BMIPP uptake was noted in 76% of patients with severe coronary stenosis, 14% of them had no perfusion defects on ^{99m}Tc-tetrofosmin images; ^{123}I-BMIPP abnormalities correlated with wall motion and ECG abnormalities reflecting recurrent and severe previous ischemia. Therefore, ^{123}I-BMIPP SPECT may be used for imaging of ischemic memory in patients presenting with acute chest pain. ^{123}I-BMIPP abnormalities were also sensitive (74%) and specific (92%) for the detection of coronary spasm.

^{123}I-BMIPP imaging has also been applied to patients with dilated cardiomyopathy. The defect in ^{123}I-BMIPP uptake correlated to the severity of LV dysfunction in some studies.[52] Other studies[53] suggested that a decrease in the uptake of ^{123}I-BMIPP in these patients indicates that they will not respond well to beta-blocker therapy.

Interpretation

Ischemic memory in LAD territory demonstrated with ^{123}I-BMIPP.

Case 18.10

History

A 63-year-old woman presented with dyspnea and lower extremity edema. She has a history of chronic obstructive pulmonary disease, obstructive sleep apnea, morbid obesity, hypertension, diabetes, and *heart failure*. She was referred for an echocardiogram to evaluate LV function and regional wall motion analysis. The transthoracic approach was technically difficult due to her lung disease and body habitus, therefore, the study was repeated following intravenous administration of an ultrasonic contrast agent, Optison (Amersham Health, Princeton, NJ). Figure C18-9 displays the apical 4-chamber views, without and with contrast, respectively.

Findings

On the apical 4-chamber view without contrast (Figure C18-10A), the endocardial border could not be adequately visualized. After ultrasonic contrast using Optison, there was better visualization of the endocardial border in the same view (Figure C18-10B). The LV systolic function was normal with an estimated LVEF of 55% to 65%. There was no evidence of regional wall motion abnormalities.

Discussion

Recent advances in echocardiography have resulted in numerous improvements in image quality, especially in patients whose body habitus made their echocardiographic evaluation suboptimal (see Chapter 16). These advances include the IV administration of ultrasound contrast agents and new imaging technology such as harmonic and pulse inversion imaging. Several echocardiographic contrast agents are now approved for use in clinical practice.

The ability to opacify cardiac and vascular structures by injecting agitated saline solution that produce strong echoes has been recognized for over 30 years. Early contrast agents, developed by encapsulating air bubbles, had a large particle size and were unable to traverse the pulmonary circulation. They were mainly used to examine the right-sided heart structures and detect intracardiac shunts. Multiple clinical studies validated their use in the detection of atrial and ventricular septal defects, and other congenital abnormalities.

Newer ultrasound contrast agents have a smaller particle size that enables them to traverse the pulmonary circulation and therefore

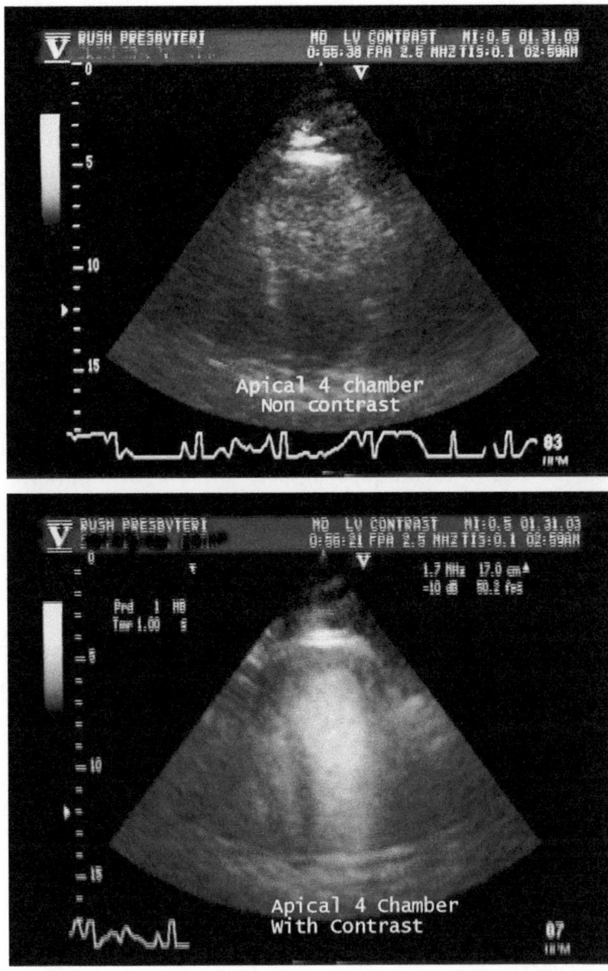

A

B

FIGURE C18-10. (A and B, courtesy of S. Feinstein, Rush University, Chicago.)

they are being used to study the left-sided heart structures. Various techniques are used to combine materials that control the bubble surface (shells) with gases that inhibit diffusion and bubble dissolution. The most commonly used agents (Optison and Albunex [albumin]) consist of air or perfluoropropane with a shell of albumin; other agents are being developed using perfluorocarbon and a shell of surfactant, galactose, or lipid.

The most common indication for contrast echocardiography in current practice is the enhancement of endocardial border delineation and LV opacification during rest and stress echocardiography in patients with suboptimal baseline echocardiograms due to nonvisualization of at least 2 segments of the myocardium.[54] In one study, contrast administration in these patients converted a nondiagnostic echocardiogram to a diagnostic study in 75% of those studied.[55] It has also been shown to enable more accurate measurement of LV volume and ejection fraction, detection of LV pseudoaneurysm formation after acute MI, and evaluating intracardiac masses such as thrombi and tumors.[54]

Obtaining adequate images to evaluate regional wall motion during stress echocardiography can be challenging in some patients due to their body habitus and excessive cardiac motion due to tachycardia and hyperventilation. The use of IV ultrasound contrast agents during stress echocardiography results in 80% to 95% improvement in endocardial border resolution,[56] and significantly improves image quality, completeness of wall segment visualization, and reviewer confidence.

Intravenous ultrasound contrast agents are currently being investigated for the use in echocardiographic evaluation of myocardial perfusion and coronary flow.[54] Meza et al.[57] compared myocardial contrast echocardiography to ^{99m}Tc-MIBI SPECT imaging for the detection of resting myocardial perfusion defects. The 2 techniques agreed in 78% of patients in the detection, size, and location of perfusion defects. Several experimental studies have shown intracoronary myocardial contrast echocardiography to be reliable in the evaluation of the area at risk for necrosis after acute coronary occlusion, regional coronary flow reserve, and collateral flow. It was also shown to be useful in assessment of viability through the demonstration of coronary microvascular capillary integrity in the setting of acute and chronic CAD.[54,58]

Interpretation

Better visualization of the endocardial borders with contrast echocardiography in an obese patient.

Case 18.11

History

A 57-year-old man was self-referred for assessment of coronary calcification by electron beam computed tomography (EBCT) because he was concerned about minor chest pain on vigorous activity. His risk factors included a strong family history for premature CAD and hyperlipidemia.

Findings

The EBCT images revealed extensive coronary calcification in the coronary arterial tree with a calcification score of 1562, which places the patient in the 99th percentile for his age (Figure C18-11A). A coronary calcium score >400 is indicative of high risk for CAD. The stress/rest SPECT images demonstrated a large, moderately severe, reversible defect in the distribution of the LAD (Figure C18-11B). Subsequent to the EBCT and SPECT MPI, the patient underwent coronary angiography, revealing a 99% stenosis of the proximal LAD with involvement in the first diagonal branch. Successful PCI was performed.

Discussion

EBCT (ultrafast CT) is a unique x-ray imaging technique that uses an electron gun to produce an electron beam that is magnetically focused to sweep a stationary tungsten target below the patient; with x-rays being captured by a stationary array of detectors above the patient. EBCT has a temporal resolution that allows imaging the beating heart with minimal motion artifact, as 30 to 40 snapshot images (50 to 100 msec each) can be captured during one or

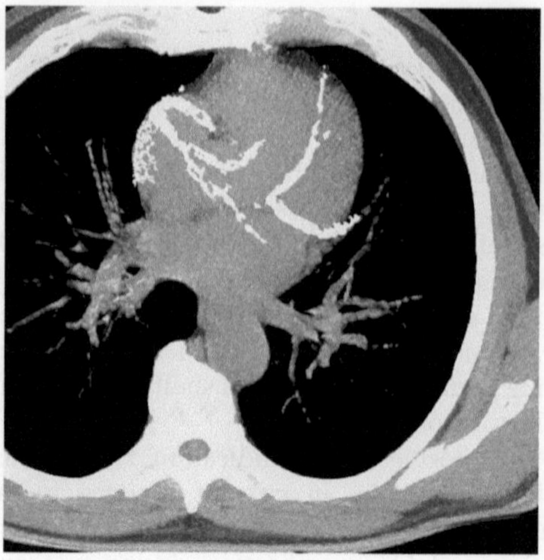

FIGURE C18-11. (A)

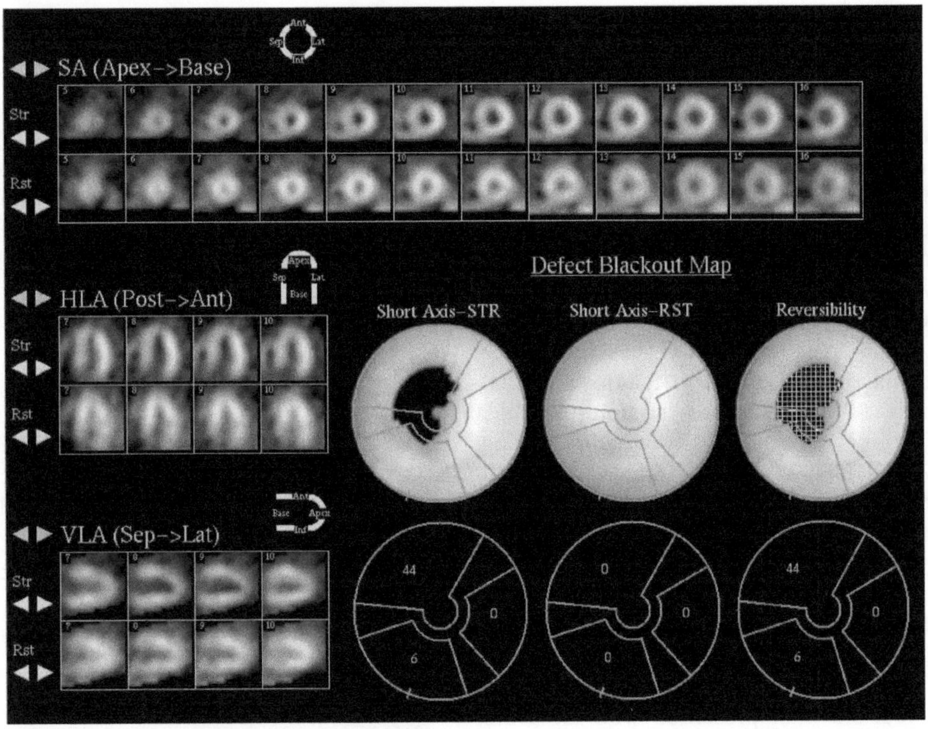

FIGURE C18-11. (B)

two breath-holding sessions. Ten minutes acquisition of images is triggered by ECG and is usually set to occur at a predefined percentage of the R-R interval, but can also be set to occur at a predefined absolute time interval after the R wave. Images are then reconstructed and displayed in tomograms or 3-D reconstruction angiography.[59]

Computed tomographic coronary angiography (CTCA) can also be performed using multislice CT scanners (MSCT); data acquisition in this method is performed in a continuous spiral fashion during a breath hold with retrospective ECG gating (see Chapter 15).

The noninvasive evaluation of CAD is the most common cardiac application of EBCT. There are several methods by which EBCT can be used for this purpose: coronary artery calcification, CTCA, and assessment of myocardial perfusion.

EBCT can noninvasively detect and quantify calcifications in coronary arteries and generate a *calcium score*. Since coronary calcification occurs as a result of atherosclerosis, an abnormal calcium score is considered evidence of CAD. Higher calcium scores correlate with age, multiple risk factors, and a greater extent of atherosclerosis. However, EBCT has been criticized for having low specificity when compared with coronary angiography.[60] In a metaanalysis of nine studies with 1662 subjects,[3,61] the pooled sensitivity of EBCT was 92% with a specificity of 51%. There is also increasing evidence that calcium scores have prognostic value in both symptomatic and asymptomatic patients. A metaanalysis of five studies[62] involving more than 4000 asymptomatic subjects revealed an increased risk of death, nonfatal MI, and revascularization if the calcium score was above the median. EBCT has also been used to further stratify patients presenting to the emergency room with acute chest pain who have normal or nondiagnostic ECG. In a study of 134 such patients[63] a calcium score of zero had a negative predictive value of

98%; on the other hand, patients with high calcium scores had a high event rate (8%) at 30 days.[63]

CTCA is a promising emerging technology with the potential for obtaining essentially noninvasive coronary angiograms. Budoff et al.[64] compared EBCT coronary angiography with conventional selective coronary angiography in 52 patients: the sensitivity and specificity of CTCA were 78% and 91%, respectively. The overall accuracy for EBCT angiography was 87%. A major limitation of CTCA was inadequate image quality, 11% of major epicardial coronary vessels were noninterpretable. MSCT offers improved image quality during CTCA. Nieman et al.[65] reported an overall sensitivity and specificity of 95% and 88%, respectively.

Assessment of myocardial perfusion offers a hemodynamic evaluation of the significance of coronary stenosis and helps guide the choice of treatment modality. EBCT was shown to have a promising potential in quantitating myocardial perfusion. Budoff et al.[66] investigated exercise EBCT imaging in 33 patients undergoing coronary angiography for evaluation of chest pain: exercise EBCT was analyzed using a global ejection fraction method and had a sensitivity of 81% and a specificity of 76%.

Interpretation

Extensive calcification on EBCT performed for a screening check-up leading to further testing by MPI and diagnosis of ischemia in the LAD territory.

Case 18.12

History

A 73-year-old man presented with an acute anterior wall MI, with markedly elevated serum levels of CK-MB and troponin levels. Coronary angiography revealed an occluded LAD and the patient underwent successful PCI with stent implantation. He developed recurrent symptoms and coronary angiography revealed reocclusion of the LAD. An MRI was ordered to determine the presence of viability in the infarcted zone.

MRI was performed 15 minutes after IV administration of 0.2 mmol/kg of gadolinium (OptiMARK, Mallinckrodt, Hazelwood, MO) using a breath-hold segmented inversion recovery FLASH pulse sequence. The delayed-enhanced MRIs are displayed in Figure C18-12.

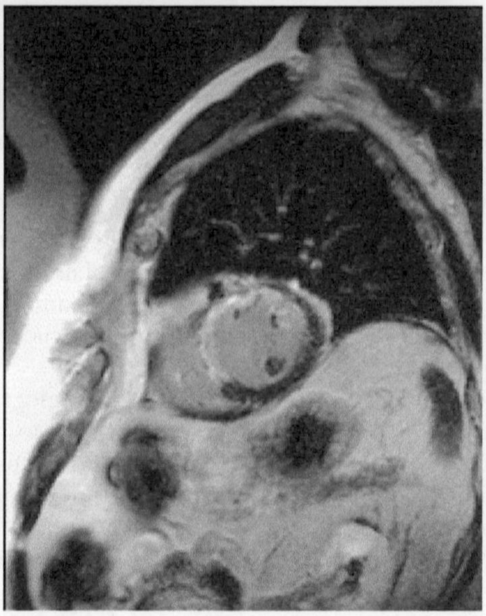

FIGURE C18-12. (Courtesy of R. Judd PhD, Duke University, Durham, NC.)

Findings

The images demonstrated extensive hyperenhancement (white) in the anterior and septal walls, indicating a large MI in the LAD distribution.

Discussion

Cardiac MRI continues to be an evolving tool in cardiovascular diseases. Several techniques are embodied in a single cardiac MR system. ECG gated, spin-echo imaging provides static images with high signal-to-noise ratio; the blood pool in this technique is black, providing sharp demarcation of the endocardium. This method is useful for anatomical imaging, and for assessing the myocardial mass, myocardial infiltration, and the area of acute infarction. ECG-referenced gradient echo imaging (cine MRI) is considered to be the gold standard in the evaluation of RV and LV size and function; it is also useful in the evaluation of intracardiac masses and valvular and shunt lesions.

Several cardiac MRI modalities can be used in the evaluation of ischemic heart disease (see Chapter 14). First-pass perfusion study using IV gadolinium has been shown to be reliable in detecting perfusion abnormalities even when they are confined to the subendocardial layer. In a study of 48 patients, an estimation of myocardial perfusion reserve index was used for the detection of compromised myocardium. Compared with coronary angiography, the sensitivity and specificity of this method was 87% and 85%, respectively.[67]

High-dose dobutamine stress testing can be used in conjunction with ultrafast cardiac MRI in a similar fashion to dobutamine stress echocardiography (DSE). In a study of 208 patients, detection of wall motion abnormalities by dobutamine stress MRI was superior to dobutamine stress echocardiography and yielded a sensitivity of 86%, and a specificity of 85% compared with coronary angiography.[68]

Direct visualization of coronary arteries using contrast-enhanced magnetic resonance angiography (MRA) is an area of rapid development. In an early study of 102 patients, the sensitivity and specificity of MRA compared with coronary angiography for the diagnosis of left main or triple vessel CAD were 100% and 85%, respectively,[69] and for the diagnosis of any CAD 93% and 42%, respectively. Cardiac MRA is also being used in the evaluation of coronary vein graft disease and restenosis after coronary angioplasty.

Another application of cardiac MRI is in the evaluation of myocardial viability. Delayed gadolinium enhancement defines areas of irreversible injury; areas that fail to hyperenhance are considered viable and display improved contractility in response to dobutamine infusion. Compared with PET, delayed hyperenhancement on MRI is a marker of scar tissue with a sensitivity of 96% and a specificity of 86%.[70] In a study of 24 patients with stable CAD and LV dysfunction, delayed hyperenhancement MRI correlated with nonviability by ^{201}Tl scintigraphy and dobutamine stress echocardiography, and the absence of hyperenhancement correlated with viability regardless of the resting contractile function.[71] The degree of enhancement can be used to predict recovery of LV function after revascularization. Quantitative analysis of regional contractile function can be performed using cardiac MRI tissue tagging in conjunction with 2-dimensional strain analysis (myocardial strain is the fractional or percentage change in the length of a contracting segment of the myocardium corrected to its original or unstressed dimension; it reflects the contraction/relaxation pattern of the myocardium). In a study of 26 subjects, the sensitivity and specificity of 2-dimensional strain analysis were 92% and 99%, respectively.[72]

Cardiac MRI is also an important tool in the evaluation of pericardial disease, congenital and valvular heart disease, cardiomyopathies, cardiac tumors, and aortic and peripheral vascular disease.

Interpretation

Anteroseptal MI demonstrated with delayed-Gd-enhanced MRI.

Case 18.13

History

A 77-year-old man with a history of CAD, including previous MI 6 years ago and CABG 2 years before admission, presented with chest pain, different in nature to his previous angina. An exercise ^{99m}Tc-MIBI/rest ^{201}Tl SPECT myocardial perfusion study was performed. He exercised for 8 minutes and 41 seconds, achieving 89% of predicted maximum HR and a

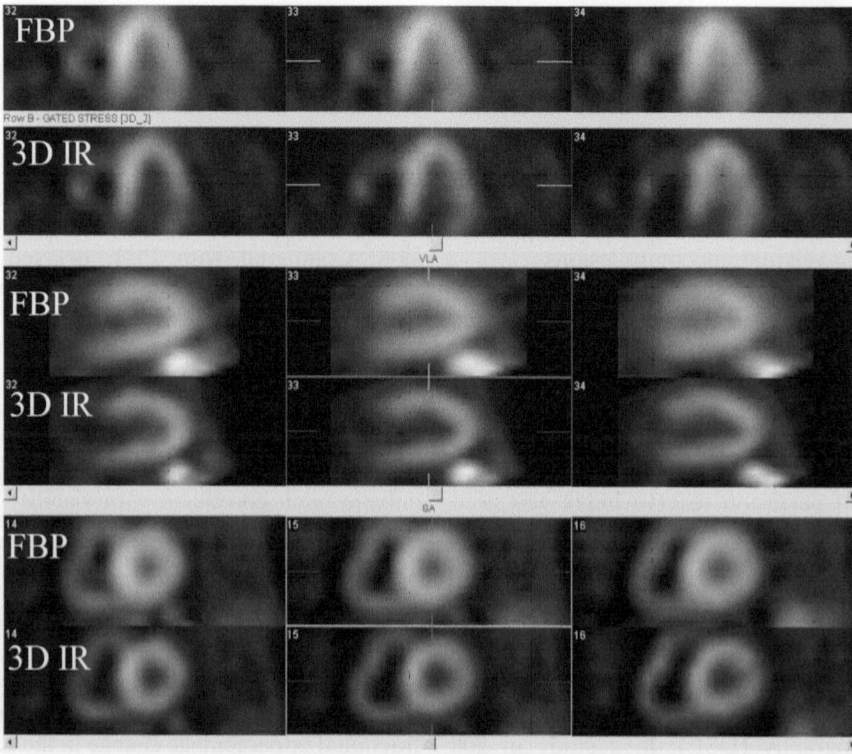

FIGURE C18-13.

pressure-rate product of 31,808. The stress SPECT perfusion images reconstructed with filtered back projection (FBP) and 3-dimensional iterative reconstruction (3-D IR) are displayed in Figure C18-13.

Findings

The stress SPECT images demonstrated a large, severe perfusion defect involving the anterolateral and inferolateral segments of the myocardium. There is also better definition of the LV borders with 3-D IR compared with FBP. Gated SPECT images revealed normal wall motion and an LVEF of 70%. Coronary angiography revealed a stenosis in the graft to the LAD as well as a new stenosis in a large branch of the LCX.

Discussion

In this example, a 3-D IR was used to process the myocardial perfusion images. IR algorithms, as opposed to conventional FBP techniques, attempt to produce an accurate representation of the distribution of the radioisotope within the myocardium by making an initial estimate of the radioactivity distribution within the heart, comparing it to the measured projection image, and making error adjustments that are then backprojected to improve the original estimate.[73] Each successive iteration creates a better estimation of the true activity distribution of the radioisotope. An added advantage of IR over conventional FBP is that these algorithms more easily incorporate attenuation correction and other compensations into the reconstruction.[74–77] IR, however, has been limited by long computational times and a higher degree of training required to process the reconstructed images.

Newer IR algorithms can be based on the ordered subsets expectation maximization (OSEM) technique, which accelerates implementation of the iterative algorithms and significantly reduces computation times.[78] The 3-dimensional reconstruction method differs from traditional 2-dimensional models in that the whole reconstruction volume is computed at once, not slice-by-slice, and therefore depth-dependent spatial resolution is more accurately accounted for. This is particularly important when considering adjacent hepatic and gastrointestinal activity.[79] In a preliminary pilot study, inferolateral defects, in particular, were better characterized in terms of extent and severity of defect with a 3-D-OSEM technique versus conventional FBP.[80]

Interpretation

Better quality SPECT images seen with IR than with FBP.

References

1. Taillefer R. New agents labeled with technetium 99m for myocardial perfusion imaging. *Can Assoc Radiol J.* 1992;43:258–266.
2. Hendel RC, McSherry B, Karimeddini M, Leppo JA. Diagnostic value of a new myocardial perfusion agent, teboroxime (SQ 30,217), utilizing a rapid planar imaging protocol: preliminary results. *J Am Coll Cardiol.* 1990;16:855–861.
3. Sitek A, Di Bella EV, Gullberg GT, Huesman RH. Removal of liver activity contamination in teboroxime dynamic cardiac SPECT imaging with the use of factor analysis. *J Nucl Cardiol.* 2002;9:197–205.
4. Garcia EV, Galt JR, Folks RD, et al. Accuracy of dynamic SPECT acquisition for ^{99m}Tc-Teboroxime myocardial perfusion imaging: Preliminary results. *J Am Coll Cardiol.* 2002;39(Suppl A):394A.
5. Chen J, Galt JR, Valentine JD, et al. Novel acquisition methods for improved image quality in ^{99m}Tc teboroxime myocardial perfusion SPECT. *J Nucl Cardiol.* 2002;9:S12.
6. Burns RJ, Iles S, Fung AY, Wright LM, Daigneault L. The Canadian exercise technetium 99m-labeled teboroxime single-photon emission computed tomographic study. Canadian Exercise Teboroxime SPECT Study Investigators. *J Nucl Cardiol.* 1995;2:117–125.
7. Vanzetto G, Fagret D, Pasqualini R, Mathieu JP, Chossat F, Machecourt J. Biodistribution, dosimetry, and safety of myocardial perfusion imaging agent ^{99m}TcN-NOET in healthy volunteers. *J Nucl Med.* 2000;41:141–148.
8. Ghezzi C, Fagret D, Arvieux CC, et al. Myocardial kinetics of Tc-N-NOET: a neutral lipophilic complex tracer of regional myocardial blood flow. *J Nucl Med.* 1995;36:1069–1077.
9. Calnon DA, Ruiz M, Vanzetto G, Watson DD, Beller GA, Glover DK. Myocardial uptake of ^{99m}Tc-N-NOET and ^{201}Tl during dobutamine infusion. comparison with adenosine stress. *Circulation.* 1999;100:1653–1659.
10. Fagret D, Marie PY, Brunotte F, et al. Myocardial perfusion imaging with technetium-^{99m}Tc NOET: comparison with thallium-201 and coronary angiography. *J Nucl Med.* 1995;36:936–943.
11. Narula J, Strauss HW. PS I love you: implications of phosphatidyl serine (PS) reversal in acute ischemic syndromes. *J Nucl Med.* 2003;44: 397–399.
12. Thimister PW, Hofstra L, Liem IH, et al. In vivo detection of cell death in the area at risk in acute myocardial infarction. *J Nucl Med.* 2003;44:391–396.
13. Hofstra L, Liem IH, Dumont EA, et al. Visualisation of cell death in vivo in patients with acute myocardial infarction. *Lancet.* 2000;356(9225): 209–212.
14. Petrov A, Acio ER, Narula N, et al. Sacrolemal phosphatedyl serine expression in ischemic myocardial syndromes can be detected by ^{99m}Tc Annexin V imaging [abstract]. *Circulation.* 2000; 102:II–544
15. Narula J, Acio ER, Narula N, et al. Annexin-V imaging for noninvasive detection of cardiac allograft rejection. *Nat Med.* 2001;7:1347–1352.
16. Narula J, Petroa, Pak KY, Lister BC, Khaw BA. Very early noninvasive detection of acute experimental nonreperfused MI with ^{99m}Tc labeled glucarate. *Circulation.* 1997;95:1577–1584.
17. Orlandi C, Crane PD, Edwards DS, et al. Early scintigraphic detection of experimental MI in dogs with technetium-99m glucaric acid. *J Nucl Med.* 1991;32:263–268.
18. Mariani G, Villa G, Rossettin PF, et al. Detection of acute myocardial infarction by ^{99m}Tc labeled D-glucararic acid imaging in patients with acute chest pain. *J Nucl Med.* 1999;540:1832–1839.
19. Okada DR, Johnson G, Liu Z, et al. Myocardial kinetics of ^{99m}Tc glucarate in low flow, hypoxia and aglycemia. *J Nucl Cardiol.* 2003;10:168–176.
20. Khaw BA, DaSilva J, Petrov A, Hartner W. Indium 111 antimyosin and ^{99m}Tc glucaric acid for noninvasive identification of oncotic and apoptotic necrosis. *J Nucl Cardiol.* 2002;9: 471–481.
21. He ZX, Cwajg E, Hwang W, et al. Myocardial blood flow and myocardial uptake of ^{201}Tl and

^{99m}Tc-sestamibi during coronary vasodilation induced by CGS-21680, a selective adenosine A(2A) receptor agonist. *Circulation.* 2000;102: 438–444.
22. Glover DK, Ruiz M, Yang JY, et al. Pharmacological stress thallium scintigraphy with 2-cyclohexylmethylidenehydrazino-adenosine (WRC-0470). A novel, short-acting adenosine A2A receptor agonist. *Circulation.* 1996;94: 1726–1732.
23. Trochu JN, Zhao G, Post H, Xu X, Belardinelli L, Belloni FL, Hintze TH. Selective A2A adenosine receptor agonist as a coronary vasodilator in conscious dogs: potential for use in myocardial perfusion imaging. *J Cardiovasc Pharmacol.* 2003;41:132–139.
24. Glover DK, Ruiz M, Takehana K, et al. Pharmacological stress myocardial perfusion imaging with the potent and selective A(2A) adenosine receptor agonists ATL193 and ATL146e administered by either intravenous infusion or bolus injection. *Circulation.* 2001;104:1181–1187.
25. Watanabe K, Sekiya M, Ikeda S, Miyagawa M, Kinoshita M, Kumano S. Comparison of adenosine triphosphate and dipyridamole in diagnosis by thallium-201 myocardial scintigraphy. *J Nucl Med.* 1997;38:577–581.
26. Takeishi Y, Takahashi N, Fujiwara S, Atsumi H, Takahashi K, Tomoike H. Myocardial tomography with technetium-99m-tetrofosmin during intravenous infusion of adenosine triphosphate. *J Nucl Med.* 1998;39:582–586.
27. He Q, Yao Z, Yu X, et al. Evaluation of ^{99m}Tc-MIBI myocardial perfusion imaging with intravenous infusion of adenosine triphosphate in diagnosis of coronary artery disease. *Chin Med J.* (Engl). 2002;115:1603–1607.
28. Geleijnse ML, Elhendy A, Fioretti PM, Roelandt JR. Dobutamine stress myocardial perfusion imaging. *J Am Coll Cardiol.* 2000;36:2017–2027.
29. Caner B, Karanfil A, Uysal U, et al. Effect of an additional atropine injection during dobutamine infusion for myocardial SPET. *Nucl Med Commun.*1997;18:567–573.
30. Santoro GM, Sciagra R, Buonamici P, et al. Head-to-head comparison of exercise stress testing, pharmacologic stress echocardiography, and perfusion tomography as first-line examination for chest pain in patients without history of coronary artery disease. *J Nucl Cardiol.* 1998;5: 19–27.
31. Schinkel AF, Elhendy A, Van Domburg RT, et al. Long-term prognostic value of dobutamine stress ^{99m}Tc-sestamibi SPECT: single-center experience with 8-year follow-up. *Radiology.* 2002;225:701–706.
32. Van Damme H, Pierard L, Gillain D, Benoit T, Rigo P, Limet R. Cardiac risk assessment before vascular surgery: a prospective study comparing clinical evaluation, dobutamine stress echocardiography, and dobutamine ^{99m}Tc sestamibi tomoscintigraphy. *Cardiovasc Surg.* 1997;5:54–64.
33. Meneguetti JC, Camargo EE, Soares J Jr, et al. Gallium-67 imaging in human heart transplantation: correlation with endomyocardial biopsy. *J Heart Transplant.* 1987;6:171–176.
34. Camargo PR, Mazzieri R, Snitcowsky R, et al. Correlation between gallium-67 imaging and endomyocardial biopsy in children with severe dilated cardiomyopathy. *Int J Cardiol.* 1990;28: 293–297.
35. O'Connell JB, Henkin RE, Robinson JA, Subramanian R, Scanlon PJ, Gunnar RM. Gallium-67 imaging in patients with dilated cardiomyopathy and biopsy-proven myocarditis. *Circulation.* 1984;70:58–62.
36. Patel AD, Iskandrian AE. MIBG imaging. *J Nucl Cardiol.* 2002 Jan–Feb;9(1):75–94.
37. Inoue H, Zipes DP. Results of sympathetic denervation in the canine heart: supersensitivity that may be arrhythmogenic. *Circulation.* 1987;Apr; 75(4):877–887.
38. Mantysaari M, Kuikka J, Hartikainen J, et al. Myocardial sympathetic nervous dysfunction detected with iodine-123-MIBG is associated with low heart rate variability after myocardial infarction. *J Nucl Med.* 1995;Jun; 36(6):956–961.
39. Inobe Y, Kugiyama K, Miyagi H, et al. Long-lasting abnormalities in cardiac sympathetic nervous system in patients with coronary spastic angina: quantitative analysis with iodine 123 metaiodobenzylguanidine myocardial scintigraphy. *Am Heart J.* 1997;Jul;134(1):112–118.
40. Yamada T, Shimonagata T, Fukunami M, et al. Comparison of the prognostic value of cardiac iodine-123 metaiodobenzylguanidine imaging and heart rate variability in patients with chronic heart failure: a prospective study. *J Am Coll Cardiol.* 2003;41:231–238.
41. Suwa M, Otake Y, Moriguchi A, et al. Iodine-123 metaiodobenzylguanidine myocardial scintigraphy for prediction of response to beta-blocker therapy in patients with dilated cardiomyopathy. *Am Heart J.* 1997;Mar; 133(3):353–358.
42. Lekakis J, Prassopoulos V, Athanassiadis P, Kostamis P, Moulopoulos S. Doxorubicin-induced cardiac neurotoxicity: study with iodine

123-labeled metaiodobenzylguanidine scintigraphy. *J Nucl Cardiol.* 1996;Jan–Feb;3(1):37–41.
43. Wilson RF, Laxson DD, Christensen BV, McGinn AL, Kubo SH. Regional differences in sympathetic reinnervation after human orthotopic cardiac transplantation. *Circulation.* 1993; Jul;88(1):165–171.
44. Langer A, Freeman MR, Josse RG, Armstrong PW. Metaiodobenzylguanidine imaging in diabetes mellitus: assessment of cardiac sympathetic denervation and its relation to autonomic dysfunction and silent myocardial ischemia. *J Am Coll Cardiol.* 1995;Mar 1;25(3):610–618.
45. Lerch H, Bartenstein P, Wichter T, et al. Sympathetic innervation of the left ventricle is impaired in arrhythmogenic right ventricular disease. *Eur J Nucl Med.* 1993;Mar;20(3):207–212.
46. Schwaiger M, Schelbert HR, Ellison D, et al. Sustained regional abnormalities in cardiac metabolism after transient ischemia in the chronic dog model. *J Am Coll Cardiol.* 1985;6: 336–347.
47. Tamaki N, Morita K, Kuge Y, Tsukamoto E. The role of fatty acids in cardiac imaging. *J Nucl Med.* 2000;41:1525–1534.
48. Tamaki N, Kawamoto M, Yonekura Y, et al. Regional metabolic abnormality in relation to perfusion and wall motion in patients with myocardial infarction: assessment with emission tomography using an iodinated branched fatty acid analog. *J Nucl Med.* 1992;33: 659–667.
49. De Geeter F, Franken PR, Knapp FF Jr, Bossuyt A. Relationship between blood flow and fatty acid metabolism in subacute myocardial infarction: a study by means of ^{99m}Tc-Sestamibi and ^{123}I-beta-methyl-iodo-phenyl pentadecanoic acid. *Eur J Nucl Med.* 1994;21:283–291.
50. Kawai Y, Tsukamoto E, Nozaki Y, Kishino K, Kohya T, Tamaki N. Use of ^{123}I-BMIPP single-photon emission tomography to estimate areas at risk following successful revascularization in patients with acute myocardial infarction. *Eur J Nucl Med.* 1998;25:1390–1395.
51. Kawai Y, Tsukamoto E, Nozaki Y, Morita K, Sakurai M, Tamaki N. Significance of reduced uptake of iodinated fatty acid analogue for the evaluation of patients with acute chest pain. [Erratum appears in *J Am Coll Cardiol.* 2002;Apr 17;39(8):1409]. *J Am Coll Cardiol.* 2001;38:1888–1894.
52. Hashimoto Y, Yamabe H, Yokoyama M. Myocardial defect detected by ^{123}I-BMIPP scintigraphy and left ventricular dysfunction in patients with idiopathic dilated cardiomyopathy. *Ann Nucl Med.* 1996;10:225–230.
53. Yoshinaga K, Tahara M, Torii H, Kihara K. Predicting the effects on patients with dilated cardiomyopathy of beta-blocker therapy, by using iodine-123 15-(p-iodophenyl)-3-R,S-methylpentadecanoic acid (BMIPP) myocardial scintigraphy. *Ann Nucl Med.* 1998;12:341–347.
54. Mulvagh SL, DeMaria AN, Feinstein SB, et al. Contrast echocardiography: current and future applications. *J Am Soc Echocardiogr.* 2000;13: 331–342.
55. Cohen JL, Cheirif J, Segar DS, et al. Improved left ventricular endocardial border delineation and opacification with OPTISON (FS069), a new echocardiographic contrast agent. Results of a phase III Multicenter Trial. *J Am Coll Cardiol.* 1998;32:746–752.
56. Porter TR, Xie F, Kricsfeld A, Chiou A, Dabestani A. Improved endocardial border resolution during dobutamine stress echocardiography with intravenous sonicated dextrose albumin. *J Am Coll Cardiol.* 1994;23:1440–1443.
57. Meza MF, Mobarek S, Sonnemaker R, et al. Myocardial contrast echocardiography in human beings: correlation of resting perfusion defects to sestamibi single photon emission computed tomography. *Am Heart J.* 1996;132:528–535.
58. Ragosta M, Camarano G, Kaul S, Powers ER, Sarembock IJ, Gimple LW. Microvascular integrity indicates myocellular viability in patients with recent myocardial infarction. New insights using myocardial contrast echocardiography. *Circulation.* 1994;89:2562–2569.
59. Gerber TC, Kuzo RS, Karstaedt N, et al. Current results and new developments of coronary angiography with use of contrast-enhanced computed tomography of the heart. *Mayo Clin Proc.* 2002;77:55–71.
60. Greenland P, Gaziano JM. Clinical practice. Selecting asymptomatic patients for coronary computed tomography or electrocardiographic exercise testing. *N Engl J Med.* 2003;349:465–473.
61. Nallamothu BK, Saint S, Bielak LF, et al. Electron-beam computed tomography in the diagnosis of coronary artery disease: a meta-analysis. *Arch Intern Med.* 2001;161:833–838.
62. O'Malley PG, Taylor AJ, Jackson JL, Doherty TM, Detrano RC. Prognostic value of coronary electron-beam computed tomography for coronary heart disease events in asymptomatic populations. *Am J Cardiol.* 2000;85:945–948.
63. McLaughlin VV, Balogh T, Rich S. Utility of electron beam computed tomography to stratify

patients presenting to the emergency room with chest pain. *Am J Cardiol.* 1999;84:327–328, A8.
64. Budoff MJ, Oudiz RJ, Zalace CP, et al. Intravenous three-dimensional coronary angiography using contrast enhanced electron beam computed tomography. *Am J Cardiol.* 1999;83:840–845.
65. Nieman K, Cademartiri F, Lemos PA, Raaijmakers R, Pattynama PM, de Feyter PJ. Reliable noninvasive coronary angiography with fast submillimeter multislice spiral computed tomography. *Circulation.* 2002;106:2051–2054.
66. Budoff MJ, Gillespie R, Georgiou D, et al. Comparison of exercise electron beam computed tomography and sestamibi in the evaluation of coronary artery disease. *Am J Cardiol.* 1998;81: 682–687.
67. Schwitter J, Nanz D, Kneifel S, et al. Assessment of myocardial perfusion in coronary artery disease by magnetic resonance: a comparison with positron emission tomography and coronary angiography. *Circulation.* 2001;103:2230–2235.
68. Nagel E, Lehmkuhl HB, Bocksch W, et al. Noninvasive diagnosis of ischemia-induced wall motion abnormalities with the use of high-dose dobutamine stress MRI: comparison with dobutamine stress echocardiography. *Circulation.* 1999;99:763–770.
69. Kim WY, Danias PG, Stuber M, et al. Coronary magnetic resonance angiography for the detection of coronary stenoses. *N Engl J Med.* 2001;345:1863–1869.
70. Klein C, Nekolla SG, Bengel FM, et al. Assessment of myocardial viability with contrast-enhanced magnetic resonance imaging: comparison with positron emission tomography. *Circulation.* 2002;105:162–167.
71. Ramani K, Judd RM, Holly TA, et al. Contrast magnetic resonance imaging in the assessment of myocardial viability in patients with stable coronary artery disease and left ventricular dysfunction. *Circulation.* 1998;98:2687–2694.
72. Gotte MJ, van Rossum AC, Twisk JWR, Kuijer JPA, Marcus JT, Visser CA. Quantification of regional contractile function after infarction: strain analysis superior to wall thickening analysis in discriminating infarct from remote myocardium. *J Am Coll Cardiol.* 2001;37:808–817.
73. Bruyant PP. Analytic and iterative reconstruction algorithms in SPECT. *J Nucl Med.* 2002;43: 1343–1358.
74. Corbett JR, Ficaro EP. Clinical review of attenuation corrected cardiac SPECT. *J Nucl Cardiol.* 1999;6:54–68.
75. Galt JR, Cullom SJ, Garcia EV. Attenuation and scatter compensation in myocardial perfusion SPECT. *Semin Nucl Med.* 1999;3:204–220.
76. Liang Z. Compensation for attenuation, scatter and detector response in SPECT reconstruction via iterative FBP methods. *Medical Physics.* 1993;20:1097–1106.
77. Maze A, LeCloirec J, Collorec R, et al. Iterative reconstruction methods for nonuniform attenuation distribution in SPECT. *J Nucl Med.* 1993;34:1204–1209.
78. Hudson H, Larkin R. Accelerated EM reconstruction using ordered subsets of projection data. *IEEE Trans on Med Imaging.* 1994;13601–13609.
79. Germano G, Chua T, Kiat H, Areeda JS, Berman DS. A quantitative phantom analysis of artifacts due to hepatic activity in technetium-99m myocardial perfusion SPECT studies. *J Nucl Med.* 1994;35:356–359.
80. Haynie J, Kite F, Barron JF, et al. Three-dimensional iterative reconstruction for SPECT myocardial perfusion imaging: initial clinical experience. *J Nucl Cardiol.* 2003;10:S84.

Index

M

P

MIX
Papier aus verantwortungsvollen Quellen
Paper from responsible sources
FSC® C105338

If you have any concerns about our products,
you can contact us on
ProductSafety@springernature.com

In case Publisher is established outside the EU,
the EU authorized representative is:
Springer Nature Customer Service Center GmbH
Europaplatz 3, 69115 Heidelberg, Germany

Printed by Libri Plureos GmbH
in Hamburg, Germany